PSYCHOMOTOR EPILEPSY

Publication Number 880

AMERICAN LECTURE SERIES®

A Monograph in

The BANNERSTONE DIVISION *of*
AMERICAN LECTURES IN LIVING CHEMISTRY

Edited by

I. NEWTON KUGELMASS, M.D., Ph.D., Sc.D
Consultant to the Department of Health and Hospitals
New York City

PSYCHOMOTOR EPILEPSY

A POLYDIMENSIONAL STUDY

By

UROŠ J. JOVANOVIĆ, M.D.

Lecturer in Psychiatry and Neurology
especially
Electroencephalography, Neurophysiology,
Psychophysiology

and

Experimental Sleep and Dream Research
Julius-Maximilians-University, Wurzburg
Germany

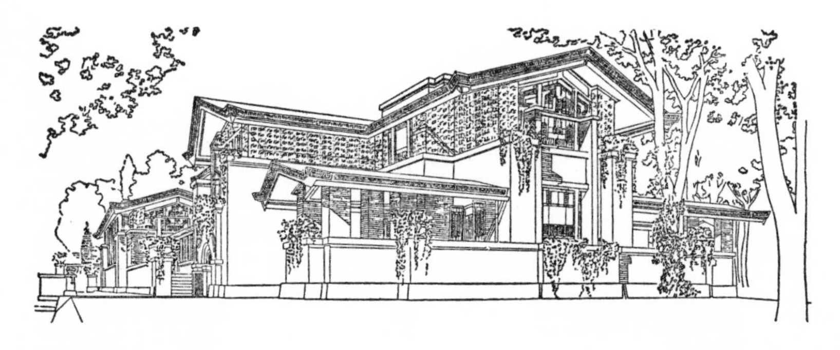

CHARLES C THOMAS • PUBLISHER
Springfield • Illinois • U.S.A.

Published and Distributed Throughout the World by
CHARLES C THOMAS • PUBLISHER
BANNERSTONE HOUSE
301-327 East Lawrence Avenue, Springfield, Illinois, U.S.A.

ISBN 0-398-02691-2
Library of Congress Catalog Card Number: 72-88481

With THOMAS BOOKS *careful attention is given to all details of manufacturing and design. It is the Publisher's desire to present books that are satisfactory as to their physical qualities and artistic possibilities and appropriate for their particular use.* THOMAS BOOKS *will be true to those laws of quality that assure a good name and good will.*

Printed in the United States of America
N-1

FOREWORD

OUR LIVING CHEMISTRY SERIES was conceived by editor and publisher to advance the newer knowledge of chemical medicine in the cause of clinical practice. The interdependence of chemistry and medicine is so great that physicians are turning to chemistry, and chemists to medicine, in order to understand the underlying basis of life processes in health and disease. Once chemical truths, proofs and convictions become foundations for clinical phenomena, key hybrid investigators clarify the bewildering panorama of biochemical progress for application in everyday practice, stimulation of experimental research and extension of postgraduate instruction. Each of our monographs thus unravels the chemical mechanisms and clinical management of many diseases that have remained relatively static in the minds of medical men for three thousand years. Our new series is charged with the *nisus élan* of chemical wisdom, supreme in choice of international authors, optimal in standards of chemical scholarship, provocative in imagination for experimental research, comprehensive in discussions of scientific medicine and authoritative in chemical perspective of human disorders.

Dr. Jovanovic of Würzburg presents a penetrating polydimensional picture of psychomotor seizures as disinhibition of excitation in the temporal lobe, the first barrier; in the medial structures of the brain, the second barrier; in the neocortical regions, the third barrier; in the lower brain stem, the fourth barrier; and in the spinal cord, the fifth barrier. There is a high incidence of structural abnormality, especially mesial temporal sclerosis. The most common focus for the clinical seizure is in the hippocampus or hippocampal gyrus. In the rudimentary form it produces dreamy states, impulsive acts and eventually acting-out behavior with clouded sensorium during the psychical seizure followed by total amnesia for the episodic behavior responsible for startling senseless criminal acts.

Psychomotor epilepsy is a biological phenomenon of great diagnostic challenge because of marked variability from patient to patient in sensory, mental, and motor manifestations. It may be primary, secondary, essential, or symptomatic, more usually combined with other patterns at any age. An aura occurs in most patients; it may be as simple as a twinge in the stomach or as complicated as a repetitive dreamlike experience. The onset is heralded by lip smacking or facial movement followed by automatism with semipurposeful bizarre behavior for several minutes. The seizure terminates abruptly with little or no postital confusion or more rarely progresses to a generalized tonic-clonic attack. The patient remains amnestic for the automation. Psychomotor status presents a confused state with persistent, inappropriate bizarre complex behavior patterns lasting for hours. Focal EEG abnormality is demonstrable in one or both temporal regions, especially during sleep. Correct recognition of psychomotor epilepsy is pathognomonic of focal neuropathology, just as in classic motor seizures with its resultant personality changes. Nevertheless, few are disabled more by psychiatric problems than by the epilepsy, and most present a good prognosis following anticonvulsant therapy or eventual surgery when drugs fail.

The precise mechanism of the temporal lobe seizure is unknown, but certain aspects of neuronal metabolism are a direct function of the threshold to seizures, intimately concerned with the focal initiation and generalized spread of seizure discharge. At the focus of irritation in the temporal lobe, the electrical stability of the surrounding neurons is impaired by acetylcholine, the excitatory transmitter substance with consequent increase in the permeability of the neuronal membrane. Increased or impaired influx of Na^+ in the neuron and depletion of intracellular K^+ lead to depolarization and increased excitability of the membrane. A repetitive spike discharge and seizure are generated locally or diffused into a major convulsion, varying directly with carbonic anhydrase in the brain and inversely with the efficacy of inhibitory mechanism. The mechanism of psychomotor seizures remains obscured by experimental difficulties in deep-seated studies of the patients. Investigators settle for what is measurable instead of measuring what they would really like to know. And we know nothing until we can measure it. Much of the research remains conceptual, for example, the search for a concept to explain a chance observation or to exploit a new technique on the one hand, or the effort to validate a concept serendipitously derived by devising proper experiments, on the other. The author's research opens mechanistic windows and therapeutic doors with intellectual delight for all who will peruse his creative art.

With accurate experiment and observation to work upon,
imagination becomes the architect of mechanistic theory.

Newton Kugelmass, M.D., Ph.D., Sc.D.
Editor

INTRODUCTION

RESEARCH dealing with all aspects of psychomotor epilepsy has encountered many problems, some of which cannot be overcome in a short time. Investigation techniques which we, and many other research workers have used, have not produced conclusive results.

Analysis of the blood serum or cerebrospinal fluid of patients with psychomotor epilepsy (as is done in almost all other diseases) does not really produce specific results.

It is not possible to produce an experimental model in completely healthy test subjects, for the purpose of biochemical research, because of the nature of the disease. It is known that psychiatric patients are sometimes treated by methods which in certain circumstances may induce epilepsy as one of the undesired sequels. However, this is hardly ever *pure* psychomotor epilepsy, but usually a type of generalized or focal seizure.

One of the most reliable techniques in biochemical research is animal experimentation; however, this does not provide particularly valuable evidence in the case of psychomotor epilespsy since here again we are usually dealing with a focal or generalized epileptic manifestation.

In recent years, the biochemical processes have been studied by producing epileptic phenomena in animal preparations. However, this method is even less suitable for studying psychomotor epilepsy. Consequently, there is no biochemical investigation technique which can give a satisfactory picture of the biochemical process which may be responsible etiologically and pathogenetically for psychomotor epilepsy. In view of these difficulties, we had to arrange the *presentation, form, scope and content* of the following study so that all the possible investigation techniques, and results therefrom, are mentioned. It is often necessary to employ *analogies,* and, from the results of other (not necessarily direct) chemical research, to draw conclusions regarding the abnormal biochemical processes before, during and after the psychomotor attack.

The symptomatology of psychomotor epilepsy is very extensive and diverse, and, about 90 percent of all epileptic symptoms assume the psychomotor form. The phenomena embrace almost every level of the mind, the motor system and the autonomic nervous system. The extraordinary diversity of this symptomatology is described in an extended introduction in chapter I.

The electroencephalogram (EEG) (chapter II) has recently been used as an indicator of many changes in the central nervous system (CNS). In many cases, reactions of the bioelectric cerebral activity are evident even before clinical symptoms are detectable. The EEG also makes it possible to demonstrate the location of psychomotor epilepsy and to distinguish this form from other types of epilepsy. We do not need to emphasize the fact that some manifestations of this disease can only be studied by special EEG recordings. The EEG has also been used for studying various chemical agents in respect of their effect in triggering psychomotor and other epileptic symptoms.

In the discussion on the EEG in patients with psychomotor epilepsy, some generally well-known facts have been mentioned. These basic points may help to simplify the text for those readers who are not directly concerned with problems of bioelectric cerebral activity in their research work.

For the same reasons as those given under symptomatology and the EEG, there is relatively detailed discussion of the morphological problems (chapter III). We believe that local biochemical studies are only possible if the convulsion focus has first been located by anatomical histological methods. The many functions of morphological structures which also play a major part in psychomotor epilepsy, also compel us to conduct parallel studies of morphology, physiology and histochemistry.

In recent years, experimental research into epilepsy, particularly microneurophysiological methods, has produced significant results. This is given due prominence in this monograph (chapter IV).

In discussing brain metabolism with regard to psychomotor epilepsy (chapter V), it has again been necessary to refer to experiments and results which are not always directly related to our problem. Since complete details of precise biochemical processes in this disease are not yet known, our observations must be extended to include related fields of study.

In the analysis of provoking and inhibiting chemical substances in respect of psychomotor attack (chapters VI and VII), it is only possible to discuss the most important drugs.

Chapter VIII deals with the model of epileptic attack and its equivalents, the argument being centered about the biochemical processes.

The mechanism of action of therapeutic substances (chapter IX) are only discussed briefly from theoretical and practical points of view. The therapy of psychomotor epilepsy is discussed in chapter X.

While discussing the subject in detail, we have not lost sight of the overall problem. The sick man is at the center of the problem, and, by bearing this in mind, we hope we have contributed to the fight against this strange disease.

CONTENTS

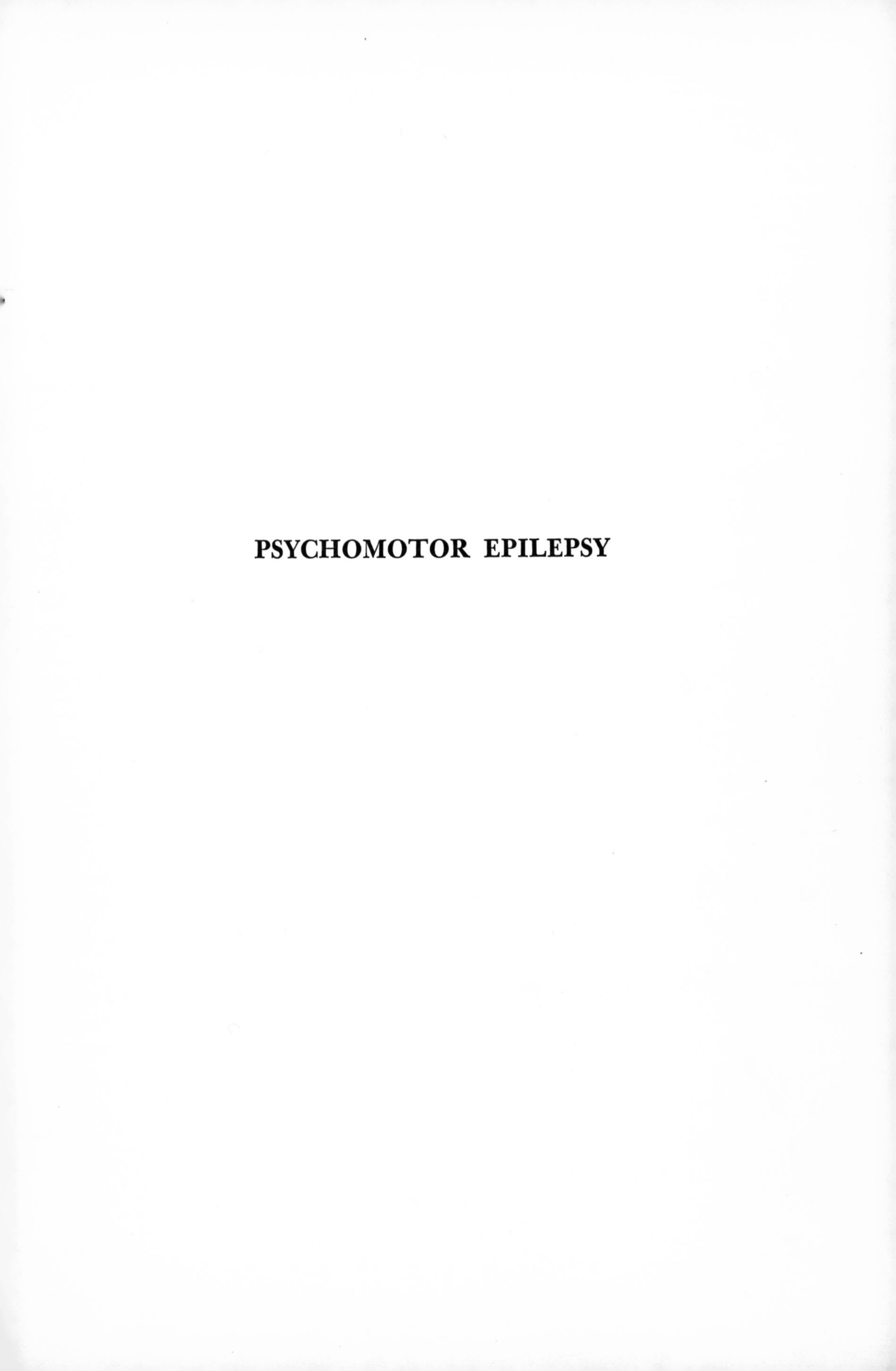

PSYCHOMOTOR EPILEPSY

CHAPTER I

CLINICAL PHENOMENOLOGY

OCCURRENCE AND COURSE

EPILEPTOGENIC NOXAE MAY produce psychomotor epilepsy in a *primary* form in originally healthy people, or the disease may develop as a *secondary* form from one of the other types of epilepsy. The primary form may occur *in isolation,* or *combined* with other forms of epilepsy; the secondary type is always *combined.*

Age is not a predisposing factor with *primary psychomotor epilepsy.* This form may occur in childhood, or at later stages in life; it may even become manifest in the elderly (Figure 1). Garsche and Schönfelder report that according to electroencephalographic and clinical criteria, it occurred in 16 of 250 cases (6.4%) of epileptic children. However, if the clinical picture is considered on its own, and the electroencephalographic findings ignored, the percentage of psychomotor epilepsy rises considerably. Bamberger and Matthes (1959) found there were psychomotor attacks in 52 of 349 children with epilepsy (15.0%), Hallen (1954 a, b; 1962) and Janz (1953 a to c; 1962; 1963) found them in 302 and 1206 epileptics (25.0%). In a large number of young patients, Matthes (1961 a, b, c) was able to detect this condition in 21% of the cases. Bamberger and Matthes (1959) and Matthes (1961) found that it did not occur predominantly in a specific age group in children, although they stress that there is a certain increase after the first ten years of life. In adults, psychomotor epilepsy is also distributed throughout almost all age groups (Figure 1). According to Gibbs and Fuster (1948), the disease peak is in the third decade of life, according to Meyer-Mickeleit (1953) it is in the third to fifth, according to Gastaut (1953) and Janz (1955) it is in the second to third (or even fourth, Janz) decade of life. According to Lennox (1951) 34.1 percent of all epileptics over the age of 40 have psychomotor attacks.

According to Lennox (1951), Hallen (1954 to 1962) and Janz (1955), every fifth epileptic has psychomotor epilepsy.

The age distribution for the onset of nocturnal epilepsy of gland mal is similar to that for the psychomotor form (Figure 2a and 2b), while matutinal epilepsy with generalized attacks is like petit mal in having a significant disease peak in the second decade of life, or between the 11th and 15th year of life (Figure 2b and 3).

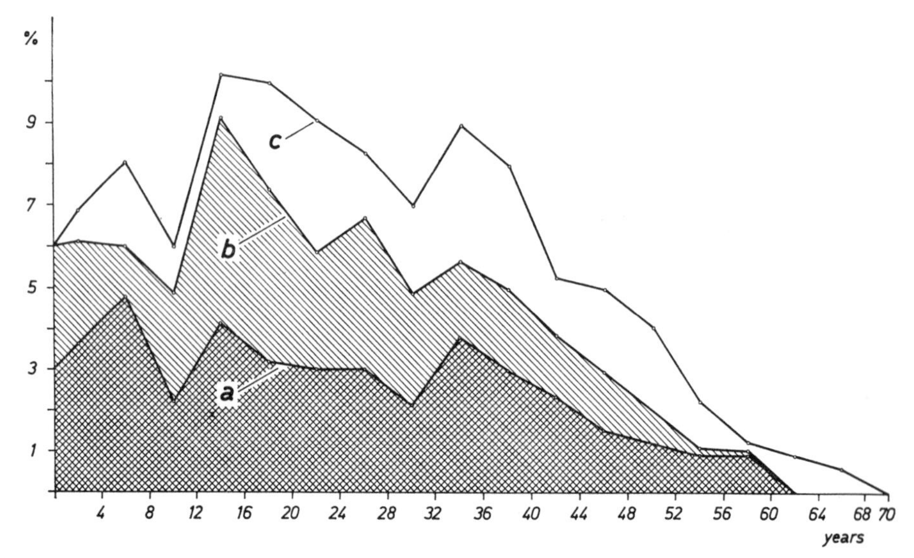

Figure 1. Age distribution, as a percentage, of 306 patients with psychomotor epilepsy, at the beginning of the disease. a.) Beginning of isolated psychomotor attacks; b.) beginning of combined psychomotor and other attacks arising from petit mal; c.) beginning of combined psychomotor and major seizures (cp. Figures 2a, 2b and 3). (From Janz, D., *Nervenarzt, 26*:20-28, 1955.)

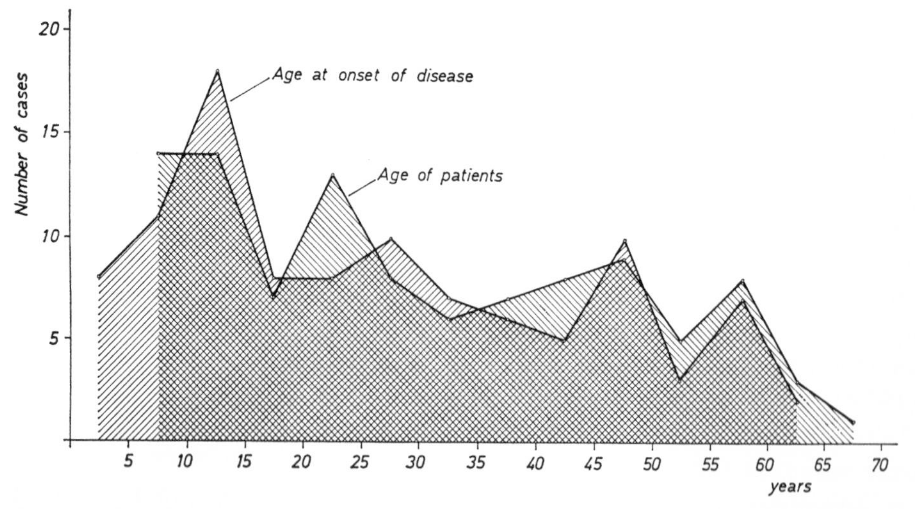

Figure 2a. Age distribution of 103 nocturnal epileptics (with isolated major seizures or with combined major and psychomotor attacks) at the time of onset of the disease and at the time of examination. There is no marked increase in prevalence in any one age group or a predisposing age. This age distribution is very similar to that in patients with isolated psychomotor attacks (cp. Figure 1). *Left vertical axis* = number of patients; *lower horizontal axis* = age in five-year groups. (From Jovanovic, U. J., and E. R. Schäfer: *Nervenarzt, 37*:290-295, 1966.)

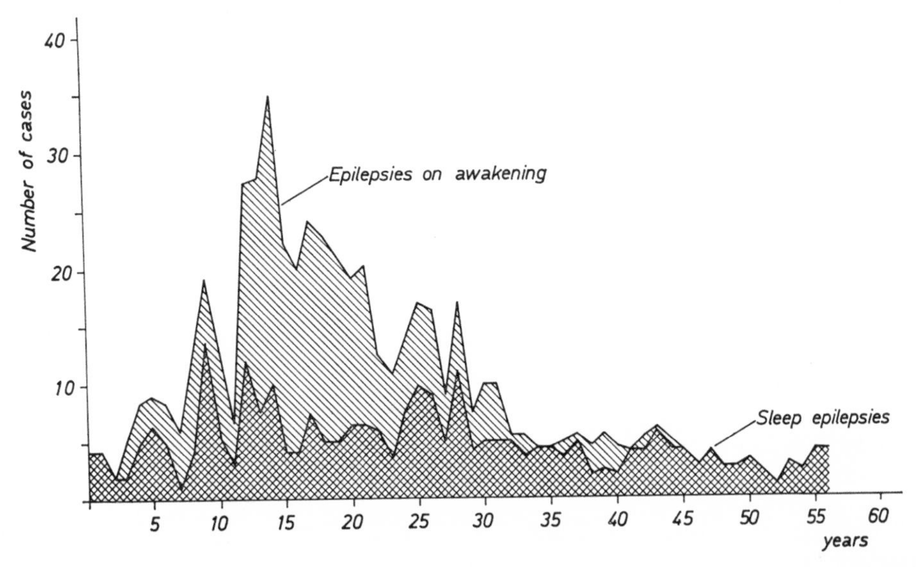

Figure 2b. Age distribution of 529 patients with idiopathic, essential (*cryptogenic*) epilepsy suffering exclusively from major seizures during sleep (nocturnal epilepsy) or in the waking state (matutinal epilepsy). The situation with these authentic grand mal forms is similar to that with the mixed (combined) epilepsies (cp. 2a and 3): the onset of nocturnal epilepsy can occur at any age, whereas the onset of matutinal epilepsy tends to occur between the ages of 11 and 15 years. (From Janz, D.: *Epilepsia, 3*:69-109, 1962.)

Psychomotor attacks are most frequently combined with grand mal. According to Lennox (1951), in two thirds of the combined forms, grand mal epilepsy began before the psychomotor attacks and in one third it began afterwards. Among 11,612 patients, Gibbs and Gibbs (1952) found 6 percent with isolated psychomotor attacks and in 17 percent these were combined with other forms of attack. According to reports from Bamberger and Matthes (1959), in one third of their patients generalized (major) seizures start before the onset of psychomotor attacks. Landolt (1960) reports that 52 of his 120 patients (43.3%) also had major attacks and 68 (56.7%) had isolated psychomotor attacks. According to Janz (1962 to 1972), Beyer and Jovanovic (1966) and Jovanovic and Schäfer (1966), in a considerable percentage of patients with psychomotor epilepsy the attacks are combined with major seizures of the nocturnal type (sleep epilepsy).

Figure 4 shows the distribution of psychomotor epilepsy in combination with other forms of epilepsy according to Janz (1962). He reports that 1,051 of 2,110 patients with grand mal (about 50%) suffered from isolated major attacks and 1,059 from combined attacks; 494 (46.7%) of these 1,059 epileptics had grand mal in combination with psychomotor seizures.

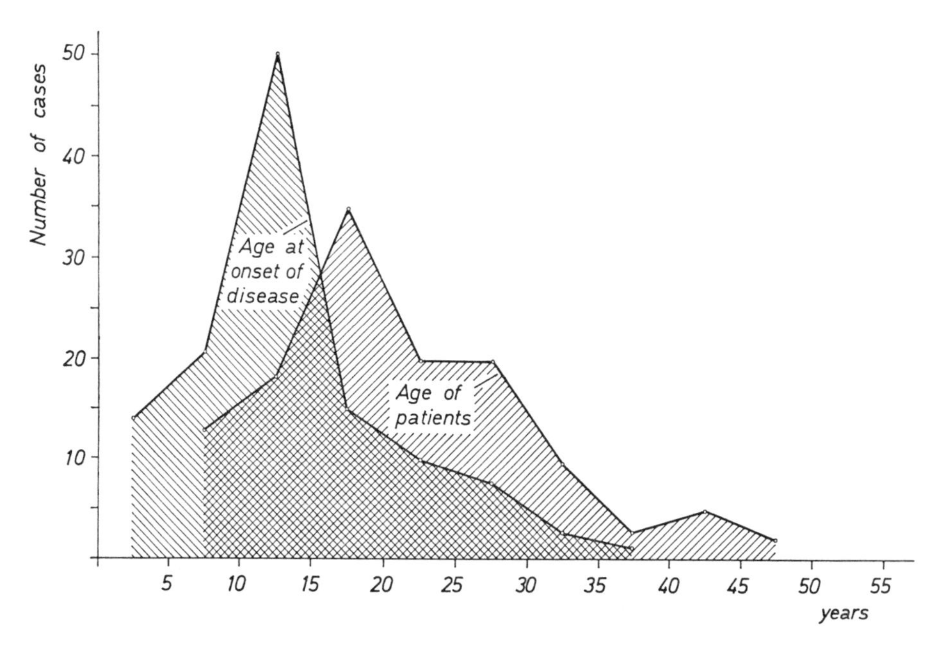

Figure 3. Age distribution of 120 matutinal epileptics (with isolated major seizures or combined with petit mal) at the time of onset of the disease (left plot) and at the time of examination (right plot). *Left vertical axis* = number of patients; *lower horizontal axis* = age in five-year groups. Compared with nocturnal and psychomotor epilepsy (cp. Figures 1, 2a and 2b) here there is a definite tendency for the disease to begin between the 11th and 15th years of life (see matutinal epilepsy in Figure 2b). (From Beyer, L., and U. J. Jovanovic, *Nervenarzt, 37*:333-336, 1966.)

Of these 494 patients, 16 percent had epilepsy on awakening (matutinal epilepsy), 26 percent had diffuse epilepsy and the largest number, 58 percent, had sleep epilepsy.

Among 103 nocturnal epileptics, Jovanovic and Schäfer (1966) found that this form was combined with psychomotor attacks in 39 cases (37.8%) and in only seven cases (6.8%) was it combined with petit mal of the centrencephalic type. On the other hand, matutinal epilepsy was combined with petit mal attacks in a large percentage of cases and with psychomotor epilepsy in very few cases. According to Janz (1962, see also 1953, 1968, 1972), the patients with grand mal in combination with petit mal, 84 percent had matutinal epilepsy (Figure 4). In 120 matutinal epileptics of grand mal Beyer and Jovanovic (1966) found major seizures combined with those of the petit mal triad in 41 cases (34.2%) and with psychomotor attacks only in 14 cases (11.6%).

This definite combination of psychomotor with nocturnal epilepsy of grand mal on the one hand, and the combination of petit mal with matu-

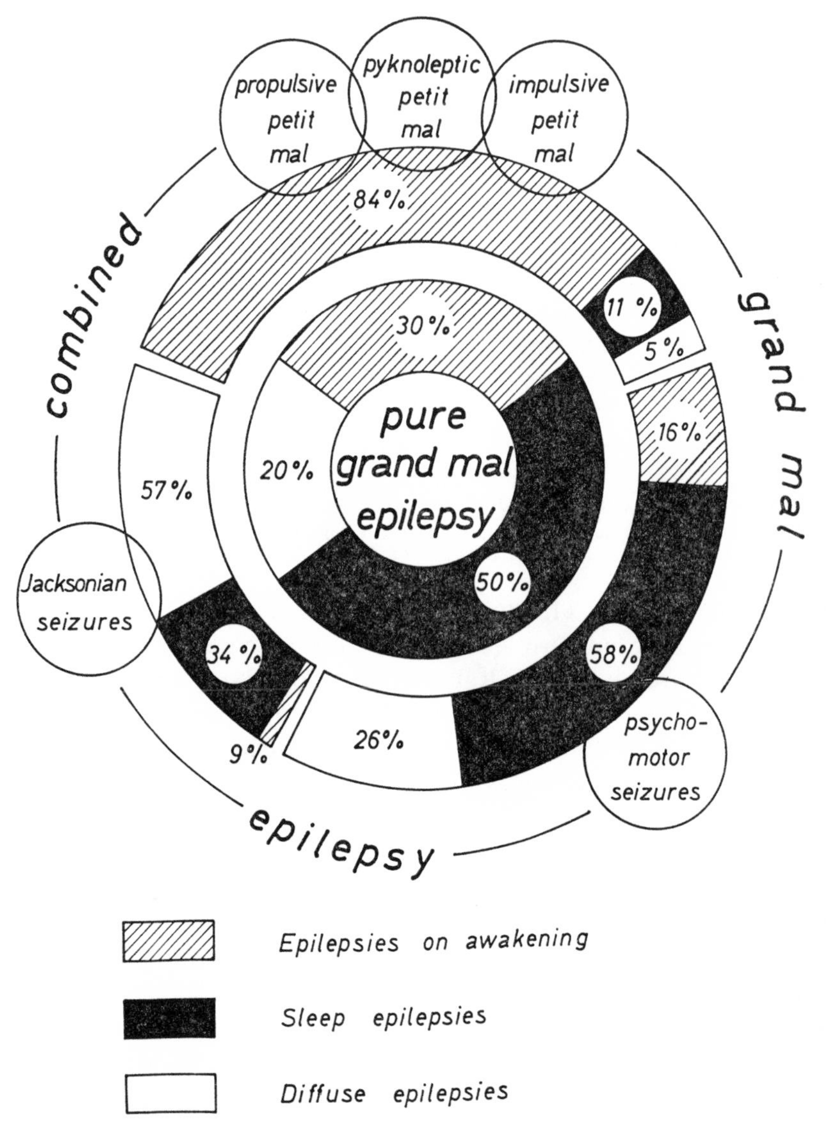

Figure 4. Distribution of the combination of seizures in 2110 grand mal epilepsies. The inner circle shows the percentage distribution of 1051 pure grand mal epilepsies (50% nocturnal epilepsy, 30% matutinal epilepsy, 20% diffuse epilepsy). The outer circle shows the distribution of the combinations of major seizures (1059 cases) with petit mal, with psychomotor attacks or with Jacksonian seizures. In the majority of cases, psychomotor epilepsy and all other forms of minor attacks described here can also occur in isolation. (From Janz, D., *Epilepsia, 3*:69-109, 1962.)

tinal epilepsy on the other, caused Jovanovic (1967 b, c) to classify the former as *temporocephalic* and the latter as *centrencephalic* forms of epilepsy (Table I).

Compared with the combination of psychomotor with grand mal epilepsy, combined occurrence of psychomotor and petit mal attacks is much less common.

Table 1. Classification of epilepsies from various points of view. According to this, psychomotor epilepsy is a temporocephalic form of epilepsy (own theory).

TABLE I
POINT OF VIEW

Combined Epilepsy	Temporocephalic Epilepsy	Centrencephalic Epilepsy	Neurophysiological and electroencehalographic
Diffuse Epilepsy Different	Sleep Epilepsy Psychomotor Epilepsy	Epilepsy on Awakening Impulsive Petit mal	Clinical (Grand mal) Clinical (Petit mal)
Combinations of Petit mal	(isolated and combined)	Retropulsive Petit mal	
Hydantoines and Barbiturates	Hydantoines and similar Compounds	Barbiturates and similar Compounds	Therapeutic

Out of more than 11,000 epileptics, Gibbs and Gibbs (1952) only found psychomotor epilepsy combined with absence in 1.2% and with Jacksonian seizures in 0.8%. Rabe (1961) found pykno-epileptic attacks combined with psychomotor epilepsy in only two out of 3,200 patients. Christian (1962) mentions the possibility of such a combination but he emphasizes that it is sometimes difficult to tell the difference between absence and a psychomotor attack and other authors have also referred to this subsequently. Doose and Scheffer (1965) admit the possibility of a combination of absence and psychomotor attacks and of a transition from the first into the second form of epilepsy. However, like Christian (1962) they point out that this borderline between two clinical forms cannot be clearly defined and it is not possible to tell where one ends and the other begins. Hedenström, v. and Dreyer (1967) described a typical case with simultaneous occurrence of psychomotor and pykno-epileptic attacks and they verified this by the EEG. Psychomotor or even focal epilepsy could arise by lateral displacement or extension of the focus which according to Penfield and Jasper (1964), is situated in the centrencephalic cerebral structures (Figure 11).

The development of the *secondary psychomotor epilepsy* from the other forms of grand mal has several possibilities (Figure 5).

Firstly, it may be associated with a severe form of grand mal-diffuse epilepsy, and become manifest in the interval between two major seizures or even occur together with grand mal seizures to round off the picture of a major attack. The second possibility is that it develops from grand mal nocturnal epilepsy or occurs as an additional factor in the transition from

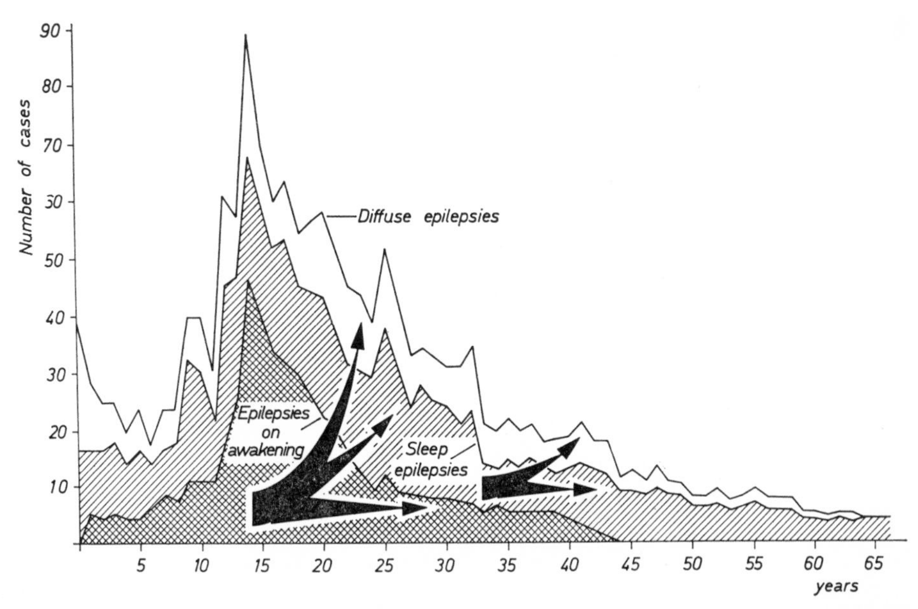

Figure 5. Disease age and course of matutinal, nocturnal and diffuse epilepsy. Nocturnal epilepsy and diffuse epilepsy have a common *finale*. Here, the psychomotor form can develop immediately or after the transition into diffuse epilepsy. Matutinal epilepsy can also combine with psychomotor epilepsy by a transition into the nocturnal type, or it can change directly into diffuse epilepsy. Psychomotor attacks can only develop after this has occurred. (From Janz, D., *Nervenarzt, 26*:20, 1955.)

nocturnal epilepsy to the diffuse form. Janz (1953, 1963, 1968) believes that, in the course of time, nocturnal epilepsy may develop from matutinal epilepsy. Here, psychomotor attacks may also occur in addition, or matutinal epilepsy may in the course of time develop into diffuse epilepsy and the psychomotor attacks be added later.

There are also several possibilities in respect to the development of psychomotor epilepsy from petit mal (Figures 6 and 7). According to Janz and Matthes (1955), Janz (1963) and also Doose (1967), the severe form of petit mal (propulsive petit mal—Blitz-Nick-Salaam spasms BNS) may end as such, but it may also develop into retropulsive petit mal (absence, pyknoepilepsy) or into psychomotor epilepsy. The second possible course of development is that from retropulsive petit mal. According to Rabe (1961) and Janz (1963), pykno-epilepsies may also heal completely as such, or may develop into impulsive petit mal (myoclonus epilepsy) or in rare cases, into psychomotor epilepsy. Finally, in time, a primary form of impulsive petit mal may also change into a psychomotor form or into grand mal (Janz 1962, 1963, 1972; Janz and Christian 1957).

The outcome of psychomotor epilepsy is unfavorable. Only in rare

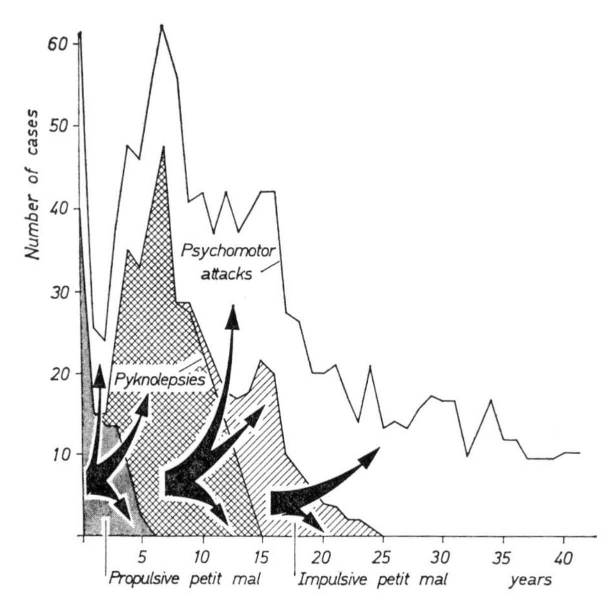

Figure 6. Development of psychomotor epilepsy from petit mal-type epilepsy. (From Janz, D., *Epilepsia, 3*:69-109, 1962.)

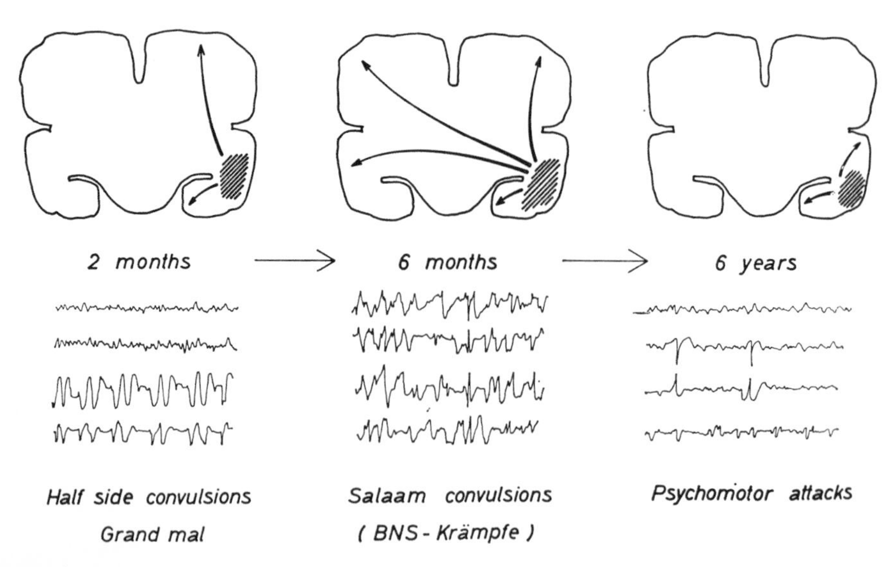

Figure 7. With increasing age, psychomotor epilepsy can develop from other forms of juvenile epilepsy. The directions of the spread of epileptic excitation in the brain are shown above, and below are corresponding changes of bioelectrical cerebral activity over the cortex. (From Doose, H.: *Forschr Neurol Psychiatr, 35*:148, 1967.)

cases is there complete recovery. Usually it develops into epileptic dementia or, in the course of time, new epileptic forms arise with major seizures which have an even more unfavorable effect on the further course of the disease. Ganshirt (1961) and Tellenbach (1965) regarded psychomotor epilepsy as the final outcome of all forms of epilepsy.

NOMENCLATURE

The classification and systematization of this very diverse form of epilepsy is very difficult. Jackson and Beevor (1890) and Jackson (1890, 1931) used the terms autonomic epilepsy, uncinate fits or dreamy state; Pette (1939) used the term autonomic epilepsy; Gibbs and Gibbs (1952) spoke of the psychomotor attack; Alliez (1952) of rhinencephalic epilepsy; Meyer-Mickeleit (1950, 1953) of twilight attacks, transient twilight state or psychomotor equivalents; Bailey (1954) of visceral epilepsy; Penfield and Jasper (1954), Symonds (1954) of temporal or temporal lobe epilepsy; Hallen (1954 a, b) and Janz (1955) of oral petit mal or oral automatisms.

A plethora of descriptions is the result of very diverse clinical phenomena or of the varied neurophysiological and neuroanatomical findings. Jovanovic (1967, d) refers to both psychomotor and nocturnal epilepsy as rhombencephalo-cortical or temporocephalic epilepsy. Of all the terms used in the literature, the best have proved to be *psychomotor epilepsy* (Gibbs et al. 1948, Gibbs and Gibbs 1952) from the clinical point of view, and *temporal* or *temporal lobe epilepsy* (Baldwin 1958, Gastaut 1954, 1963, de Jong 1957, Margerison and Corsellis 1966, Penfield and Jasper 1954) from the neurophysiological and neuroanatomical point of view.

Further difficulties are encountered when attempting to differentiate more precisely between types of psychomotor epilepsy. Compared with absence, which has few symptoms, according to Matthes (1961), psychomotor epilepsy has many clinical manifestations. The phenomenological spectrum is broad, from stereotyped automatisms to paroxysmal disturbances or re-enactions and coordinated acts. For this reason, many authors have tried to select the most important symptoms in order to carry out differentiated systematization.

Lennox (1951) proposed the *psychomotor triad:* 1.) *psychomotor attacks* (43% of a large group of patients) in the narrower sense, characterised by clouding of consciousness with or without involuntary motor activity; 2.) *automatic attacks* (32% of cases) with motor automatisms and amnesia, and 3.) *subjective (psychic) attacks* with strange psychological experiences and the nature of the attack is remembered. Beyond this, Lennox also distinguishes between two to three subgroups.

Meyer-Mickeleit (1953) regards clouding of consciousness as the principal symptoms and he divides what he calls *twilight attacks* into: 1.) *mild twilight attacks* with few symptoms: these resemble absences, but they may be accompanied by abnormal experiences (hallucinations) at the beginning of or during the attack; 2.) *motor-coordinated* attacks with automatisms, irrational acts or speech disturbances, and 3.) *tonic deviations,* twitching and disturbed physical posture or the patient may even fall.

Gastaut (1953) uses the term *temporal lobe epilepsy* and, on the basis of the results of clinical and experimental investigations, he divides it into three syndromes: 1.) *temporal psychomotor epilepsy* (superficially temporal) with lesions in individual temporal gyri. Clinically, its particular characteristics are psychosensory episodes (hallucinations, illusions, etc.) and during the attack and in the interval there are very localized foci in the EEG; 2.) *hippocampal psychomotor epilepsy,* caused both by lesions of the hippocampal gyrus and also by lesions of the Ammon's horn itself. This is the most common form. Clinically, autonomic symptoms predominate during the attacks. The EEG is characterized by typical, sporadic theta waves over all the temporal regions both unilateral and bilateral. During the attack there are temporal theta waves which show a tendency to generalize and 3.) *diencephalic psychomotor epilepsy* with lesions in the thalamus, hypothalamus and subthalamus and of the tegmentum. Here, the principal symptoms during the attack are automatisms and disturbed consciousness and, during the interval, behavioural disorders. The EEG changes are inconsistent and variable (often generalized theta and delta activity). Gastaut's classification has not as yet been accepted clinically (Christian 1960; Doose and Scheffer 1965).

Hallen (1954 a, b) defends the assertion about *oral petit mal;* he regards psychomotor phenomenon in the oral region as an obligatory symptom of an attack, in fact, as the actual paroxysmal manifestation. He assumes that foci around the amygdala and the perioamygdalar cerebral cortex are the origin of the convulsion elements. He distinguishes between: 1.) a *psychic* or purely psychomotor form; 2.) an *autonomic* form, and 3.) a *motor* form of *oral petit mal.* Janz (1955) also used this classification and undertook detailed and differentiated analysis of the attacks.

The term *oral petit mal* has been objected to for practical rather than theoretical reasons, since it might be confused with petit mal of the centrencephalic type. In view of these objections, particularly Niedermeyer's criticism (1955 a), in 1962 Hallen revised his nomenclature and referred to types of psychomotor epilepsy. Thus, Hallen's new classification of 1962 accounts for four types: 1.) *the oral type* (the oral form) is mainly characterized by uncinate fits; at the outset there are sensory-motor components in the oral region, and in rare cases autonomic sensations are also recorded;

2.) *the adversive type* with changes of body posture with pivoting about the sagittal axis; 3.) *the vocalization or dysphasic type* with speech changes and, 4.) *the pure psychomotor type,* which cannot easily be classified under one name.

Even before Hallen revised his nomenclature, Niedermeyer (1955 b) had tackled this difficult task and undertook differentiated classification. Taking account of the electroencephalographic (EEG) findings, he distinguished between six forms of psychomotor epilepsy: 1.) *the uncharacteristic form,* with unilateral or bilateral temporal, fronto-central, occipital or centrencephalic foci, temporal delta focus or theta focus, or severe dysrhythmia; 2.) *the progressive form with dementia,* with diffuse irregular convulsive activity in the EEG, centrencephalic convulsion discharges or severe diffuse slow dysrhythmia; 3.) *the psychotic form,* with unilateral or bilateral temporal convulsion focus or temporal delta focus; 4.) *the psychopathic form,* with unilateral temporal delta focus in the EEG; 5.) *the neurotic form,* with unilateral temporal convulsion focus or temporal delta focus, and 6.) *benign form,* with unilateral temporal focus, occipital focus, temporal theta focus or a normal EEG.

It is interesting that Landolt (1960, 1962, 1963a, b), who studied a very comprehensive group of patients and was able to accumulate experience with epileptics over a period of many years, undertook differential clinical analysis but did not undertake to break down psychomotor (temporal) epilepsy into smaller and more concise subgroups. On the other hand, from the course and psychopathological phenomena Landolt (1960, 1962) did attempt to give a picture of the psychomotor attack to include all the symptoms.

By *paroxysmal manifestations,* Landolt means, among other things twilight attacks. *The episodic form* then included several types and forms: 1.) *postparoxysmal twilight states* which occur after one of the paroxysms (generalized, focal psychomotor attack); 2.) *petit mal status* as an attack sui generis with long 3/sec. spike wave complexes; 3.) *productive psychotic twilight states* with forced normalization in the EEG, and 4.) *twilight states of an organic nature* without forced normalization in the electroencephalogram. However, the occasional epileptic mood does not belong to these subgroups of psychotic episodes. By *chronic disorders* Landolt means chronic psychotic changes which show many psychopathological variations but which are very difficult to classify when examined more closely. These are usually mixed states with one or more particular characteristics, with one feature or another predominating at one particular time; other characteristics predominating in turn, then disappearing.

We wish to consider psychomotor epilepsy together with its phenomenological, neuroanatomical, neurophysiological, biological and biochemical partner, nocturnal epilepsy of grand mal, and to classify them as temporocephalic forms of epilepsy (Table I).

DIFFERENTIATING TEMPOROCEPHALIC EPILEPSY FROM OTHER FORMS OF EPILEPSY

CLINICAL DISTINCTIONS BETWEEN TEMPOROCEPHALIC AND CENTRENCEPHALIC EPILEPSY ARE SUMMARIZED IN TABLE I. In temporocephalic epilepsy, the major seizures usually (or even exclusively) begin during sleep. Increasing occurrence of major seizures of this form while the patient is awake indicates rapid progression towards diffuse epilepsy (David 1955, Féré 1896, Gänshirt and Vetter 1961, Janz 1953 a to 1972, Jovanovic 1966 to 1968 e, 1972 a, d, Krischek 1962, Kruse 1964, Loiseau 1964, Vogl 1964). Psychomotor attacks are often observed while the patient is awake, but they also occur during sleep as discussed later. Since the latter are less harmful and do not take a dramatic course, the sleeping patient is often not aware of them and his relatives do not recognize them.

However, in centrencephalic epilepsy (matutinal epilepsy and petit mal) the major attacks usually occur while the patient is awake. Petit mal episodes also usually occur during the waking hours. At night they may occur during or after waking, but an insignificant number develop directly out of sleep (Jovanovic 1968 a, 1972 d).

ELECTROENCEPHALOGRAPHIC DISTINCTIONS. In a large percentage of cases of centrencephalic epilepsy, the EEG is pathological and it usually shows generalized cerebral and bilateral-symmetrical 3/sec. spike and wave complexes (Figure 9). In temporocephalic epilepsy there is a decidedly smaller percentage of pathological EEGs. The changes are manifest in the form of isolated spikes or sharp waves over the temporal cerebral regions (Figure 10). Spike and wave complexes are the exception here.

DIFFERENCES IN THE SLEEP PATTERN. The sleeping habits differ in the two forms of epilepsy. Patients with temporocephalic epilepsy go to bed early, fall asleep rapidly and peacefully, have a deep, refreshing sleep and rise immediately on waking in the morning. In contrast, patients with centrencephalic epilepsy take longer to get to sleep and they have a long, restless and superficial sleep which is unrefreshing. While the former patients have a sleep surplus, the latter (i.e. from the centrencephalic group) have a considerable sleep deficit which provokes attacks. This differing sleep pattern will be discussed again later from the biochemical point of view. The patients of the centrencephalic epilepsy group are alert during the afternoon and evening. In contrast, patients of the temporocephalic group are tired at these times, while they are lively in the morning.

DIFFERENCES BETWEEN TEMPOROCEPHALIC AND CENTRENCEPHALIC EPILEPTICS WITH REGARD TO INTELLIGENCE. This has been studied by several authors and recently discussed by Janz (1968). We should like to refer briefly to Janz's detailed psychopathological analysis in the context of temporal and centrencephalic epilepsy. He cites studies by Langdon-Down and Brain, who found that the diurnal group (mostly matutinal epileptics and petit mal patients) have an intelligence quotient (IQ) of 0.7 as against 0.6 for the nocturnal and diffuse epileptics. Patry (in Janz 1968) found an intelligence age of 13.2 in matutinal epileptics as compared with 12.2 to 12.6 in nocturnal epileptics. David (1955) also agrees that patients with matutinal epilepsy are much more intelligent. About 64 percent of his patients had received higher education. Janz (1968) also notes that the number of attacks can have an effect on the level of intelligence and he refers to the findings of Langdon-Down and Brain; in six months they recorded an average of 23 attacks in matutinal epileptics and 48 to 51 in the group with attacks arising during sleep.

Character differences. The nocturnal and psychomotor epileptics are characterized by their appearance of solidarity and social stability. They also appear conscientious, hard-working and reliable. They tend to exhibit the familiar *typical* picture (Janz 1968) of being pedantic, obstinate, dogmatic and overbearing. They are given to verbosity and nuances in speech. In contrast to the matutinal epileptic, the nocturnal epileptic tends to be introspective and hypochondriac. These characteristics are even more pronounced if there is a combination of major and psychomotor attacks. According to Leder (1966), nocturnal epileptics report twice as many autonomic symptoms as matutinal epileptics.

On the other hand, patients of the centrencephalic group are not (as generally expected) pedantic, egocentric and dogmatic. They tend to be unstable and thoughtless because they readily accept suggestion and are easily deceived, because they lack tenacity and resoluteness, and because of liberality and indolence and sometimes because of grandiosity and ostentation even to the extent of pseudology. They have strong emotions, with brief fits of bad temper, but they are easy to pacify. They often react with distrust, envy or spite, so that their behavior often seems infantile. However, they also tend to dissimulate difficulties, complaints and attacks. They also suffer from autonomic instability. Many factors may easily trigger an attack (as discussed later).

Leder (1966, 1967) carried out a detailed psychopathological investigation (blind trial) on 34 patients with isolated and combined pykno-epileptic attacks and/or matutinal grand mal, and on 55 patients with isolated and combined psychomotor attacks and/or nocturnal grand mal. He obtained the following results: 82 percent of the cases could be correctly classified with the aid of an empirically developed point scale; in 8 percent it was not possible to decide; in 10 percent, patients from the *nocturnal group* were regarded as matutinal epileptics for the test; however, *matutinal epileptics* were never regarded as nocturnal epileptics.

Differences between temporal and centrencephalic epileptics with regard to experience type. Clinically and in the Rorschach test, Leder (1966, 1967) found nocturnal and psychomotor epileptics to be apathetic, parsimonious, limited and giving an impression of being immovable and difficult to communicate with in conversation. Also, there were higher form percentages, higher perseveration percentages and lower original percentages. The patient with temporocephalic epilepsy is noted for his lack of spontaneous, emotional involvement in the events of life and for repression or suppression of emotion. The center of his range of experience is neither fantasy nor human society, but he is particularly concerned with the processes in and around his own body (Janz 1968). With regard to the temporal psychosyndrome, Landolt (1960) reports indeterminate hypochondriac complaints which also correspond to the results from the Rorschach test (Leder 1967) in nocturnal epileptics, while these complaints do not appear at all in results from matutinal epileptics. The test protocols of matutinal epileptics indicate an extravert type with a tendency to act spontaneously and sociably rather than acting independently. Thus, centrencephalic epileptics tend to be subject to passive momentary impulses and effections and always to express themselves emotionally with labile variations of mood. Tellenbach (1965) describes matutinal epileptics as having emotionally labile extravert, infantile and irascible personalities, sometimes even to the extent of fault-finding. In contrast, the nocturnal epileptic proceeds towards autonomic tyranny, independent of external factors (see also Janz 1953, 1962, 1968, 1972; Mignone et al. 1970).

Differences between the two forms of epilepsy with regard to overcoming conflict. Patients of the nocturnal group take careful note of their attacks and all the associated manifestations. According to Janz (1968) the dominant form of defense is probably found among the anacastic group of *defense mechanisms*. Bräutigam (1951) believes that the *enechetic* personality change must be regarded as a protection against increased tendency to hate and aggression. The at times exaggerated solicitude, pedantry and humility, and the pronounced sense of justice in these patients is interpreted as the product of reaction formations behind which lie contradictory tendencies of a strongly dynamic nature. Bräutigam (1951) explains that the regression to the anal stage is revealed by the typical triad of anal erotic characteristics (cleanliness, economy, love of order), in typical forms of anal resistance and in dreams in which an anal-sadistic world is manifest.

In contrast to the rigorously repressive epileptic of the temporocephalic group (Leder 1967), the centrencephalic epileptic with weak repression

(Tellenbach 1965) transforms the aggressive demands, which he is not able to repress from his consciousness, into positive features. In the test protocols menacing experiences are transformed into just the opposite and he frantically emphasizes the bright side, the good and the hopeful; thus, he employs an infantile defense mechanism to overcome his day-to-day conflicts. With forced optimism he behaves as if he is able to solve all his problems himself, as if he is free from feelings of guilt and fear, completely balanced and in harmony, and as if his attacks did not particularly interest him. Helmchen (1958) also found differences between the two groups of epileptics with regard to sexual behavior.

Differences with regard to life, orientation and social relationships. The patients of the temporocephalic group seek physical union and intimacy; this is often manifest as obtrusiveness and lack of detachment and as attachment to family and home, or hypersocial behavior (Bräutigam 1951). This author believes that these characteristics may represent a reaction formation because of fear of hostile opposition. This results in inhibitions and narrowness, and lack of polarization and expansiveness. With the difficulty in releasing the emotions, there is a growing danger of a delusional condition which occurs to excess in psychomotor epilepsy.

Patients of the matutinal group are arrogant with heightened imagination and according to Kraepelin (1913) this group also includes psychopaths who have epileptic attacks. In experimental psychology this is also referred to as psychic inflation (Janz 1968). The patient often shows ambivalent behaviour, i.e. he tends to have divergent impulses, but denies the irreconcilability of such demands. The resulting indecisiveness which pervades his everyday life both when faced with ethical, erotic or religious problems has been insurpassably portrayed by Dostojewski, and Janz (1968) goes into this in great detail.

Differences in physique and constitution are also in evidence. According to Jovanovic and Schäfer (1966), with temporocephalic epilepsy athletic, dysplastic and pyknic types predominate; patients of the centrencephalic group are most commonly asthenics, leptosomes or athletic-leptosome mixed types. This shows the extent to which epilepsy, like the individual disease groups, is a specifically biological problem and is not simply a problem of clinical symptomatology.

Predisposition to status epilepticus is decidedly greater in the temporocephalic epilepsy group than in the centrencephalic group. This and the other characteristics are discussed in detail later (cf. Janz 1964). The third, more severe form of epilepsy—diffuse epilepsy—represents a combination and distortion of the characteristics described under these ten points. In addition to these explanations, see also Matthews and Kløve (1967) and Mignone et al. (1970).

CLINICAL SYMPTOMATOLOGY OF THE PSYCHOMOTOR ATTACK

Isolated Psychomotor Epilepsy Without Grand Mal Seizures

Figure 8 shows the most common symptoms in isolated psychomotor epilepsy.

Psychic phenomena

THE CONSCIOUSNESS. Alteration of consciousness and passivity are observed in patients in the first phase of a psychomotor attack. The seizure usually begins with livid coloration of the skin, a fixed stare, salivation and disorientation. The patient does not fall; there are not usually any convulsions as occur in the major seizure. The phase of passivity lasts for a short while and then the patient begins to move. Already unconscious, he tries to orientate himself and to make contact with his surroundings; often the onset of absence is slow and accompanied by abnormal experiences, such as visual, acoustic, vestibular, olfacto-gustatory and tactile hallucinations or illusions.

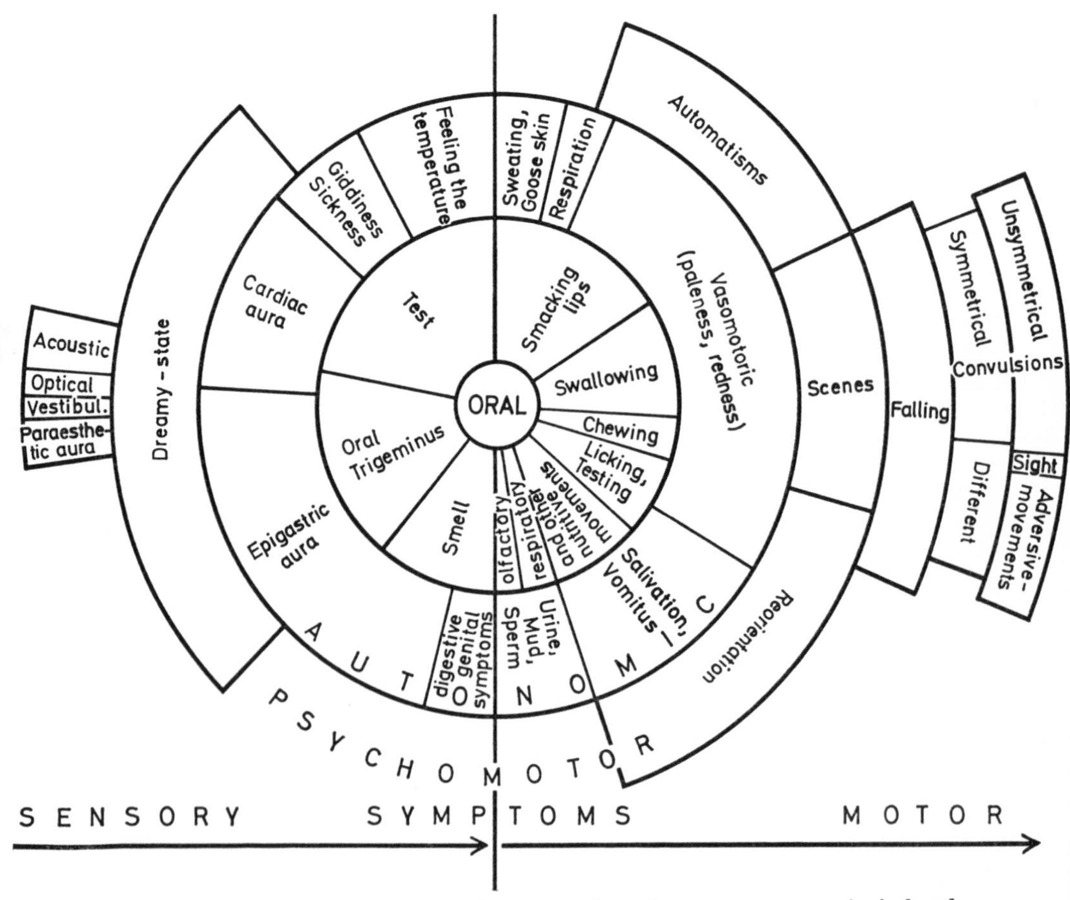

Figure 8. Brief summary of the mental, autonomic and motor symptoms in isolated psychomotor epilepsy. (From Janz, D.: *Nervenarzt, 26*:20-28, 1955.)

The *psychomotor fit,* Lennox (1951), or the *twilight attack,* Meyer-Mickeleit (1953), is often preceded by unpleasant experiences known as *aura.* In between times, the patient may come to and then lose consciousness again. This may be seen several times during an attack. At the beginning of an attack, the patients often complain of being remote or alienated from their surroundings; their sight and hearing become impaired and more distant. Thought becomes more and more difficult and slow; some waver between sleeping and waking, others experience everything as if in a film, under anaesthetic or in a dream. Some patients do not lose consciousness, or their consciousness is just a little impaired or more or less clouded.

Jackson (1899) observed a form of alteration of consciousness in patients with psychomotor attacks, which he described as a *dreamy state.* During these episodes the patient is beset with experiences and things which, according to Gowers (1902), are unlike anything normally encountered. The unusual quality of the manifestations is always apparent from the patient's dilemma when he is asked about his sensations. Answers like . . . "it is something like . . .," ". . . rather like . . ." or ". . . strange, like . . ." are evidence of the exotic nature of the experience. Sometimes specific ideas become obstrusive and the patient is then regarded as a schizophrenic. The experience is often familiar, or reminiscent of some previous event. Gowers (1902) called this phenomenon *deja vu;* Jackson (1899) referred to it as *reminiscence.* This last factor is one of the most important criteria for recognizing a psychomotor attack of the dreamy state type.

Distortion of real spatial and temporal relationships is common to nearly all cases of the dreamy state (Hallen 1954). On the other hand, with absence or major attacks the patient loses his awareness of his spatial and temporal surroundings. A further, and certainly very important criterion of the psychomotor attack is that the patient often registers the real world concurrently, but this awareness is permeated by foreign images or the feeling of things changing, the sensation of being something different. Jackson defined this state of double consciousness as *mental diplopia,* in which a *quasi parasitic state of consciousness* exists in addition to the normal consciousness. (Jackson and Stewart 1899).

Hallen (1954) distinguishes between an *illusory* and a *hallucinatory* dreamy state: 1.) In the *illusory dreamy state,* familiar objects and people seem strange to the patient, and the unreal begins to seem real. Thus, false conclusions may be reached. 2.) In the *hallucinatory dreamy state* there are no illusions about actual surroundings, but unheralded, genuine hallucinations are reported. When the attack occurs after the initial experiences, there is *retrograde amnesia.*

OPTICAL SENSATIONS. Distortion of the real surroundings is described as an *illusory* sensation. At the beginning of the attack, objects and people become less familiar, more distant, smaller and deformed in the eyes of the patient. The patient may perceive a general acceleration of walking, driving and movement. Persons and objects are misinterpreted and this may result in aggressiveness, sometimes directed towards members of the patient's own family.

The patient often reports changes in his own body. The sensation that distal limbs are shrinking or enlarging, and sensations of symmetrical changes in certain parts of the body have also been described (Hallen 1954, 1962, Lennox 1961). With visual hallucinations, objects and persons of geometric or of irregular shape may suddenly appear, although they do not really exist.

In instances of *déjà vu,* the patient may perceive places and landscapes. One of our female patients was enticed away from home for eight days into a wide but "familiar landscape" and only after these eight days did she come to herself and was able to re-orientate herself. Short *films* or entire optical re-enactions are not uncommon.

Acoustic sensations. The changes in hearing from the illusory point of view have already been mentioned. People appear suddenly to begin speaking quickly, and then get quicker and quicker. One of Hallen's patients (1954 a) was aware of a motor outside the hospital running faster and faster. During the attack he thought that the driver kept on accelerating. As the patient came to, the noise diminished and slowed, and he thought that the driver had just got out of the vehicle.

One of our female patients apparently heard water dripping from a tap with hollow echoes, as if in a cave. Flashes of light came at her from all sides and disappeared just in front of her eyes and now and again she heard a shrill ringing in her head. She had the feeling that a mountain was gaping open in front of her and that she was falling in. The episode lasted for one to two minutes before normal consciousness began to return.

With hallucinations, acoustic sensations are rarer than in the illusory dreamy state. Acoustic hallucinations occur in association with optical phenomena, but not alone. Also, the primary optical hallucinations are always incorporated into a scene or episode and are experienced by the patient as a regular course of events.

Vestibular sensations take the form of vertigo. One of Hallen's patients (1962) experienced severe vertigo as an aura; he felt that his surroundings were spinning faster and faster to the left. At the same time, he felt a desire to vomit. The aura only lasted a few seconds and then he lost consciousness, turning head and trunk towards the right and at first staring fixedly towards the right until his countenance cleared and he performed gay and abandoned turns about his own body axis. The circles became more and more like dancing and ended as pacing throughout the room. The tendency to waver to the right persisted.

OLFACTO-GUSTATORY SENSATIONS are typical of a psychomotor attack and have been observed by nearly all the authors who have dealt with this form of attack up to now. In view of the olfacto-gustatory sensations, Jackson (1899) described psychomotor attacks as *uncinate fits.* Hallen (1954, 1962) called this form *oral petit mal.*

Sensory Phenomena

As just mentioned, in the majority of cases, the sensory phenomena are manifest in the olfactory-gustatory sensory region. Sensations of taste and smell or hallucinations cause the patients to sip, lick, smack his lips, click his tongue, chew, grind his teeth, snuffle, sniff and carry out other nutritive movements associated with uninhibited sensorimotor oral function. Jackson sought the cause of these manifestations in the hippocampus or uncus hippocampi region. This hypothesis showed remarkable insight and it was later substantiated both experimentally and clinically (Hassler 1964 a, b, Landolt 1960, Lennox 1951, Margerison and Corsellis 1966, Meyer-Mickeleit 1950, 1953, Sperling and Creutzfeldt 1959).

Epigastric (stomach pains), respiratory, cardiac and tactile sensations are also familiar manifestations. Several times, pain in the epigastrium or abdomen has caused doctors to operate in the abdominal region. This form of epilepsy often occurs in children.

Moore (1946) found psychomotor epilepsy in 14 of 28 patients who reported abdominal colic. Like Moore, Livingston (1951) recorded 14 cases with abdominal complaints and psychomotor epilepsy. Hoeffer et al. (1951) studied 31 cases with pain localized in the epigastrium or around the umbilicus which had persisted for a couple of minutes or even for several hours. There was also anorexia, vomiting, diarrhea or constipation. Four of these 31 patients had already had generalized attacks from the outset, while six developed these in later life.

O'Brien and Goldensohn (1957) described a woman in whom abdominal sensations lasted for more than 24 hours. The attacks were accompanied by nausea and vomiting. During the interval or associated with the abdominal sensations there may also be other symptoms of the psychomotor attack, particularly livid facial coloration and facial rigidity. Zeskov and Hajnsek (1960) have described similar sensations in five cases. These forms are known in the literature as *abdominal epilepsy* (Gastaut and Poiner 1964, Zeskov and Hajnsek 1960).

Motor Phenomena

ORAL AUTOMATISM are the characteristic signs of motor disturbances in psychomotor epilepsy. In 75 percent of 72 patients, Meyer-Mickeleit (1953) observed motor manifestations of the mouth, tongue and jaw, including lips and similar movements of the mouth, clicking the tongue, grinding of the lower jaw, sipping (movements of the lips as if sipping something), spitting at regular and irregular intervals in one direction or another, coughing, wheezing and jaspern—the most familiar oral movements. The most common of these symptoms are: smacking lips, swallowing and chewing. Hallen (1954a) observed oral automatisms, or *nutritive re-enactions* as he calls them, in nearly all his 209 patients (100%). There was smacking of lips in 85 cases (40.7%), swallowing in 57 (27.3%), gulping in five (2.4%), sipping movements in 32 (15.3%), wiping of the mouth with inflation of cheeks in one (0.5%), drinking movements in two cases (1.0%) and oral disturbances in isolated cases.

Speech disturbances are also reported by all the authors (Hallen 1954-1962, Lennox 1951, Meyer-Mickeleit 1953, Preston and Arack 1964, and others). Our own experience correlates with that of these authors. Very often the patient utters unintelligible, meaningless phrases like: "Yes, yes, indeed, well, hallo, no, no, it can't go on like this, oh, etc." Meyer-Mickeleit (1953) reports the words of a 50-year-old gamekeeper, spoken in Latin: *"quia ex pro hobis, quia ex, ex alta pro nobis!"* The speech disturbances are often associated with acoustic hallucinations. In the literature they are referred to as speech changes, dysarthria, an amnestic aphasia, inability to understand words, paraphasic deviation, jargon aphasia, but mainly as verbal automatisms (Alajaune 1955, Castells, Fuster and Maslenikow 1957, Hecaen and Angelergues 1960, Jackson 1872 to 1899, Lennox 1950, Margerison and Corsellis 1966, Penfield 1948, Penfield and Jasper 1954, Preston and Atack 1964). Hallen (1962) demonstrated these speech aberrations in 57 (8%) of 712 patients. Castells et al. (1957) found them in five of 200 cases, Preston and Atack (1964) found them in four of 47 cases. Sometimes there is long-winded murmuring, humming and babbling, and annoying and sterotyped repetition of phrases or single words which the patient has not come across before. According to Hallen (1962) the speech may disintegrate to the extent of complete sensory aphasia with regressive degeneration. Repetition (perseveration) is a typical symptom of vocal disturbances in patients during a psychomotor attack. Neologisms are not uncommon. The patients often have the feeling that they can predict what the doctor or person they are speaking to will say. Hallen (1962) calls this kind of attack the *vocalization or dysphasic type* of psychomotor epilepsy.

Nearly all authors report *coordinated, automatic hand movements* in over 50 percent of cases. The movements may be simple, standardized and repetitive, or very varied. The patient may finger clothes or bed covers, reach for objects and fidget with things which he can reach, wipe, rub, knit, tinker, crochet, dress or undress, or feel around uncertainly for minutes on end;

these are the movements most often observed. Less common movements are plucking, tugging, scratching, scraping, smoothing, burrowing or rummaging. Here again there are stereotyped movements with rhythmic clenching and unclenching of the fists, rhythmic movements like drumming, splaying the fingers, stroking movements of one hand over the other as if to take off a glove, or clapping the hands in front of the face. Many clutch at the air as if catching flies, or gesticulate by beating their arms up and down. The possible variations of motor disturbance of the hands are too numerous to be described in detail.

According to Meyer-Mickeleit (1953), Hallen (1962) and Preston and Atack (1964), *tonic changes of posture* are also quite common. These often pass very quickly and may be overlooked because they are so transient. These tonic changes of posture are manifest as slow body and eye movements and they are usually contralateral to the convulsion focus in the EEG; they may also be homolateral, but this is less common. In many cases, the face or corner of the mouth is twisted to one side for a short time. In contrast to cortical adversive convulsions, in psychomotor epilepsy this twisting is slower, smoother and not clonic. The patient does not assume an aggressive stance and, in contrast to the adversive form, subsequently there is often complete amnesia for this episode in the attack. Deviation sometimes to the right, sometimes to the left may be observed in one and the same patient. Hallen (1962) calls this form of psychomotor epilepsy the *adversive type*.

Mimetic rigidity (the face looks expressionless and mask-like with eyes fixed straight ahead) is often recorded at the beginning of a psychomotor attack. Tonic rotation of the body has also been observed.

Changes of posture and collapse or falling are characteristic but not consistent phenomena. The upright posture is usually maintained, but Meyer-Mickeleit (1953) reports falling to the ground in about 15 percent of his cases. Here again, as with the tonic changes of posture, the process is slow. Sudden falling or collapse as occur in a major seizure, are fairly uncommon. Accordingly, here there are fewer or less serious injuries as compared with epileptic is with major attacks. Some patients incline their head forwards or lean a long way forward. Others sway backwards and forwards with the upper part of their body or lean over backwards. Many rotate or run in circles, pivoting about a sagittal axis. Twisting and circular movements largely determine the behavior in the twilight states.

Complicated, relatively ordered actions or *automatic leg movements* also occur in a large number of patients. Rhythmic, repeated movements of the legs, stamping, shuffling, trampling, tripping or skipping on the spot, are the usual manifestations. In the lying position, the patient pulls up his legs to his body alternately, kicks about or makes cycling movements. The complicated, relatively ordered actions are inappropriate. Many patients stand up and walk round the room and some stand on a table, chair or windowsill. Others try to undress and then a little while later to dress again, buttoning their shirt or blouse or pulling off their shoes. Two of Meyer-Mickeleit's patients (1953) put lighted cigarettes into their mouths the wrong way round. One patient got out of bed during the night, put on the light, dressed and wanted to go into the cellar. A boy tried to sit on the lap of the woman next to him on a train. Again and again there are reports of patients carrying out familiar activities during a psychomotor attack.

For example, many patients execute movements usually associated with eating. Women make movements as if they are washing up, knitting, crocheting or cleaning. The tailor continues to sew during the attack. In the street a patient will continue walking without passers-by noticing what has happened. It may happen that the patients regain consciousness somewhere in the town and do not know how they have got there. Among Hallen's patients (1954 a, b) there were some who had walked or travelled some considerable distance through the town. The patients may carry out extremely complicated actions in their unconscious state and often these are not fragmentary or just implied, but carried out rationally, consistently and completely. One of his patients organized a little excursion, inviting a couple of young people to go with him; he arranged for them to change buses en route and accompanied them to their destination. He conducted them right across a large city and bought more tickets, until finally he regained consciousness in a factory in the suburbs, all without the two friends with him noticing anything untoward. They had considered that minor departures from the planned program were simply amusing surprises. One of our patients was a bus driver in a medium-sized town. Suddenly he altered his usual route and drove down completely different streets and in the wrong direction. At first the passengers thought it was a detour and then they began to complain. Taking no notice of them, the driver went on and only stopped a long way outside the town, asking his passengers how he had got there.

This does not simply apply to driving and walking. The patients are capable of other complicated activities during a psychomotor attack. For example, impressive acrobatic feats like turning somersaults, vaulting, handstands, or leaping obstructions and obstacles.

Fugues should not be confused with ordered driving or walking. They may begin suddenly and be directionless, aimless and straight, sometimes ending after a few steps or a short distance. Here the patients may be in danger of walking onto or falling down on the road. They may jump into or out of a tram or bus. The episodes are violent; the patients force their way through and might become aggressive. Walking or travelling a considerable distance has often been reported in the literature (Meyer-Mickeleit 1953).

As the results of their statistical analysis of the symptoms, Bamberger and Matthes (1959) compiled 41 variations of motor automatisms, ten different autonomic symptoms and 17 different modifications of an aura. Meyer-Mickeleit (1950, 1953) found 30 different varieties of automatisms, almost 20 other motor disturbances and differentiated forms of aura which have been mentioned above.

Autonomic Phenomena

Right at the beginning of a psychomotor attack, the first symptoms are livid facial color with motor and mimic rigidity, salivation, outbreak of sweating, and singultus. Subjectively there are waves of heat in the head, an indescribable feeling starting in the stomach and rising to the neck, paroxysmal tachycardia, palpitation of the heart, gallop rhythm, changes of pulse and bright red color of the head. Hallen (1954 a) observed autonomic symptoms in the course of psychomotor attacks in 165 of 209 patients. There was increased salivation in 49 patients (23.9%), dryness in the mouth in one (0.5%), outbreak of sweating in 18 (8.6%), facial pallor in an imposing number of patients (72 cases or 34.4%), redness of face in 18 (8.6%), cyanosis of the lips in ten (4.9%) and pallor confined to the mouth in two (1.0%). He also observed goose-pimples in one patient, vomiting in nine, passage of urine in 20, discharge of feces in five, ejaculation in one, palpitation of the heart in three, increased pulse rate in 19, increased blood pressure in one, more rapid breathing in eight, singultus in five, rumbling in the stomach in one, dilated pupils in 12, constricted pupils in four and lacrimation in one patient. These findings correlate with those of Preston and Atack (1964). Nocturnal twilight attacks and psychomotor autonomic disturbances are also known to be associated with incontinence and sleep-walking. For example, Meyer-Mickeleit (1953) found sleep-walking in four of 72 cases and incontinence in 13 cases.

Autonomic phenomenon can be seen not only as one of the symptoms in classic psychomotor attacks, but also as an individual symptom or as an introduction to a more or less oligosymptomatic psychomotor reaction. The occurrence of autonomic cardiac and circulatory disorders in psychomotor epilepsy has often been mentioned or discussed in detail in the literature. Indeed, Jackson (1899) was right when he used the terms *autonomic* or *visceral epilepsy*. Lennox and Gibbs (1938) have also observed vasomotor lability with fluctuating blood pressure even during the interval, in temporal lobe epilepsy. In 100 patients with *visceral epilepsy* Mulder et al. (see Michaelis 1967) found paroxysmal cardio-respiratory disturbances in 50 percent of cases. The principal symptoms were tachycardia, labored breathing, palpitation of the heart, hyperhydrosis and attacks of hyperventilation with precordial pain and the type of symptoms also found in angina pectoris.

Penfield (1957) has described *diencephalic-autonomic epilepsy;* here the prodromal symptoms are restlessness and hot flushes and these lead into the actual attack with dark red coloration of face and arms, elevation of blood pressure up to 200/100 mm.Hg, tachycardia, increased respiratory rate, lacrimation, dilation of pupils and sweating. After the attack, the blood pressure may fall to below normal, but it will return to the mean value again a little later. Proceeding from these symptoms, work has been done to track down the neuroanatomical changes in the brain which might be responsible for both the cardiovascular manifestations and also for the psychomotor attack. Penfield and Jasper (1954) detected this type of change in the region of the third ventricle; the changes were due to a tumor which under certain circumstances intermittently compressed and hypothalamic nuclei. Cushing (see Bodechtel 1963) also found autonomic attacks with parasympathetic features with an initial fall in blood pressure which arose due to stimulation of areas in the vicinity of the ventricles. Recently Michaelis (1967) described two typical cases with *cardiac attacks* in temporal lobe epilepsy and he briefly deals with the whole problem.

Other Phenomena

We have still not covered the entire spectrum symptoms of a psychomotor attack. Attacks of laughing or crying, different kinds of anxiety state, buzzing in the head and ears as isolated symptoms, paraesthesia in the extremities and face, and trigeminal neuralgia, have also been described.

Particularly in young people and people with simple structures, we have been able to detect various symptoms before they go to sleep or immediately afterwards, symptoms which probably preceded a psychomotor attack. In all cases the EEG lead was decisive for the diagnosis, even during sleep. This is reported in Chapter II.

Psychomotor Attacks Combined with Grand Mal

Psychomotor attacks associated with generalized convulsions will be discussed briefly from the point of view of our own findings, which correlate with those reported in the literature.

The *preparoxysmal* phase begins with an *aura,* an unpleasant feeling of *air* rising from the epigastrium into the heart and neck. The patients may experience transient optical, acoustic, vestibular or olfactogustatory sensations which vary between illusory and hallucinatory.

Electroencephalographically, there is first a preparoxysmal picture of large, generalized and sharp waves from the delta or theta wave band, and quite quickly after this there is a dramatic levelling out of the entire cerebral action to a zero line for four to eight seconds. This levelling out in the EEG is followed by generalized spikes which get larger and larger with an average of 6 to 7/sec. This phenomenon may last for a further four to ten seconds. In all, the preparoxysmal phase lasts for four to 20 seconds and then it becomes paroxysmal.

The *paroxysmal* phase is known to consist of a *tonic* and a *clonic* part. Dreyer (1965) describes this phase very graphically in the following words: "Initial loss of consciousness, cry and respiratory arrest, fall, general rigidity followed by generalized clonic stage, at first constricted and later dilated unresponsive pupils and the eyes usually closed, initially pallor, later cyanosis, head bent backwards, face distorted, abdominal walls retracted, fists clenched, arms flexed at elbow and wrist, legs hyperextended and adducted with feet rotated inwards and plantar-flexed or spread toes, biting of tongue, incontinence, accompanying autonomic symptoms, rapid gasping, stertorous breathing, isolated asynchronous generalized myoclonic contractions, general relaxation, coma passing into sleep, postparoxysmal confusion and exhaustion, headaches and inability to concentrate."

According to our measurements, the tonic phase lasts about 20 to 30 seconds, the clonic about 30 to 40 seconds. In all, a generalized attack lasts about 60 seconds and, rarely, up to two minutes.

The *postparoxysmal* phase can vary in length and there may be many different symptoms. The time is spent in reorientation which may last for a few minutes, hours, days or even weeks, according to the severity of the attack and the neuroanatomical changes in the brain.

If the phase which Landolt (1962) calls *postparoxysmal twilight state* occurs, then there may be a variety of psychopathological manifestations. According to Landolt (1962), this state is associated with universal clouding of consciousness which slowly recedes (although sometimes it may persist unchanged for a fairly long period) and it is observed exclusively after generalized attacks. In addition to the clouding of consciousness and the impairment of his powers of perception, his difficulty in recollecting, the errors he makes because of incomplete temporal and spatial orientation and the incomplete orientation towards his own person (undoubtedly the principal symptom here), it is characteristic that the patient responds to elementary and primitive psychological stimuli but, under certain circumstances, does not respond to complex stimuli, and he responds with primitive reactions (flight, aggression and other basic defense and fear reactions such as piercing screams). Such primitive responses can sometimes be triggered instantly and completely by the slightest stimulus, such as a light touch. In many post-paroxysmal twilight states, there is a troubled restlessness. This may be regarded as a minimum primitive response to the situation itself.

Often the patient shows a certain awkwardness, and makes repeated attempts to reach some object. However, there are no automatic stereotypes such as are seen in twilight attacks in the generalized phase. The actions (we are still quoting Landolt) appear to be more rational and more differentiated: the personality is expressed, even if only in a primitive way, it asserts itself and has effects. According to Landolt, it is not right to speak of actual automatisms (as are found in an isolated psychomotor attack). In an earlier publication (1960) Landolt describes this condition as one of the correlatives of the generalized disorders and he regards it as an *exhaustion psychosis* closely related to the attack, and it may be regarded as the result of the attack. It is not part of the actual paroxysmal process and it usually occurs after attacks have followed one another at short intervals. It is less likely that this state would occur spontaneously, i.e. with no preceding paroxysmal episode.

FORMS, COURSE AND DURATION OF PSYCHOMOTOR SYNDROMES

Even with all that has been said up to now, we have by no means dealt with all the manifestations of the psychomotor symptom complex; to demonstrate this we must now add something further. We still have not touched upon: duration and course of brief psychomotor paroxysms; longer psychomotor episodes; the psychomotor status; the extremely important productive-psychotic manifestations with forced normalization in the EEG; the hysterical reactions in psychomotor epileptics and the chronic psychological changes in patients, the personality changes.

Brief Psychomotor Paroxysms

We, and all the other authors who have dealt with the course and duration of brief psychomotor paroxysms (Doose and Scheffer 1965, Gibbs and Gibbs 1952, Hallen 1954, 1962, v. Hedenström and Dreyer 1967, Landolt 1960 to 1963, Lennox 1950, 1951, Meyer-Mickeleit 1953, and many others) agree on a standard description of these.

Phase I: characterized by the *aura* lasting for a few seconds. After this first phase which the patient still experiences subjectively, comes the next phase.

Phase II: the phase of passivity on the part of the patient, sudden livid facial color; fixed stare straight ahead or into a corner; complete loss of consciousness; continuous staring at a by-stander; and at this moment the third phase begins. The second phase varies in length, but is usually brief: 20 seconds to one minute.

PHASE III: the phase of activity, action, perplexity and helplessness, a phase of optical, acoustic, vestibular, olfactory, gustatory and tactile illusions or hallucinations, of oral automatisms, speech disturbances, coordinated automatic hand and leg movements, tonic changes of posture, change of body attitude and further complicated, relatively ordered actions which are interpreted as attempts by the patient to orientate himself. This phase may last for one or several minutes, or even for up to half an hour.

PHASE IV: the final phase, also called the *phase of reorientation* (Hallen 1954, 1962) in which the psychomotor symptoms recede. They may subside quite quickly, in a few seconds or minutes, but often they develop into a fresh twilight phase before the patient fully regains consciousness.

For practical reasons, we would define a brief paroxysmal state as one which *does not last more than half an hour,* although biologically it is not possible to draw a dividing line.

Longer Psychomotor Episodes

According to Meyer-Mickelett (1953), longer psychomotor episodes are *twilight states* lasting for more than half-an-hour or an hour. The first and second phases are the same as those in the brief paroxysmal twilight states, while the third phase—the phase of action—may be very much prolonged. According to Landolt (1962) it may persist for days and weeks and it can be observed in patients who have never suffered any attacks. In those patients who frequently have attacks these attacks do not usually occur at all during the twilight states. The question of the absence of generalized attacks, which are replaced by the enormously prolonged twilight state, is discussed again later, and we think that this is quite an important factor in the whole biological picture of psychomotor epilepsy. In particular, we want to mention productive psychotic states and many other depressive episodes.

Psychomotor Status

All the authors recognize a definition of status epilepticus which, in the first place, cannot be regarded as complete and which, in the second place, refers more to a condition involving generalized attacks. It is defined as an accumulation of generalized epileptic attacks, between which the patient does not regain consciousness. However, loss of consciousness is not characteristic and consistent in every form of epileptic attack, so that this cannot be regarded as a complete definition.

In the literature there are only a few reports, which tend to vary, on the psychomotor status in the true sense. Hedenström, v. and Schorsch (1959) described a fairly uniform psychomotor status lasting several days. Apart from varying stages of clouding of consciousness, which was more intense on the second day, there was general motor unrest with oral and manual automatisms.

Dreyer (1962) mentions a 24-year-old man who, in one morning, suffered 110 typical attacks with tonic spasms and marked psychological changes. In the interim periods there was considerable clearing of the consciousness. Dreyer (1965) supplemented this case with another patient, although here the attacks were not so characteristic and paroxysmal. This raises the question of whether, in fact, the psychomotor status did exist, or whether they were prolonged twilight states, as described by Landolt (1960).

Kroth and Hopf (1966) described two cases. In our opinion the first case, a 15-year-old boy, did not involve a psychomotor status, but simple paroxysmal episodes in quick succession. The second case was a 34-year-old woman who had had two generalized seizures before admission to hospital. On the following day she developed a psychomotor status, which was described as follows: "Loss of consciousness, gazing to the right, head rotated to the left at first, then her lips were pushed forward, smacking of lips and definite chewing movements, at the same time slow clonic rotation of the head to the right and backwards, tongue movements, a little foaming at the mouth". Such an attack lasted for two to three minutes. These states occurred repeatedly at intervals of four to nine minutes until the next morning; for almost 24 hours. The patient was often responsive between two attacks, but her consciousness was never completely clear. In a further three hours, it was possible to overcome this status with drugs.

To summarize, it should be stressed that there must be a relatively frequent repetition of brief psychomotor attacks with all the signs of optical, acoustic, sensory, olfacto-gustatory and motor phenomena, for it to be termed *psychomotor status.* Thus, a prolonged psychomotor episode, such as Landolt (1960) describes, must not be confused with a psychomotor status. However, where a prolonged twilight state and a psychomotor status occur simultaneously it is certainly difficult to differentiate one group of symptoms from the other.

It is worth mentioning the methods used to differentiate a psychomotor status from a petit mal status. Lennox (1951) and Landolt (1960, 1962) describe the petit mal status as a special case of absences with spike and wave complexes in the attack episode. The individual complex, comprising one spike and one wave, probably represents the entire, constantly repeated course of the attack. Even in the relatively short absences there is, both clinically and electroencephalographically, a steady state in which, at most, there are quantitative changes and very few qualitative changes: a persistent state which, almost without exception, *appears abruptly and then disappears again.* To this extent, the absences with spike-wave complexes are quite distinct from the other types of attack, and in particular from twilight attacks and twilight states, and from the psychomotor status. According to Landolt (1962), in the petit mal status with 3/sec. spike-wave formations there is an enormous prolongation of the continuity of spike-wave complexes which may persist for hours and days, and thus give the impression of a twilight state.

However, the petit mal status is also easy to distinguish from the psychomotor status from the psychopathological angle. Apart from its very abrupt onset and termination and the continuous spike-wave complexes (which are not seen in psychomotor status), the petit mal status is a stuporous condition characterized by difficulty in perceiving and recollecting, strong tendency to psychological and verbal perseverations, general lack of drive and apathy, and this condition can sometimes be interrupted by psychological and physical stimuli.

Productive Psychotic Episodes

In this section we come to the problem of manifestations which do not always occur, but which are quite common in psychomotor epilepsy. There are the occasional psychotic episodes which may last for a couple of hours, or for days, weeks, months or years.

Psychopathologically and neurophysiologically, there are several distinct forms (Alsen 1965, Bonnet et al. 1959/1960, v. Ditfurth 1953, Flor-Henry 1969, 1972, Glaser 1964, Jovanovic 1966 e, Landolt, 1955, 1960, 1962, Morel 1850, Taylor 1972).

Productive Psychoses with Forced Normalization in the EEG

Sudden development of psychotic symptoms with concurrent absence of epileptic attacks and with normalization of the convulsion-specific elements in the EEG, are common to all the subforms in this group. If the psychotic episode subsides or if it is cured medicinally, then the epileptic attacks and convulsion-specific elements reappear in the electroencephalogram.

Psychopathologically, these forms resemble each other in that they have a negative orientation. Euphoric, elated, ecstatic are maniacal and uninhibited emotions are less common or disappear completely, and the dominant picture is one of depression and apathy, moroseness, touchiness and irritability, tenseness, nervousness and sometimes misery (Alsen 1965). According to Alsen, a pressing state of uneasiness can lead to an explosion of anger and to aggressive actions, and the patient may injure himself. The condition may also become manifest as poriomaniac and dipsomaniac behaviour.

In recent years Landolt (1960, 1962) has been particularly concerned with this problem and he was able to make more detailed observation of the subjects and their electroencephalographic pictures. According to this author, these are pictures of the actual *mania epileptica* which Morel (1850) described as epilepsie larvee. The clinical picture may take very many forms and those affected are sometimes extremely productive psychologically, in every respect. They may become excessively excited for a protracted period and talk or scream continuously; they are restless, constantly on the move and sometimes there is an extravagant increase in the dynamics of ideation with, at the same time, marked narrowing and sharpening of the thought processes. The same applies to the appetency. Illusions, hallucinations, absurd ideas and compulsions develop, and these must be distinguished from similar phenomena in a psychomotor attack. The patients are sometimes afraid of death, or think that the end of the world has come. However, there are also patients who feel inspired and most of them have the idea that they are thinking particularly perceptively.

Amnesia occurs in most of the cases, but this may also be absent. *However, where there is a psychotic state this amnesia has a different origin from that in a psychomotor attack.* The clouding and narrowing of consciousness during the psychotic episode is due to the fact that, in the state of excitability and complete abandon, the centripetal and reflex functions only remain for a short time, and what is perceived or understood does not register unless it is a part of the restricted realm of consciousness. According to Landolt (1962) the disorientation here is probably not the result of clouding of consciousness but is due to an abnormal heightening of perception and, in certain circumstances, the patient becomes completely engrossed in this. The psychological symptoms may vary from case to case and, in specific cases, from episode to episode.

DEPRESSIVE PRODUCTIVE PSYCHOTIC EPISODES. As an example, we shall briefly describe one of Alsen's cases (1965). This was a 26-year-old woman who had suffered originally from petit mal epilepsy and who later developed other forms of epilepsy, including psychomotor attacks. In the last two years she had experienced several short phases of depression during which there had been no attacks. About three months before the latest admission she had become extremely depressed; she complained that something inside her was missing and it was tormenting her. She did not know what was wrong with her. The ground wasn't under her feet any more, something in her head had been switched off and she was not herself any longer. She had the feeling of floating and of not belonging anywhere and she had to cry and brood over it. She could not rouse herself to do anything and she felt internal restlessness. Shortly before admission to hospital, she had cut her wrists because she could not bear the confusion any longer. Then she had felt as if she was made of glass and her body was tingling with the tension. On admission, this pyknic-cyclothymic patient showed a picture of great distress and depression.

The depressive symptoms may also occur before the first epileptic attack. Alsen (1965) cites as an example a 39-year-old woman in whom epilepsy could only be demonstrated after the first phase of depression had subsided.

PRODUCTIVE PSYCHOTIC EPISODES OF A PARANOID CHARACTER. According to Landolt (1960), this sub-form includes the *orientated* and *rational* twilight states. Several times he himself has seen cases in which the cortical EEG became normal as soon as the psychotic episode occurred and vice versa.

Tellenbach (1965) described 12 cases with centrencephalic (nine patients) or diffuse (three patients) epilepsy. Nine of these 12 cases tended to paranoid psychosis. After a completed episode with pronounced paranoid symptoms and forced normalization in the EEG, all nine cases developed into *secondary psychomotor epilepsy,* as defined by Neimanis (1962). The other cases also showed occasional signs of *de-differentiation* (Janz 1953), like patients with secondary psychomotor epilepsy. The delusional images remained nonsystematic. Usually the psychopathological syndrome developed as follows: retardation, disturbed sleep, seemingly compulsive oppression, depression, catatoni form stress, and paranoid disturbances.

Mauz (1937) has already observed that in the group of combined defective constitutions, illusions and hallucinations often occur in addition to violent motor excitation and confusion states with extreme fear or wild rage, apathetic, prolonged depression and raptuslike suicidal and aggressive fits. However, at that time the EEG was not in practical use, so that they had to depend on the clinical picture. The epileptic attacks before and after the psychotic state help to differentiate between these cases and those of other endogenous and endoform psychoses.

Alsen (1965) reported on a woman who originally had generalized and psychomotor attacks which later developed into a chronic psychosis lasting a considerable time. In 1930, at the age of 40, the patient had suffered cerebral contusion. Since 1932 the psychomotor attacks had occurred with occasional generalized convulsions. After only two more years (i.e. four years after the injury) a paranoid-hallucinatory psychosis developed; the patient died in 1961. Autopsy revealed *extremely severe contusion damage in the orbital and temporal region of the brain* and diffuse astrocytic gliosis in remote parts of the brain with the focal point in the thalamus and brain stem. Here we find a connection between psychomotor epilepsy, psychotic states of a schizophrenic nature and damage to the orbital and temporal regions of the brain. This will be discussed in detail in Chapter III.

Productive psychotic episodes of a catatonic nature. Among others, Jovanović (1966 e) has reported three cases. One of these cases was investigated thoroughly, partly for diagnostic reasons, using a polygraph during sleep. This method is reported in Chapter II.

This case involved a 26-year-old patient who had been under observation for three years. Twice he went into a classic catatonic state with *catalepsy* and *flexibilitas cerea.* These states lasted for several weeks. There were no epileptic attacks and no convulsion-specific elements in the EEG during this catatonic state, although beforehand and afterwards there were convulsions arising during sleep, with occasional twilight attacks and a convulsion-specific EEG.

Psychotic Episodes Without Forced Normalization In the EEG

According to Landolt (1960, 1962), these can be defined as *twilight states of an organic nature.* During the episode the EEG is not normal, but more pathological than before and afterwards. The psychopathological picture is typically organic in nature with mnestic disturbances, spatial and temporal disorientation, instinctive actions, difficulty in recollecting and other symptoms. According to Landolt (1965), Alsen (1965) and other authors, these conditions may be induced by toxic agents and they have arisen due to a relative overdosage of antiepileptic agents. Overdosage of antiepileptic agents may induce a pathological reaction in the EEG, in addition to causing the psychotic state. The diagnosis is simplified where there is ataxy, dysarthria, nystagmus and also, under certain circumstances, brominism with a high bromine level. The whole group shows a standard psychopathological picture and is well defined.

Hysterical Reactions and Psychomotor Epilepsy

It appears to be quite common for hysterical reactions to be related to the epileptic attacks. As early as 1874, Charcot, among others, had dealt with this problem and he referred to it in two forms: 1.) *hysterie à crises distenctes,* in which, for a certain length of time, the hysterical fits take the place of the epileptic seizures, and 2.) *hysterie à crises combinées,* in which, the epileptic and hysterical fits do not completely replace one another at intervals, and there is a combined symptom complex. Since the beginning of the last century, many authors have been concerned with this problem and it has been mentioned by Esquiriol (1838), Ball (1886), Frigerio (1899), Gowers (1902), Wilder (1931), Gibbs and Lennox (1938), Roubicek (1946), Modaud and Ajuriaguera (1948), Lennox (1950), Gibbs and Gibbs (1952) and others.

In this respect, the last 30 years have seen two significant events. Firstly, new anticonvulsant agents, the hydantoins and other preparations, have been developed and these are more reliable in curing the epileptic attacks. The second event was the discovery of the EEG which has found application in epilepsy as a relatively reliable method for research into bioelectrical cerebral activity. These two events stimulated fresh discussion among research workers about problems of epilepsy and hysterias which had been forgotten, and this altered the interpretation of these two phenomena.

To avoid going into detail on the extensive and rather controversial writings on this subject, we refer briefly to the latest discussion by Rabe (1966), since he mentions all these questions.

Rabe has observed 43 cases with epilepsy and hysterial, 21 of whom were suffering from psychomotor epilepsy. His patients comprised two groups.

The first group included 17 patients. This group was divided into two smaller subgroups. In the first subgroup, following intensive anti-epileptic treatment there were hysterical attacks, while the symptoms of epilepsy completely disappeared during the period of hysteria. If the anti-epileptic therapy was discontinued, the epileptic attacks recurred and the symptomatology of the hysterical reactions disappeared. In the second subgroup, the initial observations were of hysterical manifestations. However, in the course of time, epileptic attacks occurred as well. The hysterical symptomatology, which in some cases had existed for many years, disappeared when the epileptic attacks occurred, only to reappear as soon as the attacks were eliminated under anti-epileptic agents.

The second group of 26 patients did not differ substantially from the first. However, in this group the hysterical symptomatology did not completely replace the epileptic symptoms, although the latter were diminishing, but there was an occasional or permanent intermittent alternation between the two types of attack (hysterie à crises combinées, Charcot 1874).

A very important point has been established in connection with this problem: the convulsion-specific elements in the EEG of the epileptic disappear completely as soon as there is a hysterical fit and, conversely, convulsion elements appear in the EEG of patients as soon as the hysterical symptomatology recedes. From this, it can be concluded that hysterical attacks have an active cerebro-physiological function and that the hysterical attack has a physiological substrate in the brain as its correlative and consequently it is not a *psychogenic* manifestation (Rabe 1966).

A further point arising from Rabe's study is that in one third of the cases, the hysterical symptomatology was only a precursor of a further crisis in the clinical course, particularly in those cases given medicinal treatment. Firstly, the psychomotor attacks passed, via a hysterical reaction, into schizophrenia-like psychosis with forced normalization, according to Landolt

(1955). Secondly, the hysterical attack preceded a suicide attempt, and thirdly, the hysterical symptomatology ended in an accumulation of epileptic attacks after the medicaments had been discontinued at intervals.

Another point of decisive importance is the alternation between three states: 1.) *epilepsy* with convulsion-specific elements in the EEG; 2.) *hysterical reactions* with typical hysterical attacks (arc de cercle) and, thirdly, 3.) *psychotic episodes* with forced normalization in the EEG.

Selbach (1966), in his reply to the results and postulates of Rabe (1966) puts forward the following objections: 1.) There are certain prerequisites for the occurrence of psychogenic attacks in epileptics: a.) the presence of biologically unstable systems with damage in the final stage of differentiation (maturation disturbance); b.) an increased responsiveness to impulses, even by non-specific minimal stimuli, and c.) the dependence on the initial value. 2.) Both types of crisis have in common: a.) the same formal dynamics as multi-phase courses (build-up processes); b.) clinical courses as a primitive reaction with the aid of the extrapyramidal system. 3.) The two types of crisis differ a.) with regard to their etiology, and b.) in the extent of their autonomic correlations: *in analysing the crises, the generalized epileptic attack is considered to be a total crisis, the psychogenic attack as a partial crisis.* 4.) Because of their special characteristics, treatment of this combination of crises requires the combined effect of several factors.

However, it is possible to quote other results to refute these objections, particularly those under point three. Nayrac and Beaussart (1956 a, b) have found slower rhythms in the occipital EEG bilaterally, both in cases with epilepsy and also in those with psychogenic reactions. Roth (1962) discusses his own findings and those of other authors and comes to the conclusion that over 60 percent of prolonged rhythms in the EEG over the occipital regions of the brain occur in psychomotor epilepsy and in various hysterical and other psychogenic reactions. According to these findings: 1.) the psychogenic reactions with the typical attack, called *hysterical,* have a bioelectric correlative, and 2.) in both groups (epilepsy and neuroses) we find the same EEG changes, for example these two entities probably have certain biological, physiological and biochemical connections, which will be discussed in detail in the appropriate chapters. Apart from this, Selbach's objections (1966) are of more significance theoretically. Paal (1965) discusses this subject.

Chronic Psychic Changes in Patients with Psychomotor Epilepsy

The question of *personality change* in epilepsy seems to have been of more interest to the research worker in the last 100 years than the problems of epileptic convulsions. Originally, the investigations were all directed to the same end, to discover whether the change of personality (tenacity perseveration, pedantry, subservience, sanctimoniousness, etc.) correspond to essential epilepsy. Although as early as 1890, Féré had expressed the opinion that *idiopathic* epilepsy is only a temporary description, since from day to day more and more *essential* epilepsies were exposed as *symptomatic,* the controversy over the terms *essential, idiopathic,* and *symptomatic* has been raging for 70 years. Binswanger (1899) was strongly opposed to Féré concept and he stressed that the description *idiopathic epilepsy* covers a specific clinical course and a specific clinical concept. Redlich (1909) supported Féré's proposition and pointed out that the epileptic attack is a characteristic reaction of the brain which is triggered by various stimuli. Accordingly, the change of personality is also characteristic not only of *essential* epilepsy, but also of any other kind of epilepsy. However, Kraepelin (1913) soon rejected this idea and he maintained that the epileptic personality change was more characteristic of essential epilepsy, although he admitted that it also occurs in symptomatic epilepsy in exceptional cases.

In a statistical investigation of 1500 patients, Feuchtwanger (1930) was able to show that all changes, including character and personality changes, can occur in both essential epilepsy and in epilepsy following cerebral trauma. In an investigation carried out using 247 traumatic epileptics, Baumm (1930) found that in time, the psychological changes pass from a picture of general traumatic impairment of the brain to a picture of epileptic personality change. Fleck (1934) observed the fact that many epileptics with symptomatic epilepsy show mental changes just like those of the *essential* epileptic.

This experience was later substantiated by the discovery of Gibbs and Lennox (1937) that epileptics with psychomotor attacks and spike formations over the anterior temporal lobes exhibit an *epileptic personality* such as had previously been thought typical of the essential epileptic. In fact Stauder (1938) tried to divert the attention of scientists back to the personality change in the essential epileptic, but different, and rather contradictory results were obtained. Gibbs et al. (1948) again pointed out the personality change in epileptics with psychomotor attacks and convulsion elements in the EEG over the temporal lobe. Since then there has no longer been any doubt that, if it occurs at all, the personality change affects both *essential* and also *symptomatic* epilepsy.

Soon after this, a new fact came to light. According to studies by Hoff (1956), epileptics with fairly frequent attacks tend to show a personality change more often than those whose attacks are less frequent and fairly regular. In 338 epileptics, Hedenström, v. (1965) found a correlation between frequency of attacks and personality change. Patients with psychomotor and grand mal seizures which were manifest very frequently, showed psychological changes to a significantly greater extent than patients whose attacks occurred less often. Von Hedenström selected 161 of the 338 epileptics at random and studied the lack of psychic elasticity by means of the Rorschach test. She found that there were no differences in personality change between *essential* and *symptomatic* epilepsy. This supplementary investigation also showed that there is a positive correlation between personality change and frequency of seizures, particularly psychomotor attacks. The author also added the findings from seven patients who had been under observation for years. They had been considered to be essential epileptics and they showed clear signs of personality change; however, after death, tuberous sclerosis, tumouros vascular anomalies or chronic meningitis were found in the brain. According to extensive investigations by Gastaut et al. (1953), the cause of epilepsy, and in particular psychomotor epilepsy, is to be found in the parainal regions such as the anterior hypothalamus, uncus, amygdaloid nucleus and neighbouring cerebral structures. Subsequently, many authors have agreed with this view (this is discussed in chapter III), and so in 1957 the World Health Organization came to the conclusion "that epileptic personality change is probably linked with temporal lobe epilepsy and not with essential or centrencephalic epilepsy" (quoted from Tellez 1967).

Landolt (1962) assumes that personality change is not connected with epilepsy. It is also known to occur in other diseases. However, he adds that this *personality change is related to the pathological changes in the temporal lobe or in the limbic system.*

Tellez (1967), and other authors (Flor-Henry 1969, 1972, Taylor 1972), have discussed epilepsy and personality changes more recently.

CHAPTER II

NEUROPHYSIOLOGICAL PHENOMENOLOGY

MORPHOLOGY AND TOPOGRAPHY OF THE CONVULSION–SPECIFIC ELEMENTS (CE) IN THE ELECTROENCEPHALOGRAM (EEG)

A SERIES OF AUTHORS have dealt with the phenomenology of the convulsion-specific elements in the EEG in patients with psychomotor epilesy (Ajome-Marsan and Zivin 1970, Christian 1962, Gastaut 1953, Gastaut et al. 1959, Gibbs and Gibbs 1952, Gibbs and Lennox 1937, Jovanovic 1966 d, 1967 b, c, e, Klapetek 1963, 1964 and many others). However, in view of the volume of literature on the convulsion-specific elements (convulsion elements or CE) in epileptics of various types, it is not possible to review all this in one paper. Therefore, in the following we shall limit ourselves to a summary discussion.

Electroencephalography reveals important *morphological* and *topographical* differences between the *centrencephalic* type of epilepsy on the one hand, and the *temporocephalic* type, which also includes psychomotor attacks, on the other. These characteristics depend on the localization and, in part, on the nature of the convulsion focus (Figures 9, 10 and 11).

MORPHOLOGICALLY, in the temporocephalic type of epilepsy the form of the CE is characterized by isolated *spikes* which follow each other closely, usually *without waves,* although sometimes the spike is followed by a characteristic slower wave. The investigations of Wada and Lennox (1954) revealed spikes in 47 percent of cases, sharp waves in 31 percent of cases and slower dysrhythmic courses in 22 percent of cases. On the other hand, in a decisively high percentage of cases with centrencephalic epilepsy, there were three-per-second *spike and wave complexes* for several seconds (Figures 9 and 11).

TOPOGRAPHICALLY, in psychomotor epilepsy the spikes are localized over the temporal lobe (Figures 10 and 11), while in centrencephalic form of epilepsy the spike and wave formations are generalized and occur bilaterally and symmetrically.

In our opinion, these two differences are of major importance in the problem of psychomotor epilepsy, as we hope to show in the course of this study.

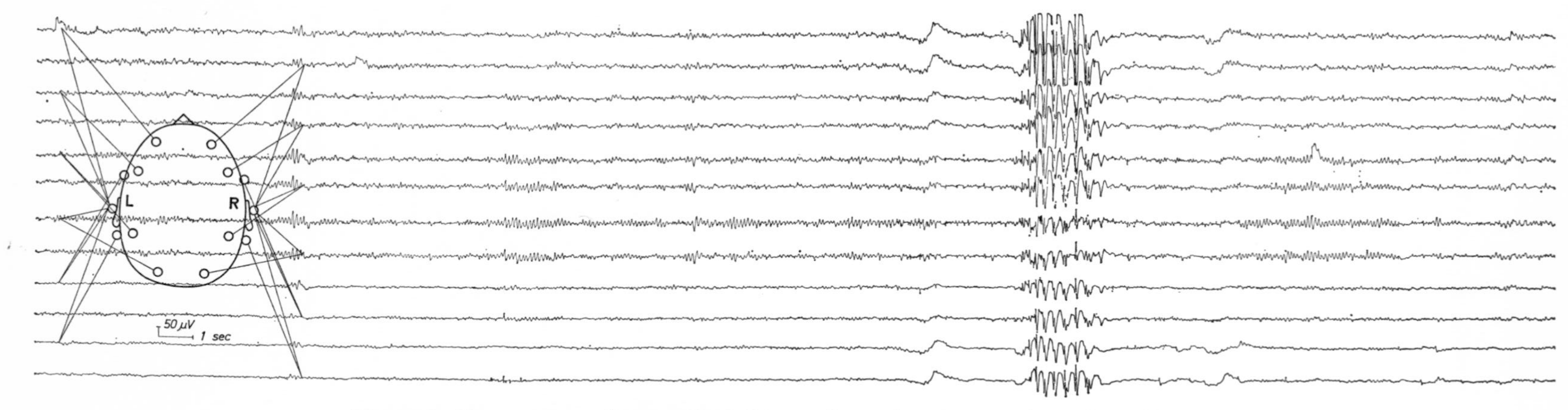

Figure 9. Abrupt onset of generalized 3/sec spike and wave complexes in a 34-year-old epileptic with grand mal of the matutinal type and absences (cp. Figure 11) (original).

THE EEG IN THE INTERVAL BETWEEN TWO ATTACKS (INTERICTAL EEG)

In psychomotor epilepsy, the interictal changes in the EEG are not consistent.

Temporal EEG changes in the EEG in the waking state only occur in 60 percent (Gastaut et al. 1955) to 70 percent Meyer-Mickeleit 1953) and even then they only appear when several leads are studied in the same patient and for a fairly long period. With routine leads, the percentage of abnormal EEG findings is very much lower. However, in a proportion of the negative cases typical changes appear in the sleeping EEG, and using this method Gibbs and Gibbs (1952) found pathological EEGs in 90 percent of the cases.

A study of the distribution of the convulsion foci in the temporal regions showed convulsive elements over the anterior parts in 83 percent of the cases, and over the central areas in 17 percent. In a series of cases with no pathological EEG findings, using deep electrodes (Kendrick and Gibbs 1957, Walker and Ribenstein 1957) it was possible to detect convulsion foci in the basal and medial parts of the temporal lobe. These electrodes together with corticographic, pharyngeal (Mac Lean 1949, Mac Lean and Arellano 1950) and sphenoidal (Pampiglione and Kerridge 1956) electrodes show that in most cases the most pronounced interictal EEG changes do not occur over the anterior and lateral regions, but in the *mediobasal and orbitofrontal regions* (Kendrick and Gibbs 1957, Mac Lean and Arellano 1950).

Using deep electrodes, Miletti (1957) usually detected a focus in the gyrus hippocampi. Of all the forms of temporal epilepsy, according to Gibbs (1951) psychomotor epilepsy occurs in 90 percent, and according to Jasper et al. (1951) and to Wada and Lennox (1954) it occurs in 50 percent.

With regard to *lateralization,* Gibbs (1951) found that the temporal EEG changes were unilateral in two-thirds of the cases and bilateral in one third of the cases. Wada and Lennox (1954) observed unilateral findings in the EEG in 85 percent of cases, Jasper et al. (1951) in 58 percent, Gastaut et al. (1955) in 53 percent and Meyer-Mickeleit (1953) in 40 percent of cases. The EEG changes in children differ considerably from those in adults (Doose 1967, Glaser and Golub 1955, Livingston 1954, Niedermeyer 1957).

From the many papers on this subject we would refer here to that of Christian (1962), since he has evaluated electroencephalographically an imposing number of patients; 712 cases (517 *idopathic* and 195 *symptomatic*). Christian found that there was a perfectly *normal* EEG in the interval in

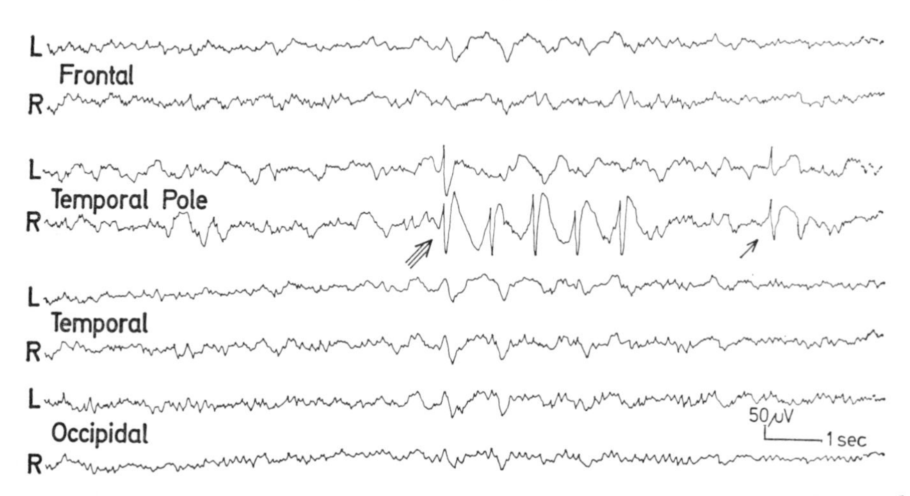

Figure 10. Isolated spikes in the temporal region in diffuse dysrhythmia in a 30-year-old epileptic with psychomotor epilepsy (cp. with Figures 9 and 11) (original).

only 12 percent of psychomotor epileptics. 85 percent of the EEG traces revealed more or less diffuse dysrhythmia.

Unilateral or bilateral convulsion foci with sharp isolated courses and spiked potentials or sharp waves or focal dysrhythmia, were shown in 60 percent in the EEG in the waking state in the cryptogenic forms, and in 38 percent in the symptomatic epilepsies. On the other hand, *temporal focal changes* or localized bioelectrical disturbances with temporal centres without specific epileptic potentials were considerably more common in the symptomatic forms (27%) than in the idiopathic forms (12%). These results correlate substantially with those of Meyer-Mickeleit (1953).

Among the cryptogenic forms, there were *strictly* unilateral foci in 34 percent of the cases; in a further 15 percent of the cases, for the most part these could only be detected over one side of the head, while *51 percent of the cases had bilateral temporal or temporobasal* convulsion foci. On the other hand, in 9 percent of the cases the position of the convulsion foci varied over the two temporal cerebral regions, at one moment being more over one, at another being more over the other temporal region. In symptomatic psychomotor epilepsies, there are *strictly* unilateral convulsion foci in 58 percent of the cases, in 11 percent of cases they are predominantly unilateral and in 31 percent of cases they are temporal and bilateral.

Where there are temporal or frontotemporal tumors, in many cases it is possible to observe conduction of epileptic discharges to the opposite side of the brain; the author assumes that this conduction takes place *via psalterium and commissura anterior.*

In patients with classic uncinate fits psychomotor attacks of the oral type

(Halles 1962), the most consistent convulsion foci are over the *anterior or mediobasal parts* of the temporal lobe. These foci are relatively well defined and are clearly bilateral. Where the clinical picture showed that the sensory disturbances or oral motor symptoms preceded a dreamy state then, in general, the focal temporo-oral dysrhythmias were more pronounced than in attacks where oral automatisms were the only, or were the predominant feature. In pure dreamy states temporal EEG changes occurred unilaterally just as often as bilaterally. With the adversive type (Hallen 1962), Christian found definite focal changes. In 80% of the cases the focus was contralateral to the direction of rotation of the head in the attack, in 15 percent of cases it was ipsilateral and in 5 percent of cases it was bilateral. Where there were speech disorders in the clinical picture (Hallen's vocalization type), the foci; if these existed, were always *left-sided* and occurred mainly over the posterior areas of the temporal lobe. With the so-called *syncopes* (Landolt 1955, 1960) or *fausses absences* (Gastaut 1951, 1953) there was nearly always a bilateral temporal convulsion focus. In psychomotor epilepsy with sympathico-vasal crises, there were also spikes over both temporal hemispheres, although more towards the temporal pole. This result correlates with the assumption of Champan et al. (1950) that the most impressive cardiovascular effects are not derived from the diencephalon but from the temporal pole.

Christian found that *in 85 percent of cases the temporal foci correlated with psychomotor epilepsy.* The corresponding data from Jasper et al. (1951) and Gibbs (1951) vary considerably from the results of Christian (1962). According to Christian, 15 percent of the cases involved pure grand mal epilepsy of mainly symptomatic origin. These 15 percent of grand mal epilepsies with a convulsion focus over the temporal lobe were all nocturnal epilepsies (Janz 1962). There were no temporal convulsion foci with matutinal epilepsies.

Extratemporal foci in addition to the temporal sites, are found in 15 to 20 percent of the cases. Hill (1949) described psychomotor attacks with circumscribed frontal foci and Jaspers et al. (1951) described them with parietal and precentral convulsion foci. The same types of attack are also known where there are frontal processes. Nevertheless, Gibbs (1951) found that psychomotor attacks were eight times more frequent where the EEG foci were in the anterior temporal lobe, as compared with in other regions of the brain (See also Lavy et al. 1972, Hutt 1972).

Summarizing all the results in the literature and our own experience with convulsion-specific elements in psychomotor epilepsy, we have the following *quantitative* and *qualitative* results:

THE EEG IS COMPLETELY NORMAL AND DOES NOT CORRELATE WITH THE CLINICAL PICTURE OF EPILEPSY OF THE PSYCHOMOTOR TYPE. In this case the

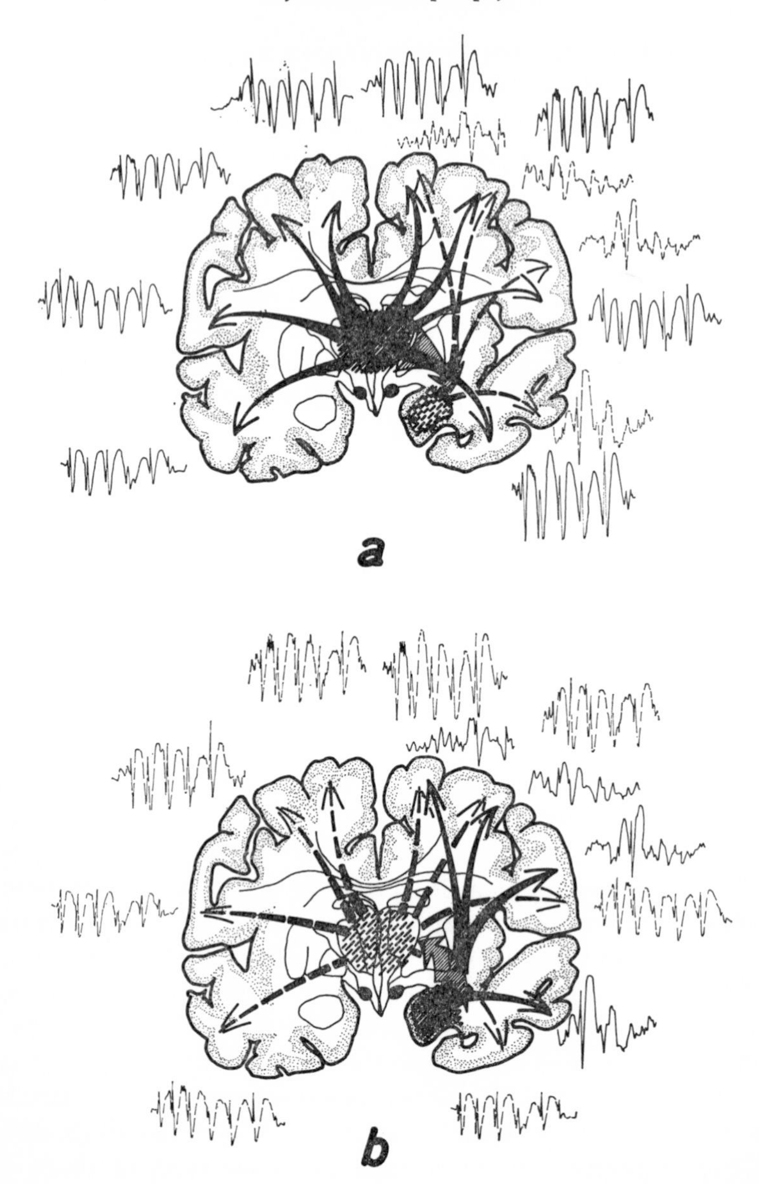

Figure 11. With a convulsion focus in the centrencephalic brain structures (a) the convulsive discharges spread simultaneously in a bilateral symmetrical way over the whole cortex, usually in the form of 3/sec spike and wave complexes. This produces convulsion elements like those illustrated in Figure 9. On the other hand, convulsion discharges from the deeper cerebral structures (b) less commonly reach the isocortex, the spikes are usually localized temporally or first appear over temporal regions of the brain and do not appear over the other cerebral structures until later. The illustration also shows the occurrence of the secondary convulsion focus after a fairly long period of illness, with secondary occurrence of convulsion potentials (broken lines) (own illustration).

convulsion focus is probably in the deeper brain structures which are not included in the cortical EEG. However, special investigations such as: EEG with pharyngeal electrodes, hyperventilation, sleep, Cardiazol, may reveal the CE.

STRICTLY UNILATERAL CONVULSION FOCI LOCALIZED OVER THE TEMPORAL LOBE OCCUR IN SYMPTOMATIC PSYCHOMOTOR EPILEPSY. In this case, the EEG in the waking state reveals isolated, more or less regular spikes proceeding from a temporal point, with or without subsequent slower waves.

A STRICTLY LOCALIZED CONVULSION FOCUS BILATERALLY OVER THE TEMPORAL REGIONS IS OBSERVED BOTH IN IDIOPATHIC (IN THE GREATEST NUMBER OF CASES) AND ALSO IN SYMPTOMATIC PSYCHOMOTOR EPILEPSIES. In the EEG there are isolated, more or less regular, smaller spikes with or without subsequent slower waves of 2 to 3/sec. In a larger percentage of cases (60 to 75%), the focus is localized or emphasized over the left temporal region.

THE TEMPORAL, UNILATERALLY LOCALIZED CONVULSION FOCUS WHICH IS NOT STRICTLY TEMPORAL, BUT WHICH EXTENDS OVER THE PRECENTRAL, PARIETAL, OCCIPITAL OR EVEN FRONTAL CEREBRAL AREAS. The maximum of the spikes is temporal; over the other cerebral regions mentioned here, instead of spikes there may be biphasic sharp waves or high waves from the theta wave band. Here, the anatomical focus is probably in the mediobasal temporal regions of the brain or in the limbic system.

THE TEMPORAL BILATERALLY LOCALIZED CONVULSION FOCUS WITH RADIATION OF SPIKES OR SHARP WAVES OVER THE REMAINING CEREBRAL REGIONS, ALTHOUGH WITH CLEAR EMPHASIS OF CE OVER THE TEMPORAL REGIONS OF THE BRAIN. Here we are dealing with a type of epilepsy of unknown origin (a larger percentage) or of symptomatic origin (a smaller percentage), where there are contusions in the basal cerebral cortex (Sperling and Creutzfeldt 1959, Landolt 1960).

STRICTLY TEMPORAL, UNILATERALLY LOCALIZED CONVULSION FOCI WITH SHARP WAVES AND SPIKES OVER ONE OF THE TEMPORAL CEREBRAL REGIONS, ALTHOUGH THE EEG REVEALS GENERAL DYSRHYTHMIA WHICH ALSO EXTENDS OVER THE REMAINING SECTIONS OF THE BRAIN. In this case we probably have symptomatic epilepsy with an anatomical focus in the lateral parts of the temporal lobe with involvement of adjacent cerebral regions or cases where the course of the disease has been fairly prolonged.

STRICTLY TEMPORAL CONVULSION FOCUS, BUT OCCURRING OVER BOTH TEMPORAL CEREBRAL REGIONS (BILATERAL) WITH ISOLATED SPIKES OVER THE TWO TEMPORAL CEREBRAL REGIONS WITH GENERAL EEG DYSRHYTHMIA WHICH ALSO INVOLVED THE REMAINING SECTIONS OF THE BRAIN. In this case we either have symptomatic epilepsy with contusions in the basal parts of the brain, or cryptogenic epilepsy where the course of the disease has been fairly prolonged.

General dysrhythmic cerebral activity with isolated, diffusely scattered spikes and occasional concentrations of the spikes over the temporal sections of the brain. In these cases we have symptomatic psychomotor epilepsy with major seizures which occur irregularly and which are not related to the diurnal rhythm, or psychomotor epilepsy of cryptogenic origin with major seizures where the course of the disease has been fairly prolonged.

Spikes which closely follow one another and which occur over all cerebral regions with or without general dysrhythmia. In this case, the anatomical focus is probably more in the medial cerebral structures, but it does not affect the neocortex or the convexity of the brain.

Spikes and wave formations occurring over all the cerebral regions with or without general dysrhythmia. The spikes do not follow one another closely as in petit mal or the other forms of centrencephalic epilepsy (i.e. 3/sec.); they occur regularly or irregularly in isolated complexes, but not closely following one another. In this case there is probably diencephalic psychomotor epilepsy (Gastaut 1953), with involvement of the limbic structures, or it may be primary psychomotor epilepsy with a bilateral convulsion focus in the limbic structures of the brain, which, in the course of time, has extended medially to involve the diencephalic structures.

Gastaut et al. (1959) have made an extensive study of the EEG findings in relation to the anatomical results.

THE EEG DURING A PSYCHOMOTOR ATTACK (ICTAL EEG)

Electroencephalographic changes during the psychomotor attacks have often been described (Christian 1962, Hill 1949, Hutt 1972, Jasper et al. 1951, Jovanovic 1969, 1970 b, Lavy et al. 1972, Lennox 1951, Meyer-Mickeleit 1953). The most extensive observations have been made by Gastaut et al. (1952) and Gastaut (1953) with 300 attacks; however, most of these attacks were provoked with pentylenetetrazol (Cardiazol®). These authors reported that in 70 percent of all attacks the epileptics showed *paroxysmal* signs of excitation in the EEG during the psychomotor attack. Sometimes, the only manifestation was flattening of the EEG curves. Occasionally this would precede the EEG seizure activity, as the preparoxysmal phase. Clinically, this is frequently accompanied by the aura. During the oral automatisms there are nearly always paroxysmal changes, sometimes in the form of typical sinusoid or slow waves with flattened peaks and diminishing frequency (Gibbs, Gibbs and Lennox 1937, 1938, Hill 1949), but at other times the electroencephalographic tracings take various forms. They are localized temporally, but are frequently bilateral, and they often show a tendency to generalize over the whole of the brain. After the actual attack, there are still non-specific *postparoxysmal* changes in the EEG accompanied by clouding of the consciousness and automatisms.

According to Gastaut (1953), the duration of the attack in the EEG is less than one minute, although Meyer-Mickeleit (1953) considered it to be longer, probably because he included part of the postparoxysmal phase in the attack.

The authors are fairly much in agreement on the characteristics of the electroencephalogram in psychomotor epilepsy *during the attack* (Christian 1962, Gastaut, 1953, 1963, Gibbs and Gibbs 1952, Jovanovic 1969, 1970 b, Landolt 1963, Meyer-Mickeleit 1953).

To summarize, the following pictures are observed:

1.) There is rarely normal cerebral activity during the clinical attack.

2.) About 20 seconds before the attack, there is a critical flattening of the cerebral activity. Immediately after this, the brain potentials become larger and larger and the sinusoidal waves of 3 to 5/sec. or 6 to 8/sec. become generalized. In addition, isolated sharp waves or spikes without a definite localization are observed. Just before the active phase of the psychomotor attack, the EEG also records muscle potentials as an indication of the tense musculature of the head and face. In the attacks itself, generalized sharp waves and spikes which closely follow one another are recorded; these disappear gradually after the attack.

3.) The spikes, which are localized unilaterally or bilaterally over the temporal cerebral regions, slowly extend over the other regions of the brain. There is dysrhythmia which is generalized but more pronounced over the temporal regions of the brain. There is no abrupt change of cerebral activity, as there is in the petit mal triad. There may be a passing phase of sharp waves which disappear again in between times. As the attack passes off, the sharp waves and spikes also fade and there is an exhaustion pause without, or with only isolated convulsion-specific elements.

4.) With the brief twilight attacks it is only possible to record transient retardation in the EEG for a few seconds, when the delta waves transform into normal cerebral activity. Such attacks usually last two to five seconds and are sometimes not diagnosed clinically, or are taken to be absences.

5.) The level of the amplitude increases over the affected point and there is a reduction of frequency which may last between 20 and 120 seconds.

6.) It may also be that the cerebral activity in psychomotor epileptics is characterized during an attack, as it is in petit mal, by spike and wave complexes (Christian 1962, Fuster et al. 1954, Jung 1957, Magnus et al. 1952, Niedermeyer 1954).

7.) On rare occasions we have observed unilateral acceleration at an electrode point over the temporal regions of the brain while isolated spikes which closely follow one another become faster and faster until the attack subsides. In this case the anatomical convulsion focus is probably in the cerebral cortex of the temporal lobe, in the lateral cortical regions. Locally, the spikes may resemble those of a Jacksonian seizure. However, they are localized temporally, not precentrally. The clinical picture is the decisive factor in the differential diagnosis, when the EEG leaves some room for doubt.

8.) Where there are fairly long psychomotor episodes lasting several days, there may be general dysrhythmia which becomes more and more pronounced and finally recedes again at the end of the clinical episode.

9.) Where psychomotor and petit mal attacks occur simultaneously, it is possible to observe isolated spikes closely following one another and also generalized, bilateral symmetrical spikes and waves of 3/sec. These elements may appear intermittently, so that the group of spike and wave formations replaces the group with isolated spikes, and vice versa (v. Hedenström and Dreyer 1967). The attack may also begin with isolated and close spikes and end with spike and wave formations.

10.) In rare cases, the cerebral activity may change only a few seconds after the beginning of the psychomotor attack.

11.) The EEG change during a psychomotor status may be intermittently dysrhythmic and normalize or almost normalize again. However, often throughout the whole status there is dysrhythmia with isolated spikes.

THE CORTICAL EEG DURING PSYCHOTIC EPISODES

This question has already been discussed in Chapter I. Landolt (1955, 1960) was one of the first to attempt to analyse this problem. This is a very important phenomenon in that the cerebral activity normalizes completely or almost completely when clinically there is a picture of a productive psychotic episode. A series of authors (Bonnet et al. 1959/1960) have discussed this problem in a joint publication. In addition to this, there have been further publications by, among others, Christian (1957), one case; Schorsch and v. Hedenström (1957), three cases, and Tellenbach (1965), 12 cases. In addition to *forced normalization in the EEG in epileptics in the waking state* during acute psychosis, Jovanović (1966 e) found renewed *forced pathological developments in the sleeping EEG* of psychotic epileptics.

In order not to repeat what was said in Chapter I, here we shall state the findings in summary form.

Where there is a psychotic psychosis in the clinical picture of an epileptic, then there is normalization of the pathological EEG observed before the psychosis developed. If the psychosis is cured by psychotropic drugs or electroshock therapy, then epileptic attacks occur again and convulsion-specific elements appear in the EEG. Here, the psychosis functions as a replacement for clinical epileptic attacks and CE in the EEG.

If epilepsy is treated very intensively with antiepileptic agents, occasionally and not uncommonly a psychosis develops with forced normalization in the EEG.

If a hysterical attack occurs, the epileptic seizures and pathological elements in the EEG disappear. If an epileptic attack recurs, the hysteria disappears and convulsion-specific elements reappear in the EEG.

NEUROPHYSIOLOGICAL AND BEHAVIOR PATTERNS PSYCHOMOTOR EPILEPSY DURING SLEEP

In our opinion, this subject is of particular importance. We did not deal with this problem in Chapter I since, for reasons of continuity, the clinical and electroencephalographic aspects of the problem should be dealt with in the same chapter. Finally, the sleep of the patients has been investigated using neurophysiological methods (Jovanović 1971a, 1972a).

Course of Sleep in the Patients

We recorded the course of sleep in epileptics by means of:

ELECTROENCEPHALOGRAPHY (EEG): to measure the depth of sleep and to check the bioelectrical convulsion discharges.

ELECTRO-OCULOGRAPHY (EOG): for checking the eye movements during sleep and in the dreaming phases.

ELECTROMYOGRAPHY (EMG): to measure the muscular contractions during sleep and an attack.

ELECTROCARDIOGRAPHY (ECG): for checking the autonomic nervous system during sleep and an attack.

RESPIROGRAPHY (RESP.): as an additional method for checking the autonomic nervous system by recording the respiratory rate.

GALVANOMETRIC OBSERVATIONS OF CUTANEOUS ACTIVITY AND OF THE GALVANIC DIRECT-CURRENT RESISTANCE OF THE SKIN. This method makes possible peripheral checks of the functional fluctuations of the sympathetic and parasympathetic nervous system.

Phallography (PhG): for recording erections during sleep, thus indicating the sleep periods.

Urography (UG): for measuring any discharge of urine during sleep or an attack.

Use of an acoustic stimulus: to verify the depth of sleep measured in the EEG.

Waking the patients from the dreaming phases: recording the content of any dreams on a tape recorder.

The course of sleep in the temporocephalic form of epilepsy, i.e. the psychomotor epileptic, differs in certain essential points from that of patients from the centrencephalic group. We shall give a brief description of the sleep of the psychomotor epileptic. Information about the sleep phenomena in other forms of epilepsy can be found in Jovanovic (1966 c, d; 1967 b, d).

The sleep was recorded during two to three nights. In certain cases the investigations sometimes lasted for up to ten nights. In all, 146 patients were studied on 356 nights, 48 of which were with psychomotor attacks.

The patients *fall asleep* significantly quicker than healthy subjects and patients from the centrencephalic group of epileptics.

The patients also *remain awake* for a shorter period than healthy people. The patients tend to remain in deeper stages of sleep.

Patients with psychomotor attacks usually complete their sleep *in the first two thirds* of the night and in the final third of the night they remain predominantly in the superficial stages of sleep. There is a *sleep excess* of between 39 and 60 percent compared with the amount of sleep taken by a normal healthy control subject.

Waking in the night is less common than with healthy subjects.

The motoricity of these patients is weaker than in control subjects, and in the autonomic nervous system the parasympathetic system is dominant. Compared with control subjects, the *dreaming phases* are also shorter.

The *dream content* is less. These results have been statistically evaluated and tested for significance.

Treating these patients with *hydantoins* makes the sleep more superficial and removes the sleep excess. *Barbiturates* do not have any effect on the course of sleep.

Convulsion-Specific Elements (CE) in the Sleep EEG

Among others, Gibbs and Gibbs (1952), Christian (1960, 1961), Ganshirt and Vetter (1961) have dealt with this subject. We shall refer briefly to our own findings (Jovanovic 1967 e).

The convulsion-specific elements seen in a relatively low percentage in the EEG during waking state, more than double during sleep. The picture of pathological EEGs during sleep may increase tenfold in comparison to the waking state.

The distribution of CE during sleep shows characteristic features. In the first hour of sleep, in psychomotor epileptics the convulsion elements appearing in the EEG represent 36.6 percent of the total number of convulsion elements for one night. In the second hour of sleep, this percentage falls to 20.8 percent, and by the third hour of sleep it has fallen to 12.4 percent. In later hours of sleep, the convulsion-specific elements occur less and less frequently (the fourth hour of sleep, 8.2 %; the fifth, 5.1%; in exceptional cases there is an increase in the sixth hour, bringing it to 10.2%; the seventh hour, 4.6%; the eighth hour, 2.1%). Accordingly, the sleeping EEG of these patients most frequently shows convulsion elements in the first hours of sleep.

On the other hand, in the sleeping EEG of contrencephalic epileptics the convulsion elements become more and more frequent from evening to morning. For example, there is between 5.8 percent and 11.2 percent in the first hour of sleep, and between 15.3 percent and 20.8 percent in the last hour of sleep. *According to this result, the EEG of centrencephalic epileptics becomes more and more pathological from evening to morning, and that of temporocephalic epileptics becomes more and more normal.*

Further analysis showed that the convulsion elements first appear in the EEG in psychomotor epilepsy while the patient is going to sleep. The deeper the subject sleeps, the more convulsion elements appear in the EEG. Where convulsion elements were already present in the EEG in the waking state, these were seen to multiply on going to sleep.

Of 48 patients, there was only one case in which it was not possible to show a pathological finding in the sleep EEG. In all the other patients, epilepsy was confirmed or diagnosed.

In sleep, the convulsion elements became more frequent towards five o'clock in the morning, i.e. just at the time that the attacks occur in sleep (nocturnal epileptics).

Morphologically, the convulsion elements can be divided into two groups. In one group there are biphasic sharp waves and in the other group isolated or continuous spikes.

Topographically, it is again possible to differentiate between two groups. In the first, the convulsion-specific elements are generalized but concentrated in the temporal-basal region. In the other group, there are temporally localized (usually left, but sometimes also right) spikes which occur uninterruptedly for 20 to 30 minutes.

Thus, using the sleeping EEG it was possible to obtain good results, particularly where the EEG in the waking state was completely normal and where the daily attacks bore a close resemblance to psychogenic attacks.

The localization over the temporal sections of the brain usually had a special significance. We fastened one of the electrodes to the mastoid process. Continual convulsion elements were recorded by this electrode, and occasionally these were emphasized over the occipital regions of the brain.

Our observations have shown that sleep is a very important method for provoking convulsion elements in psychomotor epilepsy and that the very deep sleep plays a special role here (Jovanović 1966 d).

Psychomotor and Generalized Attacks During Sleep

In the course of the investigations, we were able to record 187 psychomotor attacks during sleep without generalized convulsions, and 11 episodes which occurred at the same time as major attacks. The psychomotor attacks may last for different lengths of time:

1.) *Very brief attacks* which present in the form of pronounced twitching with or without involvement of the extremities, with smacking movements of the lips for two seconds. Following these twitching symptoms, the EEG takes on a spiked course followed by delta waves for a further four to seven seconds. These sharp waves, which on occasions also contain genuine spikes, are not localized temporally as they are in the waking state, but they are more bilateral frontal and frontotemporal. Such an attack may be repeated within a few minutes.

2.) *Brief attacks* present as twitching of the body in several places, smacking movements of the lips and subsequent sharp waves or spikes with a localization similar to that in the very brief attacks. The twitching lasts for two to four seconds, and the whole attack lasts nine to eleven seconds.

3.) *Longer attacks* with generalized flattening and hypersynchronization of the EEG waves with increasing amplitude and frequency for 12 to 20 seconds. There is then a clinical psychomotor attack with tonic deviation of the head to the left or right or forwards. This lasts seven to twelve seconds. There is smacking of the lips, licking, chewing, grinding of the teeth and speech defects for up to two minutes. The patients fidget with their clothes or bedcovers as if they were awake; they make rapid attempts to dress and undress for as long as they are still in bed. Sometimes they get up. In rare cases they are orientated for one to two seconds and fall back into the twilight attacks. Urinary and faecal incontinence only occurs in exceptional cases.

4.) *Semi-generalized attacks* have a startling onset with raising of the head and sometimes of the upper part of the body as well, and a few tonic-clonic discharges of the musculature of the upper part of the body. These discharges may often be repeated at brief intervals. In between times, the patients may try to get to sleep again and after a few seconds they are taken unawares by renewed convulsive movements. During the pauses, there are generalized spikes of 6 to 8/sec. in the EEG, and these do not show any predilection for a particular cerebral region. After the attack, the patients are in a twilight state for between one minute to one hour and they try to dress or undress, or they carry out oral automatisms. The hands make ordered knitting, rubbing or tinkering movements.

5.) *Psychomotor and generalized attacks* are the same as the attacks occurring during the waking state. There are rarely prodromal electroencephalographic signs. The onset of an attack is often startling with generalized convulsions and the elements of a psychomotor attack, which may last for up to one hour, are only recorded after the seizure. A generalized attack nearly always lasts the same length of time and this only varies between 59 and 61 seconds. The tonic phase lasts for half to two-thirds of this time.

6.) We have only recorded a *particularly long major seizure* with psychomotor disturbances; this lasted for two minutes with generalized convulsions and for over two hours as a psychomotor attack. For two hours, the 26-year old patient showed oral automatisms and hand movements with rubbing of the bedcovers, etc. Normal sleep set in after two hours, but this was frequently interrupted by brief psychomotor disturbances.

All attacks and equivalents arise during light sleep. It is an important fact that the attacks never arise out of deep sleep. Indeed this would hardly be possible since, on the nights concerned, the patients never enter a stage of deep sleep, either before or after the attack. Thus, in the evening it is possible to predict whether there will be a generalized or fairly prolonged psychomotor attack, since the patients suddenly find that they cannot sleep although normally they get to sleep much more quickly than healthy people. On the night of an epileptic attack, nearly all patients show a considerable sleep deficit. Normally only patients with the centrencephalic forms of epilepsy show such a deficit.

In patients with centrencephalic epilepsy, there are no attacks during sleep although the spikes and waves increase even if the EEG in the waking state is normal. Convulsion elements appear more often towards morning when there is already a sleep deficit.

SOMNAMBULISTIC FORM OF PSYCHOMOTOR EPILEPSY (SOMNAMBULISTIC EPILEPSY)

Although there are a few case history reports on somnambulistic episodes in psychomotor epilepsy (Meyer-Mickeleit 1953), as yet, the literature does not contain any objective results which demonstrate a psychomotor attack with sleep-walking.

The somnambulistic episodes in psychomotor epilepsy which we have recorded, were only mentioned in another connection (Jovanovic 1969, 1970 a, b).

Of the 146 epileptics investigated on 356 nights, we were able to record eight somnambulistic episodes in the course of a week in one patient. One of these is described briefly here and shown in Figure 12.

Case 1

The 28-year-old female patient had suffered from sleep-walking for ten years. She would rise from sleep, lie on the floor and continue to sleep. On one occasion she left the house, got on a bus, bought a ticket and finished up at the other end of the town. On another occasion, taking her bedclothes with her, she left the house and went under the roof of the building and slept there until morning when she was found. Another time, she got up several times in the night and telephoned friends and relatives while she was still asleep; she talked *nonsense* but they recognized her. She even phoned her employer, although she had been trying to conceal her illness from him. There were even more problems when the woman had a baby and she took the child sleep-walking with her.

There were no details about generalized attacks in the case history. In this patient, the EEG in the waking state was normal and thus it has not been possible to diagnose epilepsy; but it was assumed to be somnambulism. However, in a hospital epilepsy was suggested, and small doses of hydantoin preparations were prescribed. The symptoms during sleep did not disappear. Since there is as yet no satisfactory drug to treat somnambulism, the woman has to put up with her ailment.

At 1:33 A.M. during light sleep there was a critical flattening of the sleeping EEG curve. Still in the period where *nothing happening* is noted on the curve, there appear bilateral, symmetrical and generalized spikes breaking up the previously critical flattening of the waves. The spikes increased in size and became continuous. By 1:33.26 A.M., the patient showed motor signs (EMG in Figure 12). Within the next 34 seconds, the patient suddenly jumped out of bed and, using force, she wanted to run away quickly. The process of rising began without any definite clinical prodromal signs and, previously, there had been no psychomotor disturbances. On rising her eyes were open, her face was remarkably pallid and livid colored and her orientation instinct was good. The patient ran to the closed door and tried to open it; in doing this she did not knock into anything clumsily. When her progress was impeded she began to scream, and it was very difficult to get her back into bed. She threw herself down, first lying on her stomach and then, turning on to her right side, she began to smack her lips, lick and sniff. At first her hands were still, but after a few seconds her left hand began to rub the bedcovers rhythmically. When a few more seconds had elapsed, the patient began to make knitting movements with her eyes closed and in a few minutes she fell asleep. All this lasted for six minutes. The second sleep-walking episode was recorded at 2:40.21 A.M., the third at 4:04 A.M., the fourth at 5:00 A.M. and the fifth at 6:45.54 A.M. on different nights. On the second and third occasions, the psychomotor movements recorded were very much more pronounced and pro-

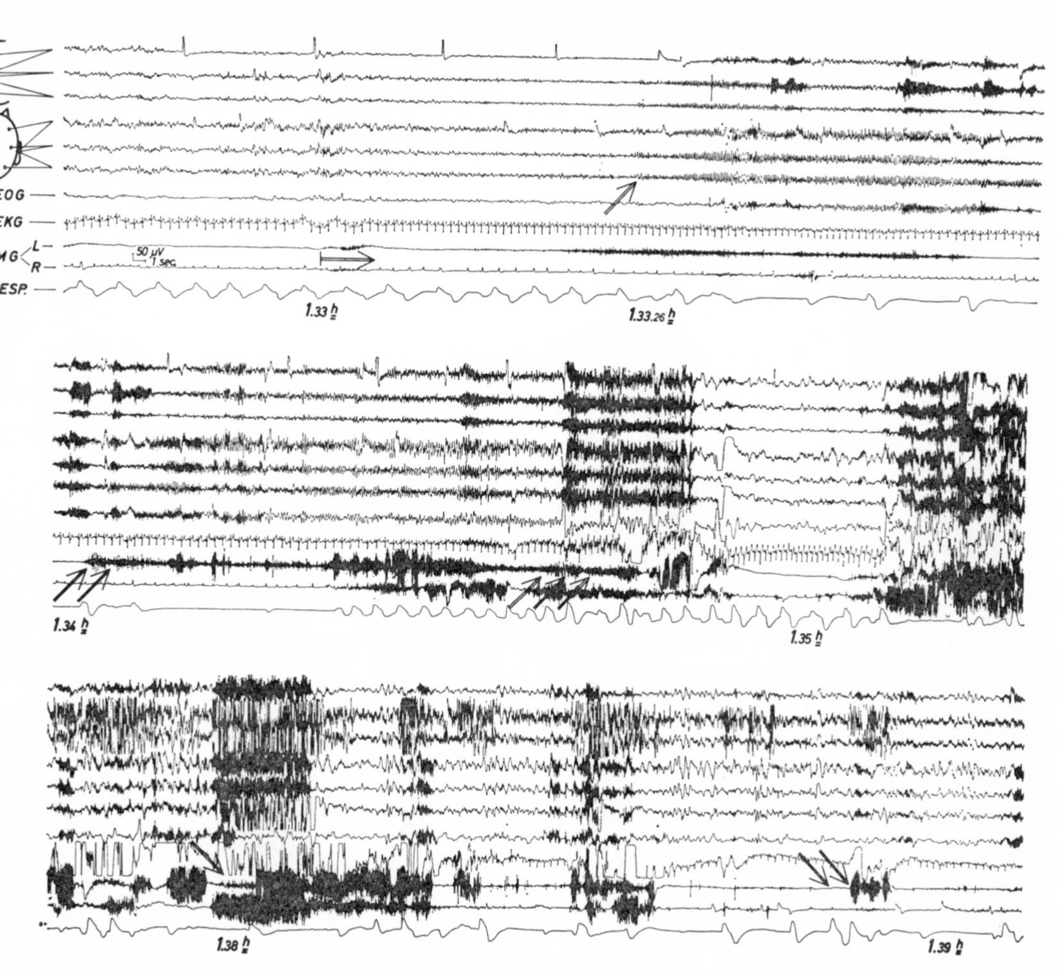

Figure 12. Somnambulistic psychomotor epilepsy. The EEG shows an attack arising out of sleep with running and sleep-walking. The first horizontal arrow (top part of the diagram) shows a critical flattening. The first arrow pointing upwards and to the right (top part of the diagram) shows where the spikes appear; these spikes get bigger and faster. The two arrows pointing upwards and to the right (center of the diagram) show where the 28-year-old female patient sat up in bed. In the middle of the center diagram there are three arrows pointing upwards and to the right. At this point the patient got up and ran away. The arrow pointing downwards and to the right (bottom left of the diagram) shows where the woman was returned to bed; at the two downward pointing arrows (bottom right of the diagram at the end) the patient lay down again and went to sleep without being aware that the attack had occurred. There was total amnesia in respect of the attack on the following day. (Original)

longed than on the first occasion. On the following morning, there was retrograde amnesia for the sleep-walking, as occurs with genuine somnambulism (see Jovanović 1969).

Clearly these attacks of sleep-walking differ from the normal type of psychomotor attack during sleep or in the waking state. A surprising factor here is the *rapidity with which the patient gets out of bed and progresses,* for example active movements without prodromal clinical signs, and the symptoms which are observed during a psychomotor attack in the daytime or in the waking state are only observed when the patient is returned to bed.

CHAPTER III

NEUROANATOMICAL AND HISTOCHEMICAL SUBSTRATE

THE TEMPORAL LOBE (LOBUS TEMPORALIS)

THIS SECTION IS CONCERNED WITH: *the problems of symptomatic epilepsy* (the disease is caused by a recognized pathological cerebral process); *epilepsy of unknown or undiagnosed origin* (so-called essential, idiopathic cryptogenic forms); *possible localizations of convulsion foci* (which morphological substrate is available for localization of the foci); *possibilities for the spread of the convulsion discharges* (which morphological-functional pathways and routes are available for the spread of excitation from the site of origin, until there is a manifest attack); *experimental anatomy and psychomotor epilepsy* (comparison of the symptoms on stimulation and excision of individual structures of the temporal lobe, with the manifest phenomena of psychomotor epilepsy), and *biochemistry of the convulsion-inducing and convulsion-promoting cerebral structures in the temporal lobe region.*

Symptomatic Psychomotor Epilepsy

In 1874, Sanders described a case with typical psychomotor attacks, with a tumor localized in the temporal pole, extending as far as the Ammon's horn and involving the nervus opticus. Hemkes (1878) observed a similar case. The tumor pervaded the entire Ammon's horn formation and extended as far as the occipital lobe. The patient presented with anxiety states, optical hallucinations and other symptoms which were later described in cases of psychomotor epilepsy. About twelve years after Hemkes, Jackson and Beevor (1890) pointed out that growing and displacing processes (tumors) in the region of the temporal lobe may induce a specific form of epilepsy with olfactory hallucinations and strange psychic experiences. They used the term *dreamy state* to describe this form.

After Gibbs, Gibbs and Lennox (1938) had defined psychomotor epilepsy as a special form of epilepsy and again pointed out the part played by the temporal lobe, intensive research work into this region of the brain began, and epileptic research work on other areas of the cerebrum rather receded into the background.

In the years which followed, Penfield and Jasper (1954) undertook surgery in epileptic patients and found changes in several regions of the temporal lobe.

At about the same time, Gastaut (1953) and Gastaut et al. (1959) carried out parallel clinical neurophysiological and neuroanatomical investigations and recognized that the temporal lobe has etiological and pathogenic significance in psychomotor epilepsy. Many other authors (Anastasopoulos 1958, Anastasopoulos and Roustonis 1964, 1967, Ganner and Stiefer 1934, John 1930, Marburg 1929, Schuster 1902, Simma 1956) found psychic behavioral peculiarities which varied but which were pronounced, in cases of temporal lobe tumors. The range of symptoms extended from schizophrenia-like and depressive pictures to severe behavioral disorders, fits and aggression.

In the last 15 to 20 years, particularly since neurosurgery has developed as a medical discipline in its own right, there have been many results showing changes in the medial parts of the temporal lobe in association with an epileptic reaction. Particular mention should be made of findings by Bailey (1951), Bailey and Gibbs (1951), Cavanagh and Meyer (1956), Earle et al. (1953), Falconer (1965), Falconer et al. (1943 to 1971), Gastaut (1956), Green et al. (1951), Haberland (1958), Krayenbühl et al. (1954), Maspers and Morossero (1954), Maspers et al. (1956), Meyer (1956), Scharenberg (1957), Scholz (1959), Scholz and Spielmeyer (1951), Sperling and Creutzfeldt (1959), Peiffer (1962, 1963, 1967), Umbach (1958, 1967), Zülch (1956). Some of the more recent findings will be discussed briefly. A comprehensive survey of the literature and discussion on the temporal lobe can be found in the paper by Sperling and Creutzfeldt (1959).

Anastasopoulos and Routsons (1967) report in detail on 11 cases with temporal lobe tumors and severe destruction of the Ammon's horn. They observed the typical psychomotor symptoms which we have already discussed in Chapter I. In cases where unilateral destruction of the Ammon's horn due to the tumor could be detected anatomically, there was a clinical picture of two to three days' clouding of consciousness, constriction of consciousness with or without associated twilight states, generalized seizures, fainting fits, olfactory and optical hallucinations, short psychomotor seizures, increased sleep requirement and drowsiness, attacks of headaches and a brief, deep sleep. The authors also described periodic hypersexuality, loss of weight, cycle anomalies, vasomotor symptoms, impaired memory and personality changes. In three patients, coma was recorded in the terminal stage.

Among other authors, Lausberg and Calatayud-Maldonado (1967) have produced valuable statistics on tumors in relation to epilepsy. According to these authors, the *incidence of attacks* in the symptomatology in broadly-based statistics on brain tumors is about 30 percent of cases. In 1,182 tumor cases, Bornmann and Schiefer (1951) found epileptic attacks in 28.5 percent of the patients. In addition, they assembled 2,888 cases from the literature and calculated that here again there were seizures in 29.9 percent. Tumors of the temporal lobe show a higher incidence of attacks (40 to 50%). in 238 cases with tumors in the temporal lobe, Pia (1953) found attacks in 124 (52.1%) cases; Penfield and Jasper (1954) found them in 62 (51.2%) of 121 cases; Castels and Maslenikov (1957) found them in 25 (43.1%) of 58 cases; Lausberg and Calatayud (1967) found them in 95 (45.9%) of 207 cases. These latter authors produced a fresh summary of the results in the literature up to the time of tehir own publication, and found epileptic attacks in 305 (49.1%) of 624 patients with tumors in the temporal lobe.

The attacks which occur where there are tumors in the temporal region are usually *psychomotor in nature.* In 95 cases with tumors in the temporal lobe, Lausberg and Calatayud-Maldonado (1967) found psychomotor attacks 49 times, generalized seizures 42 times, focal (non-temporal) attacks 28 times and combined attacks (psychomotor and generalized) 24 times. The classification reveals that among the cases with psychomotor attacks 30 patients had twilight attacks, and of these there were uncinate fits six times and autonomic attacks eight times (two of them visceral). In seven patients there were spells of dizziness of the temporal type and four times there were emotional fits.

The incidence of attacks, in relation to the type of tumor. With oligodendrogliomas the incidence of attacks is 75 percent, followed by the astrocytoms with 60 percent, intracerebral metastases with 55.6 percent, meningiomas with 48 percent, glioblastomas with 32.9 percent and other intracerebral and extracerebral tumors with about 30 percent Considering the gliomas in isolation, with regard to seizure involvement, oligodendrogliomas are first, followed by astrocytomas and glioblastomas. In 199 cases with tumors of the cerebrum, Umbach (1967) found epileptic attacks in 63.8 percent of oligodendrogliomas, in 55 percent of astrocytomas, in 44 percent of angiomas and in 38 percent of meningiomas.

Slow-growing gliomas, including six spongioblastomas, produced attacks in 67.9 percent in 59 cases and this was more than double the incidence of attacks produced by fast-growing glioblastomas, which induced attacks in 32.9 percent or 67 cases (Lausberg and Clatayud-Moldonado 1967).

According to these latter authors, *the classification of the attacks which correspond to the localization of the tumor* (with an average percentage of 45.9%) shows a particular emphasis in the temporo-*medial* regions (58%). The temporo-*frontal* regions (52%) and the temporo-*parietal* regions (49%) are also above average. Analysis of the various types of attack according to the localization of the tumor does not reveal that any particular region is predisposed to producing generalized attacks. Generalized attacks occurred in about 20 percent of cases. The focal, non-temporal attacks with about 40 percent, tended to occur in the temporo-parietal site, but never where there were temporo-medial or temporo-basal sites. Where there was a temporo-medial site, psychomotor attacks were the most common occurrence in 50 percent. The difference between this and the next in order (fronto-temporal tumors, 29%) is so great that it may be possible to draw a clinical conclusion from this. Study of the twilight attacks and the autonomic attacks in isolation revealed similar relationships.

Again from the point of view of the localization of the tumor, attacks were the initial symptoms in 46.2 percent of cases with a temporo-medial tumor site, in 30 percent with the tumor in the temporal pole and temporo-frontal position and in 25 percent with tumors in the middle of the temporal lobe and in the temporo parietal and temporo-occipital position (mean value 29% for the entire group). This classification revealed a definite relationship between the occurrence and nature of the attacks and the localization of the tumor.

Case 2

Figure 13 shows the brain of one of our patients (P.M., 27 years of age) who suffered from generalized and psychomotor attacks during the last two years, with occasional psychomotor retardation. He finally developed a status epilepticus from which he died. On the day before the final admission to hospital, the patient had been drowsy all through the day; shortly before admission, during transportation, he died while still unconscious. Death was preceded by slight twitching of the legs.

Macroscopically the brain, which was fixed in formalin, looked remarkably large. Weight 1,780 grams. The soft membranes over the convexity of the cerebrum were delicate on both sides. The gyri over both sides of the cerebral convexity were flattened and the suki between them were blurred. Sharp furrows due to constriction on the right uncus gyri hippocampi, over which the cerebral tissue protruded medially for about 1 cm. Smaller, equally sharp furrows on the left uncus gyri hippocampi, about ½ cm. deep. Traces of furrow formation at the right tonsilla of the cerebellum. The basal cerebral arteries were regular; they were fine-calibre and delicate. Close to the point of departure of the nervous trigeminus on the left side, there was a cyst the size of a small pea, filled with clear watery fluid which for the most part was surrounded by trigeminal fibres arising from the mesencephalon. There were no indications of primary traumatic changes. The anterior parts of the right temporal lobe were remarkably soft. *In the anterior third of the first and second temporal gyrus on the right side, there was whitish, liquefying tissue. This was a tumor which had reached the surface of the brain at this point.* The floor of the third ventricle was remarkably thin and it was almost translucent. The cortex of the basal parts of the right temporal lobe were not differentiated from the medulla. Here, a whitish tumor had disseminated; in one section at a height of 1 cm. occipital to the temporal pole, it included the first and the second temporal gyrus and the medulla below. The tran-

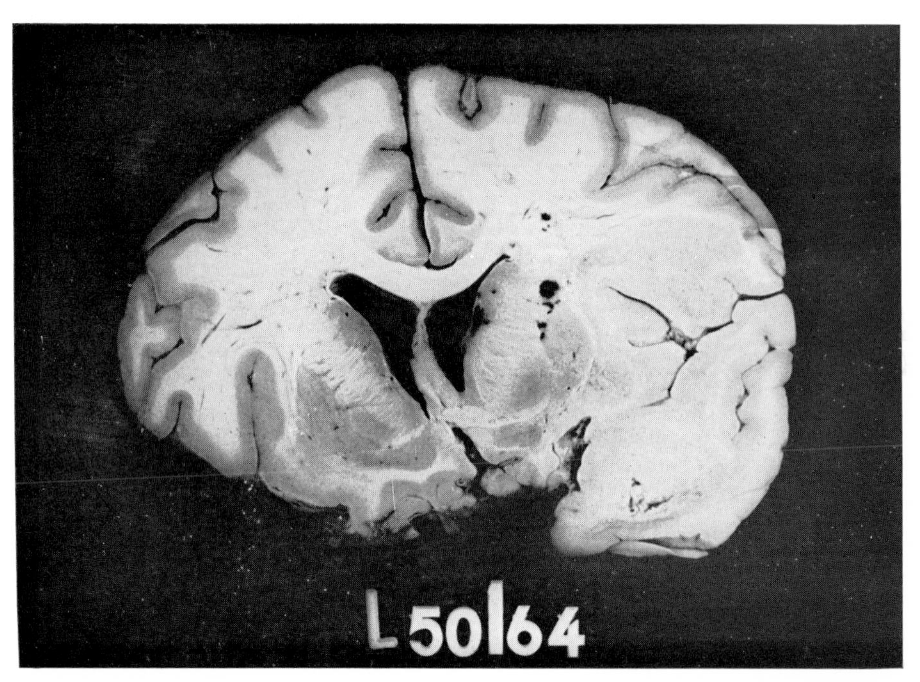

Figure 13. Local changes in the brain of a 27-year-old patient who had suffered from psychomotor and major attacks and finally died during status epilepticus (the findings are described in detail in the text). (The author is most grateful to Dr. Liebaldt of the Mental Hospital and Outpatients Department, University of Würzburg, for kindly supplying the preparation).

sition region from the frontal lobe to the parietal lobe in the neighborhood of the sylvian fissure had also succumbed to malignant change. The central ganglia were normal. There were no macroscopic findings in the cerebellum, pons and medulla oblongata. *Histologically,* there was a protoplasmatic *astrocytoma.*

Symptomatic psychomotor epilepsy not only occurs where there are tumors, but it is also seen as a result of many other cerebral processes and epileptogenic noxae (Arseni and Cristesar 1972; Blom et al. 1972; Copelman 1963; Feldman 1971; Gastaut 1971; Gibb 1971; Lugaresi et al. 1971; Martillaro et al. 1970; Mason and Cooper 1972; Rapport and Penry 1972; Ricci et al. 1972). *Perinatal, traumatic, toxic and infectious damage and damage of many other types may* induce epilepsy (Marinacci 1963, Schaefer et al. 1972, Taira et al. 1972) This will be discussed later.

Psychomotor Epilepsy of Unknown Origin

So far, we have been concerned with the topographical problems of symptomatic psychomotor epilepsy. The origin of other forms, the *cryptogenic (idiopathic)* epilepsies, presents a much greater problem.

Pathological Changes in the Brains of Patients with Psychomotor Epilepsy of Unknown Origin

With this form of epilepsy, most authors have failed to detect pathological changes in the part of the temporal lobe investigated in a quarter to a third of cases, and sometimes in an even higher percentage of patients.

Where there are positive findings the most common are *atrophies,* more or less superficial *traumatic lesions* and diffuse *glioses.* The next most frequent findings are intravital undiagnosed *tumors, microgyrias, cysts and vascular changes,* sometimes with calcification (Falconer et al. 1953, Penfield and Ward 1958). Histologically, Scharenberg (1957) has described a peculiar *amoeboid* degeneration of the astroglia; however, other authors have not regarded this as arising intravitally (see Sperling and Creutzfeldt 1959).

As with symptomatic forms, *the localization* of the lesions is again predominantly *temporo-basal and medial* in the cortex of the regio hippocampica and perifalciformis (Bailey and Bonin 1951). There are also foci in the lateral temporal gyri, but these cannot be related to the type of attack. The localized lesions which have been studied in most detail are those in the *Ammon's horn formation* (Conrad 1959, Conrad and Ule 1951, Glees and Griffith 1952, Milner 1957, Scoville et al. 1955, Ule 1954). Haberland (1958) found pathological results in only nineteen of forty-seven extirpated convulsion foci. In six cases there was sclerosis of the Amomn's horn.

Both neuroanatomical and electroencephalographic results have suggested an organic finding in the cryptogenic form of epilepsy (Hillbom 1951, Hill 1952, Mulder and Daly 1952, Rodin et al. 1957, Weil 1955).

Weil (1955) observed an increase of the temporal focal manifestations with many intercritical episodes, in six cases. In epileptics who had to be kept in hospital because of disordered social behaviour (irritability, impulsiveness, aggression) and who were kept under supervision for fairly prolonged periods, Roger and Dongier (1950) detected pathological *temporal* focal findings in 84 percent of the patients. In comparing the clinical neurophysiological and neuroanatomical symptomatology, Gastaut et al. (1959) found personality changes with *temporal* foci and a tendency to impulsive explosion in a high percentage of cases.

However, the whole problem is complicated by the fact that a focus has been found in the EEG of patients without epilepsy. In patients with abnormal behavior patterns, Hill (1952) found EEG changes in the *temporal* regions in 36 percent of his patients. The patients gave the impression of being psychopaths with social maladjustment. However, the disorders in these patients resembled those of some psychomotor epileptics with a focus in the temporal lobe. Ervin et al. (1956) emphasize that 34 of their 42 patients with *temporal foci* were referred to hospital with the clinical diagnosis schizophrenia. In these patients there were rare *idiopathic* psychomotor attacks. Kennard (1956) discusses *temporal* changes in the EEG and relates these to behavioral disorders which are frequently associated with aggressiveness. Among 62 schizophrenics *without epileptic attacks,* Kondrick and Gibbs (1957) were able to demonstrate spike activity in 100% of cases using deep electrodes over the medio-basal and orbito-temporal regions; this activity showed practically the same localization and form as in 13 control subjects with psychomotor epilepsy of known origin (see also Sem-Jacobson et al. 1956).

The difficulty in assessing psychomotor and psychopathological findings and the discovery of lesions in the temporal lobe is a result of the *anatomical and functional heterogeneity of this region.*

In spite of the difficulties, very recently there have been fairly definite pathological findings and these may be regarded as the cause of the epilepsies, even though the patients were considered to have epilepsy of unknown origin, or essential epilepsy, during their lives. From subsequent findings it can be seen that, in fact, epilepsy does not exist without corresponding organic lesions.

Neimanis (1962) observed four cases with psychomotor epilepsy and studied their neuropathological changes, and he found some very interesting connections.

Case 3

The patient suffered originally from matutinal epilepsy which is (as we pointed out in Chapter I) a centrencephalic type of epilepsy. Later, *secondary psychomotor epilepsy* developed from this first form. Morphologically, apart from slight diffuse clearing of the temporal cerebral cortex, the author found disseminated ganglion cell destruction in the uncus hippocampi sinistri and extensive deposition of corpora amylacea in the basal part of the temporal lobe periventricularly around the third ventricle and in the region of the paraventricular nuclear areas as a result of extensive boundary disturbances.

Case 4

In case 4, there was a familial epileptic affliction. Morphologically, there was an increase of the neuroglia elements in the nucleus amygdalae, slight clearing of the terminal layer in the Ammon's horn and mild, bilateral medullary gliosis in the gyrus hippocampus.

Case 5

Case 5 was 34 years old when he died in status epilepticus. He had suffered from matutinal epilepsy since he was ten years old. In his last years he had had several psychomotor attacks and once *febrile* catatonia. Morphologically, there were changes in the region of the third ventricle as a result of the boundary disturbance; there were also changes in the nucleus amygdalae and hippocampus. However, the major changes were in the basal parts of the temporal lobe and in the cerebellum.

Case 6

Case 6 had suffered from clinically major attacks for several years, and in the last few years from psychomotor epilepsy as well. Morphologically, there were changes in the Ammon's horn, in the cerebellum and periventricularly with deposition of corpora amylacea *as a result of the boundary disturbances which had taken place.*

Peiffer (1962) investigated 2,243 brains, 439 of them from patients who had suffered from epileptic attacks. In general there was *loss of color* in the Nissl preparation of the nerve cells or ischaemic nerve cell changes which preceded progressive glioproliferation. In the cortex of the cerebellum, these neuroglia reactions showed typical *aborization* along the ramifications of the damaged Purkinje cells. The nerve cell lesions were sometimes disseminated and scarcely perceptible. They were also observed to be laminar or pseudolaminar, corresponding to the cortical layering.

According to the author, there is a definite connection between the incidence of convulsion damage and the frequency of attacks. In addition to the *quantitative* picture, the *topographical* pattern is also very characteristic.

Of all the brains investigated, there were lesions in the hippocampus in 39.6 percent, in the cortex of the cerebrum in 34.6 percent, in the cerebellum in 31.8 percent, in the thalamus in 18.9 percent, in the lower oliva in 7.7 percent and in the corpus striatum in 2.5 percent of cases. Peiffer assumes the following to be direct causes of these lesions: angiospasms, mechanical stimuli, and ischaemia during a seizure. For this reason, the changes have been classified as shown above. (See also pages 71-72).

In a comparison of the lesions in the Ammon's horn, the author came to the conclusion that in non-epileptics there was Ammon's horn deficiency in only 9.4 percent of 1,881 brains, while in epileptics this occurred in 39.9 percent of 282 brains. Of all the lesions in this region, the highest percentages fall to psychomotor epilepsy: pure psychomotor epilepsy claimed 50 percent, psychomotor epilepsy combined with grand mal 46.3 percent and grand mal without psychomotor attacks 39.6 percent.

However, if lesions outside the Ammon's horn are also taken into account, for example those in the remaining structures of the temporal lobe, then there was a pathological finding in 100 percent of the cases with psychomotor epilepsy. *In typical psychomotor epilepsy and in conditions where this occurs with protracted twilight states and also where it occurs with transition to productive-psychotic episodes, a high percentage of cases show foci in the temporal lobe.*

Peiffer also mentions a very interesting finding here: the patients with psychomotor epilepsy who had shown a *personality change* during their lives, showed a high percentage of changes in the Ammon's horn. Ammon's horn sclerosis was found in 39.5 percent of them after death; this was twice as high as in other forms of epilepsy without personality change. Only 38 epileptics had a focus in the temporal lobe, but no psychomotor attacks, although they did suffer major seizures. Eighteen of these 38 patients had a focus in the Ammon's horn. However, it should be pointed out that convulsion foci in the Ammon's horn do not always lead to psychomotor epilepsy or to personality changes. In his monograph, Peiffer (1963) expands on his initial findings referred to here.

Ammon's Horn Sclerosis as a Result of Epileptic Attacks

Bauchet and Cazauveth (1825) reported on epilepsy and *Ammon's horn sclerosis* more than 140 years ago. A few decades later, Meynert (1868) put forward the suggestion that the Ammon's horn may be involved when other, remote cerebral formations are injured. Thus, if epilepsy is induced in a distant region of the brain, the Ammon's horn cannot remain unaffected since, functionally, it is connected with the other regions of the brain. Therefore, psychomotor epilepsy is not necessarily induced primarily from the hippocampus, even if anatomical changes are found there.

While Bauchet and Cazauveth (1825), Meynert (1868), Pfleger (1880), Scholz (1939 - 1959), Peiffer (1962, 1963) tend to regard Ammon's horn sclerosis as the *result* of the epileptic attacks, several other authors (Knapp 1905, 1918, Stauder 1936, 1938) have expressed the view that Ammon's horn sclerosis is not the result but the *cause* of the epilepsy. Up to the present, these two opposing positions have been consistently and vigorously defended. Many arguments have been raised in support of both of these theories.

A few recent findings will be given to support the view that Ammon's horn sclerosis is the result of epilepsy.

Quandt and Sommer (1966), Sommer and Quandt (1969) carried out experiments on 30 cats. These were performed in the same way as electroshock treatment in human patients, so that better comparisons could be made. There were changes in the cerebral formations in relation to the number of electroshock and to the site of the electrodes. By microscopic processing of the cat brains treated in this way, the authors established that there is mild acute excitation of the ganglion cells after only two electric shocks. *With an increasing number of convulsions, these changes increase both quantitatively and qualitatively.* After four electroconvulsions, the ganglion cell picture begins to show definite changes; the usual order of the normal cell-equivalents picture becomes considerably disrupted. The cellular neuroglia is increased and many ganglion cells are so damaged that they fall victim to progressive necrosis. After ten electroshock convulsions, the usual cortical stratification is completely disrupted. In particular, fronto-temporally there is pronounced clearing of the ganglion cells in the third and fifth cortical layers. Here the active neuroglia cells predominate, while almost without exception the staining ganglion cells show severe changes in their cytosome and cell nucleus; this takes the form of a severe cellular disease, such as was originally described by Nissl.

The morphological changes are concentrated in the bifrontal area through which the current passes and they behave according to the physical laws governing the propagation of an electric current.

The authors also observed changes in the behavior of the experimental animals and these corresponded to the morphological findings. Behavioral disturbances were observed after only three shocks. These consisted of abnormal *character changes* in the animals. Their orientating capacity was very much affected; they sought the protection of darkness and there was also a decrease of libido. There was a gradual decline in their appetite. These changes were intensified during seven subsequent electroconvulsions and they were not reversible, even after two months, i.e. there was an exogenous cerebral defect syndrome.

The majority of the reports on neuropathological findings are devoted to the vasomotor changes in the brain as a result of the convulsion. Even before the use of electroshock, in animal experiments, Stief and Tokay (1932) demonstrated local cerebral damage following insulin convulsions, which resembled that seen following spontaneous convulsions in man.

Hempel (1941) found that, in addition to vasomotor disorders, there were also tissue lesions in the brain, which may have been due to a change of permeability of the blood-brain barrier. Weil-Liebert (1939), Hempel (1941), Zeman (1950), Bauer and Leonhardt (1955), Bauer, Haase and Leonhardt (1956) interpreted these changes in nerve cell tissue as being the result of disturbed vasomotor reaction during the pentylenetetrazol convulsion. Echlin (1942), Alexander and Löwenbach (1944), Kreienberg and Ehrhardt (1947) have reported on changes in the cerebral tissue following electroshock. Zeman (1950) and Scholz and Jötten (1950) found that the same lesions of cerebral tissue could be produced by an electric current and by therapeutic convulsions induced by insulin and pentylenetetrazol. For the first time, these authors took into consideration the *effects of the electrical energy used.* In interpreting the morphological changes in the brain due to the effect of electroconvulsion, Scholz (1951) concluded that these must have been caused by vasomotor reaction, and he went on to say that therapeutic electroconvulsion and spontaneous convulsion induce the same vasomotor reactions and, in the case of electroshock, these are not limited to the region propagating the electrical current.

The sum total of these changes appears to be local anoxia which is not distributed uniformly throughout all the regions of the brain; the anoxia exhibits a predilection for specific sites (Scholz 1951, Quandt and Sommer 1966). In man, all these lesions of the cerebral tissue lead to a specific clinical and electroencephalographic symptomatology such as convulsion elements in the EEG, diffuse slowing of cerebral activity, isolated spontaneous convulsive seizures, ephemeral hemiparesis, aphasia, parkinsonism, lack of concentration, forgetfulness and trophic disorders in the fingers and toes (v. Baeyer 1951).

Using an electronmicroscope, Mölbert et al. (1967) carried out comparative investigations on the cerebral cortex of the cat before and after electroconvulsions, and they found that there were a series of demonstrable cellular defects as a result of the convulsion. The cortical nerve cells showed structural changes in the convulsion; these changes correspond to increased transport of RNA (ribonucleic acid) from the cell nucleus. Various transport mechanisms were observed at the convulsion membranes, and, in part, their degeneration stages as well. Changes were also found in the other cellular organelles; in particular, the structure of the mitochondria appeared to suffer partial disintegration. The vacuole content of the axosomatic synapses was also altered and, as a rule, the number of synapse vacuoles was drastically reduced. Compared with normal, the axodendritic synapses appear to undergo few changes following the convulsion.

The findings were interpreted as correlating with the number of nerve cell discharges, which is greatly increased during an epileptic convulsion. There was also discussion of the fact that, after disrupting the normal regulatory mechanisms in the neuroglia-neurone system, the convulsion makes excessive demands on the energy of cell metabolism, and thus causes structural changes.

Observations of neuroglia cells impaired by this experimental *acute* convulsion are very interesting. Here the satellites of the nerve cells, the oligodendroglia cells, showed changes similar to those of the nerve cells themselves, while the astrocytes showed completely different morphological changes in the mitochondria as the predominant finding. According to the authors, this can be attributed not only to these cells having a different function, but also to their having a different metabolism (see also Lehniger 1964, Kulenkampff 1952, Kunz and Sulcin 1947).

There are also many other findings in support of the view that Ammon's horn sclerosis is a result of epileptic attacks. Peiffer (1962, 1967, 1970) consistently found that there were fresh lesions and hemorrhage in patients who had just died during or after status epilepticus. Similar fresh lesions of the Ammon's horn had previously been found by Scholz (1959) and other authors who are cited and discussed by Peiffer. This raises the question: if Ammon's horn sclerosis is the result of epilepsy, then what is the cause?

Ammon's Horn Sclerosis as a Causal Factor of Psychomotor Epilepsy

In opposition to the view that Ammon's horn sclerosis is the secondary sequela of a convulsion (Scholz 1956, Spielmeyer 1926) it is reported that following extirpation of the entire temporal lobe including the Ammon's horn (and in these cases only the Ammon's horn showed pathological changes) the attacks ceased. The relationships between Ammon's horn sclerosis and epileptic character changes (as suggested by Sano and Malamud 1953) have often been discussed but have never been fully explained. Discussion about the origin of Ammon's horn sclerosis is still in progress.

Further arguments against the hypothesis that Ammon's horn sclerosis is the result of the epileptic attacks, are also raised by results of precision microscopy and histochemical findings from the Ammon's horn itself.

The Ammon's horn is a cortical structure with a profound degree of reduction of most layers so that the large pyramidal cells are almost all which remain; this appears to correspond to the fifth layer of the isocortex (Hassler 1964 a, b, Stephan 1964). It is an involuted gyrus (Figure 14a, 14b, and 15).The regio entorhinalis on the gyrus hippocampalis is continuous with the praesubiculum to which is connected the actual base of the Ammon's horn, the subiculum. The *fields* of the Ammon's horn itself, which are described as h_1, h_2, h_3, and h_4 by C. and O. Vogt (1937), Fleischhauer (1959), Fleischhauer and Horstmann (1957) then follow. Of these, h_4 is identical with the *terminal layer* which is bounded by the gyrus dentatus. The classification chosen by Lorente De Nó (1933, 1934) is not quite the same as the above. The descriptions are CA_1, CA_2, CA_3 and CA_4 (for histochemistry see following).

Are the Anatomic-Histological Changes in the Ammon's Horn Specific to Psychomotor Epilepsy?

According to some findings, the sclerosis found in the Ammon's horn is not specific simply to epileptics and the fields of the Ammon's horn we have mentioned are not all affected to the same extent by the sclerosis, so it seems doubtful whether this is the result of the attacks.

On the basis of experience with a fairly large quantity of autopsy material, various authors (Morel and Wildi 1956, Corsellis 1957 point out that *changes in the Ammon's horn are definitely more frequent in cases of cerebral sclerosis and other cerebral diseases, than in epileptics.*

Bratz (1920), Merritt (quoted by Hassler 1964 b) and Vogt and Vogt (1937, 1942) found defects in the *Sommer's sector* and in the terminal layer but not in the h_2 or gyrus dentatus even in progressive paralysis without epileptic attacks. There were rather similar findings in Pick's atrophy, Alzheimer's disease and senile dementia (Bratz 1920, Vogt 1942, Morel and Wildi 1956) again with no seizures. There were also localized defects of the Ammon's horn in Little's disease, various forms of idiocy and encephalitis (Peiffer 1963) without there being any epileptic attacks. However, in some cases the latter conditions have also been associated with seizures so that these results are not completely reliable as substantiating evidence. Even though these cases described by Peiffer (1963) did not happen to have any attacks, they may well have had a predisposition to seizure.

According to Hassler (1964 b), the field specificity of the Sommer's sector mentioned above cannot be attributed solely to a specific pathogenesis as a result of the epileptic attacks. This fact was also acknowledged by Scholz (1959). The field h_2 which is resistant in epileptic Ammon's horn sclerosis, is the only area, or the first area to degenerate in cases of amaurotic idiocy, without there being any attacks in the patients affected; this has been demonstrated by C. and O. Vogt (1937, 1942). Thus, Ammon's horn deficiency whatever its localization, is certainly not just the result of epileptic attacks and cannot simply be attributed to ischaemia occurring during these attacks. In animal experiments, bilateral lesions in the terminal layer and neighboring structures may actually be the *cause* of epilepsy (see Green et al. 1957). The findings of Peiffer (1962) quoted above, raise a further strong objection to ischaemia being the cause of Ammon's horn sclerosis. According to Peiffer most lesions in this region are found in cases of psychomotor epilepsy. This form of epilepsy is known not to be associated with convulsions.

Here are a few more points in connection with this problem: Hassler

(1964 b) assumes that *Ammon's horn sclerosis is not always an indicator of epilepsy and it is not simply the result of epileptic attacks.* It is more likely that the Ammon's horn plays an important part in the development of attacks. Temporal epilepsy with its special form of seizure, the psychomotor attack, is due to foci in the temporal lobe. This has been shown above (see also Meyer and Beck in Hassler 1964b). These foci *destroy neighboring structures but not the Ammon's horn itself.* The Ammon's horn, as the *most spasmophilic* structure of the brain, must obviously for the most part remain intact. It is either irritated mechanically by the foci nearby or it is impaired in its activity by disturbance of the afferent impulses. In fact, localized processes, such as a glioma in the area subcallosa, which is very remote from the Ammon's horn but within the limbic system, may provoke temporal epilepsy (Hassler and Riechert 1957, Hassler 1964 b). This also correlates with Meynert's view, put forward as early as 1868, that the Ammon's horn may also be involved when other cerebral structures became diseased. This has already been mentioned above.

The significance of the Ammon's horn in the *development* of epileptic attacks is also demonstrated by the physiological investigations of Pampiglione and Falconer (1956, 1960). By direct stimulation the Ammon's horn of epileptic patients during surgery, it was shown that *excitability of the Ammon's horn* in response to epileptic discharges is reduced by Ammon's horn sclerosis (as revealed by subsequent biopsys) (see also Hassler 1964 b). Hassler (1964 b) emphasizes that, in spite of the experimental findings mentioned above, Ammon's horn sclerosis in epileptics is of no *etiological* significance in the epilepsy. *According to this author, localized processes within the limbic system but outside the Ammon's horn itself, may be the cause of epilepsy.* There is a causal relationship between recurring epileptic attacks and cellular degeneration in h_1 and in the terminal layer in that these fields of the Ammon's horn produce particularly powerful discharges during the attacks and by doing this they probably damage themselves. Hassler's view also correlates with the findings of Jung and Tönnies (1950) and of Mölbert et al. (1967). Experimental results obtained by excision and stimulation of the structures of the limbic system demonstrate that most of the symptoms of psychomotor epilepsy arise when there are lesions of the formations outside the Ammon's horn (but symptoms are less clear when they are within).

In this discussion we have come a little nearer to discovering the etiology of the cryptogenic *(idiopathic, essential)* form of epilepsy. With this second form there is always the possibility that the lesions have not been detected even though they are present submicroscopically. This will be discussed in more detail later. *Given that Ammon's horn sclerosis is involved in the genesis of epilepsy, the cause of the sclerosis still remains to be found.*

The Significance of Perinatal and Other Brain Injuries for Psychomotor Epilepsy

We would again mention the theories on damage to the basal parts due to minor coup-contracoup episodes (Earle et al. 1953). Penfield and Jasper (1954) have summarized events in the nerve cells and neuroglia reactions in the Ammon's horn, gyrus hippocampi, nucleus amygdalae and temporal cortex under the heading *incisural sclerosis,* and pathogenetically they attributed these changes to compression of the basal temporal brain into the incisura tentorii during parturition with simultaneous compression of the afferent vessels. Haberland (1958) also takes this view.

Landolt (1960) assumes that the incidence of temporal epilepsy is, first and foremost, the result of the *exposed topographical position* of the temporal lobes. With this exposed position the cerebral region is particularly susceptible to slight damage, which would not normally be recorded. Thus, the basal surfaces and the third temporal gyrus together with the basal parts of the frontal lobe are the cerebral regions where cortical contusion foci as a result of cranial trauma are most commonly found; this is because there are inadequate protective cushions of fluid. Contusion foci are also very often found in the gyri of the first temporal lobe.

Opponents of the theory that parts of the temporal lobe are squeezed into the incisura tentorii causing *incisural sclerosis* and psychomotor epilepsy, raise the objection that this damage arises during parturition, while psychomotor epilepsy does not develop until much later in life, i.e. not in childhood (Scholz 1959, Peiffer 1962, 1963). However, Penfield and Jasper (1954) have asserted that there is a very long period of latency up to the time when the attacks begin, and this may even last for decades. During this period, there is progressive maturation of the gliose cicatrices. Gastaut (1953), Gastaut et al. (1959) developed the concept that all lesions of the temporal lobe are produced by primary cerebral damage (of whatever kind), which precedes the paroxysmal ailment.

The Predisposition of the Phyllogenetically Older Brain Structures for Convulsions

Apart from the morphological and functional heterogeneity (which will be discussed later), *mention should also be made of the different predisposition to convulsion of the phylogenetically older parts of the brain.* Servit (1962) and Peiffer (1967) deal with this problem. It was shown that the capacity to produce a generalized tonic-clonic epileptic attack can only be detected after a certain stage of development and that at an earlier stage of development there is only a certain *anarchic uncoordinated convulsive seizure* in response to an electrical stimulus, as is seen in infants and small children. In higher animals, *the convulsion threshold falls and the predis-*

position to convulsion increases. It is also very interesting that in early stages of development there is a close correlation between predisposition to convulsion and body temperature, and this becomes less and less true in higher animals. Peiffer (1967) suggests that the convulsions seen in small children during a fever may be a rudiment of this relationship to body temperature, in accordance with the biological law of curtailed phylogenesis in ontogenesis.

In the course of phylogenetic development up to man, in the higher animal species the formations of the rhinencephalon (which are most predisposed to produce convulsion) have become smaller and smaller, so that in a healthy individual they are not dangerous (Stephan 1964).

A further characteristic of the phylogenetically older cerebral formations with the greatest predisposition to produce convulsion is that they are embedded in phyloontogenetically younger cerebral tissue and enveloped by it, and they are cut off from the numerous anatomical and functional projections. *The enveloping and covering of the medial part of the temporal lobe by the convulsion-inhibiting structures of the isocortex and the central ganglia has, in our opinion, a decisive part to play in the development of the symptomatology of psychomotor epilepsy, which involves few convulsions but which is rich in psychic, emotional, sensory, autonomic and motor symptoms. This fact is one of the essential components in our model of an epileptic attack, which is presented in Chapter VIII.*

The neighboring cerebral structures must also be considered with reference to psychomotor epilepsy. Janz (1960) showed that frontal tumors frequently lead to status epilepticus and to psychomotor epilepsy. However, he found that these tumors only precipitate the symptoms by pressure on the temporal lobe.

Peiffer (1967) mentions the incidence of epilepsy where there are cerebral tumors in which the nerve cells between the tumorous tissues are still in good condition, as in oligodendrogliomas or many astrocytomas (Figure 18). However, it is known from neurophysiology (Jung and Tönnies 1950, Peiffer 1967) that the convulsion focus demonstrated in the EEG does not usually lie at the center of degenerate tissue but in the marginal area, i.e. where there are still functional nerve cells, but where the equilibrium of the complex system of excitatory and inhibitory influences on the nerve cells (normally present in the grey matter) is disrupted. If there is a tumor in the vicinity of the limbic system it stimulates these highly excitable structures and produces, among other things, psychomotor epilepsy.

Psychomotor Epilepsy as a Result of Combined Factors

In view of the exposed position of the temporal region, the damage may also be caused by other factors. In addition, Jung and Tönnies (1950), found, as did many other authors after them, that the predisposition of the hippocampus to convulsion is 10 to 12 times greater than that of the other cerebral regions. Thus, there is a *phylogenetic* reason (Lockard et al 1972, Loiseau and Beaussart 1969) for looking for the causes of epilepsy in the hippocampus. There has also been much discussion about a familial tendency; it certainly cannot be denied that this exists and it means there is a genetic component involved in the problem of etiology. Finally, we know of constitutional types of human being who react differently to this or that disease (Chevrie and Aicardi 1972; Falconer 1971; Gregoriades 1972; Hecker et al. 1972; Ross and Evans 1972; Scott et al. 1972; Show et al. 1972; Stene 1972; Tronillas and Courjon 1972). This answers the question of *disposition.* Prüll (1967) has summarized the etiological and pathogenetic factors of epilepsy:

By *disposition,* he means: 1.) *Constitution* (including cerebral angio- and chemoarchitectonics); 2.) *previous cerebral injury;* 3.) *age;* 4.) *hereditary convulsion-wave threshold* (genuine predisposition to convulsion with no realization factor); 5.) *actual psychic-somatic condition* (including triggering factors such as emotion, cycle, lack of sleep, alcohol).

In addition, we have the *exposition* with: 1.) *encephalopathies due to genetic metabolic enzymatic defects;* 2.) *foetal damage and malformation;* 3.) *circumnatal cerebral damage;* 4.) *inflammatory encephalophathies in early childhood;* 5.) *cerebral traumas;* 6.) *cerebral tumors* (endogenous, mesodermal, vascular, metastasizing, haematomas); 7.) *encephalopathies of extracranial origin* (such as restricted or disturbed utilization of O_2, glucose, electrolytes, H_2O); 8.) *cerebrovascular insufficiency* (local, generalized); 9.) *atrophic cerebral processes.*

All these factors produce a *neuronal hypersynchronous mass discharge and lead to an epileptic attack.*

Possible Localizations of Convulsion Foci

The first characteristic of the entire temporal lobe is the non-uniformity of its anatomical and functional structures. The diverse, very variable and complex symptomatology of psychomotor epilepsy is probably largely the result of these morphological and functional variations in the organic substrate of the temporal lobe. Which cerebral structures can be influenced by an epileptic focus in the temporal lobe?

Regarding simply the *medial part* itself, this again is heterogenous and this may result in different symptoms and syndromes. Morphologically, this part comprises *cortical* and *subcortical* grey structures, and functionally it covers the *olfactory system* (i.e. sensory system) and the *limbic system* (system independent of senses: Hassler 1964b, Stephan 1964).

The *lateral part* of the temporal lobe also comprises different anatomical and functional regions.

The Medial Part of the Temporal Lobe (Figure 14 a and b)

According to Hassler (1964 a), and as shown by Figure 14a, *the limbic system* comprises the fields of the *gyrus cinguli* (areas 32, 24, 23), the *Ammon's horn* with the *gyrus dentatus* and the *subiculum, praesubiculum* (27), the *regio entorhinalis* (28) and *retrosplenialis* (29), the *amygdaloid nucleus complex* (Am) and the surrounding cortex (co) together with their connecting fibres, the *cingulum,* the *fornix* and the *stria teminalis.* The limbic *system* arises from the limbic *lobe* through these connecting fibres (Mac Lean 1954 to 1962). In this way, the *"bed nucleus" of the stria terminalis,* the *corpus mamillare* and other nuclei of the *lateral hypothalamus* are incorporated in the limbic system; this also applies to the *stria medullaris thalami* with the *ganglion of habenulae* (Hb) and *interpeduncular ganglion* (Ip), and also the *anterior nuclear group of the thalamus* (Am), the *septum* (Sp) and Broca's *diagnoal fascide,* but this certainly does not include all the nuclei of the thalamus or hypothalamus (Hassler 1964a).

Rose (1926, 1927) uses the collective term *Ammon's horn formation* for the Ammon's horn, fascia dentata, tenia tecta and subiculum.

From the above description it is understandable *that psychomotor epi-*

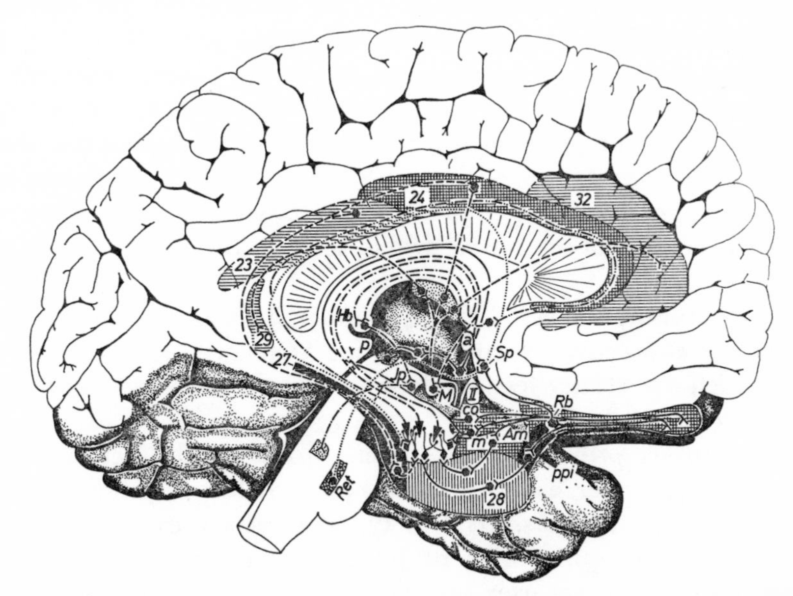

Figure 14a. Cortical and subcortical regions of the medial part of the temporal lobe with their connections to adjacent cerebral structures (see text for further explanation). (From Hassler, R., 1964a.)

lepsy is not purely and simply temporal lobe epilepsy, since the limbic structures which are involved in the symptomatology of this form of epilepsy extend as far as the medial regions of the brain and include parts of the *diencephalon.*

THE CORTICAL PARTS OF THE LIMBIC SYSTEM ARE CONTAINED (according to Stephan 1964) in the zonal region surrounding the corpus callosum and hilus of the hemispheres; the whole of this region is known as the *rhinencephalon.* Stephan believes that this term should be limited in its use since it may be misleading. Functionally, the rhinencephalon corresponds to the olfactory system, and not to the limbic system.

According to Kuhlenbeck (1927) and other authors, Gerdy (1838) was the first to realize that a circumscribed ring in the cerebral hemisphere has a special morphological and functional role. Gerdy described a *circonvolution annulaire.* This zonal boundary area was very soon divided into an inner and an outer ring (Schwalbe 1881, Zuckerkandl 1887, Retzius 1896). According to Stephan (1964), Broca's *grand lobe limbique* (1878) from which we derive the term *limbic system,* may only apply to the outer arch and does not include the hippocampus and septum. According to Broca, it consists of three sections: a rostral section *lobe olfactif,* a dorsal section *circonvolution du corps calleux* (corresponding to the gyrus cinguli) and a caudoventral section *circonvolution de l'hippocampe* (corresponding to the gyrus parahippocampi). In the limbic system of MacLean, Stephan finds that the rostral part of the *lobe olfactif* is no longer present, but the inner arch: hippocampus, fornix and septum, is certainly there.

The cortical centres in the adjoining region are almost exclusively *non-olfactory* and only the adjacent areas immediately caudal to the pedunculus olfactorius, i.e. the prepiriform and periamygdalar cortex and the olfactory bulb, are in fact *olfactory,* i.e. sensory (Stephan 1964). Stephan emphasizes that the terms *grand lobe limbique* and *limbic system* are not synonymous, since he excludes from the limbic system some of the regions in the *grand lobe limbique.*

Architectonically the vast majority of cortical regions of the limbic arch belong to the *allocortex* (we are still citing Stephan) i.e. to that group of cortices which are clearly less developed or which are very different from the typical six-layered isocortex.

The *allocortex primitivus* and *periallocortex* are distinct areas of the allocortex. The former has a thin cortex which has very few clearly distinguishable cellular layers. Its two types, palaeocortex and archicortex (hippocampus), are quite different from one another. In contrast to all other cortices, the palaeocortex does not develop over a cortical sheet. The periallocortex has many more layers, but it differs from the isocortex in that it has an often very marked, superficial medullary layer of fibres

(Meynert 1968, Stephan 1964). There is also a *proisocortex,* which, according to Vogt (1956) and Sanides (1962), can be differentiated from the isocortex and which represents a transitional formation between the genuine *isocortex* and the periallocortex (Stephan 1964).

While the olfactory system is purely palaeocortical, the limbic system is regarded as being predominantly archicortical and periarchicortical (Hassler 1964 a, b, Stephan 1964). Other cortical parts of the limbic system are septum diagonal fascicle, gyrus cinguli (the outer margin of which is not clear), hippocampus (archicortex with subiculum, cornu ammonis and fascia dentata, including precommissural hippocampus or indusem greseum), regio entorhinalis (including regio perirhinalis, praesubicularis, subgenualis) (Stephan 1964, Hassler 1964, a).

THE SUBCORTICAL PARTS OF THE LIMBIC SYSTEM INCLUDE THE REMAINING NUCLEAR REGIONS MENTIONED ABOVE: amygdaloid nucleus complex, fornix, corpora mamillaris, the lateral group of the hypothalamus, ganglion of habenulae, interpeduncular ganglion, and also the anterior nuclear group of the thalamus and septal nuclei.

The olfactory system includes the remaining formations of the rhinencephalon. Since very recently, this system has simply been described as the rhinencephalon, since the limbic system does not possess any, or only very few, direct connections with the sensory organs. The formations of the limbic system respond non-specifically, and functionally they have been grouped with the other non-specific cerebral regions (see Chapter IV).

Both the limbic and the olfactory systems have a certain part to play in psychomotor epilepsy. Both systems complicate the symptomatology of this form of epilepsy and they will be discussed in the course of this study.

The Lateral Part of the Temporal Lobe

This part extends between sylvian fissure, parietal and occipital lobe. The cranial parts are covered by the operculum. The dorsal margin is difficult to define. On the convexity a connecting line can be drawn from the ramus occipitalis of the sylvian fissure to the impressio petrosa, but on the basal plane there is no detectable border with the occipital lobe. Cytoarchitectonically, the temporo-occipital transition zone represents the parietal cortex, so that according to von Economo (1927) the caudal limit has been made more narrow. Delmas (1955) points out that an anatomical unit can only be demonstrated by macroscopical examination of the temporal lobe. Sperling and Creutzfeldt (1959) give a detailed survey of the morphological and functional anatomy, including neurophysiology, of the temporal lobe. In this present study, we are more concerned with the medial parts of this cerebral lobe.

Possible Pathways for the Spread of Pathological Excitation

When considering the discharge, spread, maintenance and detection of the convulsion elements (CE), it is particularly important to know the

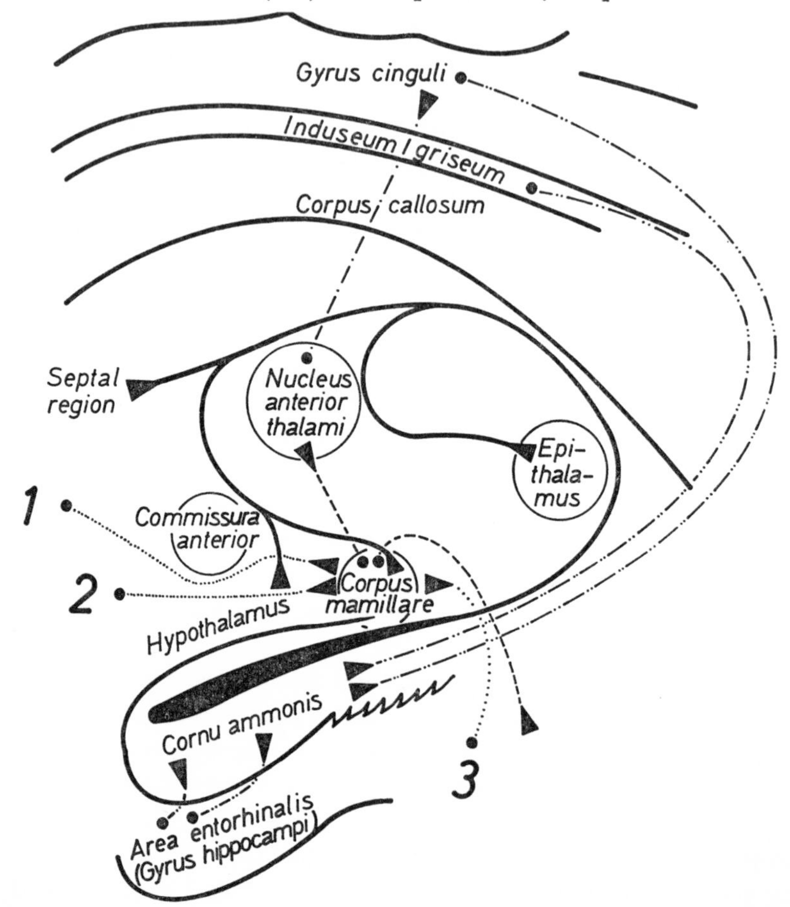

Figure 14b. Position of the Ammon's horn within the system of circuits we are interested in here. The diagram illustrates the most important afferent and efferent connections of the hippocampus.

C.A. = commissura anterior. C.M. = corpus mamillare.

● –··–·· < Afferents from the entorhinal area, gyrus cinguli and induseum griseum (from Lorente de Nó).

▬ < Fornix = efferent projection system of the hippocampus to the mamillary body with fibres to the epithalamus, septal region and sections of the hypothalamus with a low medulla content. Fibres extending to the midbrain are not shown.

● ...... < Other afferents of the mamillary body: 1 = fronto-mamillary fibres, probably coming from area 6; 2 = fibres of the basal olfactory bundle (= medical forebrain bundle = tractus olfacto-mesencephalicus) ; 3 = pedunculus mamillaris.

● ------ < Efferent system of the mamillary body = tractus mamillo-thalamicus and tractus mamillo-tegmentalis. – The thalamo-mamillary fibres running in the mamillo-thalamic tract are not shown here.

● .–.–< Thalamo-cortical fibres from the anterior thalamic nucleus to the cortical areas of the gyrus cinguli. (From Ule. G.: *Forschr Neurol Psychiat, 22*:510, 1954.)

connections which exist between the temporal lobe and other cerebral structures.

The *acoustic pathways* connect the temporal lobe with the corpus geniculatum mediale. An important factor in the propagation of excitation in psychomotor epilepsy is *the paucity of connections between the remote temporal parts and the known thalamic projections.* While there are numerous intracortical connections with frontal (fasciculus uncinatus) and occipital association tracts (Gros Clark 1948, Delmas 1955), very few connections between the temporal lobe and the thalamic regions are known (Bucy and Klüver 1955, Hartmann and Simma 1952, Sperling and Creutzfeldt 1959, Walker 1938). However, in recent years it has been discovered that there are certain functional and anatomical signs of degeneration in the thalamus after destruction of specific regions of the temporal lobe and this suggests that there must be other, as yet unknown projections between the first temporal gyrus, the medioventral nucleus of the pulvinar thalami and the corpora geniculata medalia (Chow 1950, Le Gros Clark and Northfield 1937, Simson 1953, Sperling 1957). According to the experimental results of Nauta (1956) Whitlock and Nauta (1956), all the areas of the temporal lobe have projections to the *pulvinar thalami* and to the ventral *putamen.* A few temporal fibres link the temporal lobe with the *pons* and *colliculus caudalis.* Medial temporal gyri must also be linked with *cauda nuclei caudati,* pretectal regions, *colliculus rostralis* and, via the lower thalamic region, with the *nucleus dorsomedialis thalami.* The temporal pole projects to the *colliculus rostralis,* to the *zona incerata* and to the adjacent part of the lateral tegmentum. There are also numerous afferents from the medial and lower temporal gyrus to the commissura anterior.

The functional relationships of the medial parts of the temporal lobe, i.e. the limbic system, are illustrated in the diagrams in Figures 14a and 14b.

The following authors have dealt with this problem: Cajal (1900), Rose (1926), Lorente De Nó (1933, 1934), Vogt and Vogt (1937, 1942), Klinger (1948), Ule (1954), Nauta (1956), Sperling (1967), Sperling and Creutzfeldt (1959), Hassler (1964a, b), Hernández Peón 1962 to 1965) and others.

The afferents of the *Ammon's horn formation* are derived from the area entorhinalis, the gyrus cinguli and indeseum griseum. The most important efferent projection system of the hippocampi, which are linked with one another via the psalterium, is the fornix system. According to Sprague and Meyer (1950), in the rabbit the Ammon's horn fibres terminate in the medial nuclei of the corpus mamillare and septal nucleus.

In rats, Nauta (1956) described direct hippocampal fibres to the septum region, the nuclei of the diagonal fascicle, the regio preoptica, dorsal hypothalamic fields, the thalamus (in particular the nucleus thalami anterior, the corpora mamillaria, regio supramamillaris and into the parts of the substantia grisea centralis). Later (1958) Nauta reported on the connections between the hippocampus and the mesencephalon (hippocampo-mesencephalic projections). Here there are only direct projections to the rostral part of the substantia grisea centralis. On the other hand, according to this author, there are several indirect hippocampal pathways originating in the septum, in the lateral preoptical and in the hypothalamic region, and these reach the mesencephalon via three different fibre systems: 1.) medial forebrain bundle; 2.) fasciculus retroflexus and, 3.) tractus medullotegmentalis. The circuit between the limbic system and the reticular formation is completed by ascending fibres which originate in the mesencephalon and which have numerous collaterals, some of which extend to the hippocampus.

The following authors have reported on the rhinencephalic connections with the dien-mesencephalon: Fox (1949), Mac Lardy (1950), Bürgi and Bucher (1955), Simma (1956), Simpson (1952). According to these authors, *homolateral* projections predominate throughout the fornix system. These are very important for epileptic propagation of the convulsion elements. Via the fasciculus of Vicq'd Azyr, it is also connected with the anterior nuclear groups of the thalamus which, in their turn, communicate with the gyrus cinguli.

The *amygdaloid nucleus complex,* which is situated in the depth of the uncus gyri hippocampi medial to the temporal operculum, is composed, phylogenetically, of an *older,* corticomedial nuclear group and a *younger,* basolateral nuclear group (Brockhaus 1938, Mittler 1948, Sperling and Creutzfeldt 1959).

The *projections* from the amygdaloid nucleus region to other cerebral structures have not yet been investigated in detail, although they are of great importance in the propagation and generalization of CE in epilepsies. As early as 1911, Valdenburg described a connection with the radix olfactoria. In the rabbit, direct olfactory fibres terminate in the medial amygdaloid nuclei, except in the pyriform area (Le Gros Clark and Meyer 1947). Droogleever-Fortuyn (1956), Klinger (1948) reported that there were efferent fibres to the claustrum and putamen. According to Brodal (1947), the principal efferents of the area amygdaloidea reach the hypothalamus, the septum and the regio preoptica via the tenia semicircularis (stria terminalis). In addition, Mettler (1948) describes connections with the nucleus habenulae medialis. Both amygdala are linked with one another via the commissura anterior (Fox and Schmitz 1943). Excitation from the epileptic focus in one amygdaloid group may be propagated to the other, contralateral side via this route.

Whitlok and Nauta (1956) were only able to detect a few neocortical temporo-amygdalar connections in Macacus rhesus, and these were only from the lower temporal gyrus. Ammono-amgdalar and ammono-temporo-basal pathways have not yet been definitely demonstrated anatomically (Sperling and Creutzfeldt 1959). Mac Lean et al. (1948 to 1966) describe the limbic system as a functional unit and this includes the formations mentioned above. They used the term *oral sense* which plays an important role in the symptomatology of psychomotor epilepsy, as shown by Hallen's report (see Chapter I). The oral sense is related in particular to the oral automatisms.

Experimental Anatomy and Psychomotor Epilepsy

Experiments Involving Stimulation of the Temporal Cerebral Structures

IN MAN, THE EFFECTS OF ELECTRICAL OR CHEMICAL STIMULATION OF DIFFERENT STRUCTURES, WERE VARIABLE.

Psychic responses. As regards consciousness, the response varied from slight drowsiness to unequivocal clouding of consciousness following stimulation of the uncus (Liberson et al. 1951), of the gyrus hippocampi (Kaada and Jasper 1952), and of the fornix (Ausst 1954, Hassler and Riechert 1957, Umbach and Riechert 1958). In what are already recognized as classic experiments in neurosurgery in epileptics, Penfield (1952, 1958, 1959), Penfield and Rasmussen (1951) were able to evoke dramatic, ordered subjective experiences and memories of an affective type. By stimulation of the *lateral* temporal cortex, the patients were able to recall events which they had long forgotten. The past experience was suddenly evoked in great detail, like a film strip or tape-recording. Penfield termed this evocation of past memories, which were not altered by fresh experience, *memory of experience.* After another stimulation, the patient suddenly became aware of the present; according to Penfield, this was an interpretation of the present, but not one which the patient had considered. He calls this effect the *interpreting memory.* These effects of stimuli, particularly the latter, are very similar to a twilight attack with *dejá vu* in psychomotor epilepsy. Penfield was concerned with the neurophysiology and psychopathology of memory and he named this part of the temporal lobe the *memory store.* However, shortly after this, Riechert and Umbach (1958) observed a similar course of events accompanied by affective symptoms, after stimulation of the fornix in epileptics with psychomotor epilepsy. According to these results, the lateral part of the temporal lobe is not the only memory store. However, as regards psychomotor epilepsy these latter experiments have not disproved the theories on the localization of the pathological changes.

Stimulation of corresponding fields in the lateral temporal region of the brain also produces specific sensory impressions which are also observed clinically in epilepsies as illusions or hallucinations. Helschl's transverse gyri and the area temporalis 22 may produce auditory sensations (usually indeterminate sounds) and nystagmus (Foerster 1936, Penfield and Rasmussen 1950); the first temporal gyrus also produces nystagmus (Penfield and Rasmussen 1950) and the anteromedial and basal cortex and the uncus give rise to olfactory or gustatory sensations. These sensations may be accompanied by emotions.

Sensory effects are important in that they are observed in the abdominal form of psychomotor epilepsy. The cerebral structures responsible can be localized fairly accurately by stereotactic surgery (Hassler 1968, Hassler and Walker 1970). As we are concerned with epilepsy here, we are interested in stimulation in the thalamus region (nucleus ventrocaudalis), colliculus medialis and formations of the midbrain. Abdominal sensations and changes of the gastric peristalsis can be observed after electrical stimulation of the insula (Penfield and Faulk 1955).

Motor effects in the form of *adversive movements* with a change of the muscular tone have been induced in man following stimulation in the structures of the striatum, the thalamus and the reticular formation. Ipsilateral facial contractions could also be shown in patients, following stimulation of the periamygdalar cortex (uncus) (Baldwin et al. 1954, Hassler 1964a, 1972, Hassler and Dieckmann 1970, 1972; Hassler et al. 1969a, b). These adversive movements are often found clinically in psychomotor epileptics (see Chapter I).

Autonomic effects with a change in the breathing in the form of respiratory inhibition to respiratory arrest are obtained fairly consistently following stimulation of the insular region, the temporal pole, the ventral and medial surfaces of the temporal lobe, the gyrus hippocampi (Glusman et al. 1953, Kaada and Jasper 1952, Penfield and Faulk 1955) and the uncus (Liberson et al. 1951). A few patients were able to prevent the stimulus-induced respiratory paralysis by concentrating hard (Kaada and Jasper 1952). The same authors also observed masticatory automatisms.

In animals, stimulation produces symptoms which are equally varied but which correlate more or less with those seen in man. In addition to the caution which is usually exercised when comparing effects obtained in man with those in animals. Sperling and Creutzfeldt (1959) emphasize that we must bear in mind that after electrical or chemical stimulation we are not dealing with spontaneous physiological activity. The same objections can also be raised in respect of excision experiments.

Behavioral effects, corresponding to the psychic reactions in man, were obtained in animals. These took the form of fear, flight, rage and aggression with the corresponding motor patterns, and there was also increased alertness, in the form of an *arrest reaction* following stimulation of the limbic structures and the formations of the thalamus and the midbrain (Hassler 1964 a, b, Kaada et al. 1954, Koikegami et al. 1954, Magnus and Lammers 1956). After powerful stimuli, there were attacks similar to those in psychomotor epilepsy.

Hassler (1964 a) stresses the fact that, for the most part, stimulation of the limbic structures produces uncharacteristic symptoms, in contrast to the effects of stimulating the midbrain and diencephalon. Similarly, there is no sharp distinction between stimulus and lesion effects and manifestations in convulsive attacks.

Stimulation of the medial parts of the amygdaloid nucleus complex produces rage occasionally accompanied by aggression. The manifestations are triggered by the stria terminalis, the bundle of fibres arising from the medial sections of the amygdaloid nucleus complex and leading to the hypothalamus (Hassler 1964 a). After stimulation of various cerebral structures in the cat, Hunsperger (1956, 1959) triggered responses similar to those seen in epileptics in an acute productive psychosis, with fits of depression and outbreaks of rage and aggressiveness. Rage activity can also be invoked by less stimulation of the medial thalamus and, in particular, the hypothalamus (Hess 1954). The area which produces unequivocal effects is situated lateral to the fornix in the middle and posterior hypothalamus. However, Hunsperger (1959) also produced rage activity with or without aggressiveness by stimulating the substantia grisea centralis mesencephali. The cats first tried to escape the stimulus by flight and they only became aggressive when their progress was impeded. The rage response due to stimulation of the lateral hypothalamus or excision of the medial hypothalamus is related to the intact condition of the substantia grisea centralis. Apart from these zones, rage responses could also be triggered from part of the reticular formation (Hassler 1964 a). The effects of stimulation in the Ammon's horn are very interesting in relation to Ammon's horn convulsion. Mac Lean (1949, 1952, 1957 a, b) was able to show that, following chemical stimulation of the Ammon's horn, the convulsion was accompanied by a noticeable stupor in the animal with little spontaneous movement, correction of posture or response to sensory and pain stimuli. This state of pseudo-cataleptic rigidity may deteriorate into a violent outbreak of rage with aggresiveness towards the environment but with a lack of appreciation of the situation; there may then be sudden reversion to a statuesque, motionless posture. As the induced convulsion subsides, the animal often makes unpleasant sounds and then there is a prolonged condition of seeking contact, purring, cleaning its fur and licking its body and genitals.

This is obviously a reaction similar to that occurring in man in psychomotor epilepsy, with its subsequent postparoxysmal exaustion of Ammon's horn activity.

Sensory effects in association with affective and autonomic responses were obtained from the nucleus ventrocaudalis thalami, substantia grisea centralis mesencephali, from the structures of the reticular formation and some formations of the limbic system (Hassler 1961, 1964 a, 1968).

Motor patterns with adversive movements and changes in muscular tone were induced from the gyrus cinguli, with rotation of the head in one direction and eyes in the opposite direction. Simultaneous motor responses, such as respiratory movements, were inhibited by such stimuli (Kaada 1951, 1960, Ward 1948). Rotation to the opposite side and dilatation of the pupils, are regarded as motor effects of the anterior macronucleus of the thalamus and caudatum (Montanelli and Hassler 1962, 1964). Centers for contraversive rotation and adversive movements have also been found by stimulation in the pallidum and in the nucleus entopenduncularis. There is usually rotation of the eyes or of the head to the opposite side with mydriasis and increased excitability. Rotation to the opposite side with tonization of the contralateral musculature is also obtained following stimulation of the oral ventral nucleus (nucleus anteroventralis thalami) (Hassler 1964 a). Motor effects of stimulation of the Ammon's horn are associated with affective symptoms. The results were obtained using cats, dogs and monkeys (Cadilhac 1955, Creutzfeldt 1953, Gastaut et al. 1952, Hayashi 1953, Hassler 1964 a, Kaada et al. 1953, MacLean 1954, MacLean and Delgado 1953, MacLean et al. 1955, Magnus and Lammers 1956, Wall and Davis 1951). In general, the following were observed: disturbances of behavior, suppression of the spontaneous motor activity (inhibition of movement), decrease of alertness and changes of activity; these were associated as complex symptoms following stimulation of the Ammon's horn.

Autonomic symptoms were obtained after stimulation of the area pyriformis and entorhinalis in cats and monkeys (Gastaut 1952, Gastaut et al. 1952, Hassler, 1964 a, b; Hassler and Dieckmann 1968, Kaada 1951, Kaada et al. 1949, Mac Lean and Delgado 1953, Mac Lean and Ploog 1962, Rioch and Brenner 1938, Takahashi 1951); they were complex in form, such as respiratory inhibition, salivation, dilatation of the pupils, inhibition of peristalsis, erections. In addition to this, there were complicated behavior patterns and autonomic movements such as defecation, restlessness, oral automatisms (licking, mastication, gulping, swallowing). Autonomic effects, oral automatisms, nasal secretion, uterine contractions and ovulation could be seen following stimulation of the amygdaloid nuclei, and the periamygdalaer and pyriform cortex (Baldwin et al. 1954, Gastaut et al. 1951, 1952, Hayashi 1954, Kaada et al. 1954, Koikegami and Fuse 1952,

Koikegami et al. 1952, Mac Lean and Ploog 1962, Magnus and Lammers 1956, Shealy and Peele 1957, Takahashi 1951, Vigouroux et al. 1951). In an experiment to differentiate between different parts of the amygdaloid nucleus complex, it was found that the anteromedial (phylogenetically older) nuclei which contain fibres from the olfacto-gustatory system, are mainly concerned with oral and digestive activity, while the phylogenetically younger, basolateral nuclei are responsible for the complicated general behavioral changes. As early as 1923, and on the basis of his comparative anatomical studies, Johnston had intimated at this functional division of these nuclei (see also Mac Lean and Ploog 1962). Among others, Andy and Akert (1953), Baldwin et al. (1954), Creutzfeldt (1956), Gastaut et al. (1952, 1953), Hunter (1950), Kreindler (1965) were able to produce experimental epilepsy associated with other behavioral, sensory, motor and autonomic phenomena. However, we shall be discussing experimental epilepsy in Chapter IV.

Experiments Involving Excision of the Temporal Cerebral Structures

REACTIONS HAVE OFTEN BEEN OBSERVED IN MAN. The changes depend on the degree of destruction and the extent of the cerebral formations excised.

Psychic responses are obtained after lesions in various groups of centers. A severe personality change is observed following complete amputation of both temporal lobes. There are also severe memory disturbances (Green et al. 1951, Peter et al. 1949, Terzian and Dalle Ore 1955). The symptomatology resembles that of the Klüver-Bucy syndrome in animals.

This also occurs in isolation and the intelligence is unimpaired (Wechsel-Bellervue test) after bilateral extirpation of mediobasal parts of the temporal brain, including the anterior hippocampus and gyrus hippocampi (Scoville and Milner 1957, Sperling and Creutzfeldt 1959). On the other hand, there is only temporary impairment of memory when only the anterior parts of the gyrus hippocampi are removed; thus, in essence the degree of impairment is proportional to the extent of the lesions in the uncus-gyrus-hippocampus area. Isolated bilateral removal of the uncus including the amygdaloid nuclei does not result in impairment of memory (Sperling and Creutzfeldt 1959).

Unilateral extirpation of the temporal lobe causes behavioral changes with loss of drive and emotional instability (Fox and German 1935, Hill et al. 1957, Umbach 1967).

According to Hassler (1964 b), the functional activity of the Ammon's horn clearly alters in its excision effects. Glees and Griffith 1952, Grünthal 1947, Milner 1957, Scoville et al. 1959 and Ule 1951, 1954, have shown that bilateral destruction of the Ammon's horn in man produces complete temporal and spatial disorientation, loss of responsiveness, loss of memory and dulling of the emotions. If the patient survives, he develops dementia. However, according to Hassler (1964 b), this is not primarily dementia but loss of verbal and emotional reactions and disturbance of consciousness. If it is not possible to make any contact, either verbally or by gestures, with patients with bilateral destruction of the Ammon's horn, Hassler (1964 b) believes that this acute condition is not dementia, but rather an impairment of consciousness.

Hassler (1964 b) also mentioned the irreversible comata following insulin shock; he thinks that a large proportion of these are due to severe lesions of the Ammon's horn as a result of the hypoglycaemia. In neurosurgical bilateral extirpation of the Ammon's horn, the coma occurs with immediate clouding of consciousness. This is followed by prolonged disorientation with complete loss of memory. According to Walker (1957), loss of memory may occur even in cases of unilateral lesion of the Ammon's horn. Penfield and Milner (1958) also found loss of memory following bilateral lesion of the hippocampus. Behavioral disturbances with hypersexuality are observed following bilateral amygdalotomy with removal of the periamygdalar cortex (Bailey 1954, Sawa et al. 1954).

Sensory responses are less impressive following excision. At most, various sensations and feelings of pain may be eliminated. The operations are undertaken for therapeutic purposes (Hassler 1961, 1964 a, 1968, Leonhard 1950).

The *pattern of motor activity* cannot be modified with certainty by excision. However, these operations are carried out in order to study the psychomotor system. Changes of the motor system are found after bilateral resection of the gyrus cinguli (Hassler 1964 a). This has a calming and subduing effect and the operation is done for therapeutic reasons, to curb excited and aggressive patients (LeBeau 1954). Thus it follows that these formations are involved in the acute excitation states in patients with psychomotor epilepsy.

Autonomic regulatory disorders which are more or less profound, or mainly transitory, have been observed after bilateral temporal surgery (Bengochea et al. 1954, Dott 1938, Hassler and Riechert 1957, Umbach 1959, 1967).

Changes of respiratory rate and cardiac activity may be produced after excision of the respiratory and circulatory centers in the brain stem; however, these symptoms are not always directly associated with psychomotor epilepsy (Poeck 1959, Ranke 1960).

Reduced sexual function may be observed after specific excision (or stimulation) of the limbic system. These centers are maninly localized in and around the septum (Mac Lean and Ploog 1962). Hypo- or hypersexuality is sometimes observed in epilepsy.

Looked at another way, (i.e. how successful is extirpation of the convulsion focus?) the results may not appear to be very predictable. Extirpation of an electroencephalographic convulsion focus, or a convulsion focus identified by electrical stimulation, extirpation of the temporal pole and lobe resection with or without removal of the Ammon's horn, have either had no effect or they have only resulted in temporary success. A certain time after the operation, the convulsion foci tend to develop in another region of the brain. In some cases Hassler and Riechert (1957) and Umbach (1957, 1967) have carried out fornicotomy, with only temporary success. In a female patient who had had resection of the left fornix three years previously, we observed a status epilepticus with severe psychomotor retardation and disorientation; this result was objectivised polygraphically. The psychomotor attacks were combined with frequent generalized attacks, mainly arising from sleep. The success rates for various surgical operations vary considerably, although these are greatly influenced, on the one hand, by the different indications for surgery and, on the other hand, by the different observation periods after surgery. After a $\frac{2}{3}$ resection of the diseased temporal lobe, Penfield and Flanigin (1950) achieved an improvement of the clinical picture in 50 percent of over 68 operations. Even after a prolonged observation period, 14 patients had not had any more attacks. Bailey and Gibbs (1951) report the results of 25 operations with polar resection or gyrotomies of one or more temporal convolutions; they had good results and there were fewer psychic changes after the operation than before.

On the other hand, Maspers and Marossero (1953) stress that there are even better prospects of a cure with radical unilateral surgery to include the Ammon's horn. Using unilateral radical surgery in the temporal lobe, Bailey (1954) was able to achieve freedom from attacks in 64 percent of cases, while, paradoxically, with bilateral operations this was only achieved in 23 percent of cases. Morris (1956) reported success in 78 percent of cases after unilateral radical surgery on the temporal gyri, the gyrus and uncus hippocampi and the amygdaloid nuclei. The observation period has lasted from three to nine years after the operation, so that his conclusions are not yet confirmed. With surgery involving resection of the anterior parts of the temporal lobe together with the uncus, the major part of the amygdala and the anterior parts of the hippocampus, Falconer (1965) achieved complete or almost complete freedom from attacks in 53 percent of cases, an improvement in 30 percent and no change in 17 percent (100 cases altogether). Umbach (1967) has also reported similar results (see also Rasmussen 1970).

In animals, after bilateral extirpation of the temporal lobe in rhesus monkeys, a syndrome which has now become classic, develops the Klüver-Bucy syndrome (Klüver and Bucy 1937, 1939, Klüver 1952). Symptoms include: psychic blindness, oral tendencies, hypermetamorphosis, hypersexuality with excessive masturbation, emotional disturbance, excessive tameness and fearlessness.

In all excision experiments, we must take into account the fact that 1.) the center itself may be partially or completely destroyed; or 2.) the projections to or from other cerebral formations are severed so that the symptomatology becomes manifest in many different forms.

Biochemistry of the Convulsion-Inducing and Convulsion-Provoking Formation of the Temporal Lobe

According to earlier findings, the Ammon's horn probably represents *the central* activator of psychomotor epilepsy (Creutzfeldt 1956, Hassler 1964 a, b, Janzen and Müller 1952, Janzen et al. 1951, 1954, Jung 1949, Jung and Tönnies 1950, Meyer et al. 1954).

We have already discussed this region of the chemoarchitectonics previously by briefly describing the Ammon's horn fields in h_1 h_2, h_3 and h_4 (Vogt 1937, 1942) or CA_1, CA_2, CA_3 and CA_4 (Figure 15).

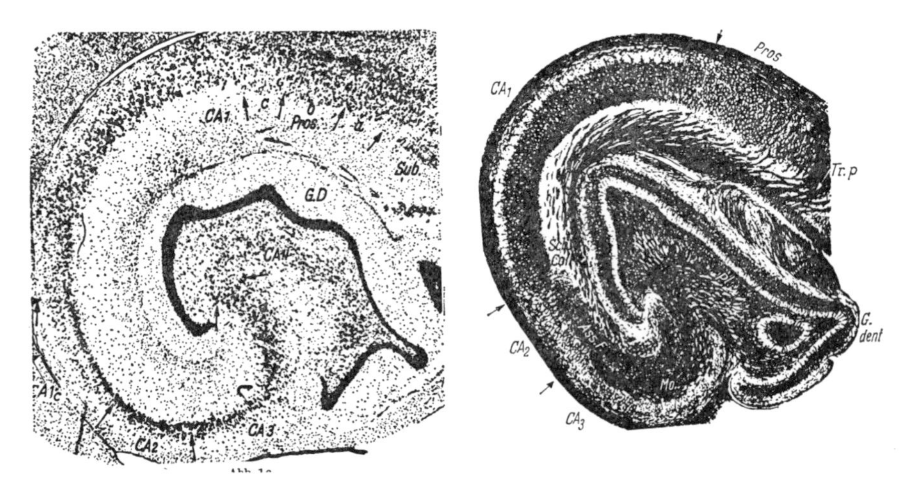

Figure 15. *Left:* Histological demonstration of the Ammon's horn fields in Macaccus. Field CA_4 is up against the gyrus dentatus (GD) which consists of a very dense margin of small cells. *Right:* Similar section through the Ammon's horn in Cajal fibre stain. Beneath the narrow cord of the gyrys dentatus (GD) in field CA_4 there is a plexiform (Pl.) fibruos layer formed from collaterals of the moosa fibres. The moosa fibres (Mo.) form a dense, dark bundle on the dendrite side of field CA_3. Field CA_2 begins at the sharp edge of the moosa fibre bundle. On the inner side of the moosa fibres there is dense fibrous layer of association fibres (Ass.F.). This only extends on the dendrite side of fields CA_3 and CA_2; it stops abruptly at the boundary between CA_2 and CA_1. Further towards the inner surface, the layer is connected to the Schaffer's collaterals (Sch.-Coll.). These collaterals extend on the dendrite side of fields CA_3, CA_2 and CA_1 and prosubiculum (Pros.). TP = tractus perforans (here, see Figure 27). (From Lorente De Nó, R.: *J Psychiol Neurol, 46:*113, 1934.)

Vogt (1936, 1942) took the view that the cyto-architectonic differences between individual cerebral structures are associated with extensive psysico-chemical differences. These physico-chemical differences were not demonstrable by the methods available when Vogt was writing 30 years ago, but modern methods have been able to confirm that he was right. Fleischhauer (1959), Fleischhauer and Horstmann (1957) produced evidence for this. From a series of investigations using different species of animal, they found that individual fields of the Ammon's horn show certain characteristics not only cyto-architectonically, but also biochemically, particularly with regard to *vitamins* and *enzymes.*

Using *dithizion* (diphenylthiocarbazone, benzeneazothioformic acid phenylhydrazide), in all animals investigated (from the hedgehog to the dog and cat) it was always the same cyto-architectonic fields which stained, while the others remained unstained or only took up a little stain.

In this way, for example, the acid *phosphatases* were found to be concentrated particularly around the base of the apical dendrites of h_3 and h_4.

On the other hand, *acetylcholinesterase* was found in h_1 nd h_2. This probably has a major part to play in the course of excitation in this formation.

There are fewer *respiratory enzymes* (succino-dehydro-genases) in h_1 and h_2 compared with field h_3 and the fascia dentata. The *oxidases* show a distribution resembling that of the *succino-dehydrogenase system.*

Other authors have demonstrated that fields h_3 and h_4 of the Ammon's horn have a high *zinc content* (Maske 1955, Hassler 1964 a). According to Timm (1958, 1961), the zinc and also the *copper* can be demonstrated with silver sulphide, and they are sharply defined. The zinc is found concentrated in the propagation regions of the neurites leading from the granular cells of the gyrus dentatus (the *moss fibres),* and their collaterals. They are in contact with the dendrites of field h_4 and, embedded in a substance which is not yet identified for certain, with the apical dendrites of field h_3. The zinc is not contained in the apical dendrites but lies at their surface (Hassler 1964 a). It is assumed that this is an enzyme containing zinc, such as *carboxypeptides or alcohol dehydrogenase.* Zinc is involved to some extent in infantile epilepsy, and this will be discussed later. A very important discovery was that during a protracted coma, insulin containing zinc produces cell deficiency in the Ammon's horn itself, sometimes typically distributed in field h_1 and in the terminal layer (Lemke 1937, Döring 1938, Hassler 1964a). Fields h_1 and h_2 are affected particularly severely after poisoning with KCN, while field h_3 suffers less damage (Fleischhauer 1959).

It is interesting to know in which structural elements of the cells the individual enzymes are found. According to microchemical analyses by Lowry et al. (1954), there are remarkably high concentrations of *lactic acid dehydrogenase* and *aldolase* in the dendrites and their branches. This is in complete contrast to the perikaryon. In the cell bodies and the base of the dendrites, there are concentrations of *fumarase, cytochrome oxidase and cholinesterase* and other enzymes. These areas also contain *nucleic acids.* In the axon there is a considerable fall in the *dehydrogenase* and *cytochrome oxidase* content, while the amount of *acetylcholine esterase* is hardly reduced microchemically. Histochemically, the cholinesterase is found in an even higher concentration here (Gerebtzoff 1960, Hassler 1964 a, b).

There is considerable metabolism of *L-methionine,* particularly in the Ammon's horn; this is also the case in the rest of the limbic cortex. It is less pronounced in the isocortex (Flanigan et al. 1957). The Ammon's horn and the area entorhinalis also contain much more *5-hydroxytryptamine (serotonin)* than in the isocortex. Thus, *reserpine* produces changes of potential in the Ammon's horn similar to those occurring under ether anaesthesia, long before any changes appear in the rest of the brain (Paasonen et al., quoted from Hassler 1964 a).

Recently, scientific interest has centered more and more on fields h_3 and h_4. Information important for the understanding of psychomotor epilepsy has been obtained by using certain antimetabolites. Many convulsion-provoking substances (see Chapter VI) including, in particular, the antimetablites of *Vitamin B,* have been under investigation (Christ et al. 1970a,b,c; Christ et al. 1971; Coggeshall and Mac Lean 1958, Coper 1966, Coper et al. 1966, 1971, 1972; Hassler et al. 1971, Hicks 1955, Niklowitz 1966, Purpura and Gonzales-Monteagudo 1960, Wooley et al. 1963). We shall now discuss some of these most important publications.

Using appropriate microscopic and electrophysiological techniques, lesions of the pyramidal cells of fields CA_3 and CA_4 of the Ammon's horn (we are using the nomenclature of the original study) were first found by Purpura and Gonzales-Monteagudo (1960) in cats following administration of antimetabolites of Vitamin B_6, *methoxy-pyridoxine,* and by Hicks (1955) and Coggeshall and MacLean (1958) in rats and mice after administration of antimetabolites of nicotinamide, *3-acetylpyridin.* In the most recent investigation, Niklowitz (1966) used optical and electron microscopy.

ADMINISTRATION OF METHOXYPYRIDOXINE: Niklowitz's aim (1966) was, firstly, to examine the acute and subacute effects of methoxypyridoxine on the structure of the *pyramidal cells of the Ammon's horn,* since at that time there had been no investigations using electromicroscopy and, secondly, he tried to obtain certain indications regarding the mode of action of *pyridoxine* and its antimetabolite methoxypridoxine on the metabolism of these cells. The experiments were carried out on 11 rabbits. The methoxypyridoxine (2-methyl-3-methoxymethyl-3-hydroxy-5-hydroxymethyl-pyridine) was administered intraperitoneally (i.p.) in single doses of 12.5 or 25 mg/kg. These doses had the same toxic effect in all animals.

BEHAVIOUR: Immediately after the injection the animals showed more rapid respiration; this normalized again in two minutes; they then became rather apathetic. After about 15 minutes the animals became restless. During this phase of intoxication the animals were very nervous. There was obviously clouding of consciousness. This phase usually lasted for five minutes and led up to the first and often most violent convulsive seizure. Just before the convulsions, the animals began powerful masticatory movements and they could be heard grinding their teeth.

A particularly violent seizure followed after 20 minutes. The principal symptoms were uncoordinated jumping movements, persistent clonic twitching of all the extremities, head in the neck bend, mouth open, spasmodic masticatory movements. Then there were extension spasms followed by rotation convulsions. The perceptible symptoms of the attack lasted for three to five minutes. The attacks were repeated at intervals of 15 to 20 minutes. Sometimes nystagmus was also observed. In the intervals, the animals showed cataleptic behaviour.

OPTICAL MICROSCOPIC FINDINGS: The early cytological changes were at first restricted to field CA_4 of the pyramidal cell band. There were also changes in isolated granular cells of the gyrus dentatus in the central apical region. After a more prolonged period the destructive effect of methoxypyridoxine also reached the pyramidal cells of the other fields. After an intoxication period of two hours in which the animals responded with violent convulsive fits and other symptoms, *about 80 percent of the pyramidal cells of fields CA_4, 20 percent of field CA_3 and only 5 percent of field CA_1 had altered microscopically, while the pyramidal cells of field CA_2 appeared not to have been damaged.* Here, there were only isolated instances of damaged and altered cells.

The author considered it particularly significant that the severe changes in field CA_4 took place very quickly (after only 10 minutes). This pattern of distribution correlated with that reported by Purpura and Gonzales-Monteagudo (1960).

The damaged cells had the character of sclerotically changed elements. The toxic changes affected both the nucleus and the entire perikaryon. The cells had shrunk and showed solidification.

OBSERVATIONS USING THE ELECTRON MICROSCOPE: The picture of the pyramidal cells of the Ammon's horn fields CA_4 and CA_3 was clearly altered by acute intoxication with methoxypyridoxine. There were changes both in the spatial arrangement and also in the structure of the organelles. The most important feature in the cells were general plasmolysis and associated changes of form and position of the organelles, intense thickening of karyoplasm and cytoplasm in contrast to the dilatation of the cisterns of the ergastoplasm, dissolution and swelling of the internal structures of the mitochondria and, lastly, the appearance of multilamellar granula in the damaged pyramidal cells. The astrocytic processes were also swollen.

Detailed comparison of the results of Niklowitz (1966) obtained after treating rabbits with methoxypyridoxine, with those of Mölbert et al. (1967) obtained by electron microscopy in the cat after experimental electroconvulsion, indicates that, in spite of the convulsions which occurred during the investigations, there are also differences in the cellular changes. Mölbert et al. refer to the findings of Niklowitz and interpret them as a primary disorder in the processing of stimuli due to functional failure of the mechanisms inhibited by excitation.

Niklowitz (1966) assumes that as a coenzyme, pyridoxine acts to control certain metabolic reactions. As a constituent of amino acid decarboxylases and amino acid transaminases, it plays an important part in protein metabolism in the body (see also Bessey 1957, Hassler 1964 a, Sinclair 1953, Snell 1953, Stepp et al. 1957, Williams et al. 1950). Another point which is of particular importance in psychomotor epilepsy is that, to a certain extent, pyridoxine also controls the mineral and water balance in the body (Diamant and Guggenheim 1957, Hartsook et al. 1958, Hsu et al. 1958, Niklowitz 1966). Pyridoxine deficiency causes *retention of potassium, sodium and chloride and reduces the capacity to excrete water* (Guggenheim 1954, Niklowitz 1966, Stebbins 1951). Niklowitz (1966) also interprets intoxication with methoxypyridoxine as a primary disorder of the normal *cell wall function,* which results in loss of turgor in the cells which finally results in plasmolysis. The pyridoxine is competitively inhibited by the antimetabolite methoxypyridoxine and thus a Vitamin B_6 deficiency arises in the cell. Inadequate metabolism in the affected cells *leads to displacement of water, sometimes within the damaged cells* (swelling of mitochondria, cistern dilatation) *and sometimes in the surrounding neuropil,* (swelling of the astrocytic processes, enlargement of the extracellular spaces). Niklowitz (1966) and Mölbert et al. (1967) agree that there is activation of the RNA of the affected nerve cells; this is also seen in certain diseases or when great demands are made of the cells (Astman 1955, Caspersson 1950). The observation that, for the most part, there are only free ribosomes in the cells while the number of polysomes is greatly reduced, indicates that there is disruption of protein synthesis (Niklowitz 1966).

Niklowitz agrees with other authors on the question of the specificity of methoxypyridoxine damage with regard to the focal disintegration of the Ammon's horn fields (Fleischhauer 1959, Fleischhauer and Horstmann

1957, Friede and Knolier 1965, Maske 1955, Ortmann 1964). Probably because of their zinc content, the fields CA_3 and CA_4 facilitate chelate formation from the active form of Vitamin B_6 and the metal ions. The suppression of pyridoxine (as an active group) from the enzymes and the enzyme blockade also has its effects on spontaneous cellular activity, and this is manifest as production of convulsive excitation. In fact, the resting membrane potential is reduced (see also Mölbert et al. 1967).

In animal experiments, the convulsive symptoms indicate that the convulsions originate in the Ammon's horn. The animals are restless before the onset of convulsions and they exhibit other hippocampal symptoms (snuffling etc.). In our opinion, the observation of changes in the pyramidal cells of the Ammon's horn before the onset of the visible convulsions, is very important (Mölbert et al. 1967, Niklowitz 1966, Purpura and Gonzales-Monteagudo 1960). On the basis of the volume changes observed, Niklowitz tends to think that disturbances of membrane function may also result in an increase of potassium concentration in the extracellular compartment. The fall of membrane potential which this would cause would then result in increased excitability.

IN CONTRAST TO THE SYMPTOMS FOLLOWING METHOXYPYRIDOXINE INTOXICATION, THE ANTIMETABOLITES OF NICOTINAMIDE, 6-AMINO-NICOTINAMIDE AND 3-ACETYLPYRIDINE ONLY INDUCE THE INTOXICATION PHENOMENA AFTER SEVERAL HOURS. According to Coper (1966, 1967, 1968), and Coper et al. (1966, 1972), numerous effects occur after different latent periods, but only a few of these are observed within the first 12 hours and recede in the same period. There are changes in the form of increased penetration of sodium ions at the nerve cell membranes. Insufficiency of the renal cells results in defective reabsorption of sodium ions. There is also disordered carbohydrate metabolism manifest as hyperglycaemia or hypoglycaemia. The mechanisms of the disorders caused by the antimetabolites of nicotinamide is similar to that occurring with the antimetabolites of pyridoxine. The function of the nicotinamide incorporated in pyridine nucleotides is the reversible addition of hydrogen at position 4 in the pyridine ring. Thus, antimetabolites of nicotinamide are substances which suppress the free vitamin in the cells or replace the vitamin incorporated in the nucleotides. The nicotinamide adenine dinucleotide (phosphate) analogous resulting from this exchange reaction are not usually capable of functioning as natural pyridine nucleotides as cofactors of hydrogen-transfer enzymes. (Christ et al. 1970a,b,c, Coper 1966, 1967, Coper et al. 1966, 1968, 1972, Niklowitz et al. 1964).

THE EFFECT OF 3-ACETYLPYRIDINE is also connected with the fields h_3 and h_4 of the Ammon's horn. After labelling this competitive metabolite with ^{14}c, autoradiographic investigations in the rat revealed that there is clearly localized storing of this substance in fields h_3 and h_4 (Hassler 1964 a). Within the nerve cells of the Ammon's horn, the codehydrases are contained in the endoplasmic reticulum. Coper and Herken (1963) and Coper et al. (1968) assume that the enzyme blockade occurs because the nicotinamide-dinucleotide-neucleosidase (DPN), which is responsible for incorporating nicotinamide into the DPN or nicotinamide-trinucleotide molecule (TPN), is not specific enough. For this reason, it also introduces related substances, such as 6-amino-nicotinic acid amide or 3-acetylpyridine into the coenzymes of the dehydrogenases. However, the same DPN-nucleosidase is not capable of releasing the anologous substances from the coenzyme again, as it normally is with nicotinamide. Hassler (1964) wonders if it is possible for this modified coenzyme to be responsible for the whole of the severe symptomatology of the intoxication, since the proportion of the 3-acetylpyridine compound of the codehydrase I in the whole brain is only 4 to 8 percent of the total codehydrase-I content. On the other hand, a much greater percentage of 3-acetylpyridine is introduced into the TPN of the codehydrase II. In the Ammon's horn of rats treated with 3-actylpyridine, 48.4 percent of the codehydrase II is modified into the compound containing 3-acetylpyridine. In the isocortex and in the remaining areas of the brain, the codehydrase II only contains 24 to 34 percent of the 3-acetylpyridine (Hassler 1964a, Herken and Neuhoff 1963).

If the nicotinic acid amide in glucose-6-phosphate dehydrogenase, which contains TPN, is replaced in vitro by 3-acetylpyridine, the oxidizing activity of this substance is reduced by 5 percent. The enzymes containing TPN which lie outside the mitochondria, are 3.26 or 2.75 times more active in the Ammon's horn than in the isocortex. Thus, after 'poisoning' these enzymes with 3-acetylpyridine, in the Ammon's horn there is considerable falling off in the production of reduction equivalents in the form of glutathion for the hydrogenation of other systems, and the supply fails to meet the demand (Hassler 1964 a, Niklowitz et al. 1964). Thus, the special action of 3-acetylpyridine in fields h_3 and h_4 of the Ammon's horn is due to the competitive blockade of dehydrogenases containing TPN, which carry out a large part of the hydrogen transfer in these structures (Hassler 1964 a).

CENTRENCEPHALIC CEREBRAL STRUCTURES

These structures are of great importance in the inhibition of epileptic excitation arising in the temporal lobe. They are a *powerful blocking system* in the center of the brain, so that the spread of excitation both to the neocortex and to the periphery can be prevented or reduced. However, since this will be discussed in the following chapters, particularly in Chapters IV and VIII, here we shall simply add a little to what has been said previously.

The pneumoencephalographic findings (PEG) have not been discussed recently. Investigations in the centrencephalic formations have shown that there are various anomalies and changes in *idiopathic* epilepsy. Important pneumoencephalographic investigations have been carried out by Gross (1931), Holzmann (1936), Laubenthal (1936), Leppien (1940), Larsby and Lindgren (1940), Dicherson (1941), Kehrer (1950, 1955), Schiermann (1952), Dicker and Nagel (1956), Krischek (1959), Huber (1957 to 1961, 1962 a, b) and others.

Data on the percentage of abnormal PEGs vary greatly, ranging from 6% (Marshal and Whitty 1952) to 80 percent (Hollzmann 1936, Larsby and Lindgren 1940). Pathological results are usually found in 40 to 50 percent of cases (see Huber 1962 b). Information about these findings can be obtained from publications by the authors mentioned. We shall simply mention the investigations by Huber (1962 b) as an example. From 1948 to 1957, he obtained the following results in 117 *essential* epilepsies, mostly young people.

Just under one third (32.5%) of the cases showed a pathological PEG. The most common changes were bilateral, lateralized (ten cases) or completely symmetrical (five cases) hydrocephalus of the lateral ventricle (15 cases or 12.8%) and an isolated enlargement of the third ventricle (13 cases or 11.1%).

There was definite *asymmetry of the lateral ventricle* in only four cases (3.4%), and *isolated external hydrocephalus* in five cases (4.2%). Also, there was a marked hydrocephalic change in the lateral ventricles (moderate hydrocephalus) with a lateral ventricle index below 3.5.

Many more changes in the internal cerebrospinal spaces (33 cases or 28.2%) compared with the external cerebrospinal spaces (eight cases or 6.8%).

In the discussion of his findings, Huber (1962 b) assumes that any psychopathological changes in the form of permanent psychic abnormality (personality change and dementia) must to a certain extent be reflected in the pneumoencephalographic findings. He refers to Gross (1931) who believed that psychic disturbances are reflected in marked external and internal hydrocephali.

In 65 cases (53 cases, personality change, 12 cases, dementia) with an average age of 29.5 years, the rates for pathological findings (43%) are more than double those for psychically *intact* patients (19.4%) with an average age of 26.4 years: in the epileptics with pronounced dementia the percentage (66.6%) was considerably higher than in the overall group of psychically changed patients.

Selbach (1954) is of the same opinion; he found an abnormal picture in 50 percent of cases.

THE REMAINING CEREBRAL STRUCTURES

We have shown in the course of this study that psychomotor epilepsy does not always develop primarily in the temporal lobe. Tellenbach (1965) also emphasizes that frontal and occipital foci develop into psychomotor epilepsy as the final stage of all forms of epilepsy. In the next chapter, we shall discuss the cerebral structures which have not been treated in detail here.

CHAPTER IV

BASIC BIOCHEMICAL AND NEUROPHYSIOLOGICAL PROCESSES IN THE CNS IN EXPERIMENTAL EPILEPSY

ELEMENTARY BIOCHEMICAL PROCESSES AT THE NERVE CELL MEMBRANES

The problem of the Nerve Cell Membrane in the More Limited Sense

TO CONSTRUCT A MODEL of an epileptic attack (see Chapter VIII), it is necessary to touch upon the elementary principles of the biochemical processes at the nerve cell membranes and incorporate these in our model. In our opinion, *epilepsy can only occur where the nerve cell membrane is damaged.* As long as the nerve cell membrane is not affected by a biochemical abnormality, another disorder may well arise, but there will not be any epileptic phenomena.

The most elementary *property* of the protoplasm of the neurons is its capacity, under certain circumstances, to respond adequately to external and internal stimuli: *irritability.* This capacity is transformed into *function* when a stimulus reaches the nerve cell from the surrounding region. The cell responds: *excitability.* However, the cell can also respond *spontaneously* (Brazier 1959, Rotschuh 1958, Schaefer 1953). The responses (excitation) may be classified basically into two groups: 1.) *Gradual, local excitation.* This can be graded and may signify a fall or rise of membrane potential (de- or hyperpolarization). 2.) *Explosive, transmitted excitation.* Once the effect of the stimulus reaches and exceeds a critical level *(the threshold)* this appears as a continuous, self-regenerating event.

When using the term regeneration, we must also mention *the ionic concentration* at the nerve cell membranes. The *resting membrane potential* of a nerve cell is closely related to the ionic composition of the intra- and extracellular fluid: within the cell there is nearly always an abundance of *potassium ions* but few *sodium ions.* The reverse is the case in the extracellular medium. The predominant anions are *sulphate* and *protein ions* within the cell and *chloride ions* outside. This distribution of ions *(polarization)* must remain fairly constant. The asymmetric distribution of charges endows the polarized nerve cell membrane with the property of being able to store electrical energy, and the membrane potential is the equivalent of this (Eccles 1953, Henatsch 1962, Muralt 1958). The lower the *membrane permeability* for the particular type of ion, the lower is the capacity of the ionic battery. The battery within the cell is called the inner battery, and that outside the cell is known as the external battery. Potassium and chloride act to produce a negative electrical charge on the inside of the membrane (Netter 1959, Stämpfli 1952, Toman and Šabelli 1969).

Since the ionic batteries threaten to discharge one another through their ionic resistances at the terminals, they need an active ionic pump for active maintenance of the membrane potential. The sodium pump is a particularly good example of this (Figure 16).

The resultant of the difference between the theoretical total potential of the membrane (about +60 mV internally) and the actual resting membrane potential (about –70mV) is a high *electrochemical gradient* of 130 mV and this has the effect of a constant and powerful in-driving force on the sodium ions which are highly concentrated in the extracellular medium. Mathematically, the passive force of diffusion inwards must be more than 100 times greater than that outwards. However, it was found by experiment that, in fact, the inward and outward flow of sodium is in a ration of about 1:1 (Hodgkin and Keynes 1955).

Thus, the active pump mechanism drives out the surplus ions which penetrate into the cell; this means that a high electrochemical gradient has to be overcome. In this way a *dynamic equilibrium* is produced (Henatsch 1962, Hodgkin and Keynes 1955, Keynes 1954). However, for the nerve cell membrane, it must be assumed that there is at least one other, independent *potassium pump* (Henatsch 1962, Shanes 1951). In addition to this, the mechanisms of many other membranes, of ions and also of nonelectrolytes must also be taken into consideration, although the nature of these has not yet been elucidated in detail (Murphy 1957, Netter 1959). *The fact that normal mechanisms at the nerve cell membranes have not been definitely explained makes it all the more difficult to carry out research into the biochemical mechanisms involved in the development of an epileptic attack.*

Furthermore, the membrane potential is very dependent on the metabolism of the cell. The energy required for driving the ionic pump is derived from cell and membrane metabolism. The chemical reactions which supply the energy are discussed in Chapter V.

For example, the membrane potential may fall to zero if it is subjected to *anoxia* (nitrogen atmosphere). Interference with the metabolism has little effect on the passive influx, but a very marked effect on the active efflux of sodium ions (Dettbarn and Stämpfli 1957, Eccles 1957, 1965, Hodgkin and Keynes 1955, Lorente de Nó 1947).

The *action potential* is of particular significance to this problem. The

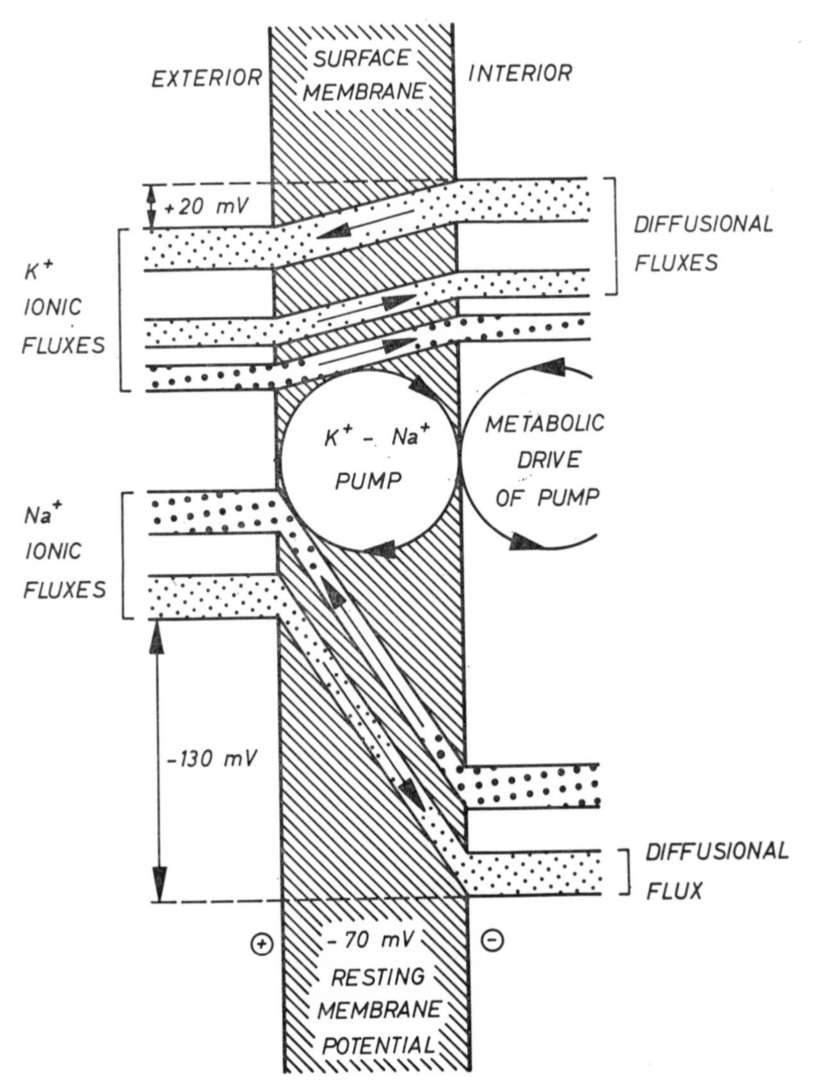

Figure 16. Diagram of K^+ and Na^+ passage across the surface membrane at rest. The slope of the ion channels in the membrane shows the steepness of the electrochemical gradients. At a resting membrane potential of –70 mV, the electrochemical gradients for K^+ and Na^+ ions correspond to potentials which are approximately 20 mV more positive and 130 mV more negative respectively than the equilibrium potentials of these ions. Ion movements by diffusion are distinct from those due to the pump. The outward diffusion of Na^+ ions is less than 1% of the inward diffusion. The width of the channels gives an approximate idea of the magnitude of the flow in each particular case. (From Eccles, J.C.: The Neurophysiology of Nerve Cells, Baltimore, Hopkins, 1957.)

action potential is much greater than simple depolarization. It does not simply require 70 mV, but the value may rise above this by some 30 to 60 mV (overshoot phenomena) (Curtis and Cole 1942, Henatsch 1962, Hodgkin and Huxley 1939, 1945). At this stage, the membrane of the neurone may be 30 to 60 mV more negative both in relation to the surroundings and also in relation to the internal environment in its own cell. Thus, the inner side of this membrane becomes positive. *We do not need to stress the absolute and relative refractory phase.* In general, it is 1 msec. (or less).

A further, very important process affecting epilepsy is the *change of ionic concentration and membrane permeability* at the onset of excitation (Hodgkin 1951, Hodgkin, Huxley and Katz 1949): 1.) In the first place, there is a *sudden increase of permeability to sodium ions* which leads to a large influx of sodium; this process controls the rise of excitation; 2.) A process, which may be termed *inactivation,* affects the *sodium-carrier system.* This arrests the initial influx of sodium, or in some circumstances it may check it from the outset, and 3.) There is a *delayed rise of the permeability to potassium ions,* and this completes the decay of excitation initiated by the process under point 2, by causing prolonged *efflux of potassium.*

The Problem of the Synapses

It has been known for some time that the synapses are a functional unit, but not a morphological unit in the strictly anatomical sense. Among others, the following properties of the synapses are of importance to our problem:

SYNAPTIC MEMBRANE ELEMENTS: (regions of the membrane beneath presynaptic terminal knobs or subsynaptic membrane elements). In the narrower sense, these are selectively active against *chemical influences,* but not, or hardly, effective against *electrical stimuli.* Normally, the responses are always gradual and they can supply the postsynaptic membrane with protracted fluctuations in potential or field changes. The responses can trigger excitatory or inhibiting postsynaptic potentials (hence, de- or hyperpolarization, Eccles 1957, 1964, Grundfest 1959).

IMPULSE-PRODUCING MEMBRANE ELEMENTS: (parts of the neuronal membrane which are distributed between the subsynaptic regions and which have the properties of a conductive membrane). In relation to the intensity, they respond to *electrical* depolarising stimuli autoregeneratively and thus produce an *explosive discharge* which is propagated in the neurities. In this way a transmitted efferent impulse (spike) is formed. This spike should not be confused with a convulsion potential.

It is known that the explosive discharge may be manifest as an *excita-*

tory postsynaptic potential (EPSP) or as an *inhibitory postsynaptic potential (IPSP)*. At this point we must mention the *inhibitability* (the possibility of inhibiting the CNS) as a property, and *inhibition* (retardation) as a function. In addition to this, we shall also mention the transmission of impulses (Figure 17).

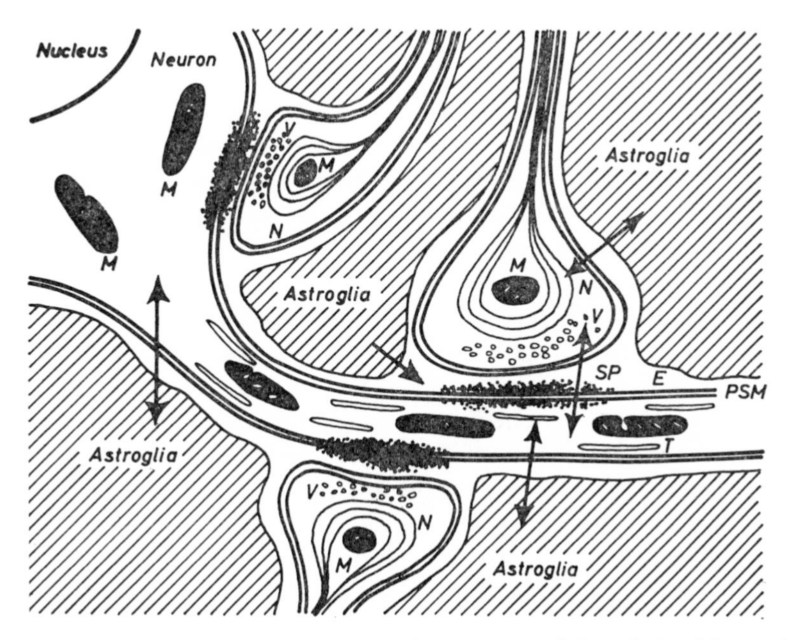

Figure 17. Diagram of the synaptic region of neurons, and its relationship to the neuroglia, which plays an important role in cerebral metabolism. The arrows show the close connections in respect of metabolic energy-producing processes and transmission processes, and substrates. In the center right of the diagram there is the end bulb of an axodendritic synapse (here, see Figure 27). E = extracellular space; M = mitochondria; N = neurofilaments; PSM = postsynaptic membrane; SP = subsynaptic gap of 200 – 300 Å; V = synaptic vesicles which contain the transmitter substance; T = cylindrical gaps in dendrites (tubuli); the neurons with axons and dendrites are surrounded by a double membrane of 25 – 30 Å. (From Prüll, G.: *Therapeutische Berichte, 39*:343-351, 1967.)

The spatial or simultaneous summation of the EPSP is an important factor. The EPSP arise simultaneously from various subsynaptic regions and produce a summed potential in the recording curve. This excitation increases with the intensity of the current used and as long as the threshold is not exceeded it is not conducted. There is simply a gradual depolarization (Coombs et al. 1955, Eccles 1964). Since the IPSP is 10 mV., the threshold is usually 10 mV. Only when this threshold is exceeded is there an explosive discharge which is transmitted.

We have now come to the point of the *inhibitory mechanisms* which must be taken as a basis of any theory about the origin of a seizure.

In principle, there are available to the CNS both *indirect* and *direct* possibilities for inhibition. Both have an important part to play in epilepsy. In psychomotor epilepsy, the second possibility (direct inhibition) is of greater significance.

Indirect synaptic inhibition (Bradley et al. 1953, Eccles 1957, 1964, Jung 1953) means that the discharges and excitatory impulses are *blocked* or completely extinguished by opposing stimuli (reflex and voluntary innervation) en route from the point of origin to the periphery. Thus, in our experience, epileptics are sometimes able to prevent an attack by competitive innervation. Focal attacks are much easier to block in this way. This inhibition can also be regarded as *secondary.*

Direct synaptic inhibition. Primarily, there are several possibilities here. The first is the inhibitory postsynaptic potential (IPSP) which is also capable of summation and may inhibit the explosive discharge to a certain extent, by opposing it (hyperpolarization of the nerve cell membrane). The IPSP has a greater latency than the EPSP and it takes rather longer to rise; its maximum amplitude never exceeds 10 mV., i.e. the membrane potential is hyperpolarized from 70 mV. to a maximum 80 mV. Thus, it never causes an explosive response; hence, it is not a mirror-image of the EPSP. Accordingly, with the IPSP the inhibitory possibilities are limited (Henatsch 1962). The second inhibitory possibility in the CNS is at the intercalated inhibitory interneurones (Eccles 1964, 1965, Jovanovic 1968 a). These act as function-reversing *pole-changers.*

Apart from these two possibilities, there are many other inhibitory processes; some of these will be mentioned again later.

The Problem of Chemical Transmitters

The transmitter substances have a major role to play, and once this has been worked out we shall be a good deal nearer to solving the problem of epilepsy.

In the first place, the ionic processes are thought to be responsible for conducting the impulses. As has already been mentioned, the permeability of the nerve cell membrane changes with an EPSP. Permeability changes have also been recorded with an IPSP. On activation of the inhibitory elementary synapses, the membrane becomes permeable, particularly to potassium ions, but also to chloride ions; other larger ions are very much held in check. A pore-size theory has recently been put forward: this postulates that not all ions are capable of passing through the membrane. When presynaptic impulses occur, the postsynaptic membrane becomes a *sieve-like structure* with different pore sizes in each case, and this permits any ions not exceeding these sizes to pass through, whatever their charge. At the *excitatory synapses,* the pores become wide enough to allow all the ions present in the internal and external medium to traverse. However, they remain narrower at the inhibitory synapses, so that ions smaller than sodium ions can pass through (mainly K^+ and Cl^-) (Eccles 1957, 1964).

There have also been biochemical and bioelectrical hypotheses in respect of synaptic transmission (Dale 1953, Eccles 1953, 1957, 1964, Fatt and Katz 1951, Feldberg 1950, Fessard and Posternak 1950, Muralt 1958, Nachmansohn 1955). The excitatory and inhibitory neurones each release a transmitter substance (excitatory or inhibitory transmitter substance) at their presynaptic terminal knobs. This diffuses across the subsynaptic gap in just under 0.5 msec. (see Figure 17) and has a chemical effect on the subsynaptic membrane elements causing the changes in permeability which are characteristic of the EPSP or IPSP. The numerous mitochondria and vesicular structures which are to be found in the terminal synaptic nodes, are direct evidence of their glandular activity (Eccles 1957, 1964). The chemical constitution of the transmitter substances is a subject of much controversy. *Acetylcholine has been suggested for the cholinergic nervous system and noradrenaline for the adrenergic nervous system.* These transmitters, which were previously thought to be effective only in the autonomic nervous system, appear to play a major role in the rest of the CNS as well; this will be further discussed in the next chapter. The cholinergic and adrenergic system (together with the serotonergic system) appear to be of

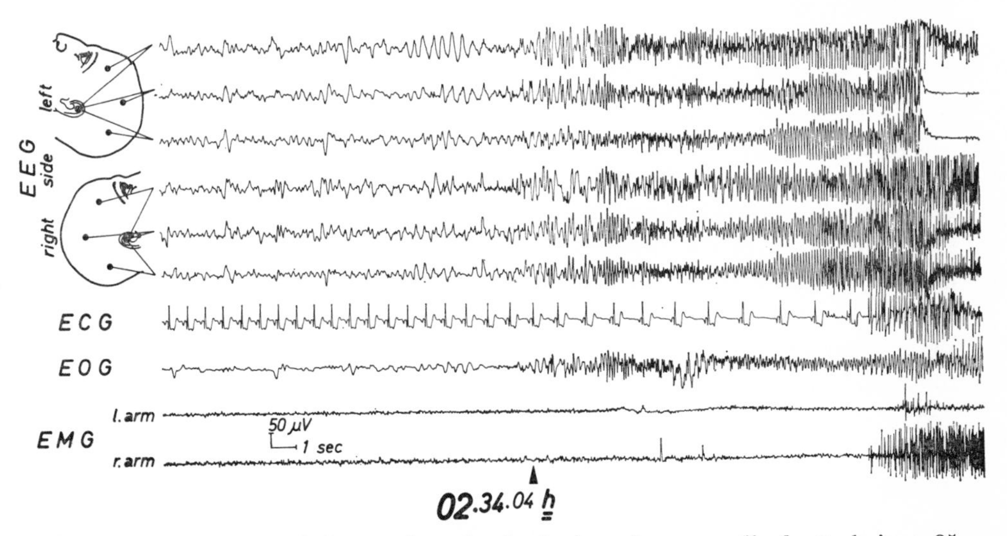

Figure 18. Immediately before and at the beginning of a generalized attack in a 25-year-old female patient with major and psychomotor attacks, bradycardia tends to develop and become dominant; this indicates that the autonomic nervous system is initially in a state of vagotonia (our own finding, original).

importance in the epileptic seizure. The predominant picture just before the seizure and at the appearance of convulsion-specific elements in the EEG is one of pronounced bradycardia (Figure 18), and this continues far on into the seizure. Since the origin of the seizure is central at the site of the damaged nerve cell membrane in the temporal lobe, it is very likely that there is a connection between the cholinergic transmitter, the focus and also the autonomic nervous system (see Chapter V).

The Specific and Non-Specific Synaptic System

After stimulation of a neuron, *primary* and *secondary* responses appear in the CNS and these can be recorded electrographically. The primary responses have a short latency (below 15 msec.) and the secondary responses have a much longer latency (30 to 80 msec.). It is assumed that the primary responses must cross a single synapse or only a small number of synapses—*monosynaptic or oligosynaptic transmission.* In contrast, there is a delay in the secondary responses because the impulses must cross a large number of synapses—*polysynaptic transmissions.* In the last 30 years, intensive research has been carried out into these two systems. It has been found that the monosynaptic or oligosynaptic mode of transmission is part of the *specific system.* The polysynaptic method of conduction and transmission is typical of the *non-specific nervous system.* At this point we should mention some other important reactions of the hippocampus, since these have not yet been referred to.

A great deal of research work has been carried out in this field in respect of the non-specific effect of stimuli. Gerard et al. (1936) found a bioelectric response in the Ammon's horn following indirect *optical stimuli.* There is known to be an epileptic response with its focus in the hippocampus as a result of the effects of optical stimuli (Kreis 1968, and other authors). Jung and Kornmüller (1938) detected the same responses following *pain stimuli* and occasionally after *acoustic stimuli* as well. There was synchronization of the bioelectrical activity over the Ammon's horn with characteristic large and regular 4 to 7/sec. waves. In later investigations by Mac Lean et al. (1952 to 1962) and Green and Arduini (1954), it was shown that these waves can also be induced in the piriform cortex and in the septal nuclei by all types of indirect and direct stimuli (see also Health and Guerrero-Figueroa 1965). Grastyán (1959) and Grastyán et al. (1956 to 1965) have also done a good deal of work on these 4 to 6/sec. waves over the hippocampus and compared them with conditioned reflexes.

A significant factor is that several or all types of stimulus induce the same response. A further connection between the hippocampus and the structures of the reticular formation was demonstrated by the discovery that, after stimuli of varying strengths at the reticular formation, over the neocortex there is a *flattening* of the curve tracing resembling Moruzzi and Magoun's *arousal reaction* (1959), and the animals become more alert (Akimoto and Creutzfeldt 1958, Albefessard 1957, Jung 1957, 1963, 1965, Monnier, 1968, Rossi and Zanchetti 1957). However, at the same time there is what appears to be a counter-reaction over the hippocampus with the large, synchronous and slow theta waves of 4 to 7/sec., which have already been mentioned (Passouant et al. 1955, Rimbaud et al. 1952, Feindel and Gloor 1954).

On the other hand, using implanted permanent electrodes it can be demonstrated in cats which are falling asleep that the tracing in the Ammon's horn becomes flatter at about the same time as the onset of sleep activity in the isocortex. On waking there are typical flat and rapid beta waves over the neocortex and slower beta waves or the theta waves referred to, over the Ammon's horn. Thus, there is a non-specific connection between the hippocampus and the neocortex, via the reticular formation.

Chemical stimulation has an effect on the neocortex and hippocampus just like that produced by indirect or direct stimulation of the reticular formation by means of an electric current. Activation of the *adrenergic* mechanism (DOPA) or the colinergic mechanism (physostigmine), causes definitie desynchronization and acceleration of the waves in the motor and sensory neocortex, while at the same time there is synchronization in the hippocampus and thalamus in the form of a theta rhythm. However, *serotonin* causes desynchronization of the isocortex, but no synchronization of the hippocampus (Monnier 1960, 1968); this is an event which must have a part to play in epilepsy (see also Chapter VIII).

EXPERIMENTAL EPILEPSY

A Brief History of the Development of the Experimental Investigations

Experimental epilepsy has a long history. As early as the third decade of the last century, research workers were trying to obtain experimental evidence about the clinical symptomatology of epilepsy. In the last 130 years, experimental work has played a major part in elucidating the biochemical processes during this strange disease, and an enormous amount of data has been collected during this period. (Bureš et al. 1952, 1953; Cereghino and Dow 1970; Chusid and Kopeloff 1969; Danilo 1883, 1889; Dolin 1938, 1952; Dow et al. 1972; Duiju van and Visser 1972; Gutnikoff 1891; Hartchenko 1942, 1948; Hutton et al. 1952; Isaacson et al. 1971; Kisselev 1964; Koenig 1972; Mutani et al. 1972; Pintilie et al. 1970; Servît 1970; Spehlmann et al. 1971; Walsh 1971).

When studying the biochemistry of convulsions, the experimenters were faced with *two* problems: *firstly,* how can we produce experimentally convulsions which resemble those which occur spontaneously in man (Busche 1957, Chang 1953, Crighel and Stoica 1961, Curtis 1940, Danillo 1883, Erickson 1940, Janzen et al. 1951, 1954, Jung and Tönnies 1950, Kreindler 1965, Ralston 1958, Ruf 1950, Schmalbach 1968 a, b, Schmalbach and Steinmann 1955, Servit and Bureš 1952 a, b, Smith and Purpura 1960, Speransky 1943, etc.), and *secondly,* what effect does such an attack have on biochemical processes in the body (Danillo 1883, 1889, Gutnikov 1891, Kisselev 1892, Lapinski 1899, 1913, Schmalbach 1968 a, Servit and Bureš 1952 a, b, Slutchevski et al. 1940, Tower 1958 a to c, 1960, Vrba 1955, 1956 a, b, 1957, Vrba et al. 1962).

Most experiments are carried out using surgery or by producing toxic chemical lesions (Bureš et al. 1952, 1953, Dolin 1938, 1952, Graschtchenkov 1935, 1936, Janzen et al. 1951, 1954, Jung and Tönnies 1950, Kreindler 1960, 1965, Mölbert et al. 1967, Naumova 1940, Niklowitz 1966, Tower 1958 a to c, Tower and Elliott 1952 a, b, 1953, Waelsch 1961, 1962, Zislina et al. 1963, Zurabashvili 1952).

Certain chemical changes in the CNS promote excitatory and others promote inhibitory processes, or there is an equilibrium between excitatory and inhibitory processes; this has been demonstrated by many authors (Eccles 1957, 1964, Jung and Tönnies 1950, Kreindler 1960, 1965, Palladin 1958, Pavlow 1919).

Elements of Experimental Methods

There are now many new neurophysiological and biochemical techniques available for studying the nervous system, and these make it possible to recognize and examine a number of biochemical features associated with basic processes in the CNS, even where there are abrupt changes such as during an epileptic attack.

Locally, in the brain, epileptic foci can be produced by various *chemical substances* or by *electric current.* The processes at the site of excitation and the development, maintenance, spread and inhibition of the convulsion elements are studied simultaneously, and immediately afterwards. The most familiar are the local foci due to direct application of *strychnine* (strychnine foci, strychninography, strychnine-neuronography) after Dusser de Barenne (Creutzfeldt 1956, Curtis 1940, Erickson 1940, Janzen and Müller 1952, Janzen, Magun and Becker 1954, Janzen, Müller and Becker, 1951, Kornmüller 1937, and others); *penicillin* (Busche 1957, Chang 1953, Crighel and Stoica 1961, Hippius et al. 1957, Ralston 1958, Schneidermann et al. 1972, and many others); *acetylcholine solution* (Brenner and Merritt 1942, Chatfield and Demsey 1942, Echlin and McDoland 1954, Forster 1945, Kristian and Courtois 1949 and many others); *mescaline* (Crighel and Stoica 1961, Kreindler 1965, and many others); *alumina cream* (Kopeloff et al. 1942, Schmalbach 1968 a, b, Schmalbach and Steinmann 1955; *cobalt* (Cereghino and Dow 1970; Dewar et al. 1972; Malzone et al. 1972). Aluminium cream is particularly suitable for producing chronic convulsion foci. Furthermore, the focus can be induced with *acetylchloride* (Morell and Florenz 1958, Torres 1960, and others) and by *local freezing* (Spermansky 1943, Stalmaster and Hanna 1972, and others).

Generalized predisposition to convulsions and generalized convulsions are most often induced in both man and animals by *Metrazol, picrotoxin* and other chemical substances, or by electric shock. However, there are still many other substances which have varying degrees of activity in provoking convulsions but which cannot be used as provocative agents (see Chapter VI). *Electroconvulsions* have been discussed in Chapters II and III.

Strychninography is particularly suitable for observing the spread of triggered discharges. Using this technique it was established that the convulsion elements (CE) do not only use the synaptic, ie. axo-neuronal route for propagation (Creutzfeldt 1956, Janzen et al. 1951, Kornmüller 1937, Kreindler 1965, Sperling and Creutzfeldt 1959).

There is yet another experimental method available. This is the *evoked potential method* in which a site in the CNS or peripheral nervous system is stimulated and then the response is observed over the particular centers (evoked potentials). Thus, for example, a stimulus is given to the reticular formation of the brain stem and the cerebral activity is recorded over the neocortex and hippocampus. However, this method is not often used in experimental epilepsy.

Combination of the chemical and electrical methods (Glezer and Jacobson 1967), makes it possible to investigate the substance used for their convulsion-provoked or convulsion-inhibiting properties, and to study predisposition to convulsion in different regions of the brain (see also Chapter V).

Development of Convulsion Elements in the CNS

The pathological or exeprimentally-induced convulsion focus (Kreindler 1965) produces *intrastimulatory and poststimulatory discharges (afterdischarges).* That is, a reactive discharge is followed continuously by further synchronous and hypersynchronous discharges which only cease when they are inhibited by the inhibitory mechanisms of the brain or when the affected neurons are fatigued. According to Kreindler (1965) the *epileptic* neurons have two, highly functional characteristics: *abnormally large potentials in the soma and dendrites and a high frequency of potentials which are propagated in the axons.* There is a close connection between the dentritic depolarization and epileptic discharges. Most of the areas in the brain fire prolonged constantly repeated spikes of high frequency. The independent activity which characterizes the *epileptic* neurons is related to their relatively prolonged dendritic depolarization and to the resulting difference of potential between soma and dendrites. The question that is always raised is how does an *epileptic* neuron obtain the energy for its very persistent and independent activity.

Using intracellular electrodes, Kreidler (1965) found progressive reduction of the hyperpolarizing waves and also progressive prolongation, i.e. *temporal summation,* of the depolarizing discharges.

At first, in an epileptic focus there is only spatial synchronization; hence, initially the convulsion potentials are small and of high frequency; however, these then become increasingly larger and slower. When the attack has developed to a pronounced degree there are high and slower courses which, in the end, become even slower until they disappear completely (silent period). A further factor repsonsible for maintaining the convulsion potentials is the constant alternation of the firing cells so that, now and again, one cell will recover and another fire.

Alternation of active neurons is not limited to one cerebral area; it also occurs in many other neighboring areas. Also, a whole series of cerebral structures may be triggered so that one is active while another is resting.

The *neuroglia* (see also Figure 17) must also be mentioned as an epileptogenic factor, not only passively (as was mentioned in Chapter III) by stimulating the neurones, but also actively as a *controlling element* (Kornmüller 1950). According to Kreindler (1965), the neuroglia play an important part in synchronizing the convulsion potentials.

Jung and Tönnies (1950) explained the maintenance of convulsion elements in a rather different way from Kreindler (see also Figure 20). According to these authors, on stimulation of the isocortex there was a *primary discharge* at the site of stimulation, directly after the stimulus. Subsequently there was a *discharge after-effect* with more or less pronounced electrical silence and periods of normal rhythms.

In general, the *primary discharge in the isocortex* comprised *short spike potentials* and *longer waves.*

With a slow sequence of stimuli there is no convulsion. The brain can compensate continuously for the actions aimed at provoking a convulsion. Where the sequence of stimuli is rapid a *self-sustaining convulsion* soon develops. After 50 to 100 stimuli, there is a striking *modification of the primary discharge.* There is a reduction in amplitude of the slow wave together with a lengthening or *double spiking.*

The discharge *after effect* consists of a period of waves which are equivalent to the spontaneous rhythms of the affected cerebral regions in amplitude and frequency.

The processes beyond the site of stimulation are also worth mentioning.

Synchronous events in the form of *remote discharges* in the other regions of the brain occur following electrical stimuli, and these are much more widespread than the regular activity. As will be discussed later, these do not only spread via the major familiar internuncial routes and pathways. The excitation resulting from the electrical stimulus runs from one field to another within the isocortex, and also from the isocortex to the allocortex and vice versa. The remote discharges resemble the primary discharge and may also be followed by an *after-effect* of normal rhythms. The *remote discharge* always lasts longer than the local primary discharge (a spike-wave complex can nearly always be detected with the former). *The allocortex of the Ammon's horn* is excited particularly readily by the various structures (and by the central ganglia). It then exhibits a typical form of remote discharge, with a large wave preceded by a peak.

Thalamic stimulation is manifest as local convulsions which do not involve the contralateral side, even though the discharges may be greater than the primary discharge at the site of stimulation.

The effects of electrical stimulation spread from the cerebral cortex into the subcortical regions and, conversely, following stimulation of the central ganglia, into the cerebral cortex.

Following stimulation of the caudatum, waves of alpha and beta frequencies in the isocortex are the first sign of *remote discharge.* Other forms of discharge are manifest in the allocortex.

Following stimulation of the intralaminar thalamus, particularly with weak stimuli, the first remote discharge is in the Ammon's horn and caudatum. With stronger stimuli the spike-wave form appears over the isocortex. The authors have established that petit mal episodes are *not only specific to the massa intermedia* (Jasper and Droogleever-Fortuyn 1947, Niedermeyer 1954), but they can also be trigger following stimulation of the lateral thalamus, the subthalamus and the corpus striatum. Similar episodes are also found with generalized electroconvulsions which are modified by administration of O_2 (Ruf 1950).

Remote discharges can be triggered particularly well in the *gyrus cinguli.* By intensifying the stimuli, the remote discharges can easily be propagated into all regions of both cerebral hemispheres. Different areas show characteristic patterns independent of structure and architectonics.

A generalized attack may occur suddenly after a high frequency stimulus and after maintaining the stimuli for several seconds. In many cases, this is preceded by local paroxysm of the Ammon's horn provoked by the isocortex, while motor discharges are still not detectable. When the paroxysm has spread to the motor cortex and other subcortical structures it is possible to see a tonic-clonic attack in the motor system. *According to these findings, the attack may remain localized in the Ammon's horn and there may be no outward manifestations; this fact must be of great importance in psychomotor epilepsy* (see Chapter VIII).

In the postconvulsive stage, initially there is no bioelectric activity at all. Then there are slow rhythms of 0.5 to 3/sec., which revert to normal rhythms with a gradual acceleration.

Spread of Epileptic Excitation

The possibilities for the propagation of convulsion discharges have been discussed in Chapter III. It appears that the convulsion potentials do not always follow this anatomical rule. At times they will appear in regions which, anatomically, they should not be able to reach from the site of the stimulus; at other times they do not use the pathways which are available. It has therefore been suggested that the convulsion discharges utilize at least *two* routes to spread and to generalize: *axo-neuronal and non-synaptic (i.e. ephaptic) pathways.*

Propagation of convulsion elements from the lateral areas of the temporal lobe is fairly limited (Creutzfeldt 1953, 1956, 1958, Creutzfeldt and Meyer-Mickeleit 1953). They only spread from the focus through the *specific* corticocortical fibres with difficulty; this occurs mainly in the isocortex. (Ajomone-Marsan et al. 1950, 1951, Segundo et al. 1955).

The discharges from the temporal pole project mainly into the piriform lobe, the periamygdalar cortex, sometimes into the medial thalamus and caudatum, and only rarely into the bordering parieto-occipital cerebral cortices.

It is possible to see a diffuse projection *from the periamygdalar cortex* and the *amygdaloid nuclei* into the thalamus, septal nuclei, the hypothalamus and subthalamus and into the mesencephalon (Creutzfeldt 1956, Feath et al. 1954, Gastaut et al. 1952, Gloor 1957, Kreindler 1965). Cortical propagation is more limited and is confined mainly to the temporal lobes (above all the hippocampus, temporo-basal cortex, temporal pole, anterior insula region and precallous cortex).

The hippocampus (Figure 19) with its relatively low convulsion threshold shows no particular tendency to propagation (Andy and Akert 1953, 1955, Creutzfeldt 1956, Health and Guerrero-Figueroa 1965, Jung 1949, Jung and Tönnies 1950, Liberson and Akert 1955, Liberson and Cadilhac 1953). Powerful projections from convulsion discharges were only observed in the region of the amygdaloid nuclei, piriform lobe, temporal pole, caudal cingular sections and, in one third of the experiments, in the occipital lobes as well (Creutzfeldt 1953, 1956, Green and Adey 1956, Green and Shimamoto 1953, Marin and Green 1953 a,b). Subcortically, there is diffuse propagation of Ammon's horn discharges into the hypothalamus (particularly into the corpora mamillaria), into the medial anterior thalamus, septal nuclei, mesencephalon and occasionally even into the cerebellum. Potentials are less often conducted in the caudatum and pallidum. In the region of the isocortex, the precentral region is *hardly ever fired,* while on rare occasions there may be a limited amount of propagation in the parietal, fronto-basal and, in particular, in the occipital regions. According to Creutzfeldt (1956), subcortical propagation of the Ammon's horn seizures takes place mainly via the fornix, although propagated convulsion potentials are still found in the diencephalon after the fornix has been severed. For this reason, Sperling and Creutzfeldt (1959) have proposed propagative pathways via the amygdaloid nuclei-stria terminalis system, and ammono-fugal pathways can be found for this in the temporo-basal cerebral cortex and amygdala. However, these authors point out that there is still no anatomical evidence for this.

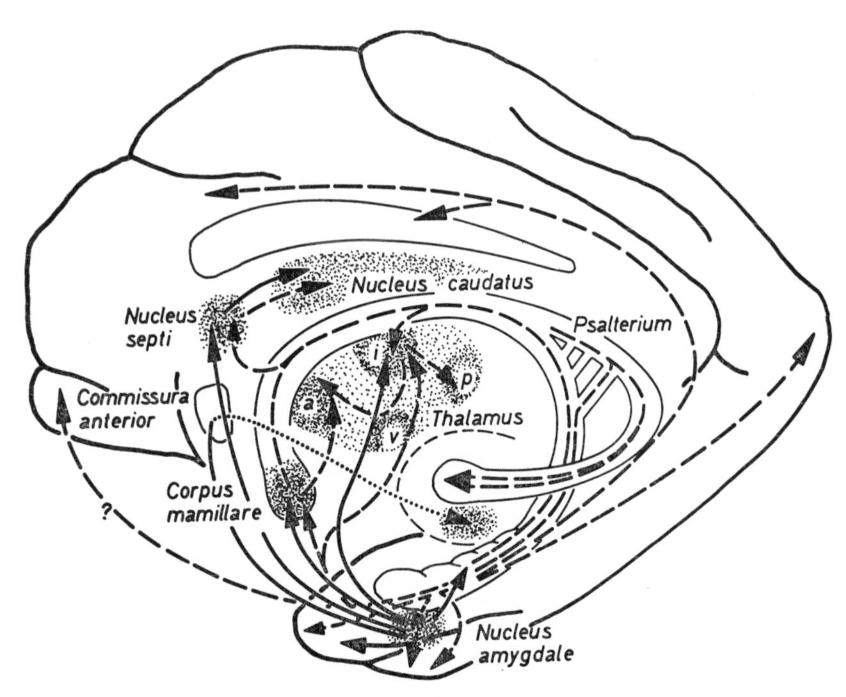

Figure 19. Diagram of the projections of Ammon's horn convulsions and temporobasal convulsions with possible projection pathways. The contralateral temporal lobe and cortical Ammon's horn are shaded. ——— = projection pathways of temporobasal convulsions (including amygdaloid nuclear area); -------- = projection pathways of Ammon's horn convulsions. (From Creutzfeldt, O.: *Schweiz Arch Neurol Psychiatr, 77:*163-194, 1956.)

Following stimulation of the hippocampal structures, Janzen, Müller and Becker (1954) found discharges in the medulla under the precentral cerebral region, as well as in the ventromedial (more) and centrolateral thalamus (less). Excitation is particularly high in the hippocampus; the discharges show a sharp form and occur continuously for a period of several seconds. Kreindler (1965) was able to confirm both these findings.

In propagating its discharges the Ammon's horn may utilize *ephaptic pathways* more than any other convulsive structure. Non-synaptic propagation is utlized in particular for radiation into the diencephalic structures. It has been suggested that convulsion discharges spread due to an increase in the volume of the nerve elements (Creutzfeldt 1956, Petsche and Monnier 1954, Petsche et al. 1956). However, Creutzfeldt's observations (1956) suggest synaptic propagation: he found that an Ammon's horn convulsion does not project into the regions named with equal intensity in all convulsion phases, but that the projection is very limited, particularly at the beginning and end. With regard to the pathogenesis of psychomotor epilepsy, it should also be mentioned that in animal experiments the Ammon's horn seizures could also be provoked by stimulation of the intralaminar thalamic nuclei, the precentral region (rarely), area striata and other subcortical cerebral structures. This means that the convulsion discharges much more readily project from other regions of the brain into the hippocampus, rather than the other way round (Feath et al. 1954, Gastaut and Roger 1955, Janzen and Müller 1953, Janzen et al. 1951, Kreindler 1965).

In man, Health and Guerrero-Figueroa (1965) found that the convulsion elements remained confined to the hippocampus for quite some time. Once they reach the septum, they are quickly propagated. According to Kreindler (1965), the focus in the amygdalo-hippocampal complex most frequently projects into the ipsilateral septum, the hypothalamus and the mesencephalic tegmentum. Stimulation of the parvocellular basal amygdaloid nuclei induces a rhythmic intrastimulatory discharge in the hippocampus like that in the lateral central amygdaloid nucleus. Stimulation of this central nucleus induces intrastimulatory discharges in the parvocellular basal amygdaloid nucleus. There is a two-track connection between these two nuclei and between the parvocellular basal amygdaloid nucleus and the hippocampus. The neocortical amygdaloid spread of the epileptic after-discharges is directed particularly to areas which are homologous with the insular and temporal lobe. Amygdaloid discharges spread to the fornix and supraoptical anterior pituitary region, to habenular stria, and nucleus medialis dorsalis thalami as has already been mentioned briefly.

According to Kreindler, with a full developed epileptic attack, the convulsive activity may extend to the cerebellum and also to the mesencephalic reticular formation. This author states that generalization of the convulsive discharges occurs mainly by intracortical and intercortical propagation, although the subcortical structures also have a significant part to play (regarding this, see Dell et al. 1953, Jasper et al. 1951, Niedermeyer 1954, Papez 1937, and many others).

The propagation of convulsive discharges from the precentral region of the brain occurs mostly in the contralateral hemisphere of the brain. However, this spread does not assume the character of an attack since it only involves isolated convulsion elements. If there are several ocn-vulsion foci (Janzen et al. 1951), then each focus is active in its own right, has its own rhythm and maintains this for as long as there are only isolated convulsion discharges. If generalization occurs, then the focus from a region other than the precentral region predominates. Contrary to expectations, according to Janzen and Müller (1952) the precentral cerebral region is not responsible for generalization of the attack. The convulsion elements first spread to other regions of the brain and from there, there is the *secondary excitation* of the precentral region. Only after this secondary excitation can there be generalization and the development of an epileptic attack in the clinical sense.

On the other hand, the *optical cortex* shows different properties from the motor region. According to Janzen and Müller (1952) and Janzen et al. (1951, 1954), the excitation following stimulation of the area striata does not show any tendency to spread to the contralateral cerebral hemisphere. However, if there is symmetrical propagaion of excitation from a region of the optical cortex to the contralateral side, then the rate of spread is considerably slower compared with the homolateral cerebral hemisphere. While the motor region requires a period of 1/100 second from one hemisphere to the other, the time from a point in the optical cortex for the same distance is several seconds. Janzen et al. assume that convulsion discharges spread in the motor cortex using an axonal pathway, while the optical cortex must use another route, which very much delays the spreading. With the optical cortex, this may involve a non-specific, i.e. polysynaptic pathway which shows a much longer latency. The focus in the area striata influences the motor region of the brain and may easily take over conduction. The motor region may then (under the influence of the optical region) trigger a peripheral convulsion while the optical region becomes fatigued. Even before the generalized convulsion has come to an end, the optical region may produce a further volley of stimuli which again affect the motor region. This fact is of great importance in *maintaining the convulsion.* In this case the convulsion is maintained by the principle of constant *reproducibility,* i.e. even during the clinical attack, part of the brain may resume its activity independently. The regions between the optical and motor cortex are not necessarily stimulated even though both these regions of the cortex are involved in convulsive activity. In the area striata, even a singular focus may lead to a generalized attack, even though it has a relatively high, perhaps the highest convulsion threshold. However, Janzen et al. report that if a focus in the precentral cerebral regions leads to a generalized attack, then the convulsion elements arising from the area striata remain unilateral, and do not become generalized. *Thus, the focus in the motor region inhibits a tendency of the other epileptic focus to generalize.* This fact is important with regard to inhibiting the attack; this will be discussed again later.

All parts of the cortex are inclined to the motor region, which transmits the function to the motor system (Janzen et al. 1951). However, it does not have a retrograde effect and it only influences the deeper parts. According to the findings of the authors mentioned, *the brain does not react as a whole.* If this principle is applied to psychomotor epilepsy, it provides a logical explanation for the simultaneous existence of *normal and parasitic consciousness* (see Chapter I).

All the cortical regions tend to propagate caudally from the focus (Janzen and Müller 1952). In this report these authors have corrected Janzen et al. (1951) somewhat. Since the experiments were carried out on rabbits, it is also possible that propagation from the area striata to the contralateral cerebral hemisphere does not readily occur because rabbits show total decussation of the optic nerves. In monkeys, for example, the discharges of the area striata are said to be much more closely related to the contralateral discharges.

The radiation of the cortical cerebral regions into subcortical areas is understandable according to the above rule about caudal spreading tending to convulsion elements.

Following stimulation of the area precentralis, there are also sharp events in the capsula interna and in the corpus callosum (Janzen and Müller 1952). In the subcortical regions of the brain, the arrival of convulsion elements does not trigger frequent spontaneous activity like that in the contralateral cortex.

Remarkably enough, the subcortical ganglia, like the nucleus ruber, substantia nigra and other extrapyramidal nuclei, show no, or only slight sympathetic excitation following stimulation in the area precentralis. In the reticular formation of Moruzzi and Magoun (1949), Janzen and Müller (1952) were only able to detect coexcitation with the motor cortex, under strictly defined conditions. The authors assume that *the reticular formation is not involved in the increased predisposition to convulsion, even where the subcortical cerebral structures are stimulated.* This question is discussed again in Chapter VIII. The precentral focus, with its different regions, very often (but not always) extends into the hippocampus-fornix system. Spreading from the precentral cortex has rarely been found in the region of the actual thalamic nuclei. When the excitation occurs in the thalamus, then in the nucleus lateralis and in the nucleus ventralis thalami. The same is also true of the intralaminar nuclei of Demsey and Morison (1942). *However, the whole situation is changed after a series of convulsions. The functional condition of the brain is now subject to the new conditions already referred to. The phenomenon of facilitation occurs, by which the excitation extends to various areas more quickly and spreads caudally until the attack is generalized.*

The subcortical regions of the brain, when stimulated, excite various neighboring structures (Janzen et al. 1954). Stimulation of the nucleus caudatus involved the internal capsule in the excitation. On stimulation of the nucleus ventralis thalami the excitation does not survive, even at the site of stimulation. However, modifications of the normal cerebral action are recorded in the subcortical region of the precentral cortex, in the hippocampus and in the area retrosplenialis. The authors stressed that it is not always possible to determine the site of the focus from the bioelectrical action of the brain. Thus, for example, in the above case it would not be assumed that there was a focus in the ventral medial thalamic nucleus because no convulsion potentials appear there, but it might be thought to be in the hippocampus. However, since the site of stimulation was known, this excluded any error. With stimuli at the boundary of the nucleus ventralis thalami and the zona incerata, a discharge survives at the site of stimulation. At first the stimulation causes *depression* of cerebral activity at the site of stimulation. From this, there develops a discharge in areas remote from the site of stimulation and, eventually, this may lead to generalization and take the form of cerebral-electrical equivalents of epileptic responses. Only at this stage, a relatively long time after the stimulus, do clinical symptoms appear.

With reference to the spreading, we should like to mention one or two more of Kreindler's findings (1965).

Chronic foci placed in *sensorimotor* regions produce functional modification of the cerebral action in the subcortical structures. This second, well-known *mirror focus* has been mentioned in more recent works on experimental epilepsy (see also Schmalbach 1968 b). Spontaneous discharges have been detected in the nucleus caudatus, globus pallidus, putamen and nucleus centralis posterior lateralis. Kreindler (1965) assumes that this spreading does not always take place along anatomical pathways, but that other possible routes of propagation are also utilized (ephaptic).

The findings in experimental epilepsy may differ somewhat. However, basically there is not a great deal of variation, since any changes usually depend on the method used. For example, a penicillin focus has different properties from a strychnine focus (Kreindler 1965). We would refer to this author's study report since it is very thorough and of great value in experimental epilepsy.

Development of an Experimental Attack

Gradual excitation and *explosive discharges* are normal and represent the basic biological function of the brain.

The first stage of a convulsion is the isolated convulsive discharges which remain fairly localized. According to Janzen and Müller (1952) and Janzen et al. (1951, 1954), particularly in the anterior neocortical regions of the brain, there are isolated biphasic discharges which persist for hours. The precentral region exhibits foci which, interestingly enough, do not show any great tendency to spread over the same hemisphere. On local stimulation of the *motor cortex,* there is a corresponding fluctuation of potential at the corresponding symmetrical point in the opposite hemisphere. This either occurs with the first convulsive discharge or very soon after. These symmetrical convulsive discharges have a lower amplitude than at the site of stimulation. After strychnine excitation, the *area striata* shows isolated convulsive discharges which tend to pass, in a few seconds, into the next stage of the convulsion. On the other hand, the strychnine focus does not show any symmetrical isolated discharges in the contralateral hemisphere of the brain.

The residual modification of the cerebral electrical activity, the *after-discharges,* is very important in the epileptic reaction (Janzen et al. 1951, 1954, Kreindler 1965). The after-discharge may be a reaction to excitation of another area, the activity of which is altered by the stimulus via a neuronal connection. The *subcortical areas* and the *allocortical structures* tend to pass into the next stage of excitation.

The second stage of the seizure as measured by the cerebral activity is the convulsion paroxysm (Janzen and Müller 1952, Janzen et al. 1951, 1954, Jung and Tönnies 1950, Kreindler 1965). As has already been mentioned for quite some time the *precentral region* only produces isolated convulsion discharges. However, the *area striata* tends to invoke a local convulsion paroxysm at once. *The subcortical regions of the brain* rapidly pass into a convulsion paroxysm following strychnine or electrical excitation.

The next stage of the convulsion is generalization of the convulsion-specific elements throughout the entire cortex of the brain. There are still no clinical manifestations of an attack (Janzen and Müller 1952, Jung and Tönnies 1950).

The generalization may produce isolated clinically manifest symptoms if the stimuli are repeated. With stimulation in the precentral area there are motor convulsions and with stimulation in the hippocampus there are psychomotor symptoms (Health and Guerro-Figueroa 1965, Janzen et al. 1951, 1954, Kreindler 1965).

Not until there is generalization of the discharges over the entire body, is there a clinical attack with tonic-clonic disturbances of the body mascula- ture and other manifest symptoms. Even then, such a seizure provoked ex- perimentally in animals by the method described is not entirely compar- able to clinical epilepsy in man.

Where there is a chronic focus (as for example with aluminium cream) the clinical attacks may be repeated at irregular intervals without any more acute stimulation. In this case, experimentally-induced epilepsy is rather like, or just like clinical epilepsy (Schmalbach 1968b, and many others). A new phenomenon develops, namely *facilitation,* which means that it is easier for the convulsion elements to spread and for the epileptic attacks to become generalized.

Inhibition of the Epileptic Discharges

Here, we are dealing with a difficult problem. There are many inhibi- tory possibilities in the brain and, as long as these are not impaired, epi- lepsy hardly ever arises. Even where there is an epileptic reaction there is a vast organization of possible means of inhibition. This collapses where there are subsidiary conditions. According to Jung and Tönnies (1950), *the normal rhythms are inhibitory processes.* Predisposition to convulsion only develops when the normal rhythms of the original system are suppressed by frequent stimuli. The above-mentioned wave of the primary discharge (in- hibitory wave) which follows the spike, becomes smaller and longer when the convulsion occurs. The breakdown of normal rhythm and the diminu- tion of the slow wave in the primary discharge is interpreted by the authors as signifying *reduced inhibitory capacity* in the brain.

A very interesting point which these authors established is that the stimuli trigger both excitatory and inhibitory processes. If the stimuli are repeated too often, the inhibitory mechanisms are the first to suffer damage or become fatigued. This prepares the ground for increased predisposition to convulsion. *Thus, in the majority of cases the convulsion is triggered by failure of the inhibitory processes, and less often by an increase in the pre- disposition to convulsion.* According to these findings, *increased* predisposi- tion of the brain to produce convulsions is only relative. This fact is one of the most important cornerstones in our model in Chapter VIII.

According to the authors mentioned above, the normal rhythms of the brain inhibit the convulsion discharge in the way in which, by regular al- ternation of the active nerve cells, they prevent too many neurons from be- coming predisposed to discharge at the same time. Thus, the normal rhythms have an order, and there is a relative equilibrium of excitation and

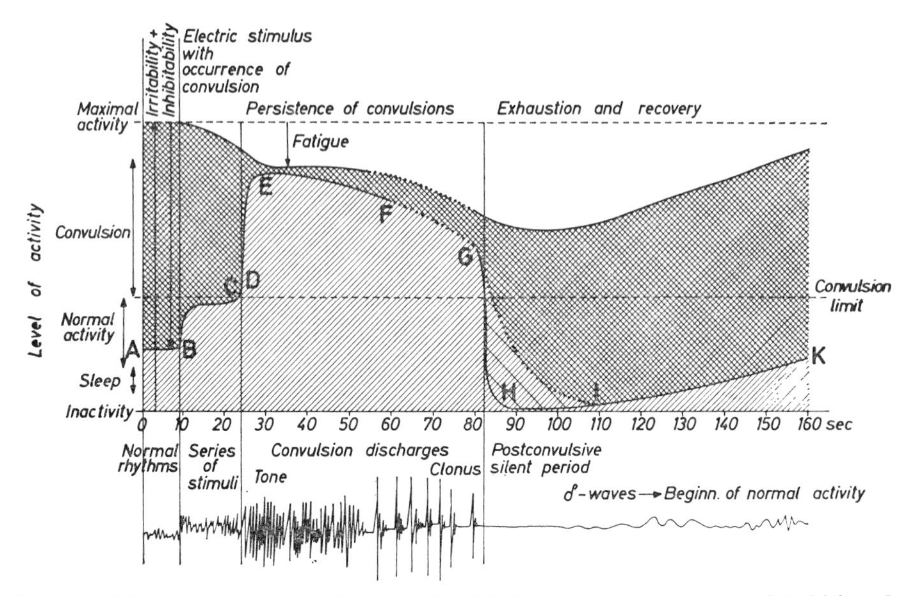

Figure 20. Diagram showing the interrelationship between excitation and inhibition during stimulation and a convulsive seizure. The upper boundary line within the / / / shading shows excitability, regarded as maximal activation of the nerve cells (potential energy). Opposing the excitability there is the inhibitory potential (shading XXX), regarded as the ability to inhibit hypernormal spread of excitation. The difference between the two gives the actual activity level (———). A and B = normal activity. At B electrical stimulation of 10/sec, at C the inhibitory potential is reduced by summated stimuli (reduction in the inhibitory threshold). Above the broken horizontal line (------) (convulsion threshold) the level of excitation ceases to be normal and a condition of convulsive discharges develops. The first convulsive discharges occur at D and this causes a rapid break-down of inhibitory potential, and thus of convulsion inhibition. E and F tonic, F and G clonic stage. Intermittent activity is shown by the dots .... There are periods of rest at times in the clonus intervals. Last clonus at G. Convulsive discharges cease, exhaustion and transition into postconvulsive rest. At first there is incomplete recovery of inhibitory potential shown by the dotted line between G and I. I and K = initially slowed delta rhythms in sleep and recovery stage. Normal physiological conditions restored with the normal rhythms. (From Jung, R. and J.F. Tönnies: *Arch Psychiat, 185*:701, 1950.)

inhibition in the central nervous system. Thus, the normal rhythms represent an important inhibitory factor. For example, in spite of the spread of synchronized discharges from the undamaged brain the effects of individual stimuli are quickly suppressed to forms of excitation which correspond to the normal rhythms in frequency, curve form and amplitude.

Only under certain circumstances, where there are certain chemical or pharmacological conditions, is it also possible to reduce the threshold of the neurons and of the synaptic transmission, and thus favor the occurrence of a convulsion.

Kreindler (1965) discusses two kinds of inhibitory mechanisms. As with normal bioelectric cerebral action, a convulsion process involves 1.) *cerebral,* and 2.) *extracerebral inhibitory mechanisms.*

The cerebral inhibitory mechanisms are part of the normal function of the brain. The author is not only thinking of inhibitory processes at the site of stimulation, but also of those in remote cerebral structures. Thus, for example, some cortical areas can moderate the excitation of others, or the subcortical ganglia can reduce excitation coming from the cortex. The inhibitory processes may also involve the cerebellum. There are many extracerebral inhibitory mechanisms involved in convulsive seizures: the rise of latency of the nociceptive spinal reflexes, powerful excitation of certain intraceptive afferents from the visceral autonomic system, spread of excitation from the reticular formation to other strucures—all have a moderating effect on subsequent convulsive episodes. Biochemical changes such as anoxia and a rise of the magnesium content in blood have also been taken into consideration by the author. In the next chapters, we shall deal with anoxia with an increase of the partial pressure of CO_2 and the inhibition of the seizure associated with this.

CHAPTER V

CEREBRAL METABOLISM AND PSYCHOMOTOR EPILEPSY

BIOCHEMICAL PROCESSES IN THE INTERVAL BETWEEN ATTACKS

IN THIS SECTION we shall discuss some of the factors involved in biochemical processes met with in epileptics or in experiments on animals, and try to relate factors to psychomotor epilepsy. We shall consider the role of: *electrolytes, water balance, oxygen, carbon dioxide and pH, carbohydrates, proteins and nucleic acids, amino acids, endogenous amines, ammonia and other products of protein metabolism, brain lipids, hormones, vitamins and enzymes* and the *blood-brain barrier.* In this section we shall deal mainly with metabolism and we shall also mention one or two points about normal cerebral metabolism. Subsequent sections in this chapter will deal with changes which are known to be closely related to epileptic episodes and their equivalents.

Electrolytes

It is extremely difficult to examine the electrolyte picture before, during and after an epileptic attack, and psychomotor epilepsy presents a particular problem here because it is often impossible to define the attack clinically. Here we shall add a little to what has already been said on this subject in Chapter IV.

It is quite obvious that if the body is to retain its functional capabilities, a state of isotonia (i.e. electrolyte homeostasis) must be maintained in both extracellular and intracellular systems. This applies particularly to the neurons. We know that osmotic pressure depends principally on the concentration and the physiological balance of the cations Na^+, K^+, Ca^{++}, Mg^{++} and the anions Cl^-, HCO_3^-, HPO_4^{--}, and in the CNS it also depends on *N-acetylaspartic acid* (Quadbeck and Helmchen 1958, Seiler 1966, Shapot 1957). According to Manery (1954), the cation concentration in dog brain, measured in microequivalents per gram moist weight is 51.8 for Na^+, 95.4 for K^+, 2.1 for Ca^{++} and 11.2 for Mg^{++}. The cations represent about 80 microequivalents/g. over and above the anions. The proportion of cations in the brain is higher than that in other organs (Shapot 1957). Naturally, this concentration may also be affected by the prevailing levels of other chemical compounds. For example, electrolyte biochemistry is closely related to the biochemistry of *acidic lipids* and *proteins.*

Apart from their stimulating and inhibiting functions (see Chapter IV) in the CNS (Höber 1925, Netter 1959, Stämpfli 1952), the cations Na^+ and K^+ also have an important part to play in cerebral metabolism. In actual fact, these two functions are closely connected (Breyer and Kanig 1970, Eccles 1953, 1964, Henatsch 1962, Hodgkin and Keynes 1955, Keynes 1954, Shanes 1951). Na^+, K^+ and Mg^{++} activate *adenosine triphosphatase (ATP-ase).* An increase of Na^+ within the neurons increases their excitability to such an extent that the convulsion threshold is lowered. In our experience, *hypernatriaemia* produces clinical convulsions and suspected convulsion elements in the EEG. Also, *adrenalectomy* is followed by increased excitability of the CNS, and a rise in the intracellular concentration of sodium. A fall of Na^+ concentration within the neurons and a rise of extracellular and serum Na^+ reduces the convulsion threshold for cortisone and cortisol, but raises the convulsion threshold for *desoxycorticosterone* (Seiler 1966). Retention of sodium ions in serum is associated with a deterioration in the clinical picture of the epileptic patient and forced excretion coincides with a clinical improvement (Schneider and Thomalske 1963). This is confirmed by post-paroxysmal diuresis with loss of sodium (Selbach et al. 1965).

Under conditions of *water retention,* the increased porousness of the neuronal membrane means that *sodium ions* tend to penetrate into the nerve cells and the aqueous sheath around the ions is stripped off. The crystal radius of sodium ions is 0.95 Ångström units (Å) and this means that they penetrate into the cells more easily than potassium ions which have a crystal radius of 1.33 Å. If sodium ions penetrate and accumulate in the neurons this may cause depolarization of the membrane (Meves 1962, Selbach et al. 1965; see also Chapter IV). Among other things, sodium ions stimulate various enzymes which are inhibited by anaesthetics and some sedative drugs (Järnefelt 1961, Le Page 1946). This may explain why some hypnotic and anesthetic drugs are capable of inhibiting an epileptic attack. Of course, there are also other inhibitory mechanisms (see Chapter IV).

Potassium ions are involved in the *oxidation of glucose. In vitro* sections of brain in a suitable medium containing glucose respire at about half the rate of the brain *in vivo.* If the proportion of potassium in relation to calcium around the tissue is increased (i.e. K^+/Ca^{++} quotient increased) or, if the brain sections are exposed to an electric current (Pogodaev 1964), then oxygen consumption increases to the level found in the brain *in vivo* (Bronk and Brink 1951, McIlwain 1953, Pogodaev 1964, Quastel 1959).

Potassium ions also increase the oxidation of *pyruvic acid, lactic acid* and *glutamic acid;* this will be discussed later. From the results described above, *in vivo* stimulation of oxidation processes by potassium ions resembles the *in vitro* stimulation of brain sections by an electric current. *In vitro* the electric current can be replaced by potassium stimulation and the responses in the experimental brain sections will be the same (McIlwain 1962, 1963, Quastel 1962). Because of this effect of potassium ions on the excitability of cerebral tissue, *hyperpotassaemia* may produce convulsions. Under conditions of *hypopotassaemia,* convulsions probably occur as a result of intracellular depletion of potassium ions (Kreindler 1965, Tower 1960).

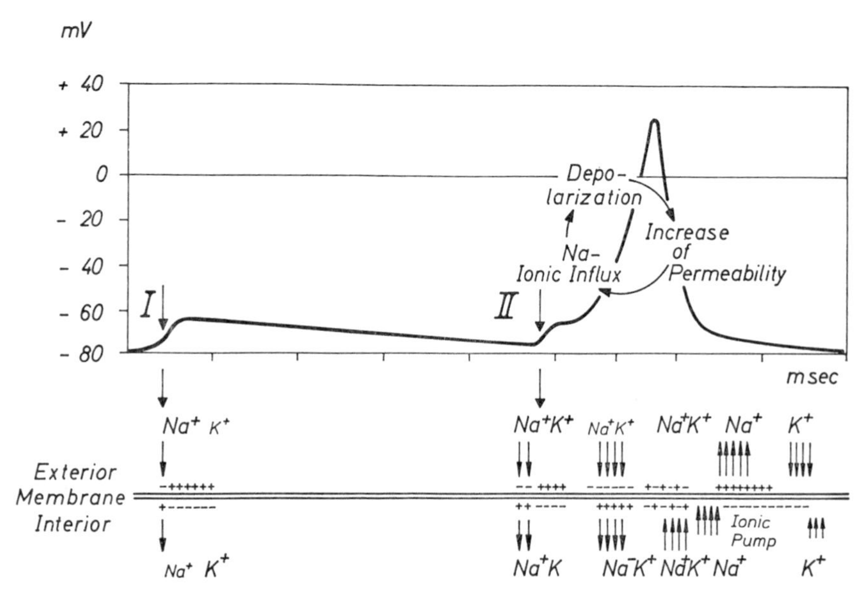

Figure 21. Excitation process and electrolyte migration in a nerve cell. There is first a breakdown of membrane potential followed by the occurrence of an action potential and finally the membrane is restored by ion transport, which requires energy (cp. Figure 16). (From Bamberger, in Prüll, G.: *Therapeutische Berichte, 39*:343-351, 1967.)

We are still not absolutely sure as to the *mechanism of action* of potassium ions on *in vivo* and *in vitro* oxidation. A change in the proportions of *adenosine diphosphate (ADP)* and *adenosine triphosphate (ATP)* or in the *ADP/ATP quotient* have been suggested. Increasing the quotient stimulates the tricarboxylic acid cycle and, in turn, this increases acetylcholine synthesis (Mann et al. 1939), increases the amount of inorganic phosphate incorporated into phospholipids and phosphoproteins (Breyer and Kanig 1970, Rossiter 1955, Shanes 1958), and promotes synthesis of glutamic acid and other amino acids from *glucose* (Kini and Quastel 1959). For example, a change of *acetylcholine glutamate* was found to be related to electrolyte shifts in epileptic reactions; this will be discussed later.

On the other hand, when applied locally, *calcium ions* inhibit these reactions. This applies both to oxidation processes and also to stimulation of the electrical activity of the brain (Bonnet and Bremer 1937, Canzanelli et al. 1942; Gosh and Quastel 1954). Hence, calcium ions antagonize the effects of K^+, and thus they may have an anticonvulsant effect. It was also found that in epileptics the serum level of ionized calcium is unstable where there are fluctuations in the diurnal cholesterol curve, in the acid-base balance, in lymphocytosis and where thymus tissue persists (Ziegler 1964). As well as causing other neurological disorders, *hypocalcaemia* produces tetany and, where there are other epileptogenic factors, epilepsy (Wolfe and Elliot 1962).

There has been a considerable amount of research into the *mechanism* of action of calcium. Ca^{++} is responsible for the release of *acetylcholine*. It is thought that an increase of intracellular calcium ions has the effect of increasing the amount of calcium at the nerve endings and this results in release of the transmitter (Hodgkin and Keynes 1957, Shanes 1958). Wooley (1958 a, b) relates the action of calcium to that of *serotonin*. According to Wooley, serotonin first combines to form a complex with a lipoid in the neuronal membrane. This complex is capable of binding Ca^{++} and, in this lipoid-soluble form, calcium is capable of diffusing through the membrane of the neuron. Once within the membrane, the complex is broken down by an enzyme and the Ca^{++} reacts with *actomyosin* and *ATP;* one of the effects of this reaction is to trigger muscular contraction. Thus, from our model of an epileptic attack (see Chapter VIII), hypocalcaemia may have an effect on psychomotor epilepsy. Binding of calcium to *citric acid* in the CNS immediately produces convulsions (Seiler 1966).

Like the other cations mentioned, *magnesium ions* are also essential nutritional factors. They antagonize the effects of calcium ions, they intensify *cholinesterase* activity and they are involved in many biochemical processes in the CNS (Del Castillo and Engbaek 1954).

However, we only know of *conditions of magnesium deficiency* in patients with chronic alcoholism (Flink 1956). Since epilepsy is sometimes seen in cases of chronic alcoholism, magnesium may play an important part here, although there is no definite evidence of this. Muscular twitching has been observed under conditions of magnesium deficiency produced experimentally (Vallee et al. 1960). It is very difficult to produce magnesium deficiency since the body has considerable reserves. However, it has been possible to induce magnesium deficiency in rats (Kruse et al. 1932, Vallee et al. 1960), and the neurons became so sensitive that even mild acoustic stimuli immediately triggered off convulsions, the process resembling *reflex epilepsy* in man (Kreis 1968). We are not yet clear about the mechanism responsible for increasing the sensitivity and reducing the stimulus threshold under conditions of magnesium deficiency, or which biochemical processes are involved. It is assumed that there are a series of enzymatic processes which are activated by magnesium. The most important reactions in which magnesium ions may play an active part are methylation of the hormones of the adrenal medulla by *catecholamine-o-methyl transferase,* formation of glutamine, conversion of *choline* into *phosphocholine* and then into *cytidine-diphosphocholine* and the break down of *ATP* by a microsomal *ATP-ase* in the brain. Since ATP-ase plays an important part in the transport of the cations K^+ and Na^+ across the neuronal membrane (McIlwain 1963), its effect in activating this mechanism is the most important function of magnesium in the CNS (Seiler 1966). Microsomal ATP-ase, which is activated by magnesium ions, is inhibited by Ca^{++}; in this respect it differs from the other *triphosphatases* present in the brain (Seiler 1966). Magnesium, sodium and potassium ions are transported physiologically by the nerve cell membrane. The passive processes by which Na^+ enters the cell and K^+ leaves the cell are actively offset by the combination of Mg^{++} and ATP. The former process is offset from within the cell and the latter from outside the cell. The ATP then breaks down into MgADP and phosphate (see also Prüll 1967).

The *trace elements* will be mentioned briefly when we discuss the role of vitamins and enzymes (See also Brunia and Buyze 1972).

Water Balance

Water metabolism has a very important part to play in epilepsy. We are not familiar with all the mechanisms responsible, but it is well-known clinically that an epileptic patient is more likely to suffer convulsions when he is *retaining water.* Actually in many hospitals a method resembling a urine concentration test is used as a means of provoking a seizure (Gänshirt and Vetter 1961, MacQuarrie 1931, 1932, Weinland 1949). The effect of water retention was recognized many years ago (Helmholtz and Keith 1930, MacQuarrie 1927, 1929, 1932, Wilder 1921).

These were stimulated attempts to treat patients by regulating their consumption of ketogenic fats (Wilder 1921). 50 years ago, research workers had already realized that *fasting days* have a favorable effect on clinical epilepsy and they are often capable of interrupting periods of recurrent attacks (Engel 1933). A low water and ketogenic fat diet has a particularly favorable effect in *epilepsy in children* (Dekaban 1966, Peterman 1924). Effective diuresis before an attack can prevent a seizure from developing, and diuresis after a series of attacks can interrupt the sequence of attacks (Engel 1933). A ketogenic diet is known to counteract water retention (Dekaban 1966, Seiler 1966). Rowntree (1926) induced tonic-clonic convulsions in dogs by *administering a large dose of water*. However, where there is pre-existing water retention, only a little water needs to be given (Engel 1933). Figures 22a, b and c show the course of attacks under therapeutically induced diuresis or under conditions of water retention.

The *mechanisms causing water retention* are well known in many other diseases but it is still not certain what mechanisms are responsible for water retention in epileptics. Selbach (1965) and Selbach et al. (1965) suggest that a general predisposition to *vagotonia and trophopaty* is responsible for water retention in epileptics. An attack is followed by acidosis and excretion of water and this produces a sympathicotonic condition which arrests the attack. Predisposition to attacks increases in epileptics in the second part of pregnancy, i.e. during a period of increased plasma volume and extravasal fluid, and reduced amounts of serum magnesium which normally stabilize the membranes (Suter and Klingman 1957).

The capacity of colloids to bind water is known to increase with the degree of colloidal dispersion. Thus, for example, an increase of finely dispersed albumins would produce water retention. The majority of findings indicate that in epileptics there is a fall (rather than an increase) *in the quantity of albumins and a rise in globulins* just before an attack. However, these findings fit into the general picture of water retention, since a fall in the albumin fraction and a rise of globulins results in an *increase of total protein in serum*. In addition to water retention, a *local lesion* of the cerebral tissue (e.g. in the hippocampus for psychomotor epilepsy, see Chapter III) is necessary for there to be convulsions. Where these local lesions are present, according to Kiyota (1961) and Quadbeck and Helmchen (1958) there is also a marked regional increase of water-binding cerebral proteins. The albumin content is mostly increased in grey matter and the alpha-globulin content in the cerebral medulla. This local alteration of cerebral proteins has the effect of reducing the convulsion threshold and of introducing other labile elements into cerebral metabolism. The fall of colloid-osmotic pressure in serum resulting from the declining concentration of finely dispersed proteins means that fluid passes from serum into tissue and this increases the pressure in the cerebral tissue. Since the nerve cell membrane is already injured in epileptics, these local changes in the protein fractions cause further damage, the depolarizations synchronize and consequently an attack occurs. Fay (1929) considered that the hydrostatic pressure in the subdural spaces stimulates the neurons mechanically; thus, predisposing to an attack. However, Höber (1925) assumed that the hypersensitivity is a function of the swelling or colloidal state of the neurons. According to Mölbert et al. (1967) and Selbach et al. (1965), this swelling of the nerve cells and the resulting *rise of permeability* reduces the threshold before an attack. As Figure 22 shows, there is always an attack if body

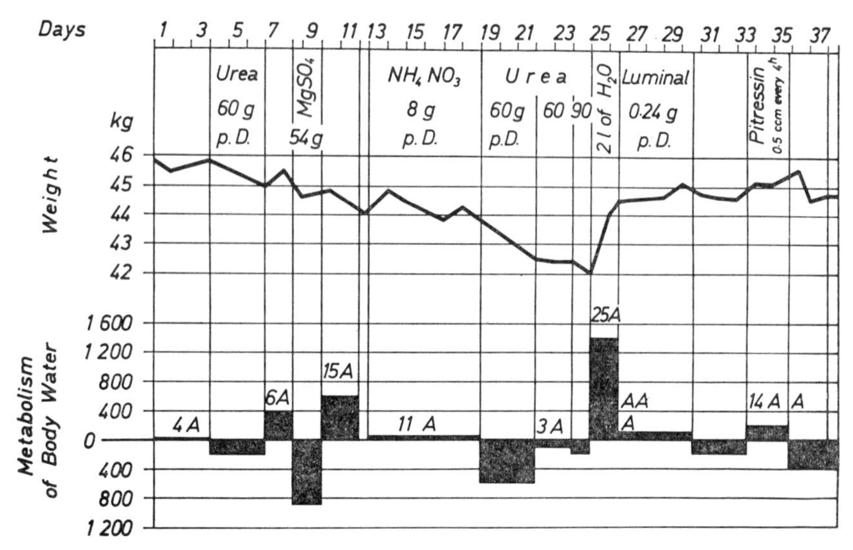

Figure 22a. Water balance in a 15-year-old girl with severe epilepsy; drug-induced diuresis was varied while her diet was kept constant (81 g protein, 83 g carbohydrate, 116 g fat). An attack (A) occurred every time her body weight increased and every time there was a marked increase of water retention. The more evidence there was of water retention, the more the attacks followed on another. (From MacQuarrie, I. et al., *Am J Dis Child, 43*:1523, 1932.)

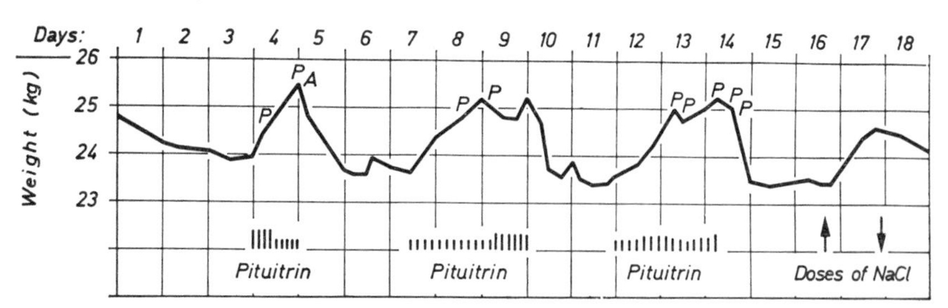

Figure 22b. Body weight and attacks under the antidiuretic effect of Pituitrin® during administration of a constant and abnormally low-salt-content diet. The attacks occur every time there is a weight increase (water retention) (P = minor; A = major attacks). (From Engel, R., *Nervenarzt, 6*:123, 1933.)

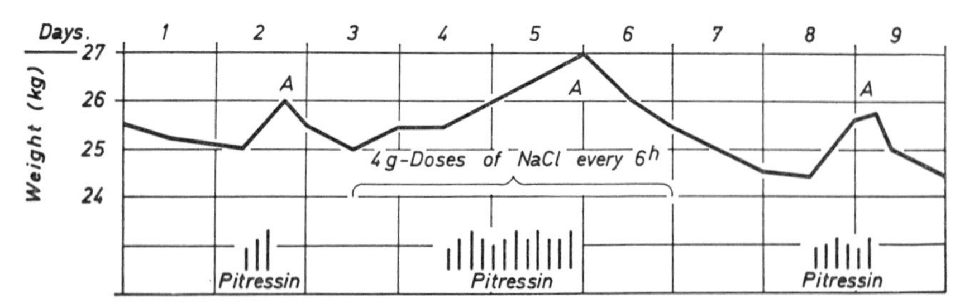

Figure 22c. Body weight and attacks in a mild case of epilepsy under the influence of Pitressin® with and without addition of sodium chloride. An attack (A) occurs every time there is a weight increase and when salt is added to the diet. (From MacQuarrie, I., and Peeler, D.B.: *J Clin Invest, 10*:932, 1931.)

weight is increased, or if medicaments are used to induce water retention in an epileptic.

In our opinion, general water retention on its own, without any local lesion of cerebral tissue, cannot produce an epileptic attack, since severe fluid retention occurs in many other diseases (e.g. renal and cardiac disease) but epileptic seizures do not occur without some other predisposing factor. Convulsions may occur, but in these diseases they only appear as late manifestations when an accumulation of metabolic products will already have produced local damage in the CNS.

Oxygen, Carbon Dioxide and pH

The role of oxygen is still not completely clear. Normally the brain consumes 20 percent of the oxygen in the human body (Kety and Schmidt 1948). It was concluded from this that oxidation provides the main source of energy for the brain. The physiological consumption of oxygen is high, and the level of consumption remains relatively constant. Major fluctuations only occur when oxidation is severely disrupted such as in a coma. Thus, for the brain to function properly the oxidation processes must be regulated very carefully (Seiler 1966). Even where oxidation processes in the CNS are regulated with some precision and where oxygen consumption is relatively stable, cerebral function may still show many different types of abnormality. Gibbs et al (1947) did not find any changes in oxygen consumption in epileptics in the interval between convulsions. Even children did not show any definite changes of oxygen consumption in the interval (Horstmann and Wegener 1966), although there may have been local changes.

According to Schmidt et al. (1945) and Tower (1960), *in vivo* oxygen consumption during the interparoxysmal phase of an epileptic attack is normal, both in experimental, chronic epilepsy induced by an injection of aluminum hydroxide and in the human epileptic focus. *In vitro* studies on brain sections from animals with epileptogenic foci induced by aluminium cream or injection of methionine sulphoximine and on brain sections from patients with a chronic epileptic focus (sections obtained surgically), did not reveal any changes in oxygen consumption or in glycolysis (McIlwain 1955, Elliott 1955). Thus, it is not possible to provide *in vitro* demonstration of permanent damage to metabolic oxidation processes in the cerebral cortex. *In vivo,* disturbed oxidation seems to be confined to the paroxysmal phase and tends (in experiments) to disappear after the attack.

However, investigations by Mison-Crighel et al. (1962) revealed that oxidation in cerebral tissue was disrupted in the interparoxysmal phase. EEG and biochemical studies of cortical scars in the cat showed that the bioelectrical elements in and near the damaged regions were associated with a reduction of *cytochrome oxidase* and *succino-dehydrogenase activity.* Convulsions were associated with similar biochemical disorders.

Experiments performed during a convulsion have demonstrated the effect of administering oxygen (Ruf 1950). Using 50 cats Ruf set out to study the effects of mechanisms which promote and those which inhibit attacks. Using leads to measure the brain potentials in the cerebral cortex, thalamus, corpus caudatum, cerebellum and medulla oblongata, with supplementary recordings of the spinal potentials and the nerve and muscle currents, and by using electroshock, this author was able to establish that convulsions induced in the cat are greatly prolonged if oxygen is given continuously at the same time. The attack begins as usual with tonic-clonic manifestations. The phase of *tonic* convulsions is greatly prolonged, and the subsequent tonic-clonic condition only begins after 100 seconds and develops into the typical clonus $2\frac{1}{2}$ minutes after the beginning of the attack. After half an hour, a convulsion focus begins to form in the cerebral cortex and this then spreads rapidly to the other cerebral hemisphere. After a single electric shock the whole attack lasts for up to one hour and 37 minutes. The condition deteriorates if Adrenaline® is also given. The convulsion patterns with a frequency of 30/sec. measured in the cerebral cortex became very dense after only half a minute. The first signs of fatigue after adrenaline usually became apparent after three minutes. The following conclusions can be drawn from these two experiments by Ruf (1950) : firstly, an epileptic attack is prolonged by administering copious quantities of oxygen since the energy requirement is increased during the attack and, secondly, an attack is hastened by giving Adrenaline and it is also curtailed because oxygen is rapidly consumed. If O_2 and Adrenaline are given together, the convulsive seizure is prolonged and this rapidly exhausts the body com-
sions can be drawn from these two experiments by Ruf (1950) : firstly, an
pletely. Prolonging of the tonic phase may be interpreted as a detrimental effect of oxygen since anticonvulsants curtail this phase and, in certain circumstances, prolong (relatively) the *clonic* phase (Pogodaev 1964).

Hyperventilation, which removes carbon dioxide, produces *alkalosis* of the blood (Bochnik 1957) and precipitates epileptic attacks, has long been one of commonest and most familiar methods for inducing attacks in epileptic and suspected epileptic patients. This was reported as early as 1926 by Foerster, who described patients in whom attacks could be induced by hyperventilation, and he used the term *hyperventilation epilepsy.* Figures reported by later authors for induction of epileptic phenomena by hyperventilation, varied from 0 to 70 percent. Epileptic attacks were induced by hyperventilation in 22 percent of cases by Hendriksen (1927), in 47.8 percent of cases by Jakusin (1927), in 15 percent of cases by Nyssen (1927), in 0 percent of cases by Gomes (1930), in 0 percent of cases by Munch-Petersen (1931), in 12 percent of cases by Forsberg (1931), in 29 percent of cases by Laruelle (1932), in 0 percent of cases by Pagniez (1933), in 70 percent of cases by Mauro (1934), in 0 percent of cases by Skobnikova (1935) and in 10 percent of cases by Janz (1937). Since the discovery of the EEG and reesarch into the different types of epilepsy, views on the effect of hyperventilation in epilepsy have altered somewhat (Christian 1968 a, Davis and Wallace 1942, Heppenstall 1944, Meyer and Waltz 1960, Niebeling 1968). Christian (1960), Beyer and Jovanović (1966) and Jovanović (1968 c) found that hyperventilation has a profound effect on grand mal of the matutinal type and on petit mal, i.e. throughout the entire group of *centrencephalic epilepsies,* while psychomotor epilepsy and the related nocturnal form of grand mal, i.e. the temporocephalic types of epilepsy, are not readily influenced by hyperventilation (Jovanović and Schäfer 1966). This explains the inconsistencies in the findings of earlier authors after using hyperventilation. Thus, psychomotor attacks cannot simply be explained on the basis of loss of CO_2 and subsequent systemic *alkalosis* with increased colloidal pressure in the cells and increased excitability of the neurons.

In discussing hyperventilation we have already touched on the effects of *CO_2*. It has long been known that CO_2 has an inhibitory effect on the cerebral predisposition to convulsion and consequently it has a favorable effect on epilepsy (Christian 1968 a, Gellhorn and Heymans 1948, Gellhorn and Yesinik 1942, Heppenstall 1944, Meyer and Waltz 1960, Selbach 1965, Selbach et al. 1965, Tower 1960, Woodbury et al. 1958 b).

Carbon dioxide is a regulated parameter with a central homoestatic effect and, since carbon dioxide rapidly passes through aqueous and lipoid layers, it is the most rapidly acting active regulator for all the cells in the body (Caspers and Speckmann 1972, Selbach et al. 1965). It is interesting to consider how cerebral metabolism is related to changes of CO_2 partial pressure (*pCO_2*) in blood and cerebral predisposition to convulsion. A rise of pCO_2 promotes synthesis of *gamma-aminobutyric acid (GABA).* At the same time, activation of *gamma-amino-decarboxylase (GAD)* normalises the cortical potentials and reduces excitatory hyperactivity in the fornix and ventral hippocampus. Addition of 5 percent CO_2 to the respiratory air relieves twilight attacks, arrests minor attacks and occasionally may even relieve status epilepticus. *Bicarbonates* also have a favorable effect on epileptic episodes (Woodbury et al. 1958 b). An epileptic with a pneumothorax and increased pCO_2 in the blood can reduce the number of attacks by chronic hyperventilation of about nine inspirations per minute or by respiring under the bedclothes. There is reduced predisposition to convulsion in patients with congenital *carbonic anhydrase (CAH)* deficiency. The number of attacks can be temporarily reduced by treatment with CAH inhibitors, e.g. with acetazolamide *(Diamox®)* due to increased CO_2 tension and *metabolic acidosis* (Penfield 1957). The same applies where the sensitivity of the respiratory center becomes normal again under treatment with *Ospolot®* (see Chapter VII), due to direct inhibition of CAH in the neurons of the brain (Selbach 1963, Selbach et al. 1965). According to Selbach et al. (1965), the carbonic anhydrase content of the diencephalon and, in particular, of the hippocampus is higher than in the rest of the nervous system. This explains the role of carbonic anhydrase in psychomotor epilepsy, where for some reason or other there are local metabolic disorders.

Experiments under conditions of low oxygen pressure at heights of 400 to 7000 m. show that administration of CO_2 delays the onset of a convulsion for up to a quarter of an hour. In experimental animals, with a lower concentration of CO_2, the convulsion threshold for electrical stimuli is increased (Caspers and Speckmann 1972, Woodbury et al. 1958 a, b).

However, if the pCO_2 falls (for instance, following hyperventilation), this destabilizes central vascular tonus and there is a tendency to vasoconstriction, reduced blood flow and local oxygen deficiency, reduced GABA, electrolyte and pH changes and a tendency for neuronal membranes to depolarize. Eventually, the excitability of the CNS increases and a partially or fully synchronized attack develops in the epileptic patient (Selbach et al. 1965).

Like the data on oxygen levels in the brain and blood of epileptic patients during the interval between attacks, figures for CO_2 content also vary considerably and the figures usually bear little relation to the last attack or a subsequent period of attacks. It is difficult to take readings continuously over long periods, particularly when dealing with patients with psychomotor epilepsy. Cumings (1960), Selbach et al. (1965) and several other authors are not aware of any such recordings, and we could not find any in the literature. Results from individual patients fluctuate. Horstmann and Wegener (1966) examined 33 epileptic children for alveolar CO_2 tension, pH of blood and excessive blood levels of bases and acids. In addition to confirming the considerable variation so typical in children, these authors obtained the following results: a prevailing tendency to hyperventilation rather than hypoventilation; in children with grand mal persistently depressed alveolar CO_2 tension interrupted by phases of hyperventilation; carbon dioxide tension became normal under administration of antiepileptic agents. Where there were interim cerebral attacks, CO_2 tension was moderately reduced, normal or even elevated. The authors concluded from this that a pathological increase of respiration is not an absolute prerequisite for precipitating an attack.

Nor do these authors believe that there is a simple connection between the degree of severity of the clinical picture and the extent of the general respiratory disorder. The pH of the blood remained the same in all the cases. Evidently, here again it is not the systemic change of CO_2 tension, but a local change which is important. Also, the decisive factor is not the absolute value, but the ratio of CO_2 concentration to the particular threshold values for the respiratory center: hence, where the nerve cell membranes of the brain or of the neurons regulating respiration are hyperpolarized, normal levels of CO_2 are no longer sufficient to maintain proper physiological function. Because of the danger of apnoic arrest, in the end it may become necessary to change over completely to tonic convulsion with maximum CO_2 flooding and acidification with cerebral vascular dilatation (Pogodaev 1964, Selbach 1965, Selbach et al. 1965).

The pH or the acid-base ratio both in blood and locally in the CNS (see Figure 28), particularly at the site of origin of the attack (the convulsion focus), is an important factor in the development of an attack. The activity of glutamic acid decarboxylase is actually optimum at pH 6.5 : thus, *intracellular acidosis promotes GABA synthesis and hence inhibits an attack.* On the other hand, the maximum activity of GABA transaminase is at pH 8.2: *thus, intracellular alkalosis promotes breakdown of GABA and hence it promotes an epileptic attack* (Roberts and Eidelberg 1960). Epileptic attacks are rare in acidotic eclampsia and typical in alkalotic eclampsia (Dubrauszky 1959, Selbach et al. 1965). Inhibiting GABA transaminase with amino-acetoacetic acid reduces the incidence of attacks. On the other hand, the condition deteriorates in schizophrenic patients (Merlis 1961). These facts are of major importance since in psychomotor epilepsy an epileptic attack occurs at one moment, and a psychosis at another, but the two hardly ever occur simultaneously. Admittedly, an elevated level of GABA does not always inhibit an epileptic attack (Wiechert and Herbst 1966), nor has it been definitely established that GABA has a reliable and unequivocal antiepileptic action or that a deficiency of GABA is always associated with epileptic attacks.

The Importance of Carbohydrates

Many authors have dealt with the general problem of carbohydrate metabolism in the brain, but there has been no conclusive explanation as to the role of carbohydrates in an epileptic attack and no one has yet produced a set of continuous recordings of carbohydrate metabolism. There are a few results, but these are concerned more with the effect of glucose on the mechanism of the attack rather than with causal relationships. Because of the enormous importance of carbohydrates in nourishing the brain we would like to discuss this subject briefly, in terms of epileptic seizures.

Glucose plays a central role in carbohydrate metabolism in the brain.

The dissimilation of glucose usually follows a definite pathway (Banga et al. 1939, Von Euler et al. 1936, Geiger 1940, Mac Farlane and Weil-Mahlerbe 1941, Malaguzzi-Valeri 1936, Meyerhof 1938, Ochoa 1941, Seiler 1966). According to these authors this proceeds in several discreet stages or reactions.

Glucose is esterified as soon as it enters the cerebral neurons, a phosphate group being transferred from adenosine triphosphate (ATP) to the glucose under the action of *hexokinase.* This forms *glucose-6-phosphate,* and, at the same time, *adenosine diphosphate (ADP)* is produced from ATP. The phosphate group is present in ATP in an active form. Together with several other energy-rich phosphates, ATP is one of the most important biological stores of energy in the CNS.

The second reaction which is continuous with the first, transforms glucose-6-phosphate into the isomer *fructose-6-phosphate.* This then receives several more phosphate groups from an ATP molecule, to produce *fructose-1, 6-diphosphate.*

Aldolase then breaks down fructose diphosphate into two trioses: *glyceraldehyde-3-phosphate* and *dihydroxyacetone phosphate.*

According to the Embden-Meyerhof principle (Meyerhof 1938, Seiler 1966), these trioses are in equilibrium with one another and if one is being utilized further supplies can be obtained continuously from the other, while fresh supplies of glucose are always needed for this process.

Phosphoglyceraldehyde is then oxidized, and the carboxyl group produced combines with phosphoric acid like an anhydrite, to form Negelein ester; this reaction takes place in the presence of the enzyme *triose-phosphate dehydrogenase,* and it involves the direct transfer of inorganic phosphate into an organic compound. The hydrogen released is transferred to *nicotinamide-adenine-dinucleotide (NAD).*

With the high energy *acylphosphate bond* in the Negelein ester, in the next stage the phosphate residue is transferred to a molecule of ADP, and this produces ATP and *phosphoglyceric acid.* This regenerates the molecule of ATP utilized during the hexokinase reaction.

Phosphoenolpyruvic acid is produced by two further reactions which play a major part in an epileptic attack, and this is also dephosphorylated by transfer of a phosphate residue to ADP. This produces *pyruvic acid,* which is important in energy metabolism and is mentioned later several times. In the presence of the catalyst *lactate dehydrogenase,* hydrogen from reduced *codehydrase I* is transferred to pyruvic acid and *lactic acid* is formed. Diagrams and a description of all these reactions can be found in Seiler (1966).

About 90 percent of the enzymes involved in glucose metabolism occur in the cytoplasm of the neurons. About 10 percent of glucose activity is associated with mitochondria (Balazs and Laguado 1959, Wu and Racker 1959).

Glucose can be formed again from any of the intermediate products of glucose metabolism mentioned above, and glycogen (which is a glucose store) is formed from many different substances (amino acids, fatty acids etc.) (Leloir et al. 1959).

Apart from the process of glucose dissimilation previously described there are also a series of non-oxidizing reactions. Under anaerobic conditions, the oxidation process is balanced by reduction of pyruvic acid to lactic acid. Lactic acid can be formed in the brain even under aerobic conditions. According to Gibbs et al. (1942), in the human brain at rest 16 percent of the glucose utilized passes into the blood as lactic acid. According to Richter and Dawson (1948), lactic acid formation in the brain is increased during stimulation and reduced during sleep and under anaesthesia. As the pH falls, lactic acid production slows down. Anaerobic glycolysis may possibly be connected with regulation of pH and blood circulation either in individual areas (which could be of importance to our problem) or in the brain as a whole (Seiler 1966). Since the pH tends towards alkalosis before an epileptic attack, it can be concluded that *before convulsions or other epileptic episodes glucose metabolism is disturbed at the pyruvic acid stage.*

Most of the pyruvic acid is oxidized further under aerobic conditions. The process responsible for this is known as the *citric acid cycle* (Krebs and Johnson 1937, Kanig 1968). The citric acid cycle is a series of reactions involving addition of water and dehydrogenation. Oxygen is not utilized at any stage (Jencke and Lynen 1960, Lipmann 1954, Lynen 1965, Seiler 1966). However, this pathway of glucose dissimilation followed by the citric acid cycle (Embden-Meyerhof) is not the only route. There is also a second, direct way of glucose oxidation (Horecker 1966), i.e. the *pentose-phosphate cycle,* although we cannot go into details of this here. Apart from those described, there are one or two more reactions involving pyruvic acid. Pyruvic acid, and all the *ketonic acids,* have an important part to play here and also in amino acid metabolism.

Abnormalities of carbohydrate metabolism in the form of familial *hypoglycaemia* cause epileptic reactions in children under two years old; these reactions produce permanent neurological defects (Cochrane et al. 1956). Hypoglycaemia may give rise to other provocative elements even in adults, and, in certain circumstances, it may induce epilepsy. For example, hypoglycaemia intensifies the effects of hyperventilation in the EEG of epileptic patients and thus it tends to provoke convulsions, whereas, the pathological effect of hyperventilation is reduced under conditions of hyperglycaemia (Davis and Wallace 1942; Kogan and Moskovich 1965).

However, the EEG changes in epileptics under hyperventilation are not directly related to the degree of elevation of the blood sugar level (Cheraskin and Ringsdorf 1963, Heppenstall 1944, Seppäläinen and Similä 1971). Since psychotic episodes often develop in patients with psychomotor epilepsy (see Chapter I), we would like to mention changes in carbohydrate metabolism occurring during psychoses.

Nucleic Acids and Proteins

The question of the involvement of nucleic acids and proteins in an epileptic attack is a very complicated one, and there are many factors to be taken into account. There are many different results and opinions on this subject and for this reason we must deal with this problem in some detail, and perhaps some of our points may stimulate further research.

We believe that the structure and function of *deoxyribonucleic acid (DNA)* in the CNS are particularly important causal factors in *essential* and symptomatic epilepsy. According to Seiler (1966) and many other authors (Oesterle and Kanig 1970, 1971), DNA is found in the chromatic parts in the nucleus of the neurons. The structure of the DNA defines the genetic code. Thus, it has a dual function: in the first place it passes on the genetic material unchanged from neuron to neuron to succeeding generations by identical duplication, and in the second place, DNA controls metabolism within the cell by supplying information for the synthesis of enzymes and structural proteins in the base sequence of the ribonucleic acid (RNA) which is formed in the cell nucleus.

It is possible that in *idiopathic* forms of epilepsy the DNA is functioning abnormally, and this is in addition to any other congenital metabolic defects (see also Chapter III).

In epilepsy DNA may also be important from another point of view. DNA is a very large molecule with a molecular weight of 6 to 10 million, RNA has a molecular weight of $\frac{1}{2}$ to 2 million, while soluble ribonucleic acids have molecular weights of 20,000 to 40,000 (Seiler 1966). If autolysis of proteins occurs during an epileptic episode (Krasnova 1960, Mison-Crighel et al. 1955, Mölbert et al. 1967, Niklowitz 1966, Pogodaev 1964, Quant and Sommer 1966), these nucleic acids may also be involved in the dispersion of colloids in and around the convulsion focus.

Ribonucleic acid (RNA) in nerve tissue has a high *guanine* and *cytosine content* (Egyhazi and Hydén 1961). On the other hand, RNA from the nuclei of the neurons is more like DNA because of its high *adenine* and *uracil content* (Edstöm 1953, 1960, Hydén 1962). One of the differences between DNA and RNA in the neurons is that the amount of DNA does not normally change while the RNA content varies considerably under different functional conditions (Kanig and Oesterle 1971, Kanig et al. 1971).

As was mentioned in Chapter III, there are considerable changes in the form of RNA released during an electrical convulsion (Mölbert et al. 1967, Quant and Sommer 1966) and after intoxication with methoxypyridoxine (Nicklowitz 1966).

According to Hydén (1959), following stimulation of the sensory and motor areas of the nervous system, the amount of RNA, protein and lipids in the affected neurons increases within physiological limits and—this is a point to stress here—*the increase is proportional to the intensity of the stimulus.* Powerful stimuli result in a pathological increase in the concentration of these substances. The biochemical levels of these substances normalize again a few hours after ending the stimulation. The ratio *adenine/uracil* in nuclear RNA has also been studied (Hydén and Egyhazi 1962). In the affected areas of the CNS, the RNA content also increases after stressing certain centers or systems and at the same time there is an increase in the ratio of adenine/guanine + cytosine (Krasnova 1960, Mison-Crighel et al. 1955, Pogodaev 1955, 1964).

To relate this to psychomotor epilepsy, we must imagine something resembling these processes occurring in the limbic system or convulsion focus; this is indicated by the results of the authors mentioned above and following.

When discussing the problem of epilepsy, it is also important to remember the differences between the nucleic acids in the neurons and in the *neuroglia* (Hamberger 1961). Under certain excitatory conditions, the neuroglia cells may often respond in the opposite way to the nerve cells. Where the demand for energy is increased, the neuroglia are capable of reducing their energy requirement in order to leave energy readily accessible to the neurons. Thus, the ATP content is high in the nerve cells and low in the neuroglia (Cummins and Hydén 1962). The metabolism (Seiler 1966) and functions (Kornmüller 1950) of the neurons and neuroglia cells are complementary, although in certain circumstances (as for example in epilepsy) this may have a detrimental effect (see also Chapter VIII).

We have not room here to go into the very complex question of the degradation and synthesis of *proteins* in the CNS, and so we would refer to the monograph on metabolism in the CNS published quite recently by Seiler (1966).

Under certain conditions (excitation, pathological processes) protein metabolism can be altered. Flexner et al (1965) found that interrupting protein synthesis by introducing *puromycin* into the hippocampi and temporal lobes may produce loss of memory which is related to the duration of inhibition. This is reminiscent of the psychic disorders which occur in patients with psychomotor epilepsy (see Chapters I and III) where the convulsion focus is situated in or near the hippocampus. Physiological stimulation by electrical means increases the nucleoproteins in the affected cells (Hydén 1959, 1960, 1962, Hydén and Egyhazi 1962, 1964).

Intensified reduction activity in the cerebral tissue was detected following electroshock (Fischer et al. 1961). There were no quantitative changes in the distribution of soluble proteins (Balley and Heald 1961), and these authors also failed to detect changes in the ratios of proteins following convulsions induced by various chemical agents. There was a slight increase in the amount of ^{32}P incorporated into phosphoproteins (Vladimirov 1953) and of ^{35}S-methionine (Palladin et al. 1957, Pogodaev 1954).

In the following sections we shall report on rather different results. For example, the spectrum of soluble cerebral proteins had altered in the neighborhood of tumors of the cerebrum (Kaps 1954) in several cases of idiopathic epilepsy (Kiyota 1961), in cerebral oedema (Kiyota 1959), in artificially elevated intracranial pressure (Ogata 1954) and in several cases of leucoencephalitis (Karcher et al. 1959). There are still no results to provide definite evidence of protein changes during psychotic episodes (Gjessing 1938, 1953, 1968, Kety 1959, Lajtha 1964) similar to those found in psychomotor epilepsy. However, these authors point out that such changes may nevertheless occur.

Many early and also some more recent authors have discussed the *changes of serum proteins in epileptics;* we can only mention a few of these authors here (Empey et al. 1932, Georgi 1925, 1927, MacQuarrie 1927, 1929, 1932, MacQuarrie and Keith 1927, 1929, MacQuarrie and Peeler 1931, MacQuarrie et al. 1932, Neri 1934, Rizzotto 1934, Rizzotto and Martinengo 1934, Teglbjaerg 1935, 1936, etc.).

De Crinis (1924, 1925) was one of the first to discuss this problem. He found a shift in the fractions of serum proteins in epileptics in the interval between attacks. He introduced the concept of *the serological equivalent of epilepsy.* He and his school argue that an attack is due to *protein breakdown toxicosis* and they observed an increase of the coarsely disperse fractions of serum protein (the *globulins*) before an attack. Georgi (1925, 1927) was unable to confirm this with any certainty. He found a slight shift of *albumins* and he thought that colloidal instability may be responsible for provoking convulsions.

Fattovich (1931, 1934) found a 50 percent increase of globulins in epileptics and Martinengo (1932) obtained the same result from three of nine epileptics he examined. Both authors were concerned with the problem of psychosis and epilepsy and they related the protein changes in both groups to the similar symptomatologies. McKenzie and McChesney (1935) observed a fall of globulins for 36 hours atfer the attack. This means that there is an increase in the *albumin/globulin quotient (A/G quotient).* These authors found nothing unusual during the intervals.

In 20 cases with epilepsy Contini (1936 b) found that during attack-free periods total protein and *fibrinogen* were slightly elevated and globulins were normal. Albumin was considerably reduced and the A/G quotient was always lower. This picture changed after an attack.

However, Frisch (1937) and Frisch and Fried (1927) reported an increase of albumins. These authors found that it was possible to reduce the predisposition to convulsion by artificially increasing the globulin level.

Lennox and Allen (cited by Klimes and Lang 1942) examined 100 epileptics and in 34 cases they found more *fibrin;* they attributed this either to increased breakdown of plasma proteins or to a disorder of liver function. Eeg-Olofsson (1940) also observed a slight increase of total protein in serum in epileptics; globulins showing the greatest change.

Klimes and Lang (1942) examined blood serum from 27 epileptics, usually during the interparoxysmal phase (before and after therapy). They based their findings on the international determinations (total protein in serum 7 to 8%; total albumins 4.9%; total globulins 2.7%); according to these figures, on average, albumin represents 62 to 65 percent of total serum protein and globulin 25 percent. In 20 of 27 patients they found an elevated level of globulin with no reduction of colloid-osmotic pressure of protein in serum.

In the 1950s, efforts were redoubled in the field of serum protein research in epileptics. Pasolini and Dede (1956) found an increase in the alpha-globulin fraction in epileptics. In the same year, Jantz (1956) reported a fall of albumins and increased globulins in traumatic psychomotor epilepsy (Figure 23). In the same year again, Honda (1956) carried out similar studies, but did not find any shift in the protein fractions in cryptogenic epilepsy.

Krupenina (1960) studied large number of epileptics by refractometry and electrophoresis. She examined 68 patients (28 men and 40 women) between 18 and 50 years of age and compared findings from these patients with those from 30 healthy test subjects between 18 and 40 years of age. Twenty-two of the epileptics were in hospital for the first time (10 cryptogenic and 12 symptomatic) and the other patients had already received treatment (usually intermittently with *Luminal*).

In the interval between attacks (Table II) there was a slight elevation of total serum protein, a reduction of the albumin fraction and an increase of the globulin fraction, and so the A/G quotient was reduced. Compared with symptomatic epilepsy (19 cases), there was a noticeable increase of α_1- and β-globulins in essential epilepsy (24 patients) although the gamma-globulins were not significantly reduced.

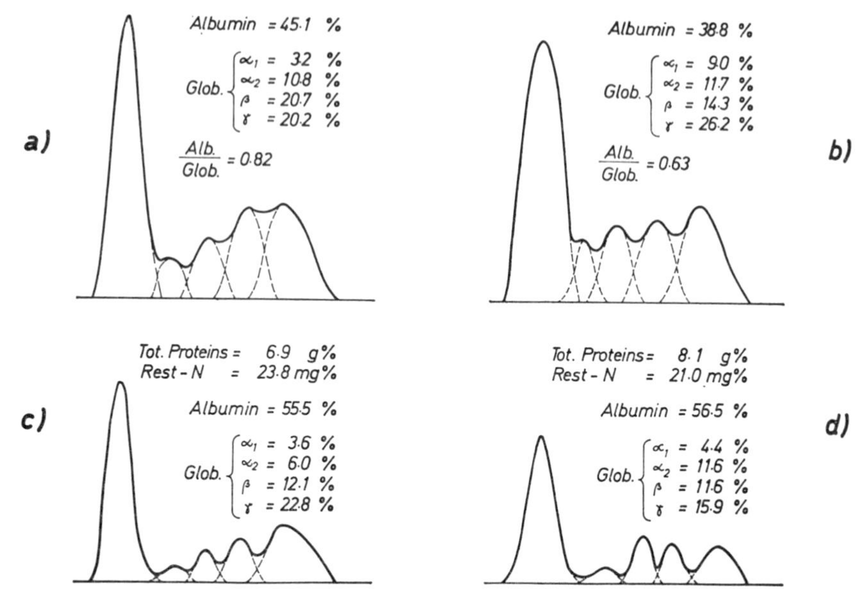

Figure 23. Comparson of changes in total proteins, albumins and globulins and serum globulin fractions in epileptics and various psychotic states. a) Serum electrophoresis in a patient with psychomotor epilepsy; b) Serum electrophoresis in an alcoholic in a state of delirium tremens; c) Serum electorphoresis in a manic patient in a state of agitation; d) Serum electrophoresis in a patient during catatonic excitation. (From Jantz, H.: *Nervenarzt, 27*:193-203, 1956.)

To summarize all the results which are known to us: 1.) in the vast majority of cases total serum proteins show a slight *increase* or tendency to increase in the interval between epileptic attacks; 2.) there is a significant fall of albumins, a substantial fall in the A/G quotient and the percentage of α_1- and α_2-globulins is substantially *increased;* 3.) according to some authors, in essential epilepsy α_1-, α_2- and β-globulins are higher and albumins lower than the corresponding values in symptomatic epilepsy.

Jovanović (1970 e, 1971 b) has examined a number of patients who suffered from epileptic attacks and has focused his attention *on the forms of attack.* Serum electrophoresis showed that there is a slight increase in serum protein, a substantial fall in the albumin fraction, an increase of *alpha-* or *beta*-globulins and a fall in the A/G quotients in *patients with psychomotor epilepsy,* and these values differed significantly from those in other forms of epilepsy. Patients with centrencephalic forms of epilepsy mostly had values which were normal or only slightly changed, while patients with diffuse epilepsy showed changes more like those found in the psychomotor form of attack. The serum protein fractions changed noticeably in patients with a tendency to develop an epileptic state, prolonged twilight attacks or psychotic episodes (Figure 24).

TABLE II. Means and ranges of variation of serum proteins and protein fractions in epileptics in the interval between attacks, before and after the attacks. (From L.B. Krupenina, 1960.)

Groups of Patients		*Number of Patients*	*Total Proteins*	*Albumins %*	*Globulins in %*				*A/G Quotients*
					α_1	α_2	β	γ	
Healthy people (Kontrol)		30	7.0±0.09 (6.47–8.1)	57.2±0.6 (51.8–63.9)	2.95±0.2 (1.7–5.0)	8.8±0.3 (6.5–11.5)	12.4±0.35 (10.0–15.3)	18.5±0.8 (15.8–20.9)	1.34±0.04 (1.07–1.7)
Epileptics (Interval)		22	7.9±0.1 (6.47–9.1)	47.1±1.0 (36.3–56.8)	6.7±0.49 (2.8–11.8)	11.1±0.5 (5.2–15.5)	14.0±0.5 (8.3–19.8)	21.1±0.7 (14.6–28.9)	0.91±0.2 (0.57–1.31)
Kind of Epilepsy	Cryptogenic	24	7.7±0.1 (6.57–8.9)	46.0±1.2 (36.3–56.8)	6.7±0.5 (3.8–11.9)	11.97±0.4 (8.0±19.8)	14.2±0.5 (8.1–19.8)	21.0±0.7 (15.1–29.5)	0.86±0.4 (0.57–1.31)
	Symptomatic	19	7.9±0.2 (6.5–9.1)	49.5±1.0 (40.9–55.8)	5.5±0.5 (2.6–11.1)	10.10±0.47 (5.2–13.7)	12.8±0.5 (8.3–18.7)	22.1–0.7 (18.4–28.9)	0.99±0.15 (0.69–1.25)
Preparoxysmal phase		18	7.8±0.1 (6.57–9.1)	44.4±0.9 (36.8–52.6)	7.8±0.6 (3.8–12.7)	12.3±0.5 (9.4–15.9)	13.6±0.4 (8.9–16.4)	21.8±0.9 (15.1–28.9)	0.8±0.1 (0.58–1.09)
Postparoxysmal phase		18	7.78±0.06 (6.4–8.9)	50.1±1.0 (43.6–57.6)	5.4±0.6 (2.6–9.8)	10.5±0.5 (6.4–13.2)	13.9±0.7 (10.0–24.2)	19.8±0.7 (19.8–0.7)	1.02±0.1 (0.6–1.35)

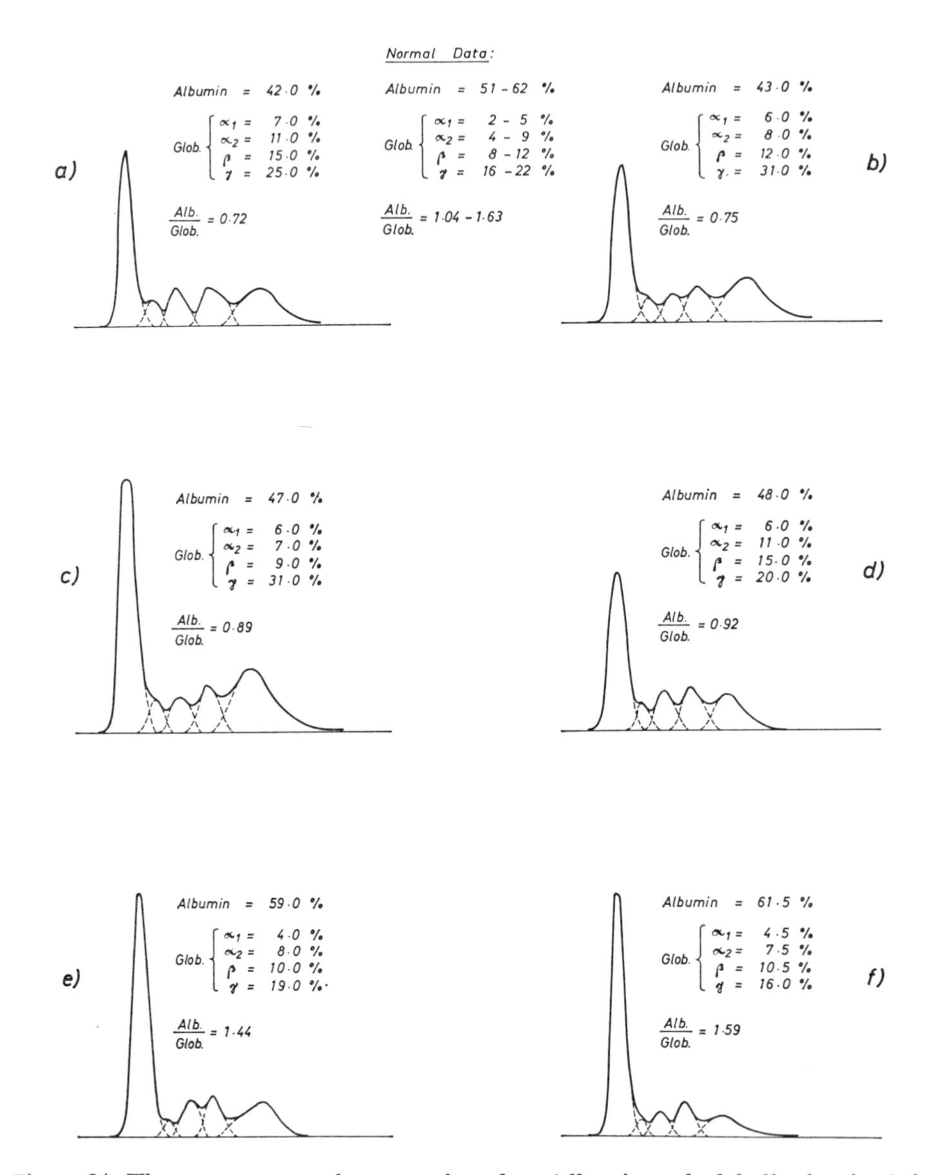

Figure 24. The top two rows show protein values (albumin and globulin fractions) in four patients with psychomotor epilepsy. In all cases albumin concentration is depressed, globulin fractions elevated (particularly alpha- and beta-globulins) and the albumin/globulin quotient is lower in the serum-electrophoregram. Results in the bottom row are from two epileptics with other forms of epilepsy. There are no serum protein changes in these patients (our own results).

Gamma-globulin fractions were elevated in cases where the serum was examined shortly before an attack. Once again there were differences between the centrencephalic group of epilepsies (where the values were much nearer the norm) and the temporocephalic forms, including psychomotor epilepsy.

Amino Acids

In the last 10 to 15 years there has been intensive research into some of the amino acids and their relation to epilepsy and, in particular, psychomotor epilepsy. However, these studies can only progress slowly since it is not really possible to examine amino acids in living human subjects, and it is known that symptoms induced in experimental animals by withdrawal or administration of some of these amino acids are not always comparable in every respect to psychomotor symptoms in man. Also, the content of natural amino acids in the brain varies considerably from species to species (Table III) and this means that the experimental procedure itself is fairly difficult (Minz 1965).

The level of free amino acid in the CNS differs considerably from that in other organs. The principal amino acids are *glutamic acid (GA)* and *aspartic acid. N-Acetyl-aspartic acid, gamma-aminobutyric acid (GABA)* and (in the human brain) *cystathionine* do not occur in any other tissue (Seiler 1966, Tallan et al. 1958).

Half of the amino acids (lysine, leucine, glutamic acid, methionine and tyrosine) are either bound, metabolized or removed from the brain *in less than one hour* (half-life) (Appel et al. 1960, Chirigos et al. 1966). This *half-life* is important experimentally since it must be related to the symptoms of the epileptic attacks.

Physiologically, amino acids have a very important part to play in the CNS. About 50 percent of the amino acid nitrogen in the brain is derived from *glutamic acid, glutamine* and *glutathion*—a petide containing glutamine (Seiler 1966). It has already been pointed out that the blood-brain barrier is usually permeable to amino acids, (Markova 1966, Seiler 1966), although there are some results which contradict this statement. Firstly, using the intravenous (i.v.) route, in experimental animals the symptoms of epilepsy could not be induced by convulsant amino acids, nor could phenomena induced by other means be inhibited by anticonvulsant amino acids (Health and Guerrero Figueroa 1965, Sinclair 1962, Wiechert and Herbst 1966). Hence, experimentally the appropriate amino acids were administered intracysternally (i.c.). Also, most of the amino acids are produced in the CNS itself and they are not supplied by the blood. About 90 percent of the GA is synthesized in the brain (Roberts et al. 1959).

TABLE III. Free amino acid concentrations in the brain of a number of experimental animals (micromol/g fresh weight) (From Singh, S.I., and L. Malhotra: *J Neurochem, 9:* 37, 1962; Stein, W.H., and S. Moore: *J Bol Chem, 211:*915, 1954; Wealsch, H.: In *Neurochemistry.* Thomas, Springfield, 1962.)

	Glu	*Glu* NH_3	*Asp*	*Asp-* NH_2	*N-Acetyl-Asp*	*γ-Amino-butiryc acid*	*Gly*	*Ala*	*Val*	*Leu*	*Ileu*	*Phe*
Cat (Total brain)	8.7	3.4	2.2	0.1	6.0	2.3	1.3	1.0	0.18	0.14	0.09	0.07
Rat (Total brain)	10.0	4.0	—	—	5.0	2.0	1.3	0.6	1.0	0.2	—	0.06
Rhesus		25.0	2.65			1.61						
Frontal lobe		26.0	2.65			1.87						
Temporal lobe		26.6	2.71			1.69						
Amygdala		23.2	2.89			1.65						
Hippocampus		17.7	2.79			1.96						
Hypothalamus		23.3	3.12			1.70						
Cerebellum	0.02		—	—	—	—	0.2	0.34	0.2	0.11	0.05	0.042
Plasma (Micro-	to						to	to	to	to	to	to
mol/ml)	0.08						0.26	0.43	0.32	0.18	0.1	0.06
	Tyr	*Try*	*His*	*Lys*	*Arg*	*Pro*	*Ser*	*Thr*	*Cys*	*Tau*	*Gluta-thion*	*Met*
Cat (Total brain)	0.06	—	0.06	0.14	0.08	0.14	0.72	0.22	0.1	2.0	0.9	0.1
Rat (Total brain)	0.1	0.03	0.08	0.02	0.2	—	1.1	1.0	—	—	—	0.08
Plasma	0.44	—	0.05	0.17	0.69	0.15	0.095	0.10	0.04	0.03	—	0.02
	to		to	to	to	to	to	to	to	to		to
	0.83		0.97	0.21	0.11	0.29	0.12	0.14	0.54	0.06		0.027

Glucose is one of the substances from which amino acids are synthesized in the brain. Most of the glucose (labelled with U-^{14}C) is not utilized directly but follows a pathway via the amino acids and hence is dissimilated in this way. More amino acids are synthesized in the CNS than in any other organ. A few minutes after ^{14}C-glucose injection, most of the glucose carbon is incorporated in amino acids, mainly in the GA, aspartic acid, alanine and GABA (Gaitonde et al. 1965, Vrba et al. 1962, Seiler 1966). CO_2 is also incorporated into the amino acids in the CNS; it is fixed by *pyruvic acid* (Bertl 1962, Moldave et al. 1953). Here we once again meet up with *pyridoxine,* which was discussed in Chapter III. Non-essential amino acids of the brain are synthesized from glucose with the aid of pyruvic acid and pyridoxine. Most amino acids can be converted into specific *alpha-ketonic acids.* The transaminases which catalyse this reaction contain heavy metal ions and pyridoxal phosphate (a phosphoric acid ester of Vitamin B_6) in the cofactor. *The amino group is transferred from glutamic acid to pyruvic acid.* Further metabolic reactions produce *alanine* from pyruvic acid and *alpha-ketoglutaric acid* from glutamic acid. In its turn, alpha-ketoglutaric acid may accept the amino group from other amino acids or bind *ammonia* in a reducing reaction (Dingman and Sporn 1959, Sporn et al. 1959, Waelsch 1962). We shall frequently mention these transaminases and glutamic acid dehydrogenase. These enzymes are considered to be responsible for many of the metabolic disorders is psychomotor epilepsy.

Both glutamic acid and gamma-aminobutyric acid are involved in the *tricarboxylic acid cycle.* A subsidiary pathway in this cycle leads from alpha-ketoglutaric acid to *succinic acid* (Figure 25).

As Figure 25 shows, GABA is very much involved in this series of reactions. On this pathway, via succinic acid, it can be oxidized to CO_2 and H_2O. The diagram shows that GABA is produced from glutamic acid by *decarboxylation.* The endogenous amines (which we shall be discussing later) can also be produced from amino acids via this pathway (Markova 1966, McIlwain 1951, 1953 a to c, McIlwain et al. 1952, McKhann et al. 1960, Müller and Langemann 1952, Pisano et al. 1957, Sporn et al. 1959, Tallan 1957).

In the last few years, the interest of research workers and biochemists studying enzyme and neural transmitters has been centered on *GA* and *GABA.*

There is still discussion on whether *glutamic acid,* in the form of its derivative GABA, has any effect in epilepsy (Health and Guerrero-Figueroa 1965, Seiler 1966, Wiechert and Herbst 1966) or whether there are perhaps other possibilities here. The success of treatment with GA and GABA varies. This variation must be attributed to the state of the blood-brain barrier. Since elevation of the serum levels of glutamic acid and GABA does not

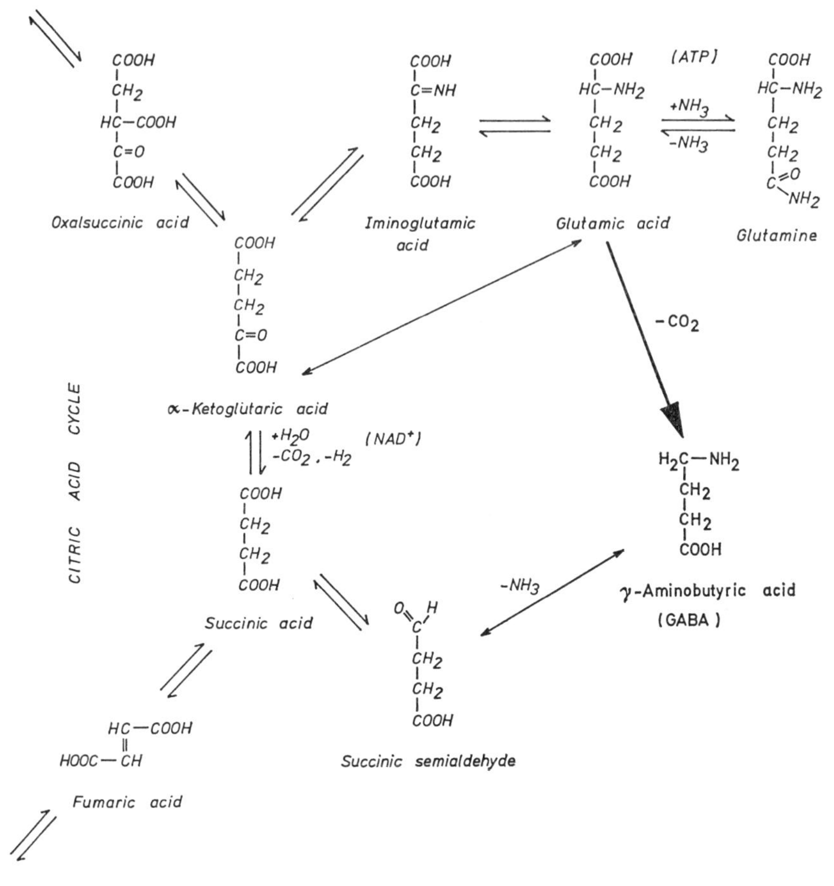

Figure 25. Gamma-aminobutyric acid shunt and GABA metabolism. Here, pyridoxal acts as the decarboxylase coenzyme. (From Seiler, N.: *Der Stoffwechsel im Zentralnervensystem*. Thieme, Stuttgart, 1966.)

cause an increase of these amino acids in the brain, it is assumed that these compounds can only assist patients in whom the blood-brain barrier is already injured (Albert et al. 1951, Chain 1959, Health and Guerrero-Figueroa 1965, Markova 1966, Sinclair 1962, Wiechert and Herbst 1966). Weil-Malherbe (1936 to 1962) and Weil-Malherbe et al. (1959, 1961) studied the problem of GA and GABA over nearly two decades and they believe that GA exerts its effect by *specific stimulation* of the synaptic nervous system. Various autonomic symptoms following administration of GA indicate that this amino acid has an adrenaline-like action, and there was a rise of adrenaline in plasma following administration of GA (Meyer-Gross and Walker 1949, Takashima et al. 1964, Weil-Malherbe 1950, Seiler 1966).

Like the endogenous amines and *substance P,* which is not yet fully understood, GABA has also been implicated in synaptic transmission (see Chapter IV) (Dale 1953, Eccles 1957, 1964, Fatt and Katz 1951, Feldberg 1950, Nachmansohn 1955, Seiler 1966). GABA proved to be one of the membrane stabilizers. It is found in the cortex, cerebellum and, in particular in the hippocampus. According to some authors (Mison-Crighel et al., 1964, 1965), its action is not as *intense* as that of some of its derivatives, for example *gamma-amino-beta-hydroxybutyric acid* and *gamma-amino-butyrylcholine.* There are changes in the glutamate-glutamine system of the cortex which appear to be attributable mainly to the reduction of GABA and glutamic acid (not always in parallel). According to Caspers (1957), GABA has a homeostatic effect on the cortical potential in cathodic polarization and as an *inhibitory transmitter* (Guerrero-Figueroa et al. 1964) it has an inhibitory effect on the transmission of stimuli. It is not so much its absolute concentration as the relative proportion in the acetylcholine-GABA ratio which causes this (Roberts and Baxter 1960). Since GABA also affects the potassium-sodium ratio, it has a normalizing and activating effect on O_2 utilization. Thus it also has a favorable effect on intracellular processes, and on the production of energy by oxidation which is the basic factor in stabilizing the nerve cell membrane and in the repolarization process. Hence, administration of GABA influences a number of physiological biochemical processes in the CNS, both in animals and in man.

The results which Price et al. (1943) obtained by treating patients with petit mal with glutamic acid stimulated a lively discussion. Glutamine and asparagine were also investigated for their therapeutic effect in epilepsy (Tower 1955, 1956, 1960). In animal experiments, additional administration of *L-asparagine* or *ATP* corrected the decline in the level of GABA. It was possible to prevent convulsive episodes by administering *methionine* (Reiner et al. 1950) or injecting *L-asparagine* or *glutamine* (Tower 1960). For example, in mice these amino acids were capable of preventing attacks induced by methionine sulphoximine, *Megimide, Metrazol* (Hawkins and Sarett 1957) or by strychnine (McLenan 1957). The inhibitory effect on convulsions induced by *methionine sulphoxide, methionine sulphoximine, Megimide®, Metrazol® or strychnine,* following administration of methionine glutamine, ATP or L-asparagine (Kreindler 1965, Mison-Crighel et al. 1962, Reiner et al. 1950, Selbach et al. 1965) must be due to an antagonistic effect which these amino acids exert against these particular convulsant agents.

According to these authors, methionine sulphoxide and methionine sulphoximine have a powerful antagonistic effect on methionine and GA (see also Chapter III). The synthesis of glutamine from glutamic acid in brain preparations can be blocked by methionine sulphoxide and methionine sulphoximine. Further inhibition can be produced by incorporating methionine into cerebral proteins. It is assumed that methionine sulphoxide and methionine sulphoximine exert their convulsant action by influencing intermediate stages in the metabolism of glutamic acid and methionine (Braganca et al. 1953, Heathcote 1949, Heathcote and Page 1950, Kolousek and Lodin 1959, Kühnau 1952, Pace and McDermott 1952, Peters and Tower 1959, Selbach et al. 1965).

We must now examine more closely some of the extremely important experiments which have been carried out with these amino acids in relation to psychomotor epilepsy, and this will provide further opportunities for discussion. Of course, it is not possible to confine our remarks simply to the biochemical processes which take place in the interval, and we shall have to deal with certain points relating to the attack itself.

Iwama and Jasper (1957) observed the normal superficial negative responses to electrical and chemical stimulation of the cerebral cortex under the action of GABA, and they established that this amino acid has an *inhibitory effect* on such brain potentials. Killam (1957) and Killam and Bain (1957) were able to induce convulsions in rats by intravenous administration of *hydrazine derivatives* including *isoniazid (INH)*. However, they were also able to demonstrate that *the attacks are accompanied by a fall in the cerebral concentration of GABA,* while the level of other amino acids is hardly affected. As compared with INH, other convulsant substances provoked rather different biochemical responses, although in both cases there was a fall of the GABA concentration in the brain. It is assumed that the drugs used do not themselves have convulsant properties but that they disrupt the synthesis of GABA. This produces convulsions due to deficiency of an amino acid responsible for preventing convulsions. The GABA deficiency may possibly also be due to increased utilization of this amino acid. This would in fact lead to a relative reduction in the concentration of GABA although there would have been no absolute fall in concentration (Sinclair 1960, 1962). This problem has yet to be solved (see also Chapter VIII).

Sinclair (1960) was able to trigger attacks in experimental animals by intraventricular injection of high doses of isoniazid. These attacks could be prevented by high doses of pyridoxine (parenteral or intraventricular). In 1962, Sinclair published a further report on the action of INH. He was able to induce typical tonic-clonic attacks in animal experiments by injecting INH into the lateral ventricle. The convulsions induced were unilateral and affected the contralateral side of the body. Like Green et al. (1957), the author assumed that these convulsions were *a result of stimulation of the rhinencephalon.* The colored injection fluid was found in one of the lateral ventricles during the animal autopsy. Convulsions following

INH could be prevented by injecting very high doses of GABA intraperitoneally. As mentioned above, GA and GABA are only effective by parenteral (but extracerebral) administration when the blood-brain barrier is damaged (see also Elliot and Jasper 1959, Quadbeck 1962). Sinclair (1962) assumes that the polythene cannulas he used (which were inserted into the animals' ventricles to administer the INH) damaged the blood-brain barrier to such an extent that GABA given by intraperitoneal injection was capable of influencing cerebral activity. Before Sinclair, Dasgupta et al. (1958) had already shown that an intraventricular injection of GABA also prevents hippocampal convulsions following isoniazid.

Much earlier than this, Cravioto et al. (1951) had demonstrated that both epileptic and hypoglycaemic convulsions in experimental animals are associated with *a fall in the cerebral concentration of free GABA*. Since both conditions (epileptic and hypoglycaemic convulsions) are characterized by a reduction of free GABA in the brain, one tends to assume that here we are dealing with a disorder of glucose and GABA metabolism (Chain 1959, Sinclair 1962). As mentioned above, most of the GABA is synthesized from glucose. Where there is an inadequate level of glucose, hypoglycaemic convulsions may be the result of a deficiency of GABA rather than the direct result of the hypoglycaemia.

Health and Guerrero-Figueroa (1965) used permanent electrodes implanted in the deeper cerebral structures in people with psychomotor epilepsy and schizophrenia to monitor the bioelectrical cerebral activity, and they were able to study some of the inhibitory effects of GABA. These anticonvulsant effects were weaker when this amino acid was introduced into the septum.

Wiechert and Herbst (1966) carried out 110 experiments on male and female dogs. They found that a tonic-clonic convulsion occurred when they injected the animals with glutamic acid. The convulsions were related to dose. Injection of a 0.2 m.molar solution elicited mild salivation after about 20 minutes, but there were no convulsions. Intracisternal injection of a 0.3 m.mol. solution of GA always induced facial convulsion after about 20 or 30 minutes and this effect was still apparent up to 24 or 36 hours after administration. This period coincides almost exactly with the fall of glutamic acid in cerebral fluid. Very high doses (of up to 0.6 m.mol.) produced spontaneous tonic-clonic cerebral convulsions preceded by facial myoclonia. These attacks finally led to status epilepticus, and unless the animals were treated, they died after one to two hours. Attacks in the facial region were accompanied by mydriasis, marked salivation, very localized coordination disorders and opisthotonus.

Aspartic acid had much less effect than glutamic acid. There were no symptoms of attacks or increased predisposition to convulsion following injection of other amino acids, such as *leucine, methionine, norvaline, valine, ATP, pyridoxine* or of isotonic saline solution.

According to Wiechert and Herbst, there were dose-related attacks following injection of *pyridoxal-5-phosphate (PYP or PAL)*. These attacks occurred after injection of a 0.03 m.mol. solution as well as after a 0.4 m.mol. solution of GA. A dose of 0.3 m.mol. PYP produced status epilepticus. The attacks were mitigated if a very high dose of GABA was administered intravenously after intracisternal injection of GA or PYP. However, if GABA was also given intracisternally, the attacks could be eliminated completely. EEGs taken at the same time correlated with the chemically induced convulsions.

At first sight these responses are rather surprising and the authors tried to explain them. They assumed that there must be an equilibrium between GA and GABA in the brain and two very important cerebral processes are involved in maintaining this equilibrium: one is the decarboxylation of glutamic acid to GABA by *glutamic acid decarboxylase,* and the other is a reversible transamination of GABA via succinate semialdehyde and alpha-ketoglutaric acid, to glutamic acid (Mellick and Bassett 1964, Roberts and Bregoff 1953, Roberts et al. 1953, Sugiura 1957) by *gamma-aminobutyryl-alpha-hydroxyglutarate transaminase (GABAT)*. Both enzymes utilize PYP as the coenzyme and the apoenzyme of GABAT shows a great affinity for PYP. The attacks follow a decline in the activity of glutamic acid decarboxylase (GAD) and result in a fall in the level of GABA which would be expected to exert an inhibitory effect.

According to Wiechert and Herbst (1966) the lack of a regulatory system for the excited neurons possibly leads to uncontrolled dissemination of the bioelectrical impulses. These authors quote Elliot and van Gelder (1958), who have discussed the extent to which GA and GABA may be neurophysiologically active substances. These authors also stressed that there must be an equilibrium between GA and GABA in the brain where there is a normal physiological balance between activity and inhibition. Karmin and Karmin (1961) also assume that an increase of GA concentration in the brain does not necessarily lead to an increase of GABA, since intracisternal injection of GA does not increase the GABA concentration. This may well explain why epileptic attacks can also be induced by GA. According to Wiechert and Herbst (1966), GA also has a direct and specific convulsant effect.

This may possibly be explained by marked, non-physiological changes in the equilibrium between glutamic acid and GABA. The increase in the symptoms of an attack after increasing the dose of GA and the occurrence of attacks similar to those which arise following injection of PYP, support the idea that the equilibrium between glutamic acid and GA is of definite physiological importance and that the attacks occur when this equilibrium is disrupted. The greater affinity of the apoenzymes of GABAT for PYP which increases the transamination reactions, results in a fall in the level of GABA in the brain and a rise in the GA concentration. The attacks can be controlled by preserving the equilibrium between these two amino acids, or by restoring the equilibrium when it has been upset. In this study, Wiechert and Herbst (1966) used GABA to restore the equilibrium which had been upset by GA, and this either prevented or alleviated the attacks.

These authors considered that the attacks produced by GA were of the *temporal type* since the oral symptoms in experimental animals following administration of GA or PYP are very similar to the oral phenomenology in human patients with psychomotor attacks.

The Endogenous Amines

We would now like to deal with some of the more important aspects of the problem of the endogenous amines and epilepsy.

Phenylalanine is known to be the *precursor* of many of these amines. An adult's daily requirement of this amino acid is 0.8 to 1.1 gram (Rose et al. 1955), and most of this is needed for protein synthesis. The remainder may be metabolized in many ways (Seiler 1966). It has not yet been established for certain whether all, or most of these reactions take place in the CNS.

As shown in Figure 26a, the most important metabolic pathway for phenylalanine is hydrolysis to *tyrosine*. This was postulated by Neubauer as early as 1909, and confirmed a few years later by Embden and Baldes (1913). However, it was not possible to demonstrate the appropriate phenylalanine hydrolase in the brain (Seiler 1966, Udenfriend and Coper 1952). The publications of Kaufmann and his colleagues (Kaufmann 1957 a, b, 1958 to 1963, Kaufmann et al. 1962) revived interest in the hydroxylation of phenylalanine. Two protein fractions are involved in the hydroxylation of phenylalanine to tyrosine: the first catalyses the hydroxylation reaction and the second protein fraction is needed to reduce the cofactor oxidized in the course of the first reaction (Kaufmann et al. 1962, Takashima et al. 1954).

Many authors have studied the pathway from tyrosine to the catecholamines in great detail (Blaschko 1939, 1942, Blaschko and Welch 1953, Gurin and Delluva 1945, Kirshner and McGoodall 1957 a, b, Leeper and Udenfriend 1956, Udenfriend et al. 1953, Udenfriend and Wyngaarden 1956, Vogt 1954). From the results it appears that hydrolysis of tyrosine produces *3,4-dihydroxyphenylalanine (DOPA)*. The enzyme which catalyzes this reaction is as yet unknown, but it is reminiscent of phenylalanine hydroxylase (Nagatsu et al. 1954, Nellhaus 1965). It would appear that

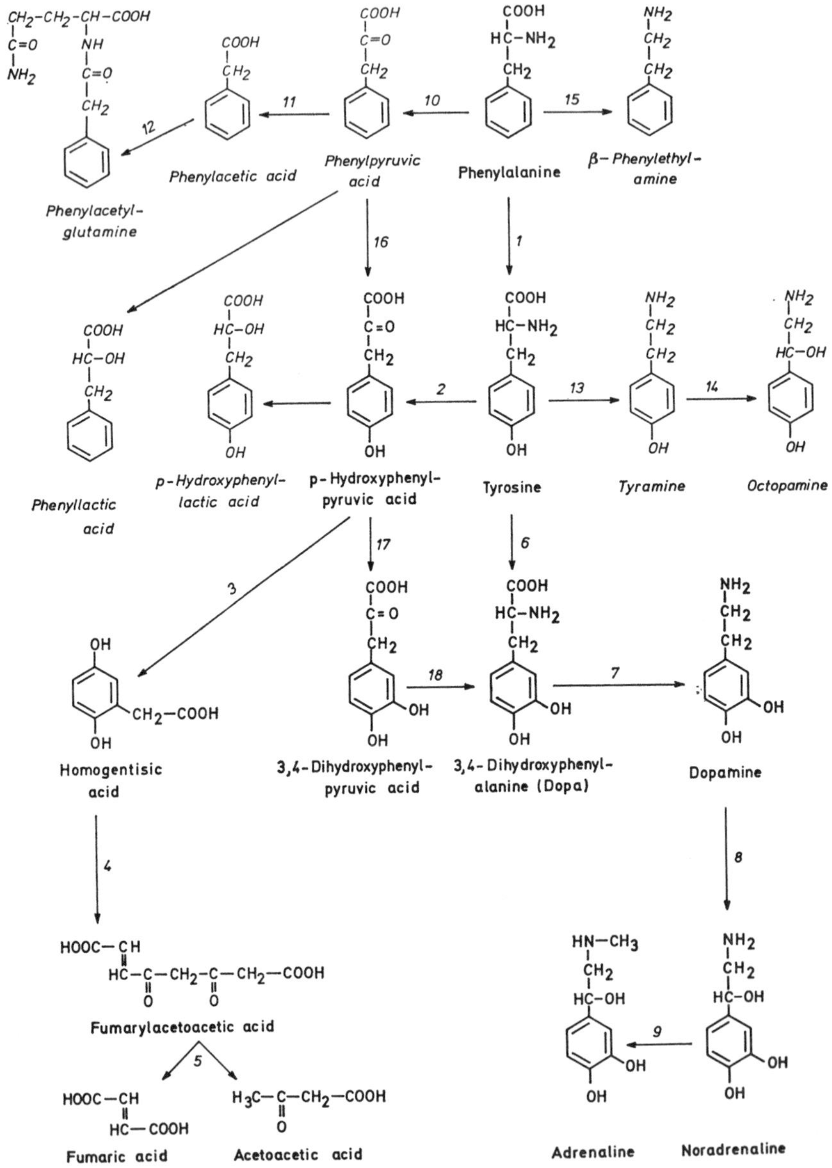

Figure 26a. The metabolic reactions of phenylalanine. (From Seiler, N.: *Der Stoffwechsel im Zentralnervensystem.* Thieme, Stuttgart, 1966.)

decarboxylation of 3,4 dihydroxyphenylalanine to *3,4-dihydroxy-beta-phenylethylanine (dopamine)* is catalyzed by a non-specific L-amino acid decarboxylase (Holtz and Heise 1938, Holtz and Westermann 1956). The same decarboxylase may also be capable of converting other aromatic L-amino acids into the corresponding amines (Seiler 1966). Pyridoxal phosphate is the coenzyme of this decarboxylase (Erspamer et al. 1961, Lorenberg et al. 1962, Werle and Aures 1959).

DOPA-decarboxylase can be found in the adrenals and other organs and in the brain (Holtz and Westermann 1956). For example, tyrosine may be hydroxylated in the brain itself. The *dopamine* produced in this way is converted into *noradrenaline* by steric hydroxylation of the side chain with the aid of beta-hydroxylase. The reaction is associated with utilization of *ascorbic acid, fumaric acid* and molecular oxygen (Kirshner 1959, Seiler 1966). According to Seiler (1966), Tower (1956) and Udenfriend and Wyngaarden (1956), beta-hydroxylase is also largely non-specific. Apart from dopamine, other beta-phenylethylamines can also be converted into the corresponding beta-phenylethanolamines. From this it would appear that noradrenaline could also be produced from *tyramine* via *octopamine*. However, this possibility has not been confirmed (Tower 1956, Udenfriend and Wyngaarden 1956), although it is interesting to note here that beta-hydroxylase has a very high activity in the hypothalamus and caudate nucleus while these regions show a low noradrenaline content (Udenfriend and Creveling 1959).

Quantitatively, methylation of noradrenaline to *Adrenaline* is not a particularly important process in the CNS, and it probably occurs in other organs ad systems. The N-methyl group of Adrenaline is derived from methionine. S-adenosyl-methionine is first produced from methionine and ATP, and the methyl group of S-adenosyl-methionine is then transferred to a series of beta-phenyl-ethanolamines by the enzyme phenyl-aminoethanol-N-methyl transferase (Axelrod 1962, Elmadjian et al. 1956, von Euler and Gaddum 1931, Keller et al. 1950, Kirshner and McGoodall 1957, Minz 1965, Seiler 1966).

It is possible that Adrenaline may be produced from phenylpyruvic acid which is hydrolysed by an intermediate reaction to 3,4-dihydroxyphenyl-pyruvic acid. This compound may then be converted into DOPA (Pogrund et al. 1955, 1961).

These endogenous *amines are involved in the pathogenesis of epilepsy* in many different ways, some of which will be discussed in Chapter IX. If phenylalanine is not metabolised in the way described above, this may produce a condition which includes epileptic manifestations. This condition, *phenylketonuria* or Fölling's disease, is known to occur in children. Phenylalanine is transaminated in the body to produce large quantities of phenylpyruvic acid. In phenylketonuria, which is frequently associated with imbecility, a whole range of partially metabolized products of phenylalanine is found in blood and urine (Armstrong and Robinson 1955, Boscott and Bickel 1953, Fölling 1934, Stein et al. 1954). The concentration of phenylalanine *in the blood* may reach 20 to 60 mg. in 100 ml.

(normally 10 mg. in 100 ml.). The enzyme which hydrolyses phenylalanine to tyrosine is absent in patients with phenylketonuria. However, a certain amount of tyrosine is still produced from phenylalanine which probably means that small quantities of the enzyme concerned are still present in some of the organs (Fellman and Devlin 1958, Jervis 1953, Udenfriend and Bessmann 1953, Wallace et al. 1957).

Epilepsy, particularly primary petit mal epilepsy, is often observed in addition to the *oligophrenia.* A secondary psychomotor form also develops. The electroencephalogram is nearly always abnormal or pathological with signs of convulsion elements (CE). The abnormalities are even more profound in the nocturnal EEG (Gross and Schulte 1968, Hsia et al. 1957, Sutherland et al. 1960). The pathogenesis of the disease is a major problem. The hypothesis that phenylalanine and many intermediate compounds would inhibit the activity of higher nerve centers (Woolf and Vulliamy 1951) may help to explain the mental retardation, but not the epilepsy. According to Allen and Schroder (1957), the disorders are caused by abnormally large amounts of phenylalanine being incorporated into body proteins due to the vast quantities of phenylalanine present.

A phenylalanine-free diet improves the clinical picture, reduces the number of epileptic attacks, and the abnormal biochemical processes disappear (Armstrong and Tyler 1955, Brickel et al. 1953, Paine et al. 1957, Sutherland et al. 1960, Woolf and Vulliamy 1951, Woolf et al. 1955, Woolf and van der Hoeven 1964, Wright and Tarjan 1957). The diagnosis may be made from this.

We must pay particular attention to the fall in the serum levels of Adrenaline and noradrenaline in these patients (Sourkes and D'Irio 1963, Weil-Malherbe 1955). A fall in the serum level of *gamma-aminobutyric acid* has also been demonstrated; this is a result of inhibition of the enzyme glutamic acid decarboxylase (Hanson 1958, Tashian 1961). Both of these facts are interesting. Inhibition of the biogenesis of *catecholamines* results in a deficiency of the anticonvulsant substances—Adrenaline and noradrenaline. The reduced level of GABA also has a convulsant effect, as we have seen above. The decline of GABA in phenylketonuria is actually regarded as the cause of the epileptic manifestations (see Minz 1965 and Seiler 1966).

However, there is yet another important factor involved in phenylketonuria. Serotonin may be implicated to some extent in the development of psychomotor epilepsy. However, in patients with phenylketonuria the concentration of serotonin is reduced because hydrolysis of trytophane is disrupted and metabolism of trytophane impaired (Armstrong and Robinson 1954, Baldridge et al. 1959, Berendes et al. 1958, Ferrari et al. 1955, Pare et al. 1957, Sandler and Close 1959). This may explain why another form of epilepsy—petit mal—is usually the first to appear in phenylketonuria, and psychomotor epilepsy only develops later as "the terminal stage, common to all forms of epilepsy" (Tellenbach 1965).

Dopamine, one of the intermediates in adrenaline synthesis, occurs in large amounts in the nucleus caudatus, putamen, pallidum, nucleus ruber and nucleus niger, and the level is not related to the concentration of DOPA and noradrenaline in the brain (Bertler and Rosengren 1959, Kanig 1969, 1971, Sano et al. 1960). Dopamine is of no immediate importance in epilepsy. It is known to have an effect in Parkinson's disease (Barbeau and Sourkes 1962, Bernheimer and Hornykiewicz 1965, Bernheimer et al. 1966, Denny-Brown 1960, Ehringer and Hornykiewicz 1960, Hassler 1938, 1953, Hornykiewicz 1962, Sorkes 1964), but epilepsy does not occur at the same time as or immediately after this disease. Probably serotonin and acetylcholine are also reduced and this limits the possible spread of hyperexcitation (see Chapter VIII).

We are still not quite certain as to the *importance of Adrenaline and noradrenaline in the pathogenesis of epilepsy* or their function in this respect.

We do not know for certain whether Adrenaline is synthesized in the brain. Apart from in the hypothalamus, the blood-brain barrier cannot be traversed by either Adrenaline or noradrenaline to any great extent (Seiler 1966, Weil-Malherbe et al. 1959, 1961). However, central effects can be induced by intravenous administration (Bonvallet et al. 1954, Jouvet 1960, Monnier 1969, Nelhaus 1965, Rothballer et al. 1956). Following topical administration of Adrenaline or noradrenaline, there was an immediate rise of blood pressure and other sympathicotonic responses (Minz and Noel 1963). The fact that Adrenaline is concentrated principally in the phylogenetically older parts of the brain is of the greatest significance in psychomotor epilepsy. From these areas Adrenaline causes desynchronization of the neocortex, an arousal reaction in experimental animals and in man, and in some instances agitation or aggressiveness (Cordeau et al. 1963, Hernández-Peón 1966, Sano 1960). The hypothalamus, the corpora quadrigemina region, the nucleus ruber, the septum pellucidum and the pons are all areas rich in Adrenaline (Jouvet 1969, 1972; Minz and Noel 1963), Around the pons, Adrenaline occurs primarily in the lateral nuclear regions.

Like the other endogenous amines, Adrenaline and noradrenaline are present *intra vitam* in the body, mainly in a bound state. There is a stable and a labile bound form, and this protects them from enzymatic attack. The CNS is also protected from any undesirable effects of these amines. The intracellular granules which store these amines and other neurogenic substances, are provided with a membrane so that to a certain extent these substances are *isolated* (Bertler et al. 1959, Blashko and Welch 1963, Eade

1958, Eliot and van Gelder 1958, Hillarp et al. 1953, Riley 1961, Whittaker 1959). The neurogenic and other active substances are stored in a temporarily inactive, bound state in the CNS and in the other organs (Burn and

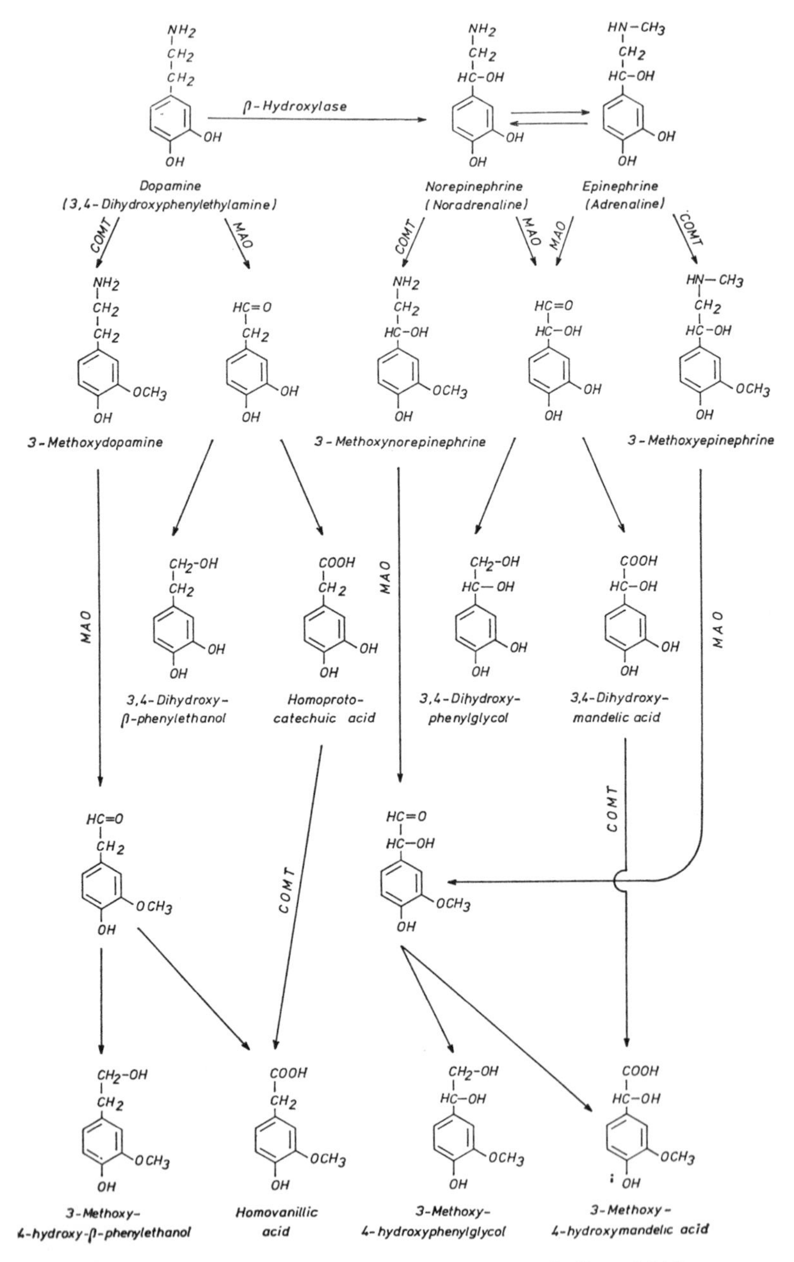

Figure 26b. Dopamine, noradrenaline and adrenaline metabolism. MAO = mono-amine-oxidase; COMT = Catechalamine — O — methyl-tranferase. From Seiler, N.: Der Staffwechsel im Zentralnervensystem, Thieme, Stuttgart, 1966).

Rand 1960, Butterworth and Mann 1957, von Euler and Hillarp 1956, Flack 1964, Koelle 1962).

Nearly all the endogenous amines (dopamine, noradrenaline, serotonin) are converted into a physiologically active chemical compound by the same enzyme—*monoamine oxidase (MAO)* (Figure 26b).

Serotonin is produced from 5-hydroxytryptophane (5-HTP) (Clark et al. 1954, Erspamer 1954, Udenfriend et al. 1953, Werle and Mennicken 1937). *Tryptophane,* the precursor of 5-HTP, can be hydrolized by the same hydrolase which converts phenylalanine into tyrosine. 5-Hydroxytryptophane is also formed in tissues which contain no phenylalanine hydrolase, e.g. in tumors and other pathological processes (Coper 1961, Coper and Melcer 1961, Dalgliesh and Dutton 1957, Gal et al. 1963, Renson et al. 1962, Schindler 1959, Seiler 1966). As we will mention later, 5-hydroxytryptophane can traverse the blood-brain barrier, where it can then be converted into 5-hydroxytryptamine (5-HT, serotonin). Table IV illustrates the serotonin content, and the activity of decarboxylases and monoamine oxidases (MAO) in different regions of the brain (see also Figure 26b).

This table shows that the activity of decarboxylase is not always high where the serotonin content is high. Thus, the serotonin content depends more on MAO activity than on the activity of decarboxylase. In the nuclei,

TABLE IV. 5-Hydroxy-tryptophan-decarboxylase and monoamine-oxidate activities and distribution of 5-hydroxytryptamine in the brain in dogs. (From Bogdansky, D.F., H. Weissbach, and S. Undenfriend. *J Neurochem, 1*:272, 1957.)

Region of brain	*Serotonin ($\mu g/g$)*	*Decarboxylase Activity Serotonin Production $\mu g/g$)*	*Monoaminoxydase Activity (Serotonin Degradation $\mu g/g$)*
Nucleus caudatus	0.72±0.2	306±37	935±200
Hypothalamus	1.7±0.3	117±25	1624±510
Septum pellucidum	1.5±0.4	109±24	1212± 58
Mesencephalon	1.0±0.2	98± 7	842±122
Thalamus	0.57±0.07	38± 7	940±164
Medulla oblongata	0.62±0.2	32± 3	1117±230
Pons	0.38±0.1	28± 7	936±110
Corp. amygdaloideum	2.1±0.4	18± 2	968± 23
Cortex pyriformis	0.94±0.08	16± 1	926±183
Hippocampus	0.64±0.04	16±3	1176± 38
Cerebellum	0.09	9	930± 87
Corpus geniculatum	—	7 to 8	707 to 844
Neocortex	0.27±0.04	7± 2	819±300
Tractus opticus	—	7± 3	701± 95
Bulbus olfactorius	0.35±0.04	5	573
Corpus callosum + Capsula interna	—	4± 1	466±120

where MAO is very active, serotonin is broken down immediately after it is released from the serotonergic neurons. Table IV also shows that the highest concentrations of serotonin are in the nucleus amygdalae, in the hypothalamus and in the septum pellucidum, i.e. in the areas which are responsible for producing psychomotor epilepsy. Monoamine oxidase activity is also high in these areas. We shall deal with all these points in Chapter VIII.

There has been much discussion on the role of serotonin in an epileptic episode and here we shall simply add a few remarks to what has already been said (Minz 1965). Both Hess (1948, 1956) and Monnier (1962) regard the autonomic part of the CNS as an *ergotropic* and a *trophotropic system* (see also Jovanović 1968 f). The *ergotropic* system is controlled by noradrenaline and the trophotropic system by serotonin (Brodie et al. 1959, Costa et al. 1962, Jouvet 1969, 1972; Monnier 1969). These two systems must be in functional equilibrim, with the trophotropic system dominant during sleep and the ergotropic system dominant in the waking state. The two systems can be examined independently by, for instance, first inhibiting MAO activity (using N-methyl-N-benzyl-propargylamine) and then simply releasing the noradrenaline in the brain (using alpha-methyl-m-tyrosine). This procedure induced a state of hyperexcitability in the test animals, indicating that autonomic function in the CNS had become *ergotropic*. However, if the level of serotonin is increased at the same time, motility is reduced and there is a tendency to trophotropism. If the level of serotonin is increased selectively, the experimental animals become mildly sedated, for example, there is a trophotropic effect (Costa et al. 1962, Matussek and Patschke 1964). Shortly after this, there is a phase of excitation which may develop into an attack (Funderbruk et al. 1962, Szimuzu et al. 1964). There have been some very contradictory results on the effects of serotonin, probably because it is not easy to release it selectively or to activate it in some other way without invoking the effects of other endogenous amines.

Functionally, the next chemical substance–*acetylcholine (ACh)*–is as important as Adrenaline, and probably more important than serotonin. The cerebral concentration of acetylcholine, bioelectrical activity and the release of acetylcholine are all very closely related (McIlwain 1955, Minz 1965, Torda 1953, Tower 1960). While ACh in rat brain at rest is 1.25 mg/g., this concentration falls to 0.87 mg/g. after stimulation. Under deep anaesthesia, the acetylcholine concentration rises to 1.76 mg/g. (Feldberg 1957, Seiler 1966, Whittaker 1959).

In the CNS the preganglionic sympathetic, the parasympathetic and the motor fibres are all *cholinergic*. Thus, ACh acts as the *neurochemical transmitter* at the synapses or nerve endings. This has already been discussed in

Chapter IV. *Adrenaline and acetylcholine* have a very similar mode of action.

However, here we must stress that acetylcholine affects the nerve endings and motor end-plate, and also the whole length of the axon (Feldberg et al. 1940, Lacwenstein and Molins 1958, Nachmansohn 1962, Nachmansohn and Feld 1947). The course of events which produces excitation can be outlined as follows: Bound acetylcholine is released by an electrical or chemical stimulus. The free ACh reacts with the receptor protein (Seiler 1966) and this alters permeability of the membrane to ions. We have explained the rest in Chapter IV. The depolarizing effect of acetylcholine was demonstrated as early as 1940 (Feldberg et al. 1940). After exerting the depolarizing effect ACh is rapidly hydrolyzed to allow the membrane to repolarize.

There has been a great deal of discussion on the extent to which the activity of acteylcholinesterase (ACh-ase) is responsible for producing an epileptic attack. In the human epileptogenic focus in the temporal lobe, there is a very marked change in acetylcholine glutamate and electrolyte metabolism. In the interparoxysmal phase, epileptics show increased cholinesterase activity and an inability to bind acetylcholine. The same metabolic defect was found experimentally in the cortex of apes, dogs and rabbits when convulsive attacks were induced by methionine sulphoximine or Megimide (Kreindler 1965, Tower 1958 b, 1960). Clinical tests have shown that inability to bind acetylcholine can be corrected by administering glutamine, GABA, L-asparagine or ATP. This type of treatment increases the amount of bound acetylcholine (Minz 1965, Tower and Elliott 1953).

The mechanisms responsible for the degradation and synthesis of acetylcholine may also be involved in inducing convulsions. (Kreindler 1965). Since acetylcholine occurs *in vivo* as an insoluble, bound form, its concentration depends on the rate of synthesis and release. During convulsive activity the rate of release is increased and this results in a higher level of ACh. Resynthesis is rapid if there is a local fall of concentration. Richter and Crossland (1949) note that one tenth of a second after electrical stimulation, the concentration of ACh, particularly bound acetylcholine, falls rapidly. It was only possible to induce convulsions with an electrical current when the level of acetylcholine in the brain had been restored. It may be that a considerable amount of acetylcholine is necessary both for cerebral activity, and for convulsive hyperactivity (McIlwain 1955). Convulsions cease when the level of ACh falls to 40% of the normal value Similar results were obtained with *Metrazol* (Crossland 1953) or picrotoxin convulsions (Stone et al. 1945). Takahashi et al. (1961) concluded that (in addition to the other factors) the level of acetylcholine must be elevated for convulsive activity to be triggered.

Antiacetylcholinesterase treatment increases the concentration of ACh and produces many functional disorders culminating in convulsions and death. The *cholinesterase inhibitor* (acetylcholinesterase inhibitors) cause convulsions and many other subjective symptoms. The most familiar cholinesterae inhibitors are the *nerve gases* (see page 341), for example fluorophosphoric acid derivatives (diisopropyl-fluorophosphate and other insecticides). These chemical substances react with the OH group of a serine moiety in the reactive group of acetylcholinesterase, forming a phosphoric acid ester instead of an acetyl ester as it would with acetylcholine (Seiler 1966). Unlike the acetyl ester this phosphoric acid ester reacts very slowly with water and is only broken down very slowly. This delays regeneration of the enzyme or blocks the enzyme completely, so that the concentration of acetylcholine rises sharply. The receptor protein is permanently occupied by any acetylcholine which is released, and this means that the neuronal membrane remains depolarized. This specific chemical lesion immediately produces convulsions and, in certain circumstances, death (Birkhäuser 1941, Mann et al. 1938, McKerracher et al. 1966, Nachmansohn and Feld 1947, Pope et al. 1952).

Histamine is regarded as a degradation product of histidine. Under physiological conditions histamine is formed from *histidine* by a specific decarboxylase. *Histidine decarboxylase* is not distributed uniformly throughout the brain. The highest concentrations are found in the hypothalamus and vermis cerebelli (Crossland and Mitchell 1956, Werle 1936, White 1959, 1960).

Histamine is of importance and interest to us in that it is thought to inhibit epileptic attacks and its precursor histidine is an important constituent of human proteins (Frieser and Frieser 1968, Kajtor 1951).

The results of Forbes et al. (1929), Schaefer (1936) and Schumacher and Wolf (1941) indicated that histamine has a vasodilator effect, and so Kajtor (1951) and other authors examined the effects of histamine on the cerebral predisposition to convulsion. Later, many authors also demonstrated and studied the changes of vessel volume and permeability of the vascular endothelium following histamine (Jovanović 1959, 1960, Sinitsky and Sologuo 1965). In 86 experiments on 27 epileptics, Kajtor (1951) was able to induce epileptic attacks with *pentylenetetrazole (Cardiazol).* Histamine was capable of interrupting or deferring these attacks, for example the attack was blocked, but the effect was only short-lived (40 to 50 seconds). *Adrenaline* injected intravenously at the same time did not abolish the effect of histamine.

When Kajtor's results (1951) are considered together with those of Gibbs et al. (1934) who discovered that there is vasoconstriction in the brain just before an attack, the significance of the vasodilator effect of histamine in the epileptic attack becomes clear (see also Sinitsky and Sologuo 1965).

Ammonia and Other Products of Protein Metabolism

There is a good deal of controversy over the role of ammonia in the genesis of epilepsy and we are still not clear as to the importance of ammonium ions in the interval between attacks. However, there are one or two very interesting results in this respect.

Studies on rat brain (Pogodaev 1964, Richter and Dawson 1948) revealed that the concentration of ammonia rose following electroshock convulsions or *Cardiazol* convulsions (Figure 31). In hibernating animals the ammonium ion concentration increases with increasing cerebral activity and continues to increase after they wake (Feinschmidt 1948). From the results of these studies, it was assumed that ammonia increases the excitability of the brain and has some part to play in an epileptic episode. Some authors actually reported an increase of ammonium ion concentration in cerebral tissue, although this was only seen at the beginning of convulsions (Benitez et al. 1954, Pogodaev 1964, Richter and Dawson 1948) and not in the interval between attacks (Figure 30 and 31). Experiments by Takahashi et al. (1961) failed to show any direct correlation between ammonia concentration and excitability in the brain, although these authors believed that the level of ammonia fell in the interval in epileptics. This correlates with the views of Krasnova (1960) and Tolkatchevskaja and Wunder (1960). They failed to detect any increase in ammonium ion concentration in the brain (or in blood) in epileptics in the interval between convulsive episodes. However, the ammonia concentration fell in the interval, and the excitability of cerebral neurons was reduced following long-term administration of ammonium salts. An intravenous infusion of ammonium acetate in patients with epileptogenic and non-epileptogenic focal lesions in the brain did not alter the excitability of the brain (Berl et al. 1961).

So these results do not indicate either that there is an increase of ammonium ions in the CNS in the interval between convulsive episodes or that the excitability of the cerebral neurons is increased following administration of high doses of nitrogen derivatives.

In most cases, examination of blood from epileptics did not reveal an elevated level of ammonia in the interparoxysmal phase, although the results of Lando and Krupenina (1962) are very different from those of other authors. Lando and Krupenina found high levels of ammonia in serum in the interparoxysmal periods in both essential and symptomatic epilepsy. In essential epilepsy, the readings varied between 126 and 935 microgram per cent, the mean value being 353 microgram per cent. In symptomatic forms of epilepsy the values were between 56 and 442 microgram per cent (mean 321 microgram per cent), while in healthy test subjects used as controls, the values varied between 84 and 226, the mean value being 186 microgram per cent. Very high levels of serum ammonium were also found in schizophrenias; this will be discussed later.

However, in contrast to Lando and Krupenina (1962), many other authors found the serum concentration of ammonia to be depressed rather than elevated (Borsunova 1952, Heirovski 1951, Krainski 1896, Krasnova 1960, Markova 1944, Pavlov and Nenski 1951, Slutchevski 1944). Both the ammonium concentration and also the levels of other products of protein metabolism indicate that protein degradation is not accelerated in the interval in epileptics (Figure 30). Studies of sulph-hydryl (-SH-) and disulphide groups (-SS-) in blood (these may arise as metabolic products of proteins from *cystine* and *cysteine*) failed to reveal any increase in activity in the interval in epileptics and it was concluded from this, by analogy, that ammonia, as one of the products of protein metabolism, could not be increased in the serum of epileptics in the interval. The presence of sulph-hydryl and disulphide groups indicates that protein metabolism is retarded in the interparoxysmal period in patients with psychomotor epilepsy. This also correlates with earlier results. (Balle-Helaers 1955, Brdička 1933, Hasselbach and Schwab 1955, Heirovski 1951, Mison-Crighel et al. 1955 to 1965, Mitew and Harisanova 1958, Petrasch and Wilschanski 1954, Pogodaev 1956, Turek and Cizinsky 1955).

Examination of urine from epileptics also indicates that protein metabolism must be retarded in the interval. Studies during the interval between attacks have been carried out by Tolkatchevskaya and Wunder (1960) and others, and we should now like to discuss their results.

Total nitrogen in urine was depressed in 12 of 21 epileptics examined, when compared with values from control subjects. In the other nine patients the values fluctuated around the lower normal limit. If epileptics with low urinary nitrogen were given 200 gram curds, 100 g. meat or 100 g. cheese, the total nitrogen in 24-hour urine became normal. After a couple of days of this treatment the urinary concentration of nitrogen increased. It is interesting to note that there was no increase of urinary nitrogen in patients whose levels had been normal before treatment.

Urea nitrogen in urine was also depressed. Relatively speaking, urea nitrogen was even more depressed than total urinary nitrogen.

The concentration of amino acid nitrogen was increased slightly or quite considerably in the urine of epileptics between two attacks according to Tolkatchevskaya and Wunder (1960). However, the amino- nitrogen levels also fluctuated in healthy subjects (Albanese and Frankston 1944, Galambos and Taus 1913, Kirk 1936), and so the authors did not attach any great significance to the increase of urinary amino-nitrogen in these patients.

The urinary polypeptide nitrogen was 19 to 50 percent higher than normal In healthy subjects the authors found absolute values of 10 to 28 percent. A figure of 85 percent was recorded in some epileptics. Thus the urinary levels of nitrogen in urea, amino acids and peptides are all elevated. This suggests that there may be a defect of protein metabolism in the epileptic. *The nitrogen level is depressed, but the amino acid nitrogen is increased slightly or considerably and the polypeptide nitrogen is increased even more.* Tolkatchevskaya and Wunder (1960) believe that one of the degradation stages in protein metabolism is retarded. This means that more nitrogen in the form of partially metabolized compounds—polypeptides—appear in the urine of epileptics.

Creatinine was found in the *urine* of epileptics by Tolkatchevskaya and Wunder (1960). They found values between zero (as in healthy people) and 600 mg. in 24-hour urine. The appearance of creatine in the urine is related to carbohydrate metabolism and it occurs when there is an inadequate concentration of carbohydrate in brain and muscles (Brentano 1931, Tolkatchevskaya 1951). Prolonged treatment of epileptics with 200 g. sugar daily or with a high carbohydrate diet may reduce or eliminate any creatinuria. Where creatinuria was only reduced after administration of sugar, it was completely eliminated by concomitant administration of glutamic acid.

Tolkatchevskaya and Wunder (1960) did not simply confine their studies to ammonia and nitrogen in urine. They also set out to examine the relationship between nitrogen and *sulphur,* since sulphur is also found in the urine as an end product of protein metabolism. Thus, as with nitrogen, determinations of sulphur salts or sulphates in the urine may give an indication of the level of protein metabolism in these patients. Under normal conditions, the amount of sulphur parallels the amount of nitrogen; the curves alter synchronously, although the absolute values for nitrogen are four or five times higher than those for total sulphur, so the ratio sulphur : nitrogen is 1 : 4 to 1 : 5. With a mixed diet, an adult excretes 15 g. nitrogen in the urine in 24 hours, but only 2.4 to 4.8 g. sulphur. According to these authors, urinary sulphur is unchanged in most epileptics. However, total nitrogen is depressed, so the sulphur-nitrogen quotient is increased to 1 : 3 or 1 : 2. Tolkachevskaya and Wunder regard the increase in the sulphur/nitrogen quotient as the result of severe disruption in the metabolism of amino acids containing sulphur. These amino acids are considered to be the source of the sulphur.

Viewed as a whole, the results of studies on the products of protein metabolism in epileptics indicate that the processes are retarded and disrupted in the interval between attacks. According to Selbach (1965) and

Selbach et al (1965) this retardation of protein metabolism alters the whole metabolic picture from an *ergotropic* to a trophotropic one and this may produce alkalosis. The situation is changed by an attack (see Chapter VIII).

Cerebral Lipids

Although about 50 percent of the dry matter of the brain consists of *lipids,* we still do not know exactly what effect these substances have in the development of an attack in psychomotor epilepsy. However, recently there have been many reports suggesting that these substances are also involved in an epileptic attack.

Apart from *cholesterol,* the complex lipids of the brain are divided into the following groups: 1.) *phospholipids,* with the subgroup phosphoglycerides (phosphatidylcholines or lecithin, phosphatidylethanolamines, phosphatidylserines, plasmalogens and cephalin B), phosphoinositides, phosphosphingosides (sphingomyelins); 2.) *glycolipids* with subgroups glycosphingosides, sulphatides (cerebroside esters of sulphuric acid), mucolipids with gangliosides and stradines; 3.) *protein-bound lipoids,* with the subgroups proteolipids, phosphatidopeptides and lipoproteins (Adams and Davison 1959, Conrforth 1959, Folch-Pi 1942, 1949, Folchi-Pi and Lees 1951, Gmellin 1824, Jatzkewitz 1958, Kishimoto and Ralin 1962, McMillan et al. 1957, Moser and Karnovsky 1959, Nicholas and Thomas 1959 a, b, Sperry et al. 1953, van Bruggen et al. 1953, Waelsch et al. 1940).

Of these groups, *lipoproteins* and *glycolipids* have recently become the center of scientific interest as regards the problem of epilepsy (Clausen 1966, Dekaban 1966 and others). A short time ago a kind of protoplasmic organelle was discovered. These organelles contain many hydrolytic enzymes, including *acidic phosphatases, acidic ribonucleases* and *cathepsin* (Koenig 1962). Earlier Duve et al. (1955) had pictured this organelle as a small neutral vesicle in a lipoprotein sheath. This sheath prevents the enclosed enzymes from wandering freely and attacking their substrates. The lysosomal enzymes can only be released by rupture of the protein barrier. According to Koenig (1962), recent histochemical and biochemical studies have shown that the majority of cerebral gangliosides, a heterogenous group of glycosphingolipids present in lysosomes, contain N-acetylneuraminic acid (N-acetylsialic acid). These cerebral gangliosides occur mostly in the cytoplasm of the neurons, neuroglia and other non-neuronal cells and they appear to be the neurosomes and gliosomes of classical neurohistology (see also de Duve 1963, de Duve and Baudhuin 1966, Siebert 1969).

However, studies using an electron microscope (Novikoff et al. 1962) indicated that the lysosomes tend to be massive organelles rather than simple vesicles. According to these and other investigations, protein-bound glycolipids are distributed uniformly throughout the lysosomes; that is to say, they are not simply found forming a peripheral sheath. As an alternative to the membrane theory Koenig (1962) suggested that cerebral lysosomes might arise from macromolecules of a hydrolytic enzyme which is bound to neuraminoglycolipidoprotein (ganglioside protein) to form a salt.

Earlier studies by McIlwain (1955), Bogoch (1962) Clausen (1966) and others reveal that *gangliosides* are involved in neural excitability. Thus, the gangliosides must be localized in the neuronal membrane and they must be involved in ion transport and other activities at the membrane. A further conclusion can be drawn from this assumption, i.e. *that various toxic substances, such as influenza virus, tetanus toxin, picrotoxin and some incompatible proteins, exert a definite metabolic effect on cerebral gangliosides.* Hence, since cerebral gangliosides occur mainly in lysosomes, these toxins must influence the release of lysosomal enzymes and consequently have a disruptive effect on cellular substrates. Basing their investigations on this assumption, Koenig and Barron (1961) and Koenig (1962) examined the neurological, histochemical and biochemical effects of a number of selected compounds which act upon the gangliosides.

These experiments and to those of Bernheimer and van Heyningen (1961), indicated that the neuraminidase which is present in certain viruses and bacteria splits off part of the neuramic acid radical form the cerebral gangliosides. Bernheimer and van Heyningen (1961) found that neuraminidase produces quite dramatic neurological symptoms when given by intrathectal injection. An intraspinal injection of neuraminidase in cats caused muscular fasciculation, tonic spasms, rhythmic myoclonia, hypertonia of the flexors and temporary paraparesis. Intracerebral injection of this enzyme into rats elicited a standard response beginning after one to two minutes and consisting of a contralateral (and sometimes also ipsilateral) tonic adversive attack. In an adversive convulsion there is often violent *circular running or rolling in the same direction.* This is important here since this phenomenon is recognized as a symptom in psychomotor epilepsy (see Chapter I).

Generalized attacks are quite common during these experiments. Preparations from *Vibrio cholerae sialidase, influenza virus neuraminidase and polyvalent influenza vaccines* are toxic. However, the toxic moeities in these preparations are thermolabile, and heating eliminates their effect on the nervous system. It is concluded from this that these effects are in fact due to the toxicity of the preparations and not to a non-specific reaction (Koenig 1962).

It was also shown by Koenig's experiments (1962) that subarachnoidal administration of low doses of neuraminidase, basic proteins and metal ions may elicit attacks and other signs of neuronal malfunction. Neurological symptoms appear to be associated with the release of lysosome-bound acid phosphatases and probably also with other hydrolases. Since these preparations activate bound acid phosphatases in the cerebral mitochondrial fraction *in vitro,* it seems likely that one of their primary effects is intravital release of lysosomal enzymes. This action appears to be catalysed by precipitation or splitting off of ganglioside-bound neuramic acid. Intravital release of lysosomal enzymes is bound to cause autolytic changes in some cell materials and this may produce various symptoms, including symptoms of psychomotor epilepsy.

Bogoch (1962) has raised certain objections to Koenig's theories (1962). However, Koenig's postulates are still important, since we are still not sure which is the primary mechanism (see also de Duve 1963, de Duve and Baudhuin 1966, Farstad 1964, Siebert 1969).

Hormones

A search of the literature has not revealed any results to suggest that hormones have a detrimental effect in psychomotor epilepsy. However, hormones many have an indirect effect since they control the most important metabolic reactions. For instance, some adrenocortical hormones stimulate the central nervous system while others inhibit it. Following injection of *ACTH* there is a rapid rise in the levels of ammonia and acetylcholine in the brain. The effects of the ammonia and acetylcholine concentrations on increased cerebral predisposition to convulsion have already been discussed. Increased bioelectrical activity in the brain following injections of ACTH has been reported (Torda 1953, Torda and Wolff 1952).

It has been shown that the intracellular concentration of sodium rises rapidly following adrenalectomy, and that there is a simultaneous increase in cerebral excitability. *Cortisone* and *cortisol* also increase the excitability of the brain, while it is depressed by *desoxycorticosterone acetate.* The fall of sodium concentration within the neurons and the increase of sodium in serum and inextracellular fluid explains the anticonvulsant effect of the desoxycorticosterone acetate when it is used in epilepsy (Careddu 1963, Seiler 1966, Woodbury et al. 1962). Successful results have been obtained with ACTH in a certain form of epilepsy (propulsive petit mal, BNS, nodding spasms, see Chapter I) (Careddu 1963, Dumermuth 1961, Gastaut and Bernard 1953, Haneke 1961, Pache and Stolecke 1962, Pache and Tröger 1967, Paludan 1961, Roser and Low 1960, Trojaborg and Plum 1960). However, the authors were not dealing here with the treatment of psychomotor epilepsy, and none of their findings indicated that this treatment had any significant effect on the psychomotor components in the attacks of propulsive *petit mal.* Thus, the mechanism of action of ACTH in the psychomotor form of epilepsy is not yet clearly understood.

Vitamins and Enzymes

In Chapter III and in nearly every section of this chapter, we have shown that vitamins and enzymes play a major part in an epileptic episode (see also Meynell 1966). We shall now deal with this problem in rather more detail. We shall not adhere to the standard classification of vitamins and enzymes as we only intend to mention those substances which are or may be of particular interest in psychomotor epilepsy.

The active compound of *Vitamin B_1 (thiamine)*—thiamine pyrophosphate—is involved in carbohydrate metabolism in the form of a *codecarboxylase.* Together with alpha-lipoic acid and coenzyme A, it converts pyruvic acid into activated acetic acid (acetylcoenzyme A). There is no direct evidence that deficiency of Vitamin B_1 on its own produces psychomotor attacks in man. Because this vitamin is involved in so many biochemical processes, it could be that a combined biochemical lesion including avitaminosis of Vitamin B_1 may produce seizures. There may be local Vitamin B_1 deficiency in the hippocampus. A deficiency of this vitamin would mean an inadequate supply of catalyst for converting pyruvic acid into the activated compound, and this would result in a build-up of pyruvic acid. As we have shown above, local accumulation of pyruvic acid in the brain produces epileptic reactions.

In view of its connection with compounds containing SH groups, particularly coenzyme A, thiamine pyrophosphate exerts certain effects on acetylcholine metabolism. Bhagat and Lockett (1962) found reduced amounts of acetylcoenzyme A and impaired synthesis of acetylcholine in cerebral extracts from animals with vitamin B_1 deficiency. However, if acetylcoenzyme A was administered, acetylcholine synthesis became normal again. A reduction of acetylcholine synthesis alters the balance of endogenous amines and, like an increase of synthesis, this may also produce psychomotor attacks.

Codecarboxylase is also involved in the conversion of alpha-ketoglutaric acid into *activated succinic acid.* This reaction is an important intermediate stage in the *citric acid cycle* (Kanig 1968).

Many disorders may be produced by B_1 avitaminosis, but we only intend to mention the symptoms which occur following the use of the *antimetabolites of thiamine* which are also capable of producing convulsions.

The most familiar antimetabolites of this vitamin are *pyrithiamine* and *oxythiamine.* These substances can induce many of the symptoms of Vitamin B_1 deficiency. Pyrithiamine inhibits the phosphorylation of thiamine (Cooper et al. 1963, Wolfe and Elliott 1962). There was a steady increase of thiamine in the brain following a single injection of 1 mg. in rats with thiamine deficiency, over an observation period of 12 days. In the other organs, after an initial rise, the level declined. Thus, the antimetabolite pyrithiamine has more activity in the brain than thiamine itself and it rapidly induces thiamine deficiency in this organ. This produces neurological symptoms in the experimental animals, including *hippocampal* convulsions, with a rapid fall in concentration of thiamine pyrophosphate in the brain (Peters 1962, Rindi et al. 1961).

Administering *neopyrithiamine* to animals also induces *hippocampal convulsions.* The mechanism involves blockade of sodium transport (Kunz 1956) due to suppression of thiamine or thiamine-like compounds which are involved in several reactions in the sodium transport system (Kunz 1956).

The thiazole ring in thiamine has an anticonvulsant effect (Lechat 1961). These properties are even more pronounced in a thiazole derivative of thiamine. This compound, which is the *sulphonate of chloroethyl thiazole* (Allgén et al. 1963, Åsander 1962, Bergener 1966, Bergener and Fritschka 1965, Charonnat et al. 1953 to 1958, Gastager et al. 1964, Giacobini and Salum 1961, Laborit et al. 1957 a, b, Lundquist 1966 a, b, Osterman et al. 1959, Petersén and Hambert 1966, Petersén and Leissner 1966, Royer et al. 1958, Salum 1963, Sattes 1964 a, b, 1966 a, b, 1967, etc.) with the chemical name 5 (2-chloroethyl) -4-methylthiazole (chlormethiazole), is known clinically as Hémineurine®, Heminevrin® or Distraneurin®. It has an anticonvulsant action on convulsions induced by electroshock, *Cardiazol, Megimide* and O_2, and also on spontaneous convulsions, both in animal experiments and in man. However, it does not have an anticonvulsant effect on strychnine or insulin convulsions. Thus, it can be seen that the action is more pronounced where administration of convulsogenic noxae has produced hippocampal convulsions. *Hémineurine* was used by Laborit et al. (1957) in status epilepticus and other authors have also reported good results in this condition (Gastager et al. 1964, Laxenaire et al. 1966, Krause 1964, Lechat 1961), in progressive myoclonus epilepsy (Petersén and Hambert 1966 a to c), in delirium tremens (Bergener 1966, Sattes 1964 a, b, 1966 a, b, 1967, Scheid 1964) and in acute mania (Gastager et al. 1964, Sattes 1964 b, 1967). However, the effect was not so pronounced in chronic epilepsies (Gastager et al. 1964, Krause 1964). In nine cases of acute status epilepticus, Krause (1964) was able to interrupt the attack in four cases with a single injection of *Distraneurin,* although a second injection was necessary in three other cases. In pre-epileptic and post-epileptic twilight states, Distraneurin was effective if the patients were agitated before the injection. Distraneurin was less effective where the epileptic psychomotor condition was less acute.

In our hospital, Sattes (1964 a to 1967) has made a particular study of threapy with Distraneurin and he has achieved very good results in acute cases of delirium tremens, status epilepticus, acute psychosis in psychomotor epilepsy and other serious conditions (acute alcohol poisoning, etc.). Our clinical experience with Distraneurin correlates with that of Sattes and the other authors mentioned above.

We shall briefly describe one of our cases to illustrate this point.

Case 7

A 49-year-old woman, W.K., was unconscious when she was admitted to hospital during the night of January 8. It was soon discovered that this patient was in status epilepticus. She was unresponsive and she suffered from adversive-tonic attacks every five or ten minutes; these attacks lasted 15 to 30 seconds. At times her state of unconsciousness deepened even more. The next day, the patient occasionally became responsive but she continued to have attacks with loss of consciousness and tonic deviations to the right, in spite of therapy with diazepins, hydantoins and Vitamin C and B. The EEG showed paroxysmal displays of either short or long groups of sharp waves and there were long periods of slow and generalized delta waves. The cerebral activity indicated a permanent twilight state with brief and frequent twilight attacks.

Distraneurin for infusion was given during the night of the January 10. After a single infusion of 500 ml., the attacks became less and less frequent and the patient became more conscious. By the January 11 the patient was fit enough to take psychological tests and on January 25 she was discharged from the hospital with a normal EEG and no clinical attacks. Since then she has been taking low doses of hydantoin preparations.

Riboflavine (Vitamin B_2) forms the prosthetic group of yellow enzymes or *flavin enzymes* which are distinguished from each other by a specific protein group (Kanig 1968, Seiler 1966). The function of yellow enzymes includes hydrogen ion transfer, and *nicotinic acid* is also involved here.

Riboflavine avitaminosis has been shown to produce *hippocampal convulsions* in animal experiments (corresponding to psychomotor epilepsy in man) (Rapoport 1964).

Nicotinic acid and *nicotinamide* are extremely important substances in the problem we are discussing and we have already mentioned them in Chapter III. *Nicotinamide* (see Formula) is a constituent of the codehydrogenases NAD (see formula) (previously called DPN) and NADP (previously called TPN, see also Chapter III). The distribution of nicotinamide and nicotinic acid in the brain and the extent to which they are involved in many of the reactions in intermediate metabolism are some indication of the enormous importance of these substances in the body. Both these vitamins occur in the brain and they come directly from the food or from the breakdown of their nucleotides. However, NAD can also be synthesized from the quinolinic acid which is produced by the metabolism of tryptophane, 60 mg. tryptophane being equivalent to 1 mg. nicotinic acid (Goldsmith 1965). Thiamine, riboflavine and pyridoxine are also necessary in this biosynthetic process (Lang 1962, McIlwain 1966, Rapoport 1964).

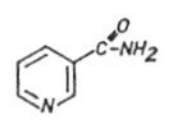

Nicotinamide

Nicotinic acid deficiency becomes particularly apparent at certain common sites, and this predilection for certain areas is an important consideration from the point of view of psychomotor epilepsy.

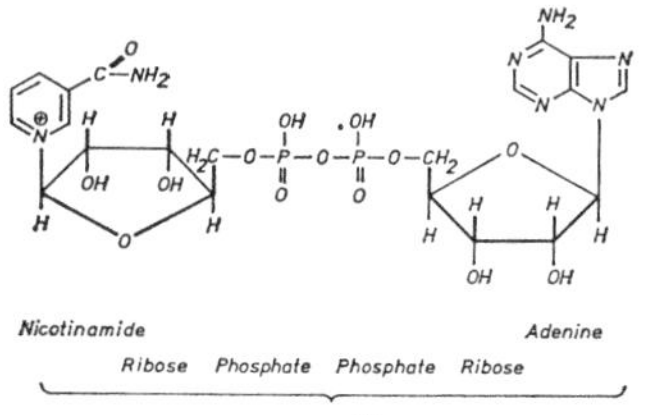

Nicotinamide Ribose Phosphate Phosphate Ribose Adenine

$NAD^{\oplus}$

The following can be added to what has already been said in Chapter III about the antimetabolites of nicotonamide.

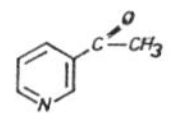

3-Acetylpyridine

The exchange of 3-acetylpyridine (3-AP see formula) for nicotinamide in NADP (nicotinamide-adenine-dinucleotide-phosphate) is most pronounced *in the hippocampus* (Kanig 1968, 1970, 1971a, b, c, 1972, Neuhoff and Herkin 1964, Willing 1964). Very interesting experimental results have been obtained in mice using ^{14}C-labelled 3-AP. A high level of radioactivity was observed in the stratum pyramidal and stratum oriens hippocampi (Figure 27). According to Eccles (1964), *there are basket cells in the stratum oriens; these have inhibitory effects and they communicate with the pyramidal cells.* This suggests that psychomotor epilepsy is induced when the inhibitory mechanisms in the limbic system are eliminated.

Brunnemann and Coper (1964 a to c), have demonstrated that compared with other enzymes in the hippocampus, glucose-6-phosphate dehydrogenase shows the highest activity. Glutathion reductase is also very active in the limbic system, particularly in the Ammon's horn (Kanig 1968). This means that the high metabolic activity in these cerebral regions can be impaired by the formation of slow reacting 3-acetylpyridine analogues of pyridine nucleotides.

We discussed the metabolism of 3-acetylpyridine in more detail in Chapter III, where we also dealt with the microscopic morphological changes in the hippocampus following administration of 3-acetylpyridine and 6-aminonicotinamide. Histochemical lesions in the hippocampus induced by 3-acetylpyridine, 6-aminonicotinamide and other antimetabolites of nicotinamide, are particularly important in psychomotor epilepsy.

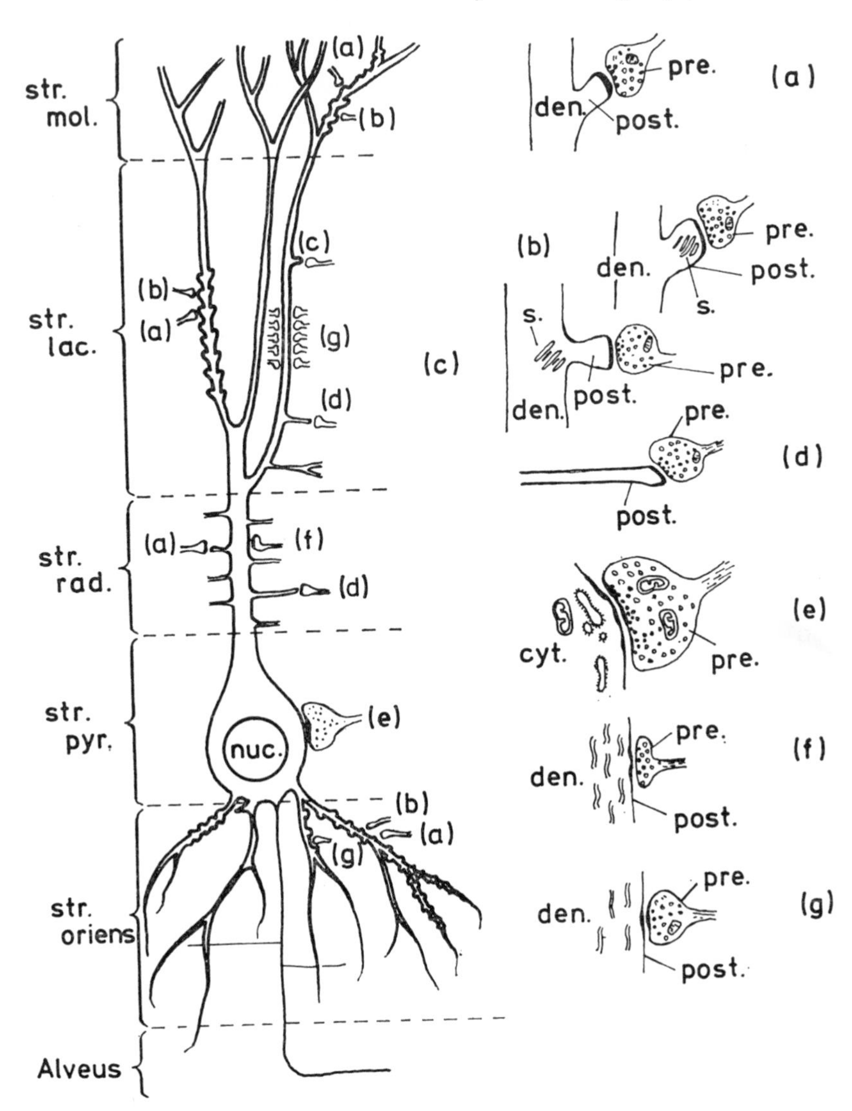

Figure 27. Diagram (not to scale) of a pyramidal neurons from field CA_1 of the Ammon's horn (see Figure 15). It shows the layers in which the various types of synaptic connections (a-g) have been observed. There are further details on the right hand side of the figure. For the sake of clarity, the various synaptic arrangements in the striatum lacunosum (str.lac.) are shown on three branches. Of course, each of these types of synaptic connection can occur on every other dendritic branch in this region. There was particularly high activity of 3-acetylpyridine in the stratum pyramidale (str.pyr.) and stratum oriens (str.oriens). Methoxypyridoxine is particularly effective on field CA_4. str.mol. = stratum molae; str.rad. = stratum radiatum; den. = dendrites; pre. = presynaptic (presynapse); post. = postsynaptic (postsynapse); cyt. = cytoplasm. (From Hamlyn, 1963. In Kanig, K.: *Die Bedeutung der B-Vitamine für das Nervensystem*. Wiss. Berichte. E. MERK A.G., Darmstadt/W. Germany, 1968.)

Quadbeck et al. (1956 to 1961) obtained some very interesting and impressive results by using nicotinic acid in animal experiments. They showed that administering aminophylline to rats altered the properties of the blood-brain barrier and permitted phosphate to pass from the blood into the brain. These authors assume that this effect on the barrier is an important factor in producing the clinical activity of this preparation. As a result of these experiments, they examined other drugs which have been used successfully for treating disorders of cerebral nutrition, for their effect on the blood-brain barrier. Among the preparations investigated, it was shown that *nicotinic acid* increased the passage of phosphate from the blood into the brain, the effect resembling that of aminophylline. They established that substances which break down the blood-brain barrier increase the predisposition to convulsion in the epileptic rat. This observation was confirmed when these authors showed that there was a definite increase in the predisposition to convulsion following aminophylline. They therefore expected that nicotinic acid would also increase the cerebral predisposition to convulsion.

In their final studies (1961), Quadbeck et al. used two groups (A and B) each of ten rats from their epileptic strain of rats. They selected animals in which an audiogenic convulsion could be induced with about 50% probability (see also Quadbeck and Röhm 1956). Before the substance was administered, these authors observed 14 convulsions in 30 individual tests in group A, and 21 convulsions in group B. Group A were given 200 mg. *nicotinic acid* per kg. body weight intraperitoneally. All the animals were subjected to the convulsion test after 30, 90 and 150 minutes. 16 convulsions occurred in control group B but there were only four convulsions in group A. The experiment was repeated after a week: this time group B was given the medicament and group A was used as the control group. Before medication, the authors observed 30 convulsions in 60 individual tests in group A and 28 convulsions in group B. After administering the drug, 20 out of 40 individual tests were positive in the control group. In group B, only one animal had a convulsion, and this was only after 210 minutes, despite the fact that this group was also given 40 individual tests. This result shows that the expected increase in the cerebral predisposition to convulsion following nicotinic acid did not occur. In fact, the predisposition to convulsion was reduced.

The authors were able to prevent convulsions, particularly the tonic components, both in the epileptic strain of rats and also in other healthy strains of rats. The outcome of this was that these authors suggested that nicotinic acid should be used as an adjuvant in the treatment of epileptic patients.

In Chapter VII we reported on the effects of *Cosaldon* (Jovanović 1970c), which contains nicotinic acid and a *xanthine derivative* (see also Jovanović 1972 b, c). We have been able to prevent symptoms of a convulsion from appearing in the EEG folowing electroshock, and, more particularly, to prevent subsequent convulsions (convulsions which occur spontaneously some days or weeks after the electroshock).

Cosaldon has also been tested and used clinically by Hackstock and Bielinski (1961) in epileptics. These authors proceeded from the assumption that a drug which has a favorable effect on the cerebral circulation may also influence an epileptic's convulsive predisposition or intensify the action of an antiepileptic agent (making it possible to reduce the dose).

In seven epileptics with essential epilepsy, three of whom were already in an advanced stage of dementia, Cosaldon was administered for an average period of one month. With these patients the attacks were so frequent that a short observation period was quite sufficient. The dose ranged from 1½ to 2½ tablets daily, divided into three separate doses and the antiepileptic therapy was reduced to one third of the previous dose. In spite of the reduced dose of antiepileptic agent, none of the patients suffered a clinical deterioration. On the contrary, the mental condition of the patient improved and they became less predisposed to convulsion. This resulted in a substantial reduction in the number of major attacks, which were replaced by a few abortive seizures or attack equivalents.

As we emphasized in Chapter III, *Vitamin B_6 (pyridoxine)* plays a most important part in the development, function and pathophysiology of psychomotor epilepsy (see also Hagberg et al. 1964). Vitamin B_6 occurs in three active forms which are distinguished from one another by the group substituted at the 4-position in the pyridine ring: *pyridoxol, pyridoxal and pyridoxamine.* Esterification with phosphoric acid at the OH group in the 5-position occurs mainly in pyridoxal, which as *pyridoxal-5'-phosphate (PAL or PYP)* represents the prosthetic group of many enzymes, among which are the amino-acid decarboxylases and amino-acid transaminases already mentioned above, and one or two enzymes involved in the metabolism of tryptophane. These enzymes are capable of producing cholic acid from tryptophane in the liver and, in the intestinal flora, they can also break down tryptophane into indole, pyruvic acid and ammonia (Kanig 1968). About 80% of the Vitamin B_6 in the brain is present in the form of pyridoxal-5-phosphate and pyridoxamine-5-phosphate. Its concentration in the brain is several hundred times higher than that in blood plasma; according to McIlwain (1966) it is 0.7 to 1.8 gamma %, and 1 gamma % in cerebrospinal fluid. Phosphorylation takes place under the influence of *pyridoxal phosphokinase* which is activated by *magnesium ions* (Killam and Bain 1957, McCormick et al. 1961). *Zinc ions* are also capable of activating this enzyme (McCormick et al. 1960). This is particularly significant in psychomotor epilepsy since the hippocampus is remarkable both for its high glutamic acid decarboxylase activity (Roberts 1960) and also for its high zinc content (McLardy 1962) (see also Chapter III). Much larger quantities of pyridoxal phosphokinase are present in the cerebral hemispheres than in the spinal cord. This phosphokinase can be inhibited by hydrazides or by deoxypyridoxol (McCormick and Snell 1961); this will be discussed later. Iproniazid and amphetamine (the 'MAO inhibitors') influence pyridoxine phosphate oxidase, an enzyme which is responsible for the oxidative deamination of pyridoximine phosphate (Wada and Snell 1961). Pyridoxamine phosphate is obviously a precursor of pyridoxal phosphate (Kanig 1968, Lyon et al. 1962, Wada and Snell 1961). Iproniazid also inhibits pyridoxal phosphokinase (McCormick and Snell 1959). Animal experiments have also shown that *thiosemicarbazide, thiocarbohydrazide* and *hydrazine* have convulsant effects, particularly in rats and mice (Fine et al. 1950, Dieke 1949, Jenny and Pfeiffer 1958, Parks et al. 1952). Pyridoxine is a very effective antidote (Bain and Wiegand 1957). Coupling the carbonyl groups of hydrazides with pyridoxal phosphate produces hydrazones (Wiegand 1956) which then block the enzymes which depend on this coenzyme (Boone et al. 1956). Hydrazides inhibit L-glutamic acid decarboxylase both *in vitro* and *in vivo* (see above). This results in the fall in the concentration of GABA in the brain, which we have already frequently mentioned.

PAL is the prosthetic group in other important enzymes: DOPA-decarboxylase (Green et al. 1945), 5-hydroxytryptophane decarboxylase (Clark et al. 1954, Buzard and Nytch 1957), diamine oxidase (Davison 1956), histidine decarboxylase (Guirard and Snell 1955) and GABA-alpha-ketoglutarate transaminase (Baxter and Roberts 1958). These enzymes are involved in the synthesis of *catecholamines* and *serotonin,* and also in the metabolism of *histamine* and *GABA* (Kanig 1968). Therefore, where the metabolism of these substances is disrupted there are also changes in the activity and concentration of Vitamin B_6, and vice versa. The fact that glutamic acid decarboxylase does not have a great affinity for pyridoxal phosphate means that this coenzyme can easily be separated from and reattached to the protein (Roberts 1963). This means that in conditions of Vitamin B_6 deficiency, CNS symptoms occur quite early.

According to Coursin (1960), there are three types of convulsions associated with Vitamin B_6 metabolism *(infantile convulsions):* 1.) convulsions due to *pyridoxine deficiency;* 2.) convulsions associated with *excessive production of pyridoxic acid,* and 3.) convulsions due to *excessive pyridoxine requirement.*

The first group includes pyridoxine-dependent convulsions in infants. These are regarded as a *genetic metabolic disorder.* In 1952 there were a series of unusual reports of convulsions in the U.S.A. in children nurtured on a low-pyridoxine diet (Moloney and Parmalee 1954). The disease affected infants between two and four months old. These babies had had a normal birth and they appeared to be developing normally, both mentally and physically until the onset of the convulsions. The clinical course developed in three stages (Coursin 1954). Firstly it seemed as if the infants had abdominal colic. Then there were episodes involving sudden screaming and straightening of the body. The infants held their heads outstretched and stared with rolling eyes. In the third stage there were generalized convulsions. There were severe convulsions six to nine times a day each lasting on average for 15 minutes. Results of clinical biochemical investigations were usually negative, apart from occasional signs of increased amounts of protein in the cerebrospinal fluid.

In searching for the cause of these complaints it was found that all the afflicted children had drunk the same milk. Obviously preparation and boiling of the milk had destroyed the pyridoxine present. The babies' illness disappeared after administration of pyridoxine. Hunt et al. (1954) reported convulsions in infants between two and four months, and also in one baby within three hours of birth. This infant showed generalized convulsions which recurred paroxysmally nearly every day during the first 13 days. The cause of these convulsions was not known at the time. The child vomited and Petrolit solution was given as an infusion because of the danger of dehydration. The infant was also given a routine multivitamin injection. The convulsions ceased immediately after the last injection, but they recurred after two days. The cause of the convulsions was not discovered until the end of the third week. By chance the same vitamin preparation was administered in another hospital and the attacks again ceased. The infant was discharged from hospital but a multivitamin preparation supplied for domiciliary use was not capable of stopping the attacks.

This preparation was analysed and it was found that it contained less pyridoxine. After that only Vitamin B_6 preparations were prescribed. Meanwhile the cause of convulsions had been discovered in other children and they had been treated with pyridoxine. So it was established that all these children had a pyridoxine-dependent condition. Their mothers had been treated with high doses of pyridoxine in the first trimester of pregnancy. Thus, the explanation was that the fetal tissue had acquired tolerance to high doses of Vitamin B_6 and hence, the children required higher and higher doses of this substance after birth. It has been suggested that the biochemical lesion is due to defective utilization of pyridoxine as a coenzyme at one of its sites of action. However, since as a coenzyme pyridoxal-5-phosphate is involved in 30 or 40 different enzyme reactions in the brain, we must undoubtedly blame a whole series of processes. Bessey et al. (1957)

pointed out that in a system of enzymes such as the pyridoxine system the bond between apoenzyme and coenzyme has only low affinity so that pyridoxal-5-phosphate shows varying sensitivity to enzymatic reactions, and this occasionally leads to relative pyridoxine withdrawal. Vitamin B_6-dependent convulsions can be eliminated both by administration of pyridoxine itself and also by administration of GABA (Cramer 1962). The vitamin requirement seems to vary according to familial disposition (Christian 1968 b, Cramer 1966, Kanig 1968), for it is remarkable that only 3 percent of children in the U.S.A. who had been given milk preparations deficient in Vitamin B_6 actually became ill. Nevertheless, in the literature there are many reports of cases of convulsions in children who responded to treatment with Vitamin B_6 preparations. Kruse (1968) recently reported on two such cases, where the diagnosis was made by administering Vitamin B_6. When the disease occurred, one child was six hours and the other three months old. These cases had been preceded by two diseases in the siblings.

The second group of diseases involving pyridoxine deficiency is not *directly* dependent on pyridoxine. Tower (1960) reported that not all of these patients can be treated with pyridoxine and according to this author, therapeutically, most of the patients are resistant to pyridoxine. However, Karmin and Karmin (1961) found that pyridoxine was capable of protecting mice from the convulsant effects of methoxypyridoxol (4-methoxymethylpyridoxol), but not from the fall in the cerebral concentration of GABA which follows methoxypyridoxol treatment. On the other hand, it is known (Kanig 1968) that an optimum concentration of GABA in the brain can be maintained by the combined effects of transaminases and decarboxylases. The pH optima for these enzymes are probably such that *acidosis increases the concentration of GABA and alkalosis reduces it.* We have emphasized that pH has an important part to play in the seizures (Selbach 1965, Selbach et al. 1965, Wolfe and Elliott 1962). So the convulsions in this second group of pyridoxine-dependent convulsions can be attributed to a change of pH following a change in the metabolic processes.

We shall only touch on one or two findings relating to the *third group:* this group includes rather older children who suffer from nodding spasms (BNS spasms) with hypsarrhythmia in the electroencephalogram (Gibbs and Gibbs 1952, Janz and Matthes 1955, Lennox 1951). Therapy with high doses of Vitamin B_6 produced neither a clinical nor a biochemical effect. However, as we have already mentioned, ACTH therapy had a favorable effect. The clinical attacks improved, the mental disorders diminished and the biochemical findings normalized. It is thought that ACTH and corticosteroids improved utilization of Vitamin B_6 or activate pyridoxal phosphokinase (Careddu 1963). Since corticosteroids promote synthesis of apoenzymes (Karlson 1963), the second possibility is neatly explained. Patients with this type of disease would then be regarded as pyridoxine-sensitive. However, Hellstöm and Vasella (1962) take the view that this disease is due to increased pyridoxine requirement.

Some alcoholics often develop convulsions 36 to 72 hours after a bout of excessive drinking, and Vitamin B_6 deficiency has been demonstrated in these patients (Lerner et al. 1958). Daily administration of high doses of Vitamin B_6 cured the convulsions in a number of patients (Lunde 1960). These patients also belong to the group with increased pyridoxine requirement.

Antimetabolites of pyridoxine frequently induce convulsions (see Chapter III). We would like to add the following to what has already been said: in experiments on mice, rats, rabbits dogs and apes, convulsions are observed 15 to 45 minutes after administering *3- or 4-desoxypyridoxol* and *omega-methoxypyridoxol* (Wolfe and Elliott 1962). Also, *toxopyrimidine* which is derived from the pyrimidine moiety of Vitamin B_1 produced convulsions which disappeared after administering pyridoxine (Stepp et al. 1952). Again in this case glutamic acid decarboxylase was inhibited, and this reduced the concentration of GABA in the brain before the convulsions occurred. Injection of 7 to 15 mg/kg. toxopyrimidine in mice induces convulsions and leads to death within three hours (Rosen et al. 1957, Sakuragi and Kummerow 1957). We have mentioned that *isonicotinic acid hydrazide (INH)* is also a pyridoxine antagonist, and long-term therapy with INH (in tuberculosis patients) sometimes causes convulsions (Biehl and Vilter 1954, Gibson and Philips 1966, Grafe 1958, Pfeiffer et al. 1956, Pleasure 1954, Quadbeck and Sartori 1957, Reilley et al. 1953, Vilter 1956, Williams and Abdulian 1956, Wolfe and Elliott 1962).

Convulsions induced by *penicillin* (see Chapter IV) have also been attributed to pyridoxine deficiency (Du Vigneaud et al. 1957). In mice, administration of 0.3 mg/g. of D,L-penicillamine i.v. produced *running fits* followed by convulsions and death (Matsuda and Makino 1961). Subsequent injection of pyridoxal is capable of preventing these convulsions.

The effect of penicillin is explained as being due to inhibition of transminase synthesis in brain and liver. Penicillin also inhibits glutamic acid decarboxylase, and this inhibitory effect can be blocked by administering pyridoxal-5-phosphate. According to Du Vigneaud et al. (1957), penicillin reacts with the carbonyl group in pyridoxal to form a thiazolidine derivative which is eliminated with the urine. Kanig (1968) has produced a most lucid report on this.

It has been postulated that, for example, D-penicillin reduces the heavy metal and alkaline earth ion concentration by mobilizing these elements. This is a most important theory in respect of psychomotor epilepsy since these trace elements, (particularly zinc and magnesium ions) are necessary for activating pyridoxal phosphate-dependent enzymes. As we mentioned above, these metal ions are found particularly in the hippocampus, and this explains the connection between penicillin and psychomotor epilepsy (see also Hamfelt 1966, Kanig 1968).

The only other vitamin worth mentioning in the context of psychomotor epilepsy is *folic acid* in relation to *3-acetylpyridine poisoning*. However, there are no reports of psychomotor attacks due to disorders in the metabolism of this vitamin, and so there is no need to go into details about the experimental findings (see in Herken and Timmler 1965, Houben et al. 1971, Jaenicke 1966, Kanig 1968, Reynolds et al. 1971, Spaans 1970, Willing et al. 1964).

For the same reason, we do not intend to discuss any of the other vitamins.

The Importance of the Blood-Brain Barrier

In the course of our discussion we have frequently mentioned substances which are not capable of traversing the *barrier between blood and cerebral tissue*. The blood-brain barrier prevents both low and high molecular weight compounds and inorganic ions from gaining access to the brain. Thus this barrier represents an important protective mechanism for maintaining the environment within in the CNS. The effect of the barrier is bilateral, i.e. the blood-brain barrier not only prevents the influx of substances from the blood, but it also tends to block the efflux of metabolites produced in the brain (Seiler 1966). It can be seen from this that the brain can only maintain its function during an attack if there is a considerable increase of rate of perfusion, since this is a prerequisite for removal of metabolites which are being produced under the abnormal conditions (Abood and Geiger 1955, Geiger et al. 1952). Under normal metabolic conditions, normal blood flow is sufficient to remove waste products and metabolites.

The blood-brain barrier is of major significance when discussing the problem of psychomotor epilepsy. A shift in the albumin-globulin fraction in epileptic patients was discussed above and we shall deal with this question again in mere detail later. Assuming that local oedema can occur in the limbic system, psychomotor epilepsy will develop. However, since a shift in the albulin-globulin fraction towards the alpha and beta-globulins represents a general change in the blood without there being general oedema, it must be assumed that *local oedema* in the temporal lobe can only occur if the brain barrier is injured at this point. Thus, with a chemical change in the blood there must also be a local lesion in the brain, and it is this that determines whether epilepsy (in particular psychomotor attacks) or some other affliction will develop.

Submicroscopic studies have shown that in experimental oedema the neuroglia cells swell but that the volume of the extracellular spaces remains unchanged (Gerschenfeld et al. 1959, Luse 1960, Torack et al. 1960). According to these findings the astroglia assume the function of special fluid spaces between blood and neuron; a function performed by the extracellular space in the other organs (Seiler 1966).

Many studies (Aird and Strait 1944, Anderson et al. 1957, Bakay 1956, Borison and Wang 1953, Van Breemen and Clemente 1955, Broman 1955, David and Brown 1959, De Robertis and Gerschenfeld 1958, Fisher et al. 1935, Hess 1955 a to c, Horstmann and Meves 1959, Kelentei and Földes 1954, Lumsden 1957, Millen and Hess 1958, Rodriguez 1955, Spatz 1934, Tschurgi 1960), particularly with electron pictures, have indicated that the brain has a maximum of 5 percent extracellular space. This small amount of extracellular space would not be particularly important in epilepsy. However, more recent results and calculations (Grüsser et al. 1968) indicate that there is about 15 percent extracellular space in the brain, and Grüsser et al. emphasize the importance of this space and its function in the therapy of epilepsy. The danger of oedema formation here must be borne in mind and attempts must be made to reduce it therapeutically.

Oedema formation is particularly likely to occur at certain common sites and lesions. For example, intensive irradiation of the skull leads to degeneration of astrocytes, and it has been shown that the permeability of the blood-brain barrier is increased at these sites (Clemente and Holst 1954). *Cerebral infections* (viruses, toxoplasmosis, bacteria) and *cerebral tumors* also cause a major disruption to the barrier (Bakay 1956, Stern and Marshall 1951). *Experimental convulsions,* stimulation of the sympathetic nervous system (electroshock) or psychological *stress* are also known to have an adverse effect on the functioning of the barrier (Bauer and Leonhardt 1955, Eichhorn 1956, Friedberg et al. 1948, Gellhorn and Kessler 1943, Jänkälä and Näätänen 1955, Jovanović 1968b, Quadbeck 1962, Quadbeck et al. 1962). Prolonged hypoxia, poisoning with haematotoxic agents (tetanus, streptococci, staphylococci) and a reduction of pH or of the pH differential between blood and brain result in increased capillary permeability in the CNS (Becker and Quadbeck 1952, Quadbeck and Randerath 1953). We have already mentioned changes occurring in the blood-brain barrier following administration of *drugs.*

For example, Quadbeck (1962) and Quadbeck et al. (1961) showed that the blood-brain barrier became more permeable following *aminophylline* (80% theophylline and 20% ethylenediamine). The barrier became permeable not only to the compound administered, but also to many other metabolites and substances which can pass in or out of cerebral tissue at the same time. Admittedly these authors have also shown that a permeability change in the blood-brain barrier can have favorable as well as adverse effects. For example, GABA cannot traverse the blood-brain barrier, but there have been reports of cases in which petit mal attacks have been substantially reduced by giving GABA, even by the oral route (Tower 1960, Kanig 1968). It has been suggested that in these cases the blood-brain barrier must be altered so that GABA can gain access to cerebral tissue via the cerebrospinal fluid.

BIOCHEMICAL PROCESSES IN THE PREPAROXYSMAL PHASE

It is difficult to study biochemical processes *directly before an attack begins* as compared with those occurring in the interval. Spontaneous epileptic attacks in man usually cannot be predicted and there is little opportunity to study them. The research worker really has to rely on good fortune here, and hence, animal experiments have assisted more towards solving this problem.

Another problem is how to define the duration of the *preparoxysmal phase*. Some biochemical changes can only be detected a few minutes or seconds before the attack, while many others can be found three to seven days before the episode. In discussing this phase we shall make a point always to mention the time of investigation in relation to the subsequent attack.

The vascular system undergoes changes immediately before an attack. Many authors have reported that the vasomotor system of the brain becomes somewhat unstable before the onset of a major seizure both in man and in experimental animals (Sinitsky and Sologuo 1965 and others).

Fattovich (1931) found that there was characteristic vasomotor constriction before an attack in epileptics and from this he assumed that there was *vasomotor diathesis in epilepsy*. The cerebral capillaries constrict and become smaller before the onset of the attack and they continue to be rather labile after the epileptic symptoms have appeared.

By taking measurements at the jugular vein, Gibbs et al. (1934) observed definite reduction of blood flow through the brain shortly before an attack in nine of ten cases with epileptic reactions. The authors interpret this as cerebral vasoconstriction preceding the attack and there is discussion as to how far this vascular reaction can be regarded as the cause of the convulsions. These authors concluded that vascular instability should be regarded more as a sequela than as a cause. Lennox (1936), Lennox et al. (1936 a, b) and other authors, some of whom we referred to in Chapter II, obtained similar results.

In the epileptic equivalents, no definite vascular changes before the attack have been reported (Vetter and Gänshirt 1962). According to Selbach et al. (1965), the bilateral spike and wave complexes and other bioelectrical elements which can be seen in the EEG a few seconds before the clinical symptoms appear are obviously adequately compensated for in normal cerebral metabolism. However a major seizure, with a maximum energy requirement of up to 50 times the normal (Bogina 1942, Ruf 1950), produces a massive increase in blood flow in the CNS and this change may be manifest at the beginning of the attack.

The extent of vasoconstriction of the cerebral vessels is very variable and there are violent fluctuations in the preparoxysmal phase, with rapid alternations between vasoconstriction and vasodilatation; this may explain any discrepancies in the results from different authors (Selbach et al. 1965). The arterial hypotension with the autonomic system exerting a maximum trophotropic effect in the decompensation phase shortly before or at the beginning of the attack, is attributed to the effect of the cholinergic mechanisms responsible for dilatation (Duesberg and Spitzbarth 1963, Selbach 1962). However, this immediately gives rise to a compensatory reversal. The vascular chemoreceptors stimulate the reticular system of the brain stem into an *ergotropic* response. This results in excessive adrenergic constriction in the network of capillaries (Fattovich 1931, Gibbs et al. 1934) and the affected area becomes anoxic (Selbach et al. 1965). So we have a labile vascular picture in which there is constriction before an attack but a change in the situation during and after the attack.

Having studied the reports on this subject we would now like to summarize the vasomotor changes which occur in the preparoxysmal phase: a few seconds before an attack there is vasoconstriction of the cerebral vessels immediately followed by vasodilatation. Renewed and possibly more profound vasoconstriction then occurs, followed by more prolonged vasodilatation, by which time the attack has already begun. During the attack the vasodilatation gradually subsides or develops into mild vasoconstriction, according to the course of the attack.

According to the authors cited above, in psychomotor attacks vasomotor changes only occur in association with major seizures. Mild psychomotor symptoms do not appear to cause general vascular changes which can be detected peripherally. However, local changes in the vascular system at the epileptic focus cannot be excluded, and these have been detected in experimental animals.

The electrolyte balance becomes unstable just before an attack. There are also fluctuations in electrolyte concentration associated with an increase of acetylcholine concentration before the epileptic episode. The release of acetylcholine in the brain produces ionic instability so that the permeability to potassium and sodium ions is increased in the postsynaptic regions of the neurons. An increase of membrane permeability has the effect of reducing the potential difference of the membrane, of increasing intracellular sodium and reducing intracellular potassium (Tower 1960).

According to Kreindler (1965) and Shanes (1958), at this stage even a small quantity of acetylcholine may synchronize the postsynaptic potentials. According to Woodbury et al (1958 a), the change in the concentration of cations in the external and internal spaces of the neurons is one of the most important events preceding epileptic convulsions. Following adrenalectomy the predisposition of the brain to convulsion increases, there are abnormal changes in the bioelectrical activity of the brain and an increase of intracellular sodium ions. Subsequent administration of adrenocorticotropic hormones reverses this process.

It is interesting to note that in animal experiments a shift in the electrolyte balance with a fall of potassium ions in the cells and an increase of intracellular sodium ions only occurs when the attacks are induced with methionine sulphoximine. These changes did not appear to occur when convulsions were induced with thiosemicarbazide (Kreindler 1965, Tower 1960). This finding may have been due to the experimental technique, since migration of ions following stimulation of the CNS has been demonstrated fairly accurately (see also Chapter IV).

Water retention is also involved in inducing an attack; this was pointed out above and is illustrated by Figures 22 a to c. It is likely that there is local swelling in the brain just before a major or psychomotor seizure since the vasomotor picture is different in healthy people or in epileptics in the interval. In addition to the authors cited in chapters II and III we would like to give a brief summary of Pogodaev's findings (1964). Using different experimental animals he found a change of pressure and of moisture content in the brain with formation of oedema following repeated attacks induced by an electric current or acoustic stimuli. This process is most important in patients who suffer from frequent attacks, where the brain does not have sufficient time to recover from the aftermath of the previous attack.

In contrast to the findings of Tower (1960) and Kreindler (1965) who reported loss of potassium before an attack, Mertens (1964) believed that this is due to excess of potassium ions in the neurons and a general tendency to retain water and certain metabolites. This would also explain the reduced excretion of potassium ions in the preparoxysmal phase. It would also be easy to tie in potassium retention with the general trophotropic (parasympathicotropic) picture in the epileptic during the preparoxysmal phase, although the predominant factor in this trophotropic autonomic picture is hyperpolarization of the nerve cell membrane. Selbach et al. (1965) regard this hyperpolarization as transitory, it being followed by incipient discharge of the action potential and depolarization, with influx of sodium ions and increased efflux of potassium. However, these authors base their views on results of blood or urine examinations and they cannot really relate this to the quite rapid *local* changes of membrane potential in the brain, without supplying experimental evidence.

Oxidation processes with a change of pH also play an important part in the preparoxysmal phase. However, there is a certain amount of discrepancy in the results here. The fact that seizures may also occur under conditions of hypoxia, hypoglycaemia and cyanide poisoning indicates that there is some change in the oxidation processes (Elliott et al. 1950). However, since hypoxia may also suppress the increased predisposition to convulsion, it is important to know which mechanisms are responsible for inducing convulsions under these hypoxic conditions.

Lennox and Gibbs (1936 a, b) and Lennox et al. (1936) found that in their patients the oxygen saturation of cerebral blood differed from that in healthy people. In 46 percent of 88 cases investigated, Lennox and Gibbs (1936 a) found reduced oxygen saturation of arterial blood, the fall being quite considerable. The oxygen saturation of arterial blood in epileptics was lower than the lowest value for normal blood. In a further 11 percent of cases the level of oxygen saturation was less than 90 percent of the norm. There was no change in partial CO_2 pressure (pCO_2). This finding correlates with that of Lennox (1936). These parameters were unchanged in cerebrospinal fluid (Lennox and Merritt 1936). Empey et al. (1932) failed to find differences in oxygen saturation and pCO_2 of the cerebrospinal fluid in their patients. The difference between hypoxia which provokes an attack (before the convulsions) and hypoxia which retards an attack (during generalized convulsions) is probably due to the change of pH. Many authors (Lennox et al. 1936 a, b, MacQuarrie et al. 1932, Selbach 1962, Selbach et al. 1965) have reported *alkalosis* in cerebral tissue and in the patient's blood before an attack, but *acidosis* during the attack. Accordingly, hypoxia can be regarded as toxic before an attack. However, toxic hypoxia may induce the attack or have a favorable effect on it (Pogodaev 1964, Woodbury et al. 1958 a, b). Acute hypoxic intoxication does not occur after the attack since the condition is prevented by the dynamic changes which restore the biological equilibrium and bring about changes in enzymatic and metabolic processes which prevent hypoxic intoxication. This will be discussed below and in Chapter VIII. However, as we pointed out in Chapters II and III even though it only occurs for a short while during an attack temporary hypoxia does in fact produce brain damage.

In animal experiments it was shown that the bioelectrical convulsion threshold of the brain is substantially increased by administering 5 to 20 percent CO_2 (anticonvulsant), but it is reduced by administering 25 to 40% CO_2 (convulsant). If administration of more than 40 percent CO_2 is continued the convulsions are again inhibited, this time because of a *toxic* increase in the cerebral convulsion threshold.

Carbohydrate metabolism is probably disturbed shortly before an attack, but we are not absolutely certain about this at the moment. We know that, as mentioned above, hypoglycaemia has an adverse effect and hyperglycaemia a favorable effect on the increased cerebral predisposition to convulsion and on the EEG of the patients.

Changes in protein metabolism in the preparoxysmal phase have been demonstrated by many authors. We can use those of Krupenina (1960) to illustrate this point briefly. This author observed serum protein changes in epileptics in the interval and shortly before an attack, and she reported on some interesting phenomena.

About nine hours before an attack, total protein in serum was a mean 7.8 percent, albumin fraction 41.8 percent, α_1-globulins 11.8 percent α_2-globulins 15.4 percent, beta-globulins 16.4 percent and gamma-globulins 14.6 percent. Thus the A/G quotient was very depressed (it being 0.72). So, compared with the interval, nine hours before convulsions occurred there was *a further fall of albumins, and a further rise of alpha- and beta-globulins, particularly of α_1-globulins, and a further fall of the A/G quotient with a further rise of total serum protein.*

About six hours before the convulsions, there was no further rise of total protein in serum, but the albumin fraction was very depressed (36.8%) and the α_1-globulins had increased further (12.3%) ; on the other hand, the α_2-globulins and beta-globulins tended to be lower than those of nine hours before. There was a substantial rise of gamma-globulins, with values fluctuating around 25.5 percent.

About four hours before the attack there were no further changes in protein fractions, except that total serum protein had increased to 8.1 g. percent, and there was a renewed rise of the albumin fraction compared with that of six hours before. The A/G quotient also began to increase and it was then 0.76 (see also Contini 1936 a, b, Eeg—Olofson 1940, Jovanović 1970 e, McKenzie and McChesney 1935, MacQuarrie 1929, Rizzotto 1934, Rizzotto and Martinengo 1934) .

It should be pointed out that the changes of serum protein in epileptics may take a different course just before an attack, and there may be a tendency for them to normalize. This indicates that the biochemical changes in the patient's body may appear much sooner than the actual clinical symptoms. The electroencephalographic changes may also appear some time before an attack (see Chapter II) .

Jovanović (1970 e) has confirmed the results of Krupenina (1960) and of the other authors mentioned above, although it must be added that this type of change of protein fractions is not observed in every form of epilepsy. In centrencephalic epilepsy the attacks usually occur when the patient is awake and there are bilateral symmetrical spike and wave formations in the

EEG. Here, there are no profound changes of protein before the attack, although gamma-globulins may be elevated for a few days before the onset of a generalized or minor attack; the other fractions and total serum protein change very little. On the other hand, *protein shifts such as those demonstrated by* Krupenina (1960) *are very prominent in psychomotor epilepsy, in diffuse epilepsy with psychomotor symptoms and in patients with epileptic attacks arising out of sleep with or without manifest psychomotor symptoms.* The basic cause of the disease (whether it is essential or symptomatic) is secondary here unless the cause is a tumor, infectious encephalitis or severe toxic brain damage where there are other symptoms apart from epilepsy. However, these cases cannot be included in this analysis.

Amino acids are also very important here. From the discussion in the beginning of this chapter it can be seen that a series of changes occur in the levels of amino acids in the interval and also shortly before an attack. We must mention in particular *glutamic acid (GA)* and *gamma-aminobutyric acid (GABA)* since these compounds are thought to be responsible for the convulsions in most cases, particularly in experimental epilepsy (Hassler et al. 1971)

According to some authors (Gershenovitch et al. 1963, Kolousek 1959a, Mison-Crighel et al. 1964, 1965, Terner et al. 1950, Tower 1960, Vrba 1955, 1957, Woodbury et al. 1958b) GABA concentration is inversely proportional to the pathological excitability of the brain and directly proportional to extracellular sodium: intracellular sodium / $Na^{ex} : Na^{in}$ /.

According to the results reported earlier, administration of GABA has an anticonvulsant effect where the convulsions are provoked by Cardiazol, acoustic stimuli, strychnine or hydrazines. *Diphenylhydantoin* medication increases the cerebral GABA content in animals. Selbach et al. (1965) have suggested that the therapeutic effect of *succinimides* (Marazzi et al. 1958) may perhaps be due to their structural similarity to GABA (see also Bamberger and Matthes 1959).

There is a certain amount of discrepancy in the results of some authors in respect of GABA and GA concentrations before an attack. Gershenovitch et al. (1963) found that both glutamines and glutamine synthesis increase in the 10-minute preconvulsive phase when convulsions are provoked by administering oxygen to animals. However, Mison-Crighel et al. (1963) found a significant fall in GA and glutamine concentrations and a rise of glutaminase within two minutes after local administration of mescaline, i.e. before convulsive activity appeared. Kolousek and Jiraček (1959 b) observed that methionine sulphoximine reduces the concentration of GA in the preparoxysmal phase due to the reaction: glutamic acid→glutamine-NH_3, and this produces a convulsive disorder. The apparent contradiction in results is probably due to the different methods used, since many authors determined the role of GABA and the GABA balance using the above-named chemical compounds (Hassler et al. 1971).

The importance of the endogenous amines in the interval between epileptic attacks was discussed above. As has been pointed out, we do not yet know all the details about the role of these amines in the development of an attack (see also Hassler et al. 1971).

In *phenylketonuria* and epilepsy (Christian 1968b), there is an increase in the concentration of phenylalanine in blood and in the level of a series of partially metabolized substances which are excreted in the urine. Apart from phenylpyruvic acid, we also find large quantities of phenylalanine, p-hydroxyphenylpyruvic acid, p-hydroxyphenyl-lactic acid and phenylacetyl-glutamine. It is reasonable to suppose that this would produce epileptic attacks, although the primary cause is not known for certain. O-tyrosine, n-tyrosine, O-hydroxy-phenylacetic acid, indolylpyruvic acid and indolyl-lactic acid are also found in epileptics with phenylketonuria (Armstrong and Robinson 1955, Boscott and Bickel 1953, Fölling 1934, Stein et al. 1954.

We do not know for certain which enzymatic reactions are involved in this abnormal type of phenylalanine metabolism. It is assumed that there is a deficiency of the enzyme which hydrolyses phenylalanine to tyrosine or that the activity of the enzyme is substantially reduced (Bessmann and Baldwin 1962, Fellmann and Devlin 1958, Jervis 1953, Udenfriend and Bessman 1953, Wallace et al. 1957).

An important point here is that with this rise of partially metabolized products, there is *a fall of Adrenaline and noradrenaline* in the patient's blood (Sourkes and D'Irio 1963, Weil-Malherbe 1955). This may indicate that the balance between the endogenous amines is disturbed in patients with phenoketonuria and epileptic symptoms; a fall in the level of Adrenaline and noradrenaline (convulsion-inhibiting substances) would wean a rise or relative *rise of serotonin and/or acetylcholine* (convulsion-provoking substances).

To some extent there is also a fall in the serotonin concentration in epilepsy and phenylketonuria. However, this does not always occur since it is possible to demonstrate selective reduction of the Adrenaline and noradrenaline concentration without any fall in the serotonin concentration (Armstrong and Robinson 1954, Baldridge et al. 1959, Ferrari et al. 1955, Jouvet 1968, Sandler and Close 1959, etc.). In other cases of epilepsy not associated with phenylketonuria there was a substantial *increase of serotonin* concentration shortly before an attack (Funderbruk et al. 1962, Szimuzu et al. 1964).

Before an attack, the *acetylcholine* concentration increases considerably. This increase of ACh concentration before the attack means that the system is unable to inactivate free acetylcholine (Kreindler 1965, Richter and Crossland 1949, Takahashi et al. 1961, Tower 1960). We can conclude from this that acetylcholine is important both before and during an attack.

The concentration of *histamine* probably remains unchanged until the onset of convulsions. We do not know what its function is before an attack. There may well be a transient rise of histamine before an attack, during the temporary periods of dilatation of cerebral blood vessels. During the attack the histamine concentration may rise. This usually occurs just as, or shortly after, convulsions begin.

The role of ammonia has been studied in some detail in the period shortly before an attack. It has been shown that there is a correlation between cerebral excitability and ammonium ion concentration in the brain, and this seems quite logical (Benitez et al. 1954, Richter and Dawson 1948). However, this correlation is not particularly significant in the period before an attack. Unlike the authors previously cited, these authors observed convulsive cerebral activity after administering ammonium salts to animals. The level of ammonium ions rose substantially during the preconvulsive phase and shortly afterwards, as soon as the convulsions were triggered off by an electric current. The same happened when the attacks were induced with picrotoxin. Sapirstein (1943) also believed that convulsions could be induced with ammonia. According to Torda (1953), ammonia must affect cerebral hyperactivity before the onset of convulsions, i.e. it *predisposes* the brain to convulsions. Torda (1953) believes that several biochemical reactions must precede the convulsions, and then these occur readily. However, these reactions have not been defined in detail or confirmed using an EEG. According to Takahashi et al. (1961) there is no correlation between the level of ammonia in the brain and increased cerebral predisposition to convulsion. These authors and some of the authors mentioned earlier assume that increased concentration of ammonia in the brain is not the cause but the result of convulsions.

Ammonia normally occurs in the brain as an end product of protein metabolism (Meister 1954) and its concentration increases whenever cerebral activity is increased even if there is no manifest convulsive activity. It may be that in epileptic attacks, shortly before convulsive activity begins, there is an abnormal biochemical reaction involving ammonia, or an abnormal metabolic reaction in which convulsant substances are formed; this problem remains to be solved. It has not yet been possible to demonstrate any causal connection between ammonia and psychomotor epilepsy. Figure 31 shows the curve of the ammonium ion concentration shortly before an attack. The ammonia concentration *in blood* shortly before the attack has not been elucidated in detail.

Hormonal changes probably occur just before an attack. There is no need to stress the fact that epileptic attacks and their equivalents often occur in female patients shortly before menstruation. Attacks occur one or two, sometimes even three or four days before menstruation, and may even develop just before the bleeding starts (Arnold 1954, Bente and Kluge 1953, Denys 1963, Griffel 1953, Grühle 1935, Helmchen et al. 1964, Mercer 1960, Pette and Janzen 1938, Selbach and Selbach 1950, Selbach 1954, Wiener 1930). It is very significant that according to these authors and in our own experience, convulsions occurring in this rhythm are recorded almost exclusively in patients with the centrencephalic type of epilepsy. Here, major attacks occurring after waking in the morning or in the afternoon during a period of relaxation, and absences and other manifestations of centrencephalic origin, are the most common. Psychomotor attacks do not correlate so well with menstruation and, clinically, such a connection is rare. Major attacks arising from sleep correlate rather better with menstruation, but nowhere near so well as does matutinal epilepsy.

Enzymes are particularly important before an epileptic attack (Pokrovsky and Pinomareva 1965 and others). Since the quantity of protein in blood and brain is elevated in an epileptic (Empey et al. 1932, Jantz 1956, Jovanović 1970e, 1971b; Klimes and Lang 1942, McKenzie and McChesney 1935, Rizzotto and Martinengo 1934, Teglbjaerg 1935, 1936, Vladimirov 1953), there must either be more rapid synthesis or less rapid degradation (inhibited) (Rittenberg et al. 1948).

A series of proteolytic enzymes have been detected in the CNS and PNS (PNS or peripheral nervous system), but we are not quite sure of their biological significance. The proteinases, *cathepsins,* have been found both in the neurons and in the neuroglia cells (Waelsch 1962). However, these are active in a relatively acid environment (at pH 3 to 6) so their activity is impaired in epileptics shortly before an attack and possibly in the interval as well. It may be that the hyperproteinaemia in patients in the interval and particularly before the attack is connected with this decline of enzyme activity. Like many other enzymes in the brain, cathepsins are probably enclosed in lysosomal particles so that their activity becomes much more pronounced after a local lesion or after general stress. In this case we are thinking in particular of a local lesion which could be an epileptic focus.

After fairly powerful electrical stimulation, activity in the PNS rises by more than 100%. There is hardly any change after weaker or brief stimulation (Ungar and Romano 1962, Ungar et al. 1957).

Neutral proteinases (optimum activity at pH 7) are also found in the CNS (Ansell and Richter 1954). The important point with these enzymes is that they require a good deal of ATP coenzyme A and oxygen for their activity. Neutral proteinases are inhibited by convulsant agents (cyanide, 2,4-dinitrophenol) (Lajtha 1964 a, b); the citric acid cycle and oxidative phosphorylation are inhibited at the same time (Marks and Lajtha 1963). Inhibition of the citric acid cycle may in itself have a convulsant effect.

The inhibitability of these enzymes has also been demonstrated with some synthetic amino acids (p-fluoro-phenylalanine, beta-2-thienyl-alanine) and these substances also inhibit protein synthesis (Steinberg and Vaugh 1956, Steinberg et al. 1956). It has been suggested that these enzymes do not break down proteins by simple hydrolysis, but that there must be intermediate stages which requires a supply of energy. The inhibition of protein synthesis and of protein metabolism by these substances seems to indicate that catabolic enzymatic processes in the attack are a reversal of the anabolic picture which prevails before an attack; however, there is no definite evidence for this.

The distribution and function of *dipeptidases and polypeptidases* in the preparoxysmal epileptic phase are not known in detail.

Blocking or inhibiting enzymatic processes or protein synthesis in the hippocampus and temporal lobes produces certain psychical changes in experimental animals, depending on the duration of inhibition. These changes closely resemble the transient changes observed in some patients just before a psychomotor attack (Flexner et al. 1965).

The *alkaline state of cerebral tissue* just before an attack also impairs the activity of other enzymes. GABA is produced from glutamic acid in the presence of the enzyme *glutamic acid-decaboxylase* which has optimum activity at pH 6.5. Thus, an alkaline environment inhibits the production of GABA. On the other hand, GABA transaminases are most active at pH 8.2. Just before an attack, conditions are favorable for GABA breakdown (transamination). Thus, there are two causes of the fall in GABA concentration before epileptic convulsions: firstly indaequate production (synthesis) and secondly accelerated breakdown. Since *decarboxylases* are relatively non-specific and are able to metabolize many amino acids an alkaline shift in the acid-base balance before an attack may also produce other metabolic abnormalities which precede the convulsions (Hanson 1958, Tahian 1961).

Metabolism of the *endogenous amines* may also be affected by these changes, and under certain conditions these amines can induce convulsions. For example, it has been found that there is a change in the activity of *cholinesterases, MAO* and other enzymes involved in the metabolism of monoamines (Appel et al. 1957, Elliott et al. 1950, Elliott and Henderson 1948, Gershoff et al. 1949, Lascăr 1958). (see also Chapter III).

The vitamins have already been discussed in detail. As we pointed out earlier, many metabolic changes occur in the interval and shortly before an attack begins. These changes, and those described in the previous chapter, are very often enough to induce convulsions and/or convulsion equivalents.

BIOCHEMICAL PROCESSES IN THE PAROXYSMAL PHASE

Some General Points Regarding the Energy Changes Which Occur in the CNS Under Conditions of Excitation and Inhibition

As mentioned above, studies of the arterio-venous system revealed significant changes in *oxygen and* pCO_2 before an attack; this was demonstrated by Kassil (1937, 1938), Martin et al. (1957), Rubel (1939) and Tchalissov et al. (1937, 1940).

Respiration in cerebral tissue is particularly important during an attack, both for *plastic processes (anabolism)* and for *energy-supplying reactions (catabolism).* Studying the activtiy of respiratroy enzymes is a particularly good way of observing the dynamic processes of the biochemical reactions in the more highly organized structures in the body (CNS). Respiratory activity *in vivo* (Benedeto et al. 1956, Cahn et al. 1957, 1958, Etling 1954, Kasimirova 1954, 1956, Kassil et al. 1936, Larrabee and Bronk 1952, Longtin 1955, Quastel 1952) or in manometric studies *in vitro* (Bondrev 1956, Dobrinina 1955, Elliott 1957, Kuschmann 1956, Mandel et al. 1955, 1957, Pogodaev 1964, Pogodaev et al. 1960) depends on the activity of basic processes in the brain or in the CNS as a whole. CNS stimulation speeds up respiration, and vice versa (McIlwain 1955, 1957).

When there is a phase of excitation which dominates the inhibitory processes, there is a rise in the concentration of *organic acids* in the brain, in particular lactic acid and pyruvic acid, and changes in the *acid-base balance* (Fedorov 1941, Gordon 1951, Martinson et al. 1956, Oeriu and Tănăseku 1958, Pogodaev 1959, Pogodaev et al. 1960, Prochorova et al. 1957, Stone 1938, Reiko et al. 1957, Vladimirova 1937).

Among other things it has been demonstrated that CNS excitation increases the rate of breakdown of energy-rich compounds containing phosphate, such as ATP, and increases the concentration of the dephosphorylation products *ADP* and *inorganic phosphorus.* Excitation processes are also linked with the break-down (dephosphorylation) of *phosphocreatine,* and this also increases the concentration of inorganic phosphorus in the CNS. The concentration of inorganic phosphorus is also increased as a result of degradation of phospholipids, phosphoproteins and ribonucleids. This process may be an indication of the degree of excitation in the CNS (Kreindler 1965, Palladin 1953, Seits 1953, 1961, Sitinski 1955, 1956, Vladimirov et al. 1964).

The relationships between the functional properties of the CNS during epileptic attacks in connection with *changes in protein metabolism* in nervous tissue, and the special properties of proteins such as *colloid-osmotic pressure, isoelectric point,* changes of *hydrophilic properties* and of *adsorp-*

tive capacity, have been studied by Barmina (1957), Gorodiskaya et al. (1941), Ivanenko and Dunaeva (1955), Kiyota (1961), Pappius and Elliott (1956), Pogodaev (1954 to 1964), Pogodaev et al. (1960), Schurminski (1957), Schwarz and Yanoff (1965), Tower (1960), Tower and Elliott (1952 a, b, 1953), Varipaeva (1957, 1958), Voinar (1935), Vrba (1955, 1956, 1957), Vrba et al. (1962).

Protein metabolism is affected by the physiological processes in the brain during an attack. During a phase of excitation, catabolic processes dominate the synthetic processes, while when the inhibitory processes are dominant in the brain catabolism is retarded or arrested in order to allow the processes of resynthesis to take precedence (Giatonde and Richter 1956, Kreindler 1965, Palladin 1959, 1962, Palladin and Vladimirov 1955, Richter 1958, 1959, Schwarz and Yanoff 1965, Waelsch 1961).

When dealing with protein metabolism, we must also mention the problem of the effect of *amino acids* in an attack (Berl et al. 1959, Biel and Vilter 1954, Dawson 1953, Haber and Saidel 1948, Hydén 1943, Killam 1957, 1958, Killam and Bain 1957, Kuchinskas and Du Vigneaud 1957, Mison-Chrighel et al 1964, 1965, Roberts et al. 1953, Sinclair 1960, 1962, Suguira 1957, Tashian 1961, Wiechert and Herbst 1966).

The *endogenous amines* are also important substances in epileptic episodes; the metabolism and function of these amines is quite similar to that of the amino acids (Bertaccini 1959, Costa-Foru 1961, Feldberg 1957, Geiger 1957, Kreindler 1965, McIlwain 1955, McIntosh and Oborin 1953, McKerracher et al. 1966, Pope et al. 1947, Uzunov et al. 1961).

Increased activity in the nerve cells (excitation) is characterized by increased *proteolytic enzyme* activity with formation of nitrogenous metabolic products (Fomin 1928, Geiger et al. 1953, Gorodiskaya 1926, Pferdmann and Feinschmidt 1932, Pogodaev et al. 1956, 1957, 1959, 1960, Pokrovsky and Smirnova 1965, Smirnova 1941a, Soula 1912, 1913, Vrba 1956, 1957, Walsne et al. 1958).

Although there is some argument about the role of *ammonia* in the interval and we are not yet certain as to its role directly before an attack, the metabolism of this compound during an attack is thought to be very important. In fact, the ammonia concentration is regarded as an extremely important indicator of the basic functions of the CNS *in vivo* at any given moment (Kolousek et al. 1959, Okumura 1960, Richter and Dawson 1948, Takagaki et al. 1957, 1961, Vladimirova 1953, 1961, Vrba 1956).

An attack affects the entire body and all the metabolic processes. All the changes mentioned above are linked with activation and/or inhibition of enzymes, hormones and vitamins (Careddu 1963, Kanig 1968, Lang 1962, McIlwain 1966, Neuhoff and Herkin 1964, Rapoport 1964, Seiler 1966,

Willing 1954, Wolfe and Elliott 1962). The processes change before an attack, and then also change during and after the attack.

Before we deal with these problems in detail, we should like to mention several points regarding the course of an experimental attack.

Most research workers classify convulsive episodes in animal experiments into: 1.) tonic phase, 2.) clonic phase, 3.) locomotor phase, and 4.) coma or exhaustion phase (Froklis 1953, 1958, Glasov 1940, Grashtchenkov and Fiedelholz 1934, Ilina 1953, Keit 1950, Kogan 1927, Livencev 1952, Sereiski 1946, Servit and Buresch 1952 a). Some Russian authors (including Pogodaev 1964, Hartchenko 1942, Livencev 1952, Servit and Bureš 1952 b) have added several points to these, when classifying the epileptic phases manifest in animal experiments.

Pogodaev (1964) has been carrying out biochemical and physiological experiments using different species of animal (more than 5,000 animals) over a period of twenty years and has produced many valuable results. He has divided the visible symptoms of an epileptic attack induced by electric current, acoustic stimuli or by chemicals into several phases:

He called *the first phase* the *initial clonus* (see also Servit and Bureš 1952 a, b); in rats this lasts for 3.18 seconds (s ± 0.71). Livencev (1952) uses the term *initial epileptic spasm,* and apparently he has in mind here the same phase as the initial clonus of Servit and Bureš (1952 a, b), Pogodaev (1964) and Pogodaev et al. (1956, 1959, 1960 a, b, 1961). This initial tonus consists of a few twitches before the next phase begins.

According to Pogodaev (1964), *the second, tonic phase* corresponds to the classic tonic phase in man and in animals; in experiments on rats, this phase lasts 8.35 seconds (s ± 0.97).

The third phase is the clonic phase: this is slightly longer, lasting 19.4 seconds (s ± 2.93). This is essentially the same as the clonic phases of epileptic convulsions described earlier.

According to Pogodaev, *the fourth phase* is the phase of motor automatisms (the *locomotor phase*) in which the experimental animals exhibit rhythmic twitching of the hind limbs which resembles running movements, and hence, the name *locomotor* (in Russian: *beg na meste*). This lasts 23.0 seconds (s ± 5.31). Many authors include this in the clonic phase (Frolkis 1953, Grashtchenkov 1935, Hartchenko 1942, Ilina 1953, Speransky 1932, Steblov 1932, 1936).

The fifth phase is the *coma* or *exhaustion phase,* characterized by absolute rest and complete areflexia. In rats this lasts 18.2 seconds (s ± 7.11).

The sixth and last phase is a period of *muscular rigidity;* this phase is very protracted (128 ± 12.4 seconds) and there is little scatter compared with the fifth phase. Unlike the fifth phase there are very weak reflexes in this final phase. Coordination of movement is disturbed and bodily function is still not restored (Civilko 1947, Davidov 1950, Ilina 1953, Juchlov 1952, Kreindler 1955, 1965, Pogodaev 1954, 1957, 1959 1963 a to c, Pogodaev and Krasnova 1954, 1955, 1956, Pogodaev and Mehmedova 1957, Pogodaev and Turova 1959, Pogodaev et al. 1956, 1959, 1960 a, b, 1961, Sedina 1945, Shebrin 1949).

In each of these phases there are different energy and biochemical changes. These changes will be discussed now.

Electrolyte Changes

Microcombustion techniques have shown that during convulsions, and even right at the beginning of an attack induced by electric current or *Metrazol,* in rats and rabbits there is a fall in the concentration of intracellular potassium ions compared with normal brain samples (Colfer and Essex 1947). The same or similar changes were found after inducing convulsions with acoustic stimuli. The concentration of potassium ions within the cell returns to normal within three hours. Experiments carried out by Cicardo (1945), Adams et al. (1952), Mison-Crighel et al. (1955), Breyer and Kanig (1970) confirmed the results of Colfer and Essex (1947).

Differences resembling those found in experimental animals could not be demonstrated in samples taken from epileptogenic areas of human cortex or from non-epileptogenic sections of human brain (Pappius and Elliott 1954). According to these authors, there were no significant differences between sodium and potassium ion concentrations inside and outside the neurons.

Also, the differences seen in rats and rabbits after inducing convulsions by local administration of mescaline could not be demonstrated in cats (Mison-Crighel et al. 1964).

According to Woodbury et al. (1958 a, b) the absolute concentration is not so important as the ratio of electrolytes to one another. For example, Woodbury et al. (1958 a, b) did not detect any definite intracellular ionic changes in epileptic animals, while there was a reduction in the differences between extracellular and intracellular potassium ions and the ratio of extracellular to intracellular sodium ions was reduced. These findings reflect a rise in the intracellular sodium ion concentration and a rise in the concentration of extracellular potassium ions, or to put it another way, *a relative deficiency of intracellular potassium ions.*

These findings indicate that: during excitation, depending on the strength and intensity of the stimulus, there is a flow of ions in opposite directions across the nerve cell membrane, but the neurons are not exhausted right at the start of epileptic convulsions. In the coma phase there is temporary bioelectrical exhaustion of the nerve cells. However, in a certain sense this exhaustion is a very important retarding process.

The Oxidizing Activity in Cerebral Tissue

The apnoea of an epileptic is inspiratory or expiratory, according to the phase of respiration at the onset of the attack (Frolkis 1958). In minor attacks it begins after a latent period of 0.5 to 2.5 seconds after the 3/sec. spike-wave complex, i.e. there is delayed autonomic synchronization (Bogacz and Yanicelli 1962, Selbach et al. 1965). However, in major attacks it begins immediately and it is in fact the first symptom of sudden and complete synchronization (Selbach et al. 1965). This apnoea affects the respiratory conditions in the brain and according to the latest concepts on neural regulation of respiration (Wyss 1964) it acts in the primary autonomic *ergotropic* sympathetic matrix to arrest the activity of the motor inspiratory aggregate in the bulbus medullae oblongatae (lateral part of the reticular formation). According to Selbach et al. (1965) this is the site of action of the pCO_2 and an acute condition develops in the epileptic patient which threatens the automania of the respiratory center; this condition develops for two reasons: firstly, these authors believe that a maturation defect throughout the *ergotropic* system, i.e. reduced sensitivity of the regulating substrates reduces the sensitivity of the respiratory center to CO_2, and pathologically impaired sensitivity of the respiratory center together with a general trophotropic tendency with hypersomnia and obesity explains why attacks arise out of sleep in patients with Pickwickian syndrome, in spite of the increase of pCO_2 (Herberg 1965, Jovanović 1969, Selbach 1965). Secondly, there is a relative fall in production of the specific activator, CO_2. Maximal production of and saturation with this and other activators which occur under crisis conditions according to the *all or nothing law* and which are promoted by the tonic convulsions, represent the life-saving consequences of periodic reorganization of a physiological surface activity, and this even occurs in the *ergotropic* substrates of the respiratory center. *Trophotropic overweight and instability are characteristics of the epileptic metabolism and its effects on CNS function and it is these two factors which determine the symptoms and therapy in epileptic patients.*

There are several objections to this theory, which was put forward by Selbach and Selbach (1950), Selbach (1965) and Selbach et al. (1965) based on Rosenthal's principles of oscillation (1864); however, we cannot discuss these objections here. For example, we do not know whether a person who suffers accidental brain injury does in fact necessarily have "a maturation defect throughout the ergotropic system" from the outset, nor are we sure if the respiration of epileptics is in fact controlled in this way, i.e. during crises (see Chapter VIII).

The results of animal experiments (Pogodaev and Krasnova 1955) have shown that the epileptic spasm mentioned above, or the *initial clonus,* occurs at the moment the electric current reaches the experimental animal. At the moment this initial clonus subsides, the *tonic component* of the attack intensifies and the oxygen saturation of arterial blood falls. This was also reported by Lennox et al. (1936), Lennox and Gibbs (1936 a, b) and Lennox and Merritt (1936) just before an attack. During the *next phase* of the attack oxygenation of the blood is increased although according to Pogodaev and Krasnova (1955) it does not return to the initial level or reach the level achieved during the *locomotor phase.* By assaying the oxygen with a Krebs oxygenometer (Pogodaev and Krasnova 1955, Pogodaev 1964) it has been shown that the oxygen saturation of arterial blood is reduced by 40% to 60% both during electroshock in humans (psychoses) and also during electroconvulsions in experimental animals (experimental epilepsy).

The powerful motoricity during the clonic phase does not parallel the fall of oxygen saturation in arterial blood. Oxygenation only increases after a couple of minutes. *Abortive attacks and some psychomotor attacks which are protracted and not very violent, are characterized by the fact that the fall of oxygen saturation lasts a little longer than in generalized attacks.* However, after this type of protracted attack there may be an enormous rise of oxygen saturation, which may then become abnormally high (Pogodaev 1964).

During the convulsions there is a significant *increase in the blood supply* to the brain, *particularly to the regions which are responsible for producing the attack.* Circulation of blood is delayed in these regions (Empey et al. 1932, Frolkis 1958, Gänshirt et al. 1959, Gellhorn 1953, Gibbs et al. 1940, Kassil 1938, Lennox and Gibbs 1936 a, b, Lennox et al. 1936, Penfield and Erikson 1949).

During an attack, experimental animals need 20 to 50 times more oxygen than control animals and much more carbon dioxide is produced (Bogina 1942, Meistrach 1948, Ruf 1950). If the brain is forcibly respired there is both dissociation of the oxygen concentration in arterial and venous blood and dissociation of the oxygen supply and the actual oxygen consumption in the brain (Geiger and Magnes 1947, Kassil 1938, Mosinger 1957, Pogodaev 1964, Pogodaev et al. 1956, Schmidt et al. 1945).

Immediately before an attack begins, the oxygen level in the brain becomes unstable (Lennox and Gibbs 1936 a, b, Lennox et al. 1936, Word et al. 1948). Polarographic studies have shown that the oxygen content of cerebral tissue falls rapidly at the beginning of an attack, indicating increased oxygen consumption (Davies and Remond 1947).

Pogodaev (1964) obtained some interesting results when he set out to determine the *respiratory activity* of the brain in the *initial phase* in experimental animals (rats). In this phase overall respiratory activity in the brain is higher than in control animals. After 40 minutes incubation period, oxygen consumption of cerebral homogenates was higher than in the brain sections from control animals, by 28 percent in the cerebral hemispheres, by 26 percent in the brain stem, by 50 percent in the medulla oblogata and by 12 percent in the cerebellum.

Further assays revealed that in rats, in the initial phase oxygen consumption was higher than that of control animals, by 49 percent in the cortex, by 54 percent in the vicinity of the subcortex (subcortical ganglia) and by 164 percent in the brain stem. The values were 7 percent lower than those of the controls in the cerebellum.

If the animals were stimulated with small pulses for two minutes before the attack was induced, at the beginning of the attack oxygen consumption was increased by 76 percent in the cortex of the cerebral hemispheres, by 62 percent in the subcortex and by 51 percent in the brain stem. Once again oxygen consumption in the cerebellum was lower than in the control animals, although only by 1 percent.

Using rabbits, Pogodaev (1964) was able to show that oxygen consumption in the brain is higher in the *initial clonic phase* than in the later tonic phase: the difference was 45 percent in the cerebral hemispheres, 37 percent in the subcortex, 48 percent in the medulla oblongata, 22 percent in the brain stem and 22 percent in the cerebellum.

Compared with control animals, respiratory activity *in the tonic phase* in rabbits was 35 percent higher in the brain stem and 18 percent higher in the cerebellum, while in the cortex it was 19 percent lower than normal and 31 percent lower than in the clonic phase. Respiratory activity in the subcortex and in the medulla oblongata was very much the same.

In the clonic phase in rats, the respiratory activity increased by 42 percent in the cortex, by 33 percent in the subcortex, by 67 percent in the brain stem, by 51 percent in the cerebellum and by 93 percent in the spinal medulla, compared with values from control animals.

In the locomotor phase, respiratory activity in the experimental animals was lower than in the controls, by 30 percent in the cortex, by 47 percent in the subcortex and by 58 percent in the spinal medulla.

Following this, Pogodaev (1964) performed experiments on rabbits to study oxygen consumption in the central region of the brain, rhinencephalon, reticular formation of the medulla oblongata and in the rest of the medulla oblongata after removing the reticular formation, hypothalamus, Ammon's horn and corpora quadrigemina. The results showed that the activity of the central region in experimental animals in the clonic phase is 29 percent higher than in control animals; there was no difference in the rhinencephalon; it was 26.5 percent higher in the reticular formation of the medulla oblongata and 16.3 percent (not significantly) higher in the hypothalamus than in control animals. After removing the reticular formation, respiratory activity in the medulla oblongata was much the same as normal.

To summarize, we can say that respiratory activity in the brain is highest in the clonic phase, rather less pronounced in the tonic phase and lowest in the locomotor phase. In the *coma* phase, oxygen consumption in the brain is practically normal (Figure 28).

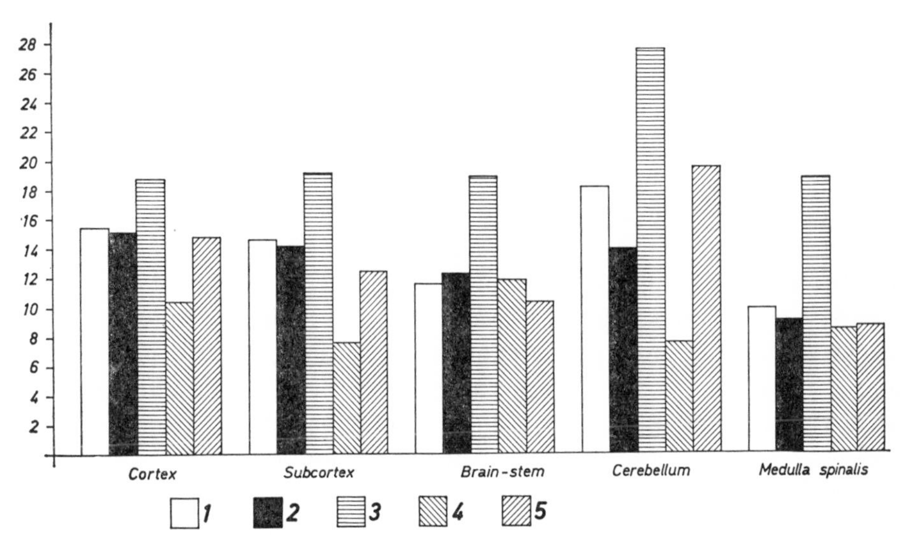

Figure 28. Oxygen consumption in various parts of the rat brain during an epileptic attack triggered electrically (in microlitres per 100 mg fresh cerebral tissue after 40 minutes incubation) 1 = control animals; 2 = tonic phase; 3 = clonic phase; 4 = locomotor phase "beg na meste"; 5 = after awakening from the coma. (From Pogodaev, K.I.: *Biohimija Epileptičeskovo Pristupa,* Moscow, 1964.)

The problem is more complex when attacks occur at frequent intervals with one attack closely following another. During the first few attacks the oxygen saturation of arterial blood is lower than in later attacks, particularly in the tonic and clonic phases. The more attacks there are, the higher is the oxygen saturation of the blood, so that after the first few attacks it may become abnormally high (Pogodaev 1964). This may explain any discrepancies in the results, since the number of attacks is not always specified when oxygen saturation is determined.

The reverse is true of oxygen consumption during a repeat attack. Measuring this parameter using Warburg's manometer apparatus, after 40 minutes incubation period oxygen consumption in the brain was higher in the clonic phase of the first attack (22% higher in the hemispheres and 21% higher in the brain stem) compared with the clonic phase of the tenth attack. *Thus, the respiratory activity of the brain declines as the number of repeat attacks increases.* The activity of the neurons which are causally responsible for the convulsions is reduced because protein metabolism and respiratory activity are reduced, and this attenuates the excitatory processes. Attenuation of the explosive convulsions may also produce other attack equivalents (see Chapter VIII). Following a succession of attacks in animals, the course of the attack changes; this supports the view that some cerebral structures cease to function in the course of the disease or during an experiment, particularly when one attack follows another in quick succession. As we can demonstrate with our model (see Chapter VIII), this may then alter the function of one of the inhibiting barriers.

After repeated attacks in experimental animals, Pogodaev (1964) found that the subsequent exhaustion phase was longer and more profound; the body needs more and more time and (relative) rest before it can recover and become fully functional again. When there is no exhausion phase (coma), the outcome is fatal. Actually there is a limit to the number of attacks which will prolong the exhaustion phase, and after many convulsions the exhaustion phase begins to get shorter again. Studies of the individual structures in the brain show that repeated attacks *wear out* the CNS. The first part to be damaged in psychomotor epilepsy is the hippocampus (see also Chapter III).

Acid-Base Balance

First we shall mention the changes in the levels of organic acids in the brain and blood during an attack. Most experiments set out to determine *uric acid and pyruvic acid,* but some have dealt with *citric acid, malic acid and amino* acids and some other acids derived from the breakdown of proteins (Epstein 1947, Stefanenko 1953, Vladimirov and Epstein 1939, Pogodaev 1964). These and other authors (Dusser Barenne 1954, Klein and Olsen 1947, Pogodaev 1960, Stone et al. 1945, Vladimirova 1937) found that the concentration of organic acids in the brain increased during experimental convulsions.

Pogodaev (1964) obtained some interesting results by determining these acids on the basis of the number of carboxyl groups. *In the initial phase* in rats, carboxyl groups in the cortex were increased by 81 percent, in the brain stem by 211 percent and in the cerebellum by 50 percent, compared with control animals.

At the beginning of the tonic phase, the concentration of carboxyl groups in the cortex was no higher, but in the brain stem it was 74 percent higher and in the cerebellum 27 percent higher than in the controls. *At the end of the tonic phase* in rats, the concentration in the cortex was significantly lower (by 20%) than in control animals. On the other hand, in the brain stem the carboxyl groups were increased by 80 percent, and in the cerebellum by 33 percent compared with the controls.

Comparison of the values in the initial and tonic phases showed that during the initial phase the concentration of organic acids in cortex and cerebellum is much higher than in the tonic phase. On the other hand, the concentration of organic acids in the brain stem was higher during the tonic phase than in the initial phase (Figure 29).

Determination of carboxyl groups in the *clonic phase* of an attack in

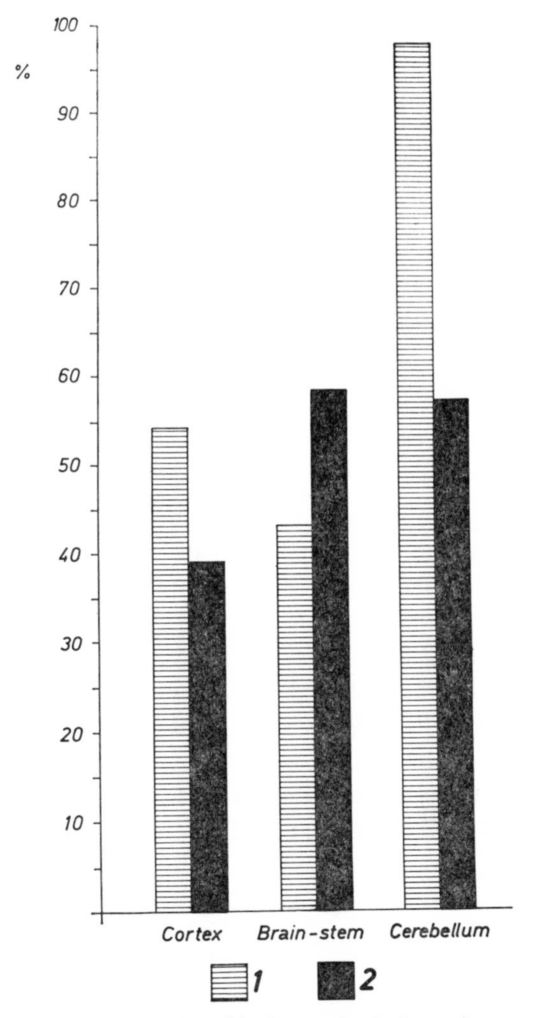

Figure 29. Concentration of organic acids in cerebral tissue in rats during the initial and tonic phase of an attack triggered electrically (in mg/equivalents to 100 g fresh tissue) 1 = initial phase; 2 = tonic phase (From Pogodaev, K.I., 1964.)

rats gave the following results: in the cortex they were elevated by 78 percent, in the subcortex by 83 percent, in the brain stem by 110 percent, and in the cerebellum by 112 percent compared with the control animals ($p < 0.01$). *In the locomotor phase* and during the *coma* the situation was reversed, i.e. the concentration of organic acids or carboxyl groups in rat brain was depressed.

Determination of pH in rats revealed a significant fall in the *initial phase* compared with the controls (fall or increase in acidity). According to Pogodaev (1964), *in the tonic phase* there was a further fall of pH, particularly in the subcortex and brain stem, but also in the cerebellum. In *the clonic phase,* the pH showed a further tendency to become acidotic in the cortex, subcortex, brain stem and cerebellum. *In the locomotor phase* the pH was practically normal. The pH normalizes in the coma and 40 minutes after the coma it is still normal, or it tends to be alkalotic; alkalosis is also found in the interval following repeated attacks (Figure 28).

A check in dogs showed that during the clonic phase of an attack the pH shifted 0.1 to 0.2 units towards the acid side in the cortex, subcortex, diencephalon, midbrain and medulla oblongata. After the attack, again in dogs, the pH became alkaline, particularly if there were repeated attacks.

According to Pogodaev et al. (1959), *determination of the isoelectric point of proteins* in rats showed that in the locomotor phase the pH is still 0.05 lower than in control animals. Particularly in the medulla oblongata, the isoelectric point of proteins was pH 4.24 in the locomotor phase, and pH 4.50 as the coma phase subsided. Thus, during the locomotor phase there was acidosis of 0.26 pH units compared with the coma phase. In the other cerebral regions the isoelectric point of proteins or the pH responded as they did in the medulla oblongata in the epileptic phases mentioned.

Studies on the isoelectric point of proteins where there were repeated attacks (Mekler et al. 1959, Pogodaev 1964) revealed results similar to those in an isolated attack, although there were also certain shifts.

In the clonic phase there was a shift of pH 0.1 towards the acid side in the pyramidal cells of the central region; in other cells of the cortex this shift was also 0.1; in the plasma of the neurons it was 0.25; in the nuclei it was 0.11 and in the nucleoli it was pH 0.14. Viewing the tissue as a whole, during the clonic phase there were acid shifts of pH 0.08 in the Ammon's horn, pH 0.23 in the medulla oblongata and pH 0.16 in the cerebellum.

The situation is reversed where there are repeated attacks with a *fatal outcome; there is relative alkalosis during the attack.* After the attacks have been repeated some 24 or 25 times in rats the pH changes by 0.3, in doves it changes by 0.9 after 20 attacks, by 0.86 in fish after 16 to 18 convulsions, and by 0.81 in frogs after nine attacks. Pogodaev (1964) concluded from these results that there is a limit to the time that the body is able to inhibit (retard) an attack by acidosis, and eventually status epilepticus develops during which patients in hospital or animals during an experiment, must be given acids.

Carbohydrates and Adenosine Triphosphate (ATP)

The change in the oxidizing activity of the brain discussed above is also associated with a change in glucose metabolism during an epileptic attack.

Apart from this resulting in additional production of CO_2, lactic acid and other organic acids, there may also be release of acetylcholine and other active substances (Elliott 1955). Increased oxygen consumption in cerebral tissue during convulsions is essential for keeping the organism alive, and it also causes other metabolic changes. Without these metabolic changes associated with the increased oxygen consumption, the bioelectrical activity of the cortex is depressed (Gibbs et al. 1947, Jasper and Erikson 1941, Kreindler et al. 1963 b, Mison-Crighel et al. 1963).

On the other hand, glucose can be utilized by means of energy-rich phosphate bonds. Oxygen deficiency in the brain will lead to disruption of phosphorus metabolism in the course of an attack. Production and reconstruction of ATP is absolutely essential for accumulating functional energy and for biosynthesis of amino acids, peptides, proteins, phospholipids, acetylcholine and glycogen (Palldin 1954, Strickland 1956).

In generalized convulsions induced by electric current, acoustic stimuli, absinth oil, camphor, picrotoxin, caffeine, Metrazol, strychnine, oramine and sulphopyridine, *there is a fall in the cerebral glucose and glycogen concentration* (Klein and Olsen 1947, Kreindler 1947). The ratio between cerebral glucose and glucose in the blood is upset. On the other hand, the amount of lactic acid in the brain increases and this reduces the pH. The fall in pH and its tendency towards acidity has an anticonvulsant effect and this may have an important part to play during convulsions.

Consumption of oxygen and glucose is much higher than the supply of these substances and this leads to a fall in the concentration of energy-rich biochemical compounds (such as phosphocreatine and ATP) (Gurdjan et al. 1947, Mison-Crighel 1957, Pogodaev 1954). These energy-rich substances are utilized in the brain right at the beginning of convulsive activity in the body, and the reserves in cerebral tissue are rapidly used up. This may be paralleled by characteristic bioelectrical patterns (Dawson and Richter 1950, Kreindler 1965). In the first 15 seconds of convulsions, there are changes in the bioelectrical potentials in the brain, and also a shift in the levels of phosphocreatine and ATP. At the end of convulsions induced by electric current, picrotoxin, Metrazol and amidopyrine, Mison-Crighel

(1957) observed a rise of lactic acid and fall of phosphocreatine in experimental animals.

In vitro studies on sections taken from the cerebral cortex revealed quantitative and qualitative changes (Gore and McIlwain 1952) : there was increased oxygen and glucose consumption and accelerated break-down of phosphocreatine. However, these changes only occurred where the attacks were induced by electric current, and they were not seen after administering picrotoxin, Metrazol or caffeine (Anguiano and McIlwain 1951). This means that some caution must be exercised when drawing analogies between biochemical changes found in experiments and the changes which occur during spontaneous attacks. A different biochemical situation prevailed after convulsions had ceased.

In contrast, Rosengardt et al. (1955) did not observe any changes in ATP, creatine or inorganic phosphates during electroconvulsions. However, the most important features in the results of Bakashov et al. (1958), Rosengardt and Maslova (1956) and Goifond and Richter (1956) correlate with those of Anguiana and McIlwain (1951).

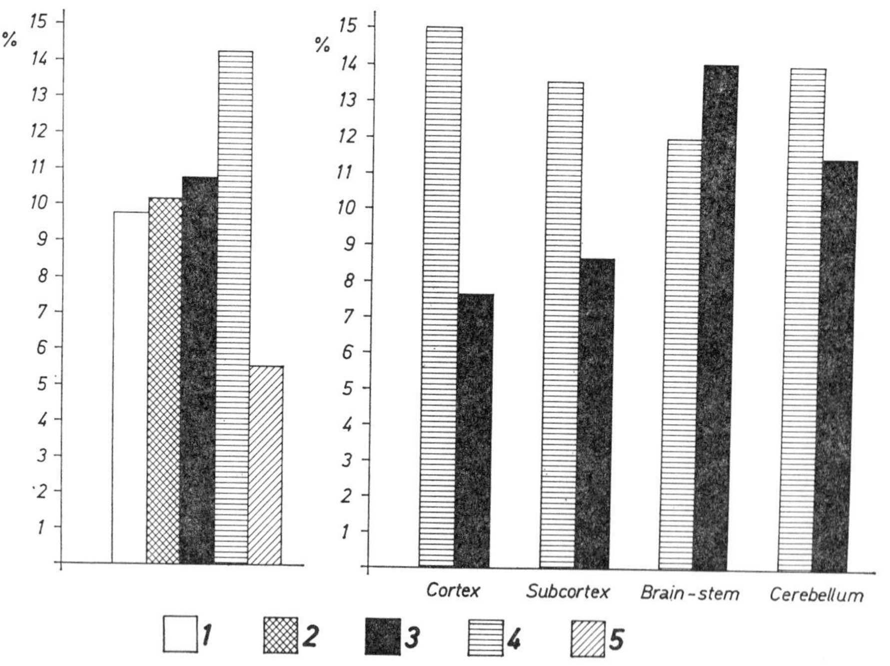

Figure 30. *Left:* Concentration of inorganic phosphorous as a metabolic product in cerebral tissue of the rat. The rats were decapitated at different stages of an epileptic attack triggered electrically. *Right:* Concentration of inorganic phosphorus in various parts of rat brain; the rats were decapitated in the clonic and in the tonic phase of an epileptic attack triggered by an electrical current (phosphorus in mg% of fresh cerebral tissue) 1 = control animals; 2 = initial phase; 3 = tonic phase; 4 = clonic phase; 5 = immediately after awakening from the coma. (From Pogodaev, K.I., 1964.)

The increase of *inorganic phosphorus* in the brain during excitation is not so much due to break-down of ATP and phosphoric acid as to splitting of other phosphate compounds, such as phosphopeptides, ribonucleic acids, ribonucleids and phospholipoids.

Pogodaev's experiments (1964) revealed a general rise of inorganic phosphorus during the initial and tonic phases of epilepsy, and a substantial rise to 45 percent above the normal concentration during the clonic phase. However, by the end of the postparoxysmal coma the concentration of inorganic phosphorus had fallen by 44 percent compared with the initial level (Figure 30, left).

Pogodaev interprets this phenomenon as being due to an increased rate of resynthesis of protoplasm. This process would have been impaired during the attack and would now be regaining momentum.

There is more inorganic phosphorus present in the clonic phase than in the tonic phase: e.g. it is 95 percent higher in the cortex and 55 percent higher in the subcortex. On the other hand, in the brain stem inorganic phosphorus is 15 percent higher in the tonic phase (Figure 30, right).

Further tests on 18 rabbits by Pogodaev (1964) revealed different results for different areas of the brain. In the tonic phase, the inorganic phosphorus content was practically the same in the frontal and occipital lobes (about 8%), while in the clonic phase the phosphorus in the frontal lobe had increased to 15 percent and in the occipital lobe to 11.4 percent. The relative increase of inorganic phosphorus in the clonic phase as compared with the tonic phase is 78 percent frontally and 48 percent occipitally. In the other cerebral regions, in the tonic phase inorganic phosphorus was higher than in the frontal or occipital lobes, so that there was no significant difference between clonic and tonic phases.

The adenosine triphosphate content in the tonic phase was practically the same in the frontal and occipital lobes (about 8.5%). In the clonic phase ATP had fallen to 6 percent in the frontal lobe and increased to 10 percent in the occipital lobe. In the other cerebral areas examined, the ATP concentration was rather higher during the tonic phase than in the clonic; it was 14 percent higher in the midbrain, 9 percent higher in the medulla oblongata and 4 percent higher in the diencephalon. These results correlate with the findings of authors cited by Pogodaev (1964).

Protein Metabolism and Some Problems Regarding Energy

In the rat, there was no change in the *moisture content of cerebral tissue,* either in the cortex or in other cerebral structures examined, following a single attack or during the coma (Pogodaev 1960, 1964). Kudravčeva and Kudravčeva (1950) and Goshev (1955) obtained similar results using rabbits and the moisture content remained the same even after several isolated attacks.

Belezko et al. (1936) found that the *capacity of cerebral tissue to swell* may be increased by excitation, particularly in the clonic phase of an epileptic attack. This swelling is associated with forced break-down of protein, and it persists even where there is predominant inhibition (coma stage) and it is just as pronounced when protein catabolism is reduced.

Where there are frequently recurring attacks, cerebral oedema develops, and proteins must be involved in the local changes here (see Chapter III).

The brain increases in size (Gortner 1933) and swelling occurs in individual areas of the brain. We must again return to Pogodaev's experiments (1964). He found that in different species of animal the degree of swelling and the number of convulsions vary. First, by measuring brain sections from experimental animals, he made the general observation that swelling is more pronounced than in control animals. Where there is a single, isolated attack, cerebral swelling is more pronounced during the exhaustion phase than during the attack. After ten convulsive episodes, cerebral enlargement was more pronounced than after one attack. The changes were particularly marked in the cortex where the swelling after ten attacks was 27 to 57 percent more than after one attack. After an interval of two days, the ability of the brain to swell on inducing attacks was greater than in animals in which several attacks had been induced without interruption; there was 43 percent more swelling in the cortex, 36 percent more in the subcortex, 31 percent more in the brain stem and 19 percent more in the cerebellum.

Studies on ribonucleic acid (RNA) in the pyramidal cells of the precentral region revealed that the RNA content increases after one attack, but that after 24 attacks it is very depressed (Mölbert et al. 1967, Pogodaev 1960, 1961, 1963, 1964, Turova 1963). When RNA is destroyed the exhaustion phase is always prolonged. If further attacks occur there is no corresponding increase in the length of the exhaustion phase; it becomes shorter or disappears altogether, resynthesis of RNA ceases and the mechanisms responsible for inhibiting the attacks are impaired or fail altogether. Finally the experimental animal dies.

Protein metabolism during an epileptic attack can be studied by means of radioactive amino acids, such as methionine, tyrosine and glycine, labelled with ^{14}C or ^{35}S (Borsook and Deasy 1951, Palladin 1956, 1962, Palladin and Vladimirov 1955). These experiments showed that cerebral activity is increased by excitation and this is linked with increased regeneration of protein.

Other results (Gaitonde and Richter 1956, Rosengardt et al. 1956) indicate that during an epileptic attack there is no more than a slight increase in the rate of incorporation of amino acids (observed using radioactive labelled methionine) into proteins. However, with these authors the interval observed between two induced attacks varied in length.

Pogodaev (1964) studied the changes in proteins and amino acids in various phases of an attack and at different times during the convulsion-free interval.

In the the first series of experiments (methionine with ^{35}S), rats were stimulated for three minutes (one second stimulation, 30 seconds pause). This type of intermittent stimulation failed to produce any change in methionine metabolism. With more powerful stimulation there was a slight increase of methionine metabolism; the increase was greater in the cortex than in the subcortex and brain stem. With repeated stimulation and induction of three consecutive attacks, methionine metabolism altered considerably, but only in the cortex and brain stem. After four to six convulsions there was further activation of methionine metabolism in the cortex, subcortex and brain stem (activity was increased 2 to 2.6 times) and the level of *radioactivity in cerebral proteins also increased* ($p < 0.05$).

In a second series of experiments, Pogodaev (1964) used radiotyrosine. After a single stimulation of the animals there was no substantial change in the level of radioactivity in cerebral proteins. The ^{14}C-labelled tyrosine was incorporated into cerebral proteins to the same extent as in the controls. Examination of the protein-free filtrate of blood did not reveal any difference in the level of radioactive contamination. Two hours after administering tyrosine, seven attacks were induced at intervals of seven minutes. The activity of cerebral tyrosine increased 3.2 times, but it was only 1.9 times higher in plasma proteins. Radioactive contamination of cerebral protein was very much greater than that of the protein-free filtrate.

After seven attacks at intervals of two minutes, the activity of cerebral proteins was 2.1 times higher than in the controls. Examination of the blood revealed a similar picture, where the activity of the proteins was 2.6 times higher ($p < 0.05$).

After three consecutive attacks, *the level of inorganic phosphorus* increased by 73 percent. With three attacks at 30-minutes intervals there was no change in the level of inorganic phosphorus. Thus, changes in the results depend on the frequency and intensity of the attacks. Protein metabolism also depends on the nature and intensity of the attacks.

Inorganic phosphorus, creatine phosphorus and adenosine triphosphate were examined in 37 rats following one, two and seven attacks, the animals being decapitated in the locomotor phase. These studies showed that the concentration of these substances changes in relation to the number of consecutive attacks. Inorganic phosphorus increases and creatine phosphorus and ATP decrease with successive attacks ($p < 0.01$).

^{15}N was used to examine *the process of incorporation of ammonia into proteins* in animals during repeated attacks, and some interesting results were obtained (Geiger et al. 1960, Plischevski 1955, Pogodaev 1964). The picture with regard to cerebral and blood proteins depends on the functional condition of the experimental animal. For instance, there is 3.5 percent more bound ^{15}N in the coma than during the attacks. A similar picture emerges in the liver: 2.8 perment more in the coma than during attacks. On the other hand, in blood the situation is reversed: there was 2.8 percent less ^{15}N in proteins during the coma than during the attacks. *These results show that the coma following an attack is characterized by an increase of bound (labelled) ammonia in the brain and in the liver.* At the same time, the amount of nitrogen in the protein-free filtrate is reduced. During excitation of the neurons in an attack, the capacity of brain and liver to bind ammonia is reduced, and more bound ammonia is found in the protein-free filtrate than in blood proteins. During the coma, the ammonia-binding activity in cerebral tissue is 160 percent more intense than in the liver. The same is true during a profound attack. Thus, both during phases of excitation and of inhibition, the ammonia-binding and releasing activities in the brain are greater than in the liver.

According to Pogodaev (1964), ammonia binding is due to binding to the carboxyl groups in proteins, rather than to incorporated into protein, because if the latter were the case the binding effect in the liver would have exceeded that in the brain. The binding of ammonia to the carboxyl groups of proteins is an important function of proteins and it is associated with the molecular-disperse property which may also be involved in energy function in the brain.

In addition to observations made using ^{15}N, experiments have also been carried out using ^{32}P. The metabolic activity reflected by incorporation of ^{32}P during convulsive paroxysms has actually been used as an index for assessing the level of convulsive activity (Volanschi et al. 1961). During convulsions induced by electroshock in cats, there was a significant rise in the amount of ^{32}P incorporated into most cortical and subcortical structures (anterior and posterior regions of the cortex, nucleus, caudatus, hypothalamus, mesencephalon, cerebellum). Highest values were found in the neocortex and mesencephalon. In contrast to the results in adult cats, electroshock in two-week-old cats did not significantly alter the level of ^{32}P incorporation into most phylogenetically younger cortical and subcortical structures, although there were some changes in the mesencephalon, hypothalamus and hippocampus. There was a significant level of ^{32}P incorporation into these latter cerebral structures. Electroshock in adult and newborn guinea pigs produced a significant and substantial rise in the amount of ^{32}P incorporated into the various cortical and subcortical structures.

Haematological studies in epileptics revealed some interesting protein shifts compared with the picture in the interval and shortly before attacks (Krupenina 1960). Compared with results obtained before attacks, serum protein was depressed during an attack. The albumin fraction was substantially elevated, fluctuating between 53.1 and 71.1%. There was no further rise of alpha-globulins, but beta-globulins continued to rise slightly. Gamma-globulins returned to normal. It is significant that the albumin/globulin quotient did not fall below 1 in any case. It varied between 1.13 and 2.4. *During status epilepticus* there was a pronounced shift in serum proteins compared with the picture before the status and during an isolated attack (Krupenina 1960).

Total serum protein did not increase *in symptomatic epilepsy,* although the percentage of protein in serum was slightly elevated after a status which had lasted several days or weeks. The albumin fraction was usually higher than 50 percent, but it could fall as low as 40 percent where there were frequent attacks or fairly prolonged status asthmaticus. The same picture emerged with alpha-globulins. Beta-globulins were normal, but in some cases there was a rise of gamma-globulins. An A/G quotient of more than 1 was recorded in cases where the status was not prolonged and attacks occurred less often; an A/G quotient of way below 1 was recorded in cases where there were very frequent attacks and a status of several days duration (in one case it was 0.69 and in another 0.67).

In essential epilepsy total serum protein was markedly elevated during the status, while in some cases the albumin fraction was very depressed (down as far as 36.4%). There were increases of alpha-globulin concentration, and even sharper increases of gamma globulins, which were up as much as 40 percent in some cases. The A/G quotient did not always improve, compared with the situation before the status. In fact in some patients it actually fell (0.57 and 0.65). These results of Krupenina (1960) showed that there are differences between the results during and before the status, there are also differences between results in essential and in symptomatic epilepsy. Although these differences may appear to be rational, they are not easy to explain. It may be that essential epileptics are born with the type of metabolic defects (Prüll 1967) which only develop later in symptomatic epileptics. Our results (Jovanović 1970e, 1971b) correlate in their essential details with those of Krupenina (1960).

Shifts of total protein and protein fractions during an attack, as compared with the picture before convulsions and in the interval, are particularly important since during an attack there is a tendency for the preexisting alkalosis (Figures 28 and 30), to develop into acidosis (Figure 28). At the beginning of an attack there is a rise of finely dispersed albumins and a fall of coarsely despersed globulins and the A/G quotient rises practically to normal. These processes must have a part to play in inhibiting an attack, *although it is hardly apparent during status epilepticus* (see Figure 30 and Chapter VIII).

Amino Acids and Their Derivatives During an Attack

Here, we shall simply discuss a few supplementary findings with regard to the amino acid picture during *the attack itself.* Although amino acid metabolism has not been thoroughly studied, there are certain points which we must mention.

In the cortex of the cat, in epileptogenic lesions produced by freezing a small region with ethyl chloride there were changes in the concentrations of *glutamic acid (GA), glutamine and glutathion* during paroxysmal bioelectric activity. The level of gamma-aminobutyric acid (GABA) remained constant (Berl et al. 1959). On the other hand, there was a 50 percent fall in the concentration of GA at the beginning of convulsive activity, and the concentration of glutamic acid was also depressed where convulsions were induced by strychnine and fluorine acetate (Dawson 1953, Haber and Saidel 1948). Thus the authors were not able to demonstrate a fall in the concentration of GABA during convulsions, although many authors have done so.

Following local administration of mescaline, there was an important change in the epileptic focus involving the *glutamate-GABA system,* but this was not a specific change in the activity at the focus since the same changes were observed throughout the cortex (Mison-Crighel et al. 1964). Following local administration of mescaline, glutaminase activity increased significantly to reach initial activity in the tenth minute of epileptic discharge.

According to Vrba (1956, 1957), cerebral activity stimulated by prolonged muscular activity is associated with a fall of amino-nitrogen in cerebral proteins and an increase of free glutamines and glutamic acid. However, there is some disparity in the results here (Hyden 1957, 1958).

The total amount of amino-nitrogen in the brain declines immediately after an epileptic attack and then rises again after ten epileptic attacks, although qualitative differences may occur (Wertheimer-Luca 1957, 1958).

At the end of an attack induced by electric current, the glutathion concentration falls, but the level becomes normal again within 15 minutes of the end of convulsions. A *rise of ascrobic acid* has also been observed.

It is best to *study the glutamate-GABA system* with convulsions induced by pyridoxine deficiency or by antimetabolites of pyridoxine. As we explained in Chapter III and previously in this chapter, deoxypyridoxine and methoxypyridoxine block the activity of pyridoxine, and bring about certain changes in amino acid metabolism. The same or similar changes in amino acid metabolism, particularly in the glutamine-GABA system, are also induced by thiosemicarbazides, semicarbazides, isoniazids (Biel and Vilter 1954) and penicillin-amines (Killam 1957, Kuchinskas and Du Vigneaud 1957).

Where there are *repeated attacks* further changes occur in the brains of experimental animals. For example, after three repeated convulsions the total nitrogen content of the brain falls by 8 percent and by 3 percent after nine attacks. The *sulphur content* falls by 26 percent after three attacks (determined as sulph-hydryl groups) and by 68 percent after nine consecutive attacks. The N/S ratio (nitrogen-sulphur quotient) is reduced after a number of attacks: by 25 percent after three attacks and by 256 percent after nine attacks. The elevated level of sulphur indicates that there is considerable breakdown of amino acids containing sulphur and this is also shown by the sharp fall of cystine and cysteine in cerebral tissue after repeated attacks (Krasnova and Pogodaev 1959). Since the activity of proteinases is depressed following repeated attacks we must assume that the enzymes for SH-groups have a specific activating effect (Goldstein 1938, 1955). There are also other findings indicating that cystine and cysteine are actively involved in the processes of epileptic attacks; this has already been discussed. Cystine has an antiepileptic effect and it is used in the treatment of epilepsy (Andreev 1956, 1958, Novlanskaya 1956).

Endogenous Amines and Other Neuromodulators in an Attack

The effects of *serotonin* and *acetylcholine* during an attack have been studied in far greater detail than those of other amines and neuromodulators. A rise of serotonin in the brain has been reported during convulsions induced by electric current (Bertaccini 1959, Laborit et al. 1947). The concentration of copper ions was also determined (Costa-Foru 1961). After Metrazol convulsions metabolism of *lipids* and *nucleic acids* was also intensified, and there was an increase of serotonin (Geiger 1957). Breakdown of acetylcholine is vastly accelerated during epileptic convulsions. According to Kreindler (1965) the onset of convulsions may depend on the difference between the rates of breakdown and resynthesis of acetylcholine. The time interval between breakdown and resynthesis of acetylcholine is similar to that between breakdown and resynthesis of phosphocreatine; this applies to the metabolic changes which precede convulsions. However, there is a quantitative difference between the amounts of acetylcholine and phosphocreatine metabolized; 500 times more phosphocreatine is metabolized (McIlwain 1955).

Kreindler (1965) states that, following administration of methionine sulphoximine to cats, dogs and rabbits typical epileptiform anomalies appear in the EEG but there were no histopathological changes in respect of acetylcholine. Samples of cortex taken 18 to 24 hours after administering methionine sulphoximine, and after the onset of convulsions, revealed anomalies which were the same as those observed in samples of cerebral tissue from human subjects, i.e. there was defective binding of acetylcholine. This has been discussed previously.

According to McIntosh and Oborin (1953) there is close correlation between the level of acetylcholine in the brain and cortical bioelectrical activity. Feldberg (1957) found that bioelectrical activity in the brain correlated with the release of acetylcholine. The acetylcholine system is essential for convulsive activity to occur in the cortex and some subcortical structures, and it is particularly active at the convulsion focus. The rise of cholinesterase activity at an epileptic focus as compared with non-epileptic regions of the cortex is also an indication that acetylcholine is an essential component in convulsive activity (Pope et al. 1947, Tower and Elliott 1952 a, b). This rise of cholinesterase activity in the epileptogenic focus may also be interpreted as a compensatory mechanism, and it may possibly be the result of the increased level of free acetylcholine during convulsive activity (Kreindler 1965).

Cholinesterase activity is also increased both where there is a definite mirror focus, and in the symmetrically equivalent cortical or subcortical regions of the brain in which a mirror focus is not yet detectable. Cholinesterase activity normalizes when the primary focus is removed, although it remains unchanged in the cortical mirror focus (Pope et al. 1947). Uzunov et al. (1961) and Atzev (1962) found that the activity of convulsions induced by atebrin depends on cholinesterase activity. We have discussed acetylcholine activity in relation to electrolyte balance earlier in this chapter.

Enzyme Activity

Pogodaev's results (1964) indicate that even *in the initial phase* of an isolated attack the *activity of proteolytic enzymes* is substantially higher than in control rats. Protein degradation as measured by non-protein nitrogen (NPN) increases at the beginning of an attack by 41 percent in the cortex, by 81 percent in the subcortex (thalamus and subcortical ganglia) and by 61 percent in the brain stem caudal of the thalamus ($p < 0.01$). However, the increase of 13 percent in the cerbellum is not significant.

As measured by the carboxyl groups, the activity of proteolytic enzymes in rats in the initial phase is 119 percent higher in the cortex, 87 percent higher in the brain stem and 28 percent higher in the cerebellum, compared with control animals.

The picture is different in the *tonic phase.* The activity of proteolytic enzymes was depressed by 21.5 percent in the cortex, but it was 21.5 percent higher in the subcortex, 38 percent higher in the brain stem and 13 percent higher in the cerebellum, compared with the controls.

After autolysis of brain homogenates from dogs, in the tonic phase enzymatic activity was 18 percent lower in the cortex ($p < 0.05$), but it was 17 percent higher than in the controls in the subcortex, 21 percent higher in the brain stem and 14 percent higher in the cerebellum, ($p < 0.05$). Interesting pictures emerged from the results for activity of proteolytic enzymes in the rat before and during the tonic phase and as the coma phase subsided. In the tonic phase enzymatic activity increased by 29.5 percent in the brain stem, by 62 percent in the cerebellum and by 11 percent in the cortex. After the coma phase had ended the values approached those from control animals or there was overcompensation in the opposite direction.

NPN was 29 percent higher in the initial phases as compared with in the tonic phase in the cortex of rats. The reverse obtained in the brain stem: 33 percent higher in the tonic phase compared with that in the initial phase of an attack. In the other regions of the brain NPN was somewhat higher in the initial phase than in the tonic phase: 17 percent higher in the subcortex and 12.5 percent higher in the cerebellum.

Comparison of NPN in the brain stem and in the cortex during the tonic and initial phases, showed that it was 70 percent higher in the brain stem during the tonic phase, although in the initial stage NPN was only 9 percent higher in the cortex than in the brain stem. *Thus, in the tonic phase the activity of proteolytic enzymes is much higher in the brain stem than in the cortex. In the initial phase, the activity of these enzymes is only slightly higher in the cortex than in the brain stem.*

A further experiment by Pogodaev (1964) showed that lipids are not changed during the initial and tonic phases. There was very little change in cerebral lipids, even where there were repeated attacks. Thus, the free nitrogen (NPN) found in the brain is derived from cerebral protein, not from cerebral lipids. The rise of proteolytic activity is not due to a slowing of cerebral blood flow (Krasnova and Pogodaev 1959, Pomisslova 1949, Vladimirova 1937 to 1961).

According to Pogodaev (1964), during an attack the activity of proteolytic enzymes is highest during the *clonic phase* (Figure 31), and it is much higher than in control animals, particularly in the cortex, subcortex, brain stem and cerebellum. However, these changes in proteolytic enzymes were no longer to be found after the end of the *coma phase*.

For instance, *in the clonic phase* in rats, NPN before autolysis was 50 percent higher in the cortex, 31 percent higher in the subcortex, 131 percent higher in the brain stem and 43 percent higher in the cerebellum. Similar results were also obtained in rabbits: NPN was elevated by 58.5 percent in the cortex, by 29.5 percent in the subcortex, by 17 percent in the brain stem and by 21.2 percent in the cerebellum, compared with control animals.

Proteinase activity in the clonic phase was higher than in control animals. The optic, temporal and frontal lobes (the precentral region) were compared with the subcortex, mid-brain, medulla oblongata and cerebellum, in dogs. The results showed a 67 percent rise of NPN in the cortical structure during the clonic phase. Following autolysis this was reduced to 40 percent.

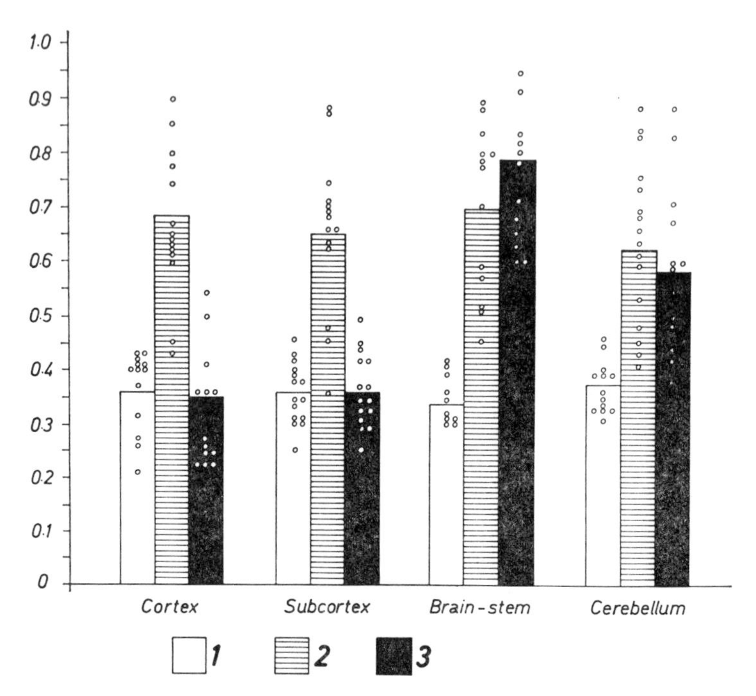

Figure 31. The dynamics of free ammonia in various parts of rat brain in the tonic and clonic phase of an epileptic attack triggered by an electrical current (in mg% of fresh cerebral tissue). 1 = control animals; 2 = clonic phase; 3 = tonic phase. (From Pogodaev, K.I.: *Biohimija Epileptičeskovo Pristupa,* Moscow, 1964.)

In the precentral region NPN was increased by 116 percent before and by 83 percent after autolysis, by 92 percent before and 87 percent after autolysis in the subcortex, by 39 percent before and 96 percent after autolysis in the mesencephalon and by 97 percent before and 91 percent after autolysis in the medulla oblongata. On the other hand, in the cerebellum the concentration of NPN was reduced by 47 percent before and by 11 percent after autolysis, as compared with the level of NPN in control animals.

In the clonic phase, the activity of proteolytic enzymes in the precentral region is double that in the optical cortex. Comparison of the activity of proteolytic enzymes in the entire frontal lobe with that in the occipital lobe revealed that activity is twice as high in the frontal lobe as in the optical cortex.

It is also interesting to examine the results from rabbits. The enzymatic activity increased by 70 percent before and 50 percent after antolysis in the frontal lobe, by 55 percent before and —14 percent after autolysis in the occipital lobe, by 33 percent and 32 percent respectively in the diencephalon, by 88 percent and 49 percent respectively in the corpus caudatum and by 45 percent before and 80 percent after autolysis in the Ammon's horn, as compared with control animals. Thus, as in rats, proteinase activity in rabbits during the clonic phase is higher in the frontal lobe than in the optic lobe.

Now, if we consider the findings in respect of carboxyl groups, in rabbits the proteolytic enzymes during the clonic phase are again much more active than in control animals. However, there are some differences.

In an isolated attack, during the clonic phase the carboxyl groups were elevated by 27 percent in the frontal lobe, by 43 percent in the thalamus, by 81 percent in the corpus caudatum, by 31 percent in the Ammon's horn and by 36 percent in the region of the quandrigeminal bodies, compared with control animals. There were no changes in the optical cortex or pons.

Compared with the controls, the activity of proteinases was 113 percent higher in the frontal lobe, 23 percent higher in the thalamus, 95 percent higher in the corpus caudatum, 255 percent higher in the Ammon's horn and 436 percent higher in the corpora quadrigemina. No differences were found in the optical cortex or pons.

In a further experiment, Pogodaev (1964) compared the level of free ammonia in rats during an attack with that in control animals, and he found it was 4.2 times higher in the brain in the test group of animals during the clonic phase. However, by the end of the tonic phase it had only increased 1.7 times. In the coma phase the level of free ammonia in the brain in the test animals was more than 50 percent lower than in the clonic phase. In the coma, free ammonia was still 2.5 times higher in test animals than in the controls.

In a subsequent series of experiments, free ammonia was determined in the brains of animals by using special diffusion methods (Rose and Brown, 1954). Pogodaev used 45 rats weighing 150 g. (s ± 5).

As Figure 31 shows, during the clonic phase, as compared with control animals, the level of free ammonia increased in all parts of the brain examined. In the cortex and subcortex the level of ammonia was substantially higher than at the beginning of the tonic phase. In the tonic phase ammonia was only increased (in terms of the controls) in the brain stem and cerebellum. There was no great difference between the levels in these two areas in the tonic and clonic phases. All Pogodaev's results (1964) correlate with those of Vrba (1956, 1957).

The picture is different where there are *repeated epileptic convulsions.* After ten convulsions, the activity of proteolytic enzymes rose by 118 percent in the cerebral hemispheres and by 123 percent in the brain stem (during autolysis). One hour after the final attack the activity of proteolytic enzymes was very much reduced; in the hemispheres it was 66 percent lower and in the brain stem 72.4 percent lower than immediately after the attack. However, NPN was still high one hour after the attack: it was 14 percent higher in the hemispheres and 5 percent higher in the brain stem (Pogodaev 1964). According to Britanishki (1947) and Frolkis (1958), the level of ammonia, which remains elevated for as much as an hour after the final attack, can be explained by a reduced rate of removal, since blood flow is reduced to a minimum.

About 24 hours after the final attack, the cerebral haemodynamics and the NPN level return to normal (Pogodaev 1964). This may explain the discrepancies in the results of different authors. The important point here is the time at which the ammonia level was determined: during the attack, shortly before, shortly after or not until 24 hours after the attack.

Autolysis of cerebral tissue is higher in experimental animals sacrificed in the clonic phase of the first attack than in animals sacrificed in the clonic phase of the tenth attack. Thus, in the course of time, where there are several convulsions autolytic activity in cerebral tissue is reduced.

Krasnova and Pogodaev (1959) found that the ratio glutamine-nitrogen: free ammonia nitrogen ($N\text{-}NH_2 : N\text{-}NH_3$) is reduced during an attack: it is 6.18 in test animals as compared with 18.4 in control animals. This quotient normalizes again after the attack in test animals, rising to 17.6. Thus, the NPN produced during an attack is mainly due to ammonia.

Hormonal Changes and Vitamin Activity

Hormonal changes and vitamin activity in the context of epileptic episodes were discussed in detail in the beginning of this chapter.

BIOCHEMICAL PROCESSES IN THE POSTPAROXYSMAL PHASE

In this section we shall add a few remarks to what has already been said in earlier sections of this chapter. After an epileptic attack has run its course, there is reversal of the biochemical changes, as already described.

The most marked *change is in the concentration and function of electrolytes* after an attack. For instance, directly after experimentally induced convulsions, there is an increase of magnesium ions in the renal and splenic vessels (Mison-Crighel et al. 1955). It has been suggested that these magnesium ions are responsible for reconducting the calcium ions back to the surface of the membrane after the attack. In this way, both these ions may inhibit the convulsions (Flink 1956, Gordon and Waelsch 1955, Kreindler 1965, Miranescu 1908).

The concentration and function of other cations also change immediately after an attack. There is a migration of sodium ions out of the nerve cells, and of potassium ions into the cells and this compensates for the potassium deficiency in the cells. The permeability of the membrane is also altered and this prevents further convulsions.

The oxidation processes begin to change right at the beginning of an attack. As a result of the apnoea mentioned above the predominant picture becomes one of acidosis. Right up until the end of convulsions there is increased respiratory and metabolic acidosis which has the effect of inhibiting the attack.

According to Davies et al. (1944) and Pogodaev (1964), during an attack, and particularly as it is subsiding (locomotor and comatous phases), there is a significant fall of oxygen pressure in the grey matter of the cortex. According to Kreindler (1965), this fall of cerebral O_2 may be the result of increased utilization which cannot be compensated for by increased blood flow. The fall of oxygen pressure in the brain is accompanied by a high level of metabolic activity (Ward et al. 1948) and, according to Kreindler (1965) and Pogodaev (1964), this leads to oxygen deficiency in the brain which, in turn, results in accumulation of acids. The brain then needs even more oxygen because, in addition to maintaining the normal metabolic processes of oxidation, it has to neutralize these acids. However, oxygen supply is not particularly high immediately after an attack so that the state of acidosis prevails for some time after the attack, and this has the function of inhibiting the next attack.

According to Dunlop (1957 a, b), Gellhorn and Heymann (1948), Gellhorn and Yesinick (1942), Pollock and Bain (1950), Pogodaev (1964), Selbach et al. (1965) and other authors, CO_2 reduces the excitability of the neurons and thus checks the convulsions. Of course, the acidosis alters a whole series of enzymatic processes which also have an inhibitory effect on the attack.

The changes in the oxidation processes after an attack are also linked with a *change of carbohydrate metabolism.* It is interesting to consider the way in which the body compensates for hypoglycaemia, which may develop before an attack, but which certainly occurs during an attack. According to Dawson (1953), the body utilizes glutamic and gamma-aminobutyric acids as a compensatory mechanism in carbohydrate metabolism. As we mentioned above, amino acids may be synthesized from glucose, and vice versa. As we have pointed out, before an attack there is a fall in the levels of these amino acids in the brain so that they must then be synthesized from carbohydrates. However, if the pH alters and acidosis develops this speeds up the synthesis of amino acids in the brain and these amino acids then affect carbohydrate metabolism. After the attack there is a rise in the blood sugar level (Kreindler 1965).

One of the important metabolic changes after an attack is the change in *cerebral and serum proteins.* De Crinis (1924, 1925), Contini (1936b),

Mc Kenzie and Mc Chesney (1935) and many of the other authors mentioned above have been able to show that after an attack there is a shift of protein fractions in blood opposite to that which occurs before the attack. There is a reduction of total proteins, and increase of albumins, and the level of globulins falls to normal; there is also a reduction in the levels of fibrin and fibrinogen and a general trend towards normalization. Water balance is adjusted by increased diuresis.

More recent authors, such as Jantz (1956), Krupenina (1960), Jovanović (1970 e), have confirmed the results of these earlier research workers. However, it must be stressed that both in this case and in the case of other metabolic processes (carbohydrate metabolism, amino acid metabolism, etc.), status epilepticus, psychomotor attacks or attack equivalents usually fail to normalize the metabolic changes which prevailed before the episodes. As Figure 24 (case "a") shows, serum proteins show further changes in the electrophoregram, although the patient here was in status epilepticus when the blood was sampled. The change in serum protein was maintained over more than a week during which there were frequent major and psychomotor epileptic attacks. This may be one of the reasons why this patient (with status epilepticus and psychomotor attacks) developed a series of psychotic symptoms more often than other patients (with major attacks occurring in the waking state, petit mal attacks). Thus, development of psychotic symptoms produces what epileptic equivalents and attacks cannot induce, i.e. metabolic normalization.

We have already mentioned the effect on *amino acid metabolism,* of the changes which occur in the metabolic picture immediately after an attack. The acidosis promotes the activity of glutamic acid decarboxylase and more GABA is formed. GABA then has an inhibitory effect on the convulsions. The concentration of GABA in the brain is increased since more is formed from glutamic acid and the rate of degradation is also reduced, since the processes which increase the formation of GABA also inhibit its degradation by inhibiting GABA transaminase. Not only does GABA have a homeostatic effect on the cortical potential (Caspers 1957) but it also brings about normalization of endogenous amines.

The normalization in the concentration of *endogenous amines* mentioned above has the effect of normalizing the other metabolic processes.

The level of free acetylcholine also returns to normal (Kreindler et al. 1957). Normalization of cerebral acetylcholine has an inhibitory effect on the brain and it also has the effect of normalizing amino acids and electrolytes. In turn, the amino acids bring about better binding of free acetylcholine, so that here we have a series of normalizing processes. Elliott (1955) assumes that convulsive activity only subsides when the reserves of acetylcholine are exhausted. Subsequent resynthesis of acetylcholine to readjust the level to normal takes place with the aid of carbohydrate metabolism and ATP (De Robertis et al. 1963, Hebb et al. 1956, 1958, Kreindler 1965, Waelsch 1961).

Where the concentration and activity of acetylcholine is reduced, we believe that there is an increase of Adrenaline and noradrenaline, and possibly of serotonin as well, in the exhaustion phase. This combination of concentration and activity of endogenous amines may have an anticonvulsant effect. However, if there is no increase of noradrenaline, adrenaline and serotonin (which may, in fact, happen) then there must be some other mechanism for inhibiting the attacks. Finally, not all kinds of attack are inhibited in the same way.

Figure 36 shows how the *degradation products of proteins* and their concentration in brain and blood, alter after an attack. However, very often it is difficult to distinguish between cause and effect which regard to these changes, and so great caution must be exercised when assessing changes in the metabolic products of proteins and other biochemical substances. One thing that seems certain is that during the attacks, there is a trend towards catabolism, and this leads to many other changes. However, in the last phases of an attack, anabolic biochemical processes begin to increase (see Pogodaev 1964).

COMPARISON OF BIOCHEMICAL PROCESSES IN PSYCHOMOTOR EPILEPSY AND PSYCHOSES

Some General Remarks

There are three important factors which justify our comparing the biochemical findings in psychomotor epilepsy with those in psychoses.

Firstly, earlier research workers (Bleuler 1911, 1925, 1954, 1957, Gjessing 1935, 1953, 1968, Kraepelin 1898, 1900, 1909, Padovani 1935, Penacchietti 1935, 1936, Pilcz 1901, Poli 1942, Stössel 1942) had already noticed that epilepsy, particularly psychomotor epilepsy, may suddenly develop into psychosis; this was discussed in Chapter I.

Secondly, many neurophysiologists have found (see Chapters II and III) that the same dysrhythmic changes of bioelectrical cerebral activity derived from the deeper cerebral formations (septum pellicidum, hippocampus) may occur in both psychomotor epilepsy and in psychoses (schizophrenia). These dysrhythmias in the EEG of deeper cerebral structures may be induced by the same biochemical agents in both of these diseases (see also Chapter VI). Also, in epileptics with forced normalization in the cortical EEG (see Chapters II and III) there may be dysrhythmias in the bioelectrical cerebral activity derived from these deeper regions of the brain.

Thirdly, during our discussion in this chapter, again and again we come across biochemical findings in psychomotor epilepsy which parallel those occurring during psychotic manifestations of known organic origin, or of unknown origin.

These three points suggest to us that psychosis could be a biological equivalent of epilepsy, and vice versa, and we must now ask ourselves how closely are these two groups of diseases related to one another.

In respect of psychoses, we shall only discuss the biochemical findings which have an important bearing on the problem in hand, and we shall refer particularly to publications which are probably less well-known in the English-speaking parts of the world.

As early as 1935, Gjessing observed that there was retention of *water* and *electrolytes* during periodic catatonia and he examined the possibility of *retention psychoses.* Jouschtschenko (1911), Gulotta (1931), Hoskins (1937), Fischer (1933, 1954), Herzberg (1937), Arutunov (1937), Polischtchuk (1937 to 1947), Sereiski and Schneersohn (1937), Sereiski and Rothstein (1938), Sereiski and Lando (1946) believed that they had detected *retardation of oxidation processes* in psychoses, which must be causally connected with the occurrence of psychotic symptoms. There was also a change in glutathion metabolism.

Like the authors mentioned above, Tchalissov (1958, 1960), Natalevitch (1958, 1960), Ephimovitch (1958) and others found *the processes of phosphorylation were retarded* in psychoses, and this was again causally related to these psychoses.

Later results point to a *change in carbohydrate metabolism* (Altschule 1953, Drury and Marran-Ridge 1925, Henry and Mangum 1925, Kitay and Altschule 1952, Lorenz 1922, Löwendahl and Valatin 1941, Mann 1925, McFarland and Goldstein 1938, Papadopulos 1960, Raphael et al. 1928, Thompson and Aste-Salazar 1939, Wortis et al. 1940) in psychoses. Recently this biochemical abnormality has received special attention (see Polischtchuk and Sobolevskaya 1947).

Bettzieche (1930), Fattovich (1933), Markovits (1934), Lingjaerde (1933 to 1937), Davidson (1933), Cassiano (1935), Desani (1935), Padovani (1935), Vitello (1935), Amico (1936), Gunner (1936), Penta (1937), Poli (1942), Skuin (1948), Köersher (1948), Rassin (1949) and more recent authors have laid particular emphasis on the *protein changes* in endogenous psychoses; these include disruption of protein synthesis. Degradation products and *pigments* are formed and these then have a toxic effect. A *haemolytic syndrome* has also been considered as a possibility here (Jahn and Greving 1936).

Because of the clinical and biochemical difficulties, research into these problems has had to be carried out in the same way as the study of epilepsy —research workers have to induce psychoses experimentally and then compare these with spontaneous psychotic conditions (Baruk 1931, Buscaino

1923 to 1933, Buscaino and De Giacomo 1930, Claude and Baruk 1928, De Giacomo 1930, Harrefeld and Kok 1935, Leach et al. 1956, Leuner 1962, Natboom 1934).

A significant factor in these studies is that chemical substances capable of inducing a psychosis are also capable of inducing epileptic symptoms.

According to the results of Buscaino (1923 to 1933) and De Giacomo (1930), the picture of experimental psychosis, and its intensity and similarity to a spontaneous psychotic episode depend on the radical group of the chemical substance which has been used to induce the experimental psychosis. For example, a psychosis can be induced very readily with *amines* which have a *complicated cyclic ring* in their chemical structure. The symptom complex of experimental psychoses may, for instance, resemble spontaneous schizophrenia if there is a cyclic amine in the inductor. Using radioactive labelled mescaline, Block (1953) demonstrated that the duration of the hallucinogenic effect depends on the time taken for the formation, accumulation and degradation of the protein moeities of mescaline in the liver. He concluded from this that schizophrenia is a chronic disorder due to *intoxication with aminoproteins.* Normally there would be a protective mechanism to neutralize these amines as soon as they become active in the body. This protective mechanism would be the responsibility of an *amine oxidase* which would have the task of breaking down and inhibiting complex hallucinogenic cyclic amines as soon as they were formed.

However, Marazzi and Hart (1955) emphasize that hallucinogenic chemical agents have certain structural similarities to *Adrenaline* and hence, they exert their effect on the synapses of the neurons. Of the hallucinogens which are used for experimental psychoses, *lysergic acid diethylamide (LSD)* has some particularly interesting properties: extremely low doses are sufficient to induce a psychosis with particular psychopathological symptoms which probably arise due to the effect of this substance on the parietal region of the brain and the diencephalon (Bercel et al. 1956). LSD is more like *tryptophane* and some *polypeptides* than adrenaline, and this introduces a new aspect of the problem. According to Bercel et al., in certain circumstances the body is capable of synthesizing LSD spontaneously from tryptophane and other similar substances, and this may produce a spontaneous psychical condition. Blickensdorfer (1953) assumes that exogenous LSD and spontaneously synthesized LSD both combine with an agent in the body to form a substance which exerts a psychotic effect. However, he is not sure whether this agent has an etiological or pathogenetic role (Kanig 1966, 1969, 1971, Monnier 1969).

With regard to LSD, Gaddum (1953), Page (1954), and Wooley and Shaw (1954) stress that this substance is a *serotonin* antagonist and they believe that serotonin has a role as an antipsychotic. However, other authors

(Evarts 1956, Koerscher 1932, Sjoerdsma et al. 1956, etc.) have found that the action of LSD and *bufotenine* (N.N. dimethyl-4-hydroxy-tryptamine) is analogous to the action of serotonin and that all of these may have a psychotic effect. Stoll (1947), Gaddum (1953), Wooley and Shaw (1954), Schwarz et al. (1956), Sjoerdsma et al. (1956) go on to suggest that *adrenochrome* must also have a part to play in the mechanism of action of LSD. Adrenochrome may also be involved in the action of mescaline (Fischer 1954).

Tchalissov et al. (1937 a, b) succeeded in maintaining experimental catatonia by giving *bulbocapnine*. The symptomatology of this catatonia resembled that of a corresponding form of spontaneous schizophrenia. The same intermediate metabolism was found in both experimental and spontaneous catatonia.

These experiments led to a thorough study of intermediate metabolism, particularly in schizophrenias, with the research workers on the look out for chemical agents which could induce spontaneous psychoses.

Heath et al. (1957, 1958) and Heath and Leach (1962) succeeded in isolating a protein fraction, *seruloplasmin,* from the plasma of schizophrenics. This substance, called *taraxein,* resembles the gamma-globulins and when administered to healthy test subjects it induces psychic symptoms similar to those observed in schizophrenic patients. At the same time in the deeper cerebral structures there were signs of dysrhythmic bioelectrical activity like those which have already been mentioned. This dysrhythmic cerebral activity is observed in particular in the septum pellucidum and in the hippocampus (Arnold and Hofmann 1968, Bergen et al. 1962, Coppen 1968, Frohmann et al. 1962, Health and Guerrero-Figueroa 1965, Kety 1968, Penell and Sarsvis 1962, Richter 1968, Robins et al. 1964, Sandres et al. 1962, Seiler 1966, Siegel 1959, Vartanian 1968, Wolfsohn 1960). This substance also produces catatonic symptoms when administered to animals.

The discovery of taraxein has stimulated a flood of research work. Martens (1957) succeeded in isolating ceruloplasmin from schizophrenics and he compared its action with the effect of ceruloplasmin from healthy people. Ceruloplasmin from schizophrenics induces psychotic symptoms when it is administered to healthy people, but the ceruloplasmin isolated from healthy subjects does not induce any psychic phenomena following administration to other healthy test subjects. Therefore, there is a psychotropic property associated with the ceruloplasmin of schizophrenics.

Associated with metabolic disorders in psychoses, particularly disorders of protein metabolism, it was found that, as mentioned above, *degradation products were being retained;* this produces intoxication. This led mainly to closer examination of *nitrogen* since elevated nitrogen levels in blood serum are found right at the beginning of a psychotic episode (Arutunov 1937, Glasov 1937, Küppers 1932, Lando 1957, 1960, Polischtchuk 1937 to

1947, Polischtchuk and Sobolevskaya 1947, Protopopov 1946, Riebling 1939, Scheid 1937, Schriyver and Schriyver-Herzberger 1932, Wolfsohn 1960).

Apart from the increase of aromatic compounds in the serum of patients with schizophrenia, retention of aromatic compounds in the *brain* and *cerebrospinal fluid* has also been reported by Buscaino (1923 to 1933), Tchalissov and Wolfsohn (1940), Polischtchuk (1947), Leschtchinski and Bordskij (1947), Protopopov and Polischtchuk (1948), Gorodkova (1953), Poroschina (1955), Kemali and Romano (1956). Kemali and Romano (1956) reported on a disruption of *indole metabolism,* and this correlates readily with the findings in experimental psychoses.

A change in the *sulphur content in serum and urine* and formation of *thiocyanates* in schizophrenics was found as a result of the disturbances of protein and amino acid metabolism (Jouschtschenko 1911, Kaufmann 1941, Leschtschinski and Brodskij 1947, Polischtchuk 1937, Protopopov 1946, Schmain and Arutunov 1936, Skuin 1939, 1948, Tchalissov 1958, 1960, Wolfsohn 1960), and Wolfsohn (1960) observed a rise in the blood level of *uric acid* in schizophrenic patients.

We also have some results on metabolic changes in *cerebral lipids* (Farstad 1964, Lehmann-Facius 1937). Recently there has been considerable interest in *false regulation of the enzymatic system* in psychoses (Arnold and Hofmann 1968, Chapman and Wolff 1959, Coppen 1968, Looney and Childs 1934, Shevko 1960, Wolfsohn 1960), and there has already been some talk of *enzymopathies* or *enzymopathic psychoses* with a familial predisposition (Arnold and Hofmann 1968).

We shall discuss all these problems in detail in the next few pages, where we have tried to use the same presentation as for epilepsy. The interval in psychomotor epilepsy corresponds to the interval between two attacks of schizophrenia or between two phases in manic depressive psychosis; the preparoxysmal phase in epilepsy corresponds to the onset of the acute symptomatology in psychoses (initial stage); the paroxysmal phase in epilepsy corresponds to the development of the acute symptomatology in psychoses (acute stage); the postparoxysmal stage in epilepsy corresponds to the subsidence of the acute symptomatology in psychoses (remission stage). Chronic psychoses and psychoses which lead to mental deficiencies are compared with chronic states and similar conditions in epilepsy.

Changes in Electrolytes

There has not yet been any thorough research into these electrolyte changes in psychoses, which can be compared with those occurring in psychomotor epilepsy. Nevertheless it would be relevant to attempt to draw a comparison here. However, all we shall do is to mention a very topical subject.

Very recently, *lithium* has been introduced into the treatment of manic depressive psychoses (Angst and Weis 1968, Baastrup and Schou 1967, Cade 1949, Lauter 1969, Schou 1967, Schou and Baastrup 1967). It has been suggested that lithium salts are rather different from other psychotrophic drugs, since they have a biological mechanism of action. Lithium salts are capable of influencing the mechanism of catecholamine metabolism, and this leads to binding, e.g. of excess noradrenaline, and eliminates the cause of clinical psychotic symptoms. Some authors also believe that lithium salts affect the mechanism of action of serotonin. Serotonin is involved in both psychoses and psychomotor epilepsy (see Chapters VI and VIII). If the hypothesis on the influence of lithium on serotonin metabolism proves to be correct, then this will go some way towards explaining its role in epilepsy.

The fact that, apart from other side effects, an overdose of lithium leads to epileptic attacks is also an indication that lithium is involved in the mechanism of epilepsy. Thus, lithium must exert some effect on the water and electrolyte balance and this brings about certain metabolic changes.

This example illustrates that even if the developmental mechanisms responsible for producing psychoses and epilepsy are not the same, they are certainly similar and, symptomatically, there may be transitions from one to the other. However, after the acute symptomatology has subsided the two groups of diseases become less alike, until, with the onset of a further acute condition, they once again tend to resemble one another.

Water Balance

As with electrolytes, the reason for the change in water balance in psychoses has not yet been explained. There have been reports of water retention in acute and chronic psychoses (Gjessing 1968). The classic school of psychiatry has already dealt with this problem, but it is not always possible to distinguish here between causes and effects.

As we shall discuss later, there are changes in serum and cerebral proteins in psychotic states as well as in psychomotor epilepsy. The changes are very much the same, although not identical. Where there is slight hyperproteinaemia, slight hypoalbuminaemia and slight to more pronounced hyperglobulinaemia, water retention must also be a possibility. However, this water retention could arise simply as a result of these protein changes.

In certain cases of acute catatonia, acute paranoid-hallucinatory schizophrenia and stuporous depression, there may be total metabolic changes and the patient may refuse to eat. Again in these cases it is not possible to assess for certain the causes of water retention since a refusal to eat may lead to further metabolic changes.

The water balance must also depend on the symptoms of a disease. In a catatonic stuporous patient it is assumed that the prevailing condition is one of vagotonia and there will be a greater tendency for water retention to occur. On the other hand, a manic and paranoid hallucinatory condition will tend to be associated more with sympathicotonia and this will result in forced excretion of water. In any case, care must be exercized when drawing comparisons between psychosis and epilepsy here.

Oxidation Processes and pH

Many authors have tackled the problem of oxidation processes in psychoses. The hypnoid state in the psychopathology of schizophrenias is regarded as the result of a blockade of the oxidizing enzyme system by by-products of metabolism. Buscaino (1933) found this type of change in the striatum and thalamus of his patients and he was able to demonstrate reduced *cytochromic* activity. Aschbi (1960) observed reduced *carbonic anhydrase* activity in the frontal lobe in his patients. According to Jelinski (1960), the serum of schizophrenics in a mentally deficient condition indicates *inhibited oxygen consumption* in the brain. This process is associated with an accumulation of toxic substances in blood and brain, and these toxins are capable of suppressing oxygen utilization and consumption in cerebral tissue. The serum develops such toxicity that it is capable of prolonging the disease for 30 to 40 years. This toxicity resembles cobra toxin (Much and Holzmann 1960) or rosta lupinusa (Max 1922).

The reduction of oxidation processes in schizophrenics was detected very early by a number of authors, including Omorikov (1909). There is a rise in the urinary levels of partially oxidized metabolic products (Docenko et al. 1960). Blood oxygen may also be elevated and cerebral oxygen reduced. (Tchalissov 1937, Wolfsohn 1928, 1932, 1940).

Looney and Childs (1934), Tchalissov et al. (1937, Protopopov (1946) and others were able to show that the reduction of oxidation processes in psychoses has an effect on intermediate metabolism of the brain. According to Shevko (1960) a reduction of oxidation processes is often associated with an acceleration of peroxidizing acidification, a fall of pH in blood and brain and formation of some peroxide products which inhibit respiration. Also, this is coupled with a retardation of Adrenaline metabolism, which leads to formation of toxic substances in brain and blood.

Shevko (1956, 1958, 1960) has dealt in detail with the problem of oxidation processes and, by way of an example, we should like briefly to discuss some of his results. He examined more than 1000 schizophrenic patients at various stages of the disease; he studied: the activity of *catalase,* peroxides, carbohydrate metabolism and the polarographic properties of the protein fractions from blood serum.

Catalase is known to be one of the haemoprotein enzymes and its function is to catalyse the breakdown of hydrogen peroxide (Fieser and Fieser 1968). According to Shevko's reports (1960), at the initial stage of the disease catalase activity is elevated in most of the patients and reduced in a few patients. However, catalase becomes unstable at the stage when the symptomatology is pronounced, and in a chronic stage of the disease it will be significantly impaired. A forced schizophrenic symptomatology results in a reduction in the rate of reaction of catalase, an increase of peroxides and reduced serum haemoglobin.

The change of catalase activity in the serum of schizophrenics leads the author to re-examine the effect of many different factors. Thus, he assumes that, among other things, there must be various humoral changes in the patient's blood which impair catalase activity. According to Shevko (1960), at the stage when the schizophrenic symptomatology is pronounced, substances with *anticatalatic properties* are formed in the blood, and these become particularly effective when the activity of the enzyme increases. Thus, at the initial stage there is first activation of the enzyme and this then causes anticatalatic substances to be formed and these substances then inhibit the catalase. This inhibition causes the clinical picture to deteriorate, and so we have a vicious circle. Catalase only catalyses the break-down of hydrogen peroxide. Other peroxides are not broken down by catalase (Fieser and Fieser 1968), and for this reason, it is not possible to draw any overall conclusions about the oxidation processes and their effects, simply from catalase activity.

The activity of *peroxidase* may be elevated or depressed in schizophrenics (Kukoleva 1957, Shevko 1960, Wolfovski 1958). In the initial stage it is usually activated and at the stage of pronounced schizophrenic symptoms it is inhibited. Peroxidase may be activated by chromoprotein activity.

Catalase and peroxidase activity normalize when the schizophrenia is subsiding (Bach 1950, Brams 1955, Dolenko 1958, Paritchenko 1958, Shevko 1960, Soreni 1945, Tchalissov 1960, Vladimirov and Kolotilova 1947, Wolfovski 1958).

All the results we have come across so far seem to indicate that there is a *disturbance of peroxidizing oxidation* in schizophrenics and this results in the formation of undesired chemical products. These lead to deterioration of the clinical picture, which in turn causes further biochemical changes. The change in peroxidizing oxidation in schizophrenics is of great importance in epilepsy, particularly in psychomotor epilepsy. In fact, an *alkalotic tendency* in brain and blood has often been discussed with regard to psychomotor epilepsy. On the other hand, the metabolic disorders met with in psychoses lead to *acidosis*. Thus, the *alkalosis of the epileptic may be corrected either by an epileptic attack or by a psychotic episode.*

Carbohydrate Metabolism

Many authors have studied *carbohydrate metabolism* in psychoses, since there are often various types of abnormality to be found. The chemical topography of the cortex in schizophrenics had been worked out as early as 1932 on the basis of results obtained up to then (Gorodiska 1932) ; this is now known as *lactacidogenic topography*. Similarly, Embden examined the distribution of hexose monophosphate in muscles in 1912. The *lactacidogens* in the brain consist of a mixture of *glucose-6-monophosphate* and *fructose-6-monophosphate*. Postmortem examination of the cortices from 20 schizophrenics revealed a higher concentration of lactacidogen in the right hemisphere of the cerebrum than in the left (Tchalissov 1960) .

Persistent *hyperglycaemia* has been observed in patients with catatonia (Lorenz 1922, Schesterikova et al. 1960, Seiler 1966) , paranoid-hallucinatory schizophrenia (Herny and Mangum 1925, Kovaleva 1960, Papadopulos 1960) , periodic endogenous depression (Drury and Farran-Ridge 1925, Haimovitch and Podka-Mennii 1960, Kovaleva 1960) , and during the depressive phase of manic depressive psychosis (Drury and Farran-Ridge 1925, Henry and Mangum 1925, Kovaleva 1960, Lorenz 1922, McCowan and Quastel 1931, Raphael and Parsons 1921, Raphael et al. 1928, Tchalissov 1960) . Flat tolerance curves are found during the manic phase of manic-depression and these indicate abnormal glucose tolerance (Henry and Mangum 1925, Mann 1925, McFarland and Goldstein 1938) . As the clinical picture improves, the glucose tolerance curves nomalize (Altschule 1953, Mann 1925, McFarland and Goldstein 1938) .

Investigations of other sugar constituents of blood (products of glucose metabolism) , such as lactic acid, alpha-keto acids (Buscaino and Rapisarda 1948, Dawson et al. 1954, Hennemann et al. 1954) , ketones (Kitay and Altschule 1952, Lövendahl and Valatin 1941, Northcote 1932, Thomson and Aste-Salazar 1939, Wortis et al. 1940) and one or two other substances, indicate that there is defective utilization of glucose here, possibly at the hexose-6-monophosphate or pyruvic acid stage. Less CO_2 is produced directly from ^{14}C glucose *in vivo* in the brains of chronic psychotic patients than in healthy test subjects (Sacks 1957, 1959) . We feel that this point is very important and so we should like to discuss one or two results in rather more detail.

Papadopulos (1960) studied the first bout in 29 acute schizophrenics and from the glycaemic curves he found a pathological course in all patients following glucose tolerance tests; 50 percent of cases were very abnormal. Examinations after six months, one and two years showed that some of the patients still had pathological glucose tolerance curves.

Kovaleva (1960) compared glucose tolerance curves from schizophrenics and manic-depressive patients. In 119 of 132 schizophrenics she found a *hyperglycaemic curve* with impaired glucose tolerance. The results were normal in the other 13 patients. In the manic phase of manic-depression, utilization of available glucose was decidedly better than in schizophrenics. Kovaleva interprets this difference in schizophrenics as being related to the initial condition of the autonomic nervous system: the parasympathetic system is functionally dominant in schizophrenics and the sympathetic system in the manic phase of manic-depression.

Natalevitch (1960) studied glucose tolerance in schizophrenic patients with either an autistic or a catatonic syndrome, and he came up with some interesting results. The results of his studies on hyperglycaemia following administration of glucose were basically the same as those of the other authors referred to above. However, his findings indicate that the blood levels of ATP and diphosphoglyceric acid are depressed in catatonic patients, and there is also a slight elevation of glucose phosphate and inorganic phosphorus, i.e. *elevation of the substances from the first stage of glycolysis and depression of substances from later stages of glucose metabolism.* The depressed level of ATP can be interpreted as the result either of further rapid degradation or of inadequate (re)synthesis. The author considers the second possibility to be the more likely. Inadequate or delayed (re)synthesis of ATP is seen as the result of the catatonic condition rather than its cause.

Tchalissov (1960) has tackled the problem of disorders of glucose metabolism in psychoses and he has tried to explain these. According to Tchalissov, the metabolic processes undergo a change when the first psychotic symptoms appear. This change is reflected primarily in a reduction of fatty particles which results in loss of body weight. However, if the patient does not lose weight, these fatty particles are deposited at different, abnormal sites. The author attributes this deposition of fat or weight loss to disorders of energy metabolism. According to Tchalissov (1960), the principal metabolic disorders and the origin of the clinical symptomatology occur at a common site, i.e. the brain. However, both symptoms and metabolic disorders spread throughout the body so that a study of these processes cannot be confined simply to the brain.

The most recent investigations (Haikin and Gontcharova 1954, Kanig 1969, Seiler 1966) show that there is very active synthesis of glycogen in the brain, and the processes are only a little slower than in the liver. Breakdown of polysaccharides in the brain occurs under the action of *phosphorylase* and *amylase* (Raschba 1948). The most important reaction is the hydrolysis of polysaccharides under the action of amylase.

According to Tchalissov (1960), in healthy people there is a greater concentration of amylase in the blood leaving the brain than in that flowing into the brain. However, the blood amylase concentration is labile in schizophrenics and there is no difference between the concentration of this enzyme in blood entering and blood leaving the brain. The author concludes from this that carbohydrate metabolism is less intense in schizophrenics than in the brain of a healthy person.

Haikina and Gontcharova (1954) found that the level of polysaccharide metabolism in the brain depends on the lability of the cerebral functions.

According to Blochin (1951), the increase of polysaccharide metabolism coincides with a rise in conditioned reflex functions of the CNS with an accumulation of lactic acid and phosphorus.

Richter (1957) does not believe that there is any conclusive evidence of changes in glucose metabolism in the brain in schizophrenics, but there are many findings to contradict his view.

Lingjaerde (1953) reports that there is a carbohydrate deficiency, particularly in the initial phase in schizophrenia, and that both brain and liver are important here. According to the results of Altschule (1953), Altschule et al. (1957) and Hennemann et al. (1954), the blood levels of pyruvic acid, citric acid, alpha-keto-glutaric acid and inorganic phosphorus are normal in schizophrenics. However, the concentrations of sugar and lactic acid are higher than in healthy people.

Following administration of 100 g. glucose to patients there was a rise in the blood sugar concentration, a sharp rise of uric and pyruvic acids, a fall of citric acid and alpha-ketoglutaric acid and prolonged depression of inorganic phosphorus. According to the above-named authors, these changes depend on the organic changes in the brain, even in the initial phase. Altschule et al. (1957) demonstrated that, irrespective of any change in the clinical picture, *chlorpromazine* and *reserpine* do not alter the pathological glycogen curve following administration of 100 g. glucose. The authors conclude from this that the *psychotropic drugs do not have any effect on the basic mechanism responsible for producing schizophrenia.*

This can also be applied to the action of antiepileptic agents; this will be discussed in Chapters VII, VIII and IX.

Other authors (Friedman et al. 1954, Henneman et al. 1954, 1955) have studied the glycogen level and the metabolic products of glycogen following administration of insulin or adrenaline (Altschule 1953, Hennemann et al. 1955, Lingjaerde 1953). These findings also revealed pathological changes in glucose metabolism following test administrations of sugar.

Schevko et al. (1953) tried to find some connection between glucose in the brain and ATP in blood. To do this, they examined 35 schizophrenics and 30 epileptics and they found changes in fundamental biochemical processes which were associated with a change of ATP activity in blood, in the cortex of schizophrenics. As the symptoms became more intense in these patients, there was a more profound change of ATP in blood, and vice versa.

All the research work mentioned above and also studies by Haimovitch and Podkameni (1960), Staub and Traugott (1926, 1927), Skuin (1939), Sereiskii and Lando (1946), Hennemann et al. (1954), Lando et al. (1954), Padovani (1954), Tatarenko (1954), Haimovitch (1956), Popov (1957), Papadopulos (1960), Schesterikova et al. (1960) and many other authors, indicate that there are disorders of carbohydrate metabolism in schizophrenics and in other patients with endogenous psychoses; the picture is one of hyperglycaemia, particularly if a glucose tolerance test is performed.

There are more parallels between the hyperglycaemic curve following a glucose tolerance test and the clinical symptoms in schizophrenics in the initial stage of the acute phase rather than in a later phase of the disease. When the acute schizophrenic symptomatology is developed, the hyperglycaemic curve always correlates with the clinical symptoms, while there is not always correlation with the hyperglycaemic curve when the acute clinical symptoms are subsiding. In the majority of cases, the hyperglycaemic curve persists, even when the clinical symptomatology has subsided; in a smaller number of patients, both clinical picture and metabolic disorders normalize simultaneously.

In order to abridge the reports of many authors, we have summarized the results. The *hypoglycaemia, vagotonia and alkalosis* of the epileptic means that the initial metabolic picture that he displays can be altered either by an epileptic attack or by acute schizophrenic symptomatology. If his symptoms assume a schizophrenia-like picture, then he immediately develops *hyperglycaemia, sympathicotonia and acidosis.* These processes lead to deterioration of the schizophrenic symptoms but protect the epileptic from an attack. When the schizophrenic symptomatology disappears, this abnormal condition subsides. The hyperglycaemia normalizes, the acidosis is compensated for, and there is no longer a prevalent state of sympathicotonia. Thus, here the schizophrenic symptoms have replaced an epileptic attack, but achieved just what the attack would have achieved. We do not know when and how an epileptic will be *predisposed* to schizophrenic symptoms rather than to an epileptic attack but, as we stressed before, these symptoms seem to occur more often in epileptics with a focus in the limbic system, i.e. in psychomotor epilepsy. They occur more rarely in other forms of epilepsy where the focus wanders laterally, from the medical region (see Chapter III).

Characteristics of Protein Metabolism

Many authors have studied proteins in the brain, blood and urine of psychotic patients. Certain abnormalities of both carbohydrate and protein metabolism have been found in schizophrenic patients and other psychotic patients and we shall now discuss these points (see also Figure 23).

Polischtchuk (1937, 1939 a, b), Skuin (1939, 1948) Wolfsohn (1940), Lando (1946, 1957), Rasin (1949), Lando and Seleva (1952), Buscaino (1953), Honda (1956), Jantz (1956) Lando (1960), Tchalissov (1960) and other authors have shown that there are certain metabolic changes in schizophrenia. First there is the general point that the serum level of protein is rather higher in schizophrenics than in healthy people (Lapteva 1956). Buscaino (1953) and Honda (1956) only found this elevation in the acute stage of the disease. According to some authors (Buchner and Gabsch 1956, Collens and Banovitch 1955, Genes 1955, Lapteva 1956, Schesterikova et al. 1960, Wolfsohn 1960) the albumins are relatively depressed and the globulins elevated. Since even in healthy people the serum level of proteins and the relation of protein fractions to one another may be altered, we would like to draw one or two comparisons from the literature.

Kelmischkeut and Sigrist (1960) set out to compare the changes in serum protein concentrations in healthy and sick people in the course of growing up and aging. They based their conclusions on their own findings and on those of Buscaino (1953), Denissova (1956), Lapteva (1956), Rudoj (1956), Lando (1960). For the purpose of their study Kelmischkeut and Sigrist (1960) established two large groups which were then divided into subgroups. The first group comprised younger healthy and sick people and the second group older healthy and sick people. The results are shown in Tables V and VI. As Table V shows, the concentration of total protein in serum is significantly lower in healthy people between 40 and 50 years of age than in people between 20 and 25 years of age. However, this does not apply to sick people; in fact, the reverse is the case and there is a rise rather than a fall of the serum protein concentration in older patients.

The albumin fraction declines with age in both healthy and sick people: there is a greater reduction in the first group, by 6 percent; from 62.7 percent to 56.7 percent. The reduction in the second group was 3.1 percent; from 60.9 percent to 57.8 percent. The A/G quotient was also depressed.

There are higher levels of both total globulins and globulin fractions in adults compared with younger people. There is no difference here between values for healthy and sick people. According to these authors, the globulins represent 37.3 percent of the total protein in younger healthy people and 43.3 percent in older people between 40 and 50 years of age. The globulin fraction in young patients was 39.1 percent and 42.2 percent in older patients. In young healthy test subjects 3.16 g. percent globulin was found in 100 ml. serum and in older people between 40 and 50 years of age this figure was 3.40 g percent. Corresponding values for sick people were 3.07 g. percent and 3.52 g. percent. Alpha-globulins increase more with the age of the patient than do beta-globulins (Table XI). Gamma-globulins do not change during growth or aging in either healthy or sick people.

TABLE V. Concentrations of serum protein fractions in two groups of healthy people and patients of different ages. The results from young healthy people are compared with those from older healthy subjects, and results from young patients are compared with those from older patients(cp. Table VI). (From Kelmischkeit, E.G., and A.G. Sigrist: *Obmen Vesôstv pri Psihičkih Zabolevanijah.* Moscow, Medgiz, 1960, p. 87.)

		Group of Test Subjects							
	Proteins	*Healthy People*				*Psychotic People*			
		M_1	M_2	M_2-M_1	*Significance*	M_1	M_2	M_2-M_1	*Significance*
Fractions of Proteins (%)	Albumins	62.7	56.7	—10	4.0	60.9	57.8	— 5	1.7
		±0.4	±1.2			±1.4	±1.1		
	α-	8.0	10.1	±26	2.2	11.0	13.2	+20	1.4
	Globulins	±0.5	±0.8			±0.9	±1.3		
	β-	9.7	11.7	±21	2.3	9.6	11.4	+19	1.7
	Globulins	±0.5	±0.7			±0.6	±0.9		
	γ-	19.6	21.5	±10	2.3	18.4	17.7	— 4	0.4
	Globulins	±0.4	±0.7			±1.3	±1.2		
	A/G-	1.70	1.30	—24	5.0	1.60	1.40	—13	1.5
	Quotient	±0.03	±0.07			±0.11	±0.06		
	Total	8.45	7.85	— 7	6.1	7.86	8.35	+ 6	2,3
	Proteins	±0.09	±0.05			±0.17	±0.12		
Concentration of Prot.	Albumins	5.29	4.45	—16	8.1	4.79	4.83	+0.8	0.2
		±0.07	±0.08			±0.15	±0.11		
	α-	0.68	0.79	+16	1.5	0.86	1.10	+28	1.8
	Globulins	±0.04	±0.06			±0.07	±0.11		
	β-	0.82	0.92	+12	1.4	0.76	0.95	+25	2.0
	Globulins	+0.04	±0.06			±0.05	±0.08		
	γ-	1.66	1.69	+ 2	0.4	1.45	1.47	+ 1	0.1
	Globulins	±0.05	±0.06			±0.12	±0.1		

M_1 = People between 20 and 25 years of Age;
M_2 = People between 40 and 50 years of Age;
Significance = Significance Level (Probability)

Table VI also shows that younger patients exhibit a 38 percent rise of alpha globulins compared with 26 percent in younger healthy subjects. The rise of α-globulins in older patients compared with older healthy subjects is 32 percent and 39 percent respectively. The differences in the falls of γ-globulins are not so marked in old and young, healthy and sick subjects. According to these authors, the protein changes in the sick can be clearly distinguished from the changes which take place as a result of the aging process.

Wolfsohn (1960) also studied serum proteins in schizophrenics and his results are very interesting. He examined 100 patients before, during and after therapy and demonstrated that there are changes in serum proteins during the disease and during the recovery period.

Right up to the beginning of therapy, the serum protein concentration showed a wide scatter—from slight depression to marked elevation, with a mean at around normal. In the course of treatment, there was a trend to-

TABLE VI. Concentration of serum protein fractions from healthy people and patients of different age groups. Here, young healthy people are compared with young patients, and healthy old people are compared with old patients. (From the authors of Table V.)

	Proteins	*Groups of Test Subjects* — *Younger People (20-25 Years of Age)* M_1	M_2	M_2-M_1	*Significance*	*Older People (40-50 Years of Age)* M_1	M_2	M_2-M_1	*Significance*
Fractions (%)	Albumins	62.8	60.9	— 3	1.2	56.8	57.8	— 2	0.6
		±0.8	±1.4			±1.2	±1.1		
	α-	8.0	60.9	+38	2.9	10.0	13.2	+32	2.1
	Globulins	±0.5	±1.4			±0.8	±1.3		
	β-	9.7	9.6	— 1	0.1	11.7	11.4	— 3	0.3
	Globulins	±0.5	±0.9			±0.8	±1.3		
	γ-	19.6	18.4	— 6	0.9	21.5	17.7	—18	2.7
	Globulins	±0.4	±1.3			±0.7	±1.2		
Concentration in g/%	Albumins	5.29	4.79	— 9	3.0	4.46	4.83	+ 9	2.8
		±0.07	±0.15			±0.08	±0.11		
	α-	0.68	0.86	+26	2.0	0.18	0.99	+39	2.5
	Globulins	±0.04	±0.07			±0.05	±0.11		
	β-	0.82	0.76	— 7	1.3	0.92	0.85	— 8	0.3
	Globulins	±0.04	±0.05			±0.04	±0.02		
	γ-	1.66	1.45	—12	1.6	1.69	1.47	—13	1.9
	Globulins	±0.05	±0.12			±0.06	±0.10		
	Total	8.45	7.86	— 7	3.3	7.86	8.35	+ 6	3.8
	Proteins	±0.08	±7.86			±0.15	±0.12		

M_1 = Healthy People
M_2 = Patients (Psychosis)

wards a reduction of the serum protein concentration in all groups. In the group where the therapeutic results were good, the difference in the levels before and after therapy was greater than in patients where treatment was ineffective.

The initial levels of serum proteins were the same in all groups, whether or not therapy was effective. The A/G quotient was elevated at the onset of the disease in both groups, although it was much higher in the group which did not respond well to treatment later. This quotient fell during treatment, in the group which responded well to treatment. This reduction was statistically significant ($p < 0.05$). Thus, according to Wolfsohn (1960) there was only a slight rise in blood proteins (and alpha-globulins) at the beginning of the disease. Unlike the other authors mentioned, Wolfsohn did not find any fall in the A/G quotient at the beginning of treatment; there was actually a rise (see Table VII).

Schesterikova et al (1960) found *dysproteinaemia,* i.e. a fall of albumins and a rise of globulins, in all schizophrenics examined; this condition was present both in patients who were resistant and in those who were not resistant to insulin therapy (see Table VIII). At the beginning of the

TABLE VII. Changes of serum protein in schizophrenic patients before and during treatment, with and without therapeutic success. (From Wolfson, N.M., 1960.)

Proteins	*Therapy*					
	Successful			*Resistent*		
	Before	*During*	*Difference*	*Before*	*During*	*Difference*
Total	7.17±0.28	6.97±0.21	—0.20	7.44±0.29	7.21±0.48	—0.23
Proteins	(6.0—9.9)	(5.2—8.4)	±0.35	(4.8—9.4)	(4.5—9.6)	±0.56
Albumins	5.08±0.25	4.72±0.18	—0.36	5.31±0.31	5.35±0.37	+0.04
	(3.8—7.7)	(2.9—6.5)	±0.31	(2.3—8.0)	(3.4—6.9)	±0.49
Globulins	2.07±0.09	2.13±0.06	+0.06	2.07±0.69	1.94±0.13	—0.13
	(1.2—3.0)	(1.4—3.5)	±0.11	(1.0—3.1)	(1.2—2.8)	±0.70
A/G-Quotient	2.52±0.18	2.20±0.14	—0.33	2.90±0.36	2.70±0.20	—0.20
	(1.3—5.1)	(1.1—4.4)	±0.23	(1.5—8.5)	(1.5—4.0)	±0.41

disease there was no great shift in the proteins. At the stage in which the symptoms were developing there was a rise of total protein and then a fall of albumins, a rise of β-globulins and later on a rise of α-globulins. These authors found that the A/G quotient is depressed and their results do not correlate with those of Wolfsohn (1960) (see Table VII).

Tschumburidze (1960) examined 142 schizophrenics between 18 and 35 years of age with various forms of the disease at the acute (68 patients) and chronic stages (74 patients).

In acute catatonic patients there were rises of total protein and globulins, particularly β-globulins. The α_1, α_2 and gamma-globulin fractions were at the upper normal limit or a little above. According to Tschumburidze, the elevation of β-globulins is involved in formation of antitoxins and this indicates a toxic condition in schizophrenics. This supports the theory of the toxic nature of catatonia.

In the other forms of schizophrenia, there was hyperglobulinaemia at the expense of the α_1 and α_2 fractions. Beta- and gamma-globulins were at, or a little above, the upper normal limits.

In cases which responded well to treatment (26 of 36 patients), the total protein concentration was 8.2 to 15.2 g.% (mean 11.7 g.%) in the period before insulin shock, i.e. it was elevated as compared with the initial value. During the shock there was a further rise of 4.6 to 7.2 g. percent. In most of the patients there was a tendency for the parameter to normalize immediately after treatment. There was a change in the albumin fraction corresponding to the change in total protein. However, the globulins responded rather differently. There was a fall of α_1- and α_2-globulins until after the shock and then, some time after the shock, they rose again slightly, although the levels did not approach those recorded before treatment.

At the end of treatment there was either complete normalization of proteins or a tendency for the values to normalize. In patients who did not respond well to treatment there was no great change in proteins at first.

TABLE VIII. Changes of total proteins and protein fractions in the serum of schizrophrenics during insulin treatment. The results are compared with those from other mental patients. (From Schesterikova, P.T., Ignatova, N.I., and Schuhhalter, W.M., 1960.)

Diagnosis	*Success of Therapy*	*Number of Cases*	*Albumins* %	Globulins in %				*A/G Quotient*
				α_1	α_2	β	γ	
Schizophrenia	Resistent	18	52.2±2.28 (37.6–67.5)	5.14±0.48 (2.5–8.1)	7.9±1.24 (3.4–14.2)	16.5±1.53 (6.1–28.6)	18.2±1.91 (9.3–15.2)	1.18±0.11 (0.66–2.13)
	Successful	21	55.4±1.39 (41.7–66.5)	4.9±0.84 (1.8–12.5)	6.3±0.93 (2.2–15.0)	16.3±0.98 (7.8–24.2)	19.2±1.33 (10.9–29.0)	1.22±0.07 (0.61–1.96)
Other psychotic Patients	Resistent	6	54.7±2.20 (40.8–62.4)	3.1±0.3 (2.8–3.4)	6.6±2.6 (4.0–9.2)	19.2±1.21 (15.2–23.8)	16.1±2.42 (7.9–22.7)	1.26±0.14 (0.69–1.66)
	Successful	6	52.8±3.66 (40.7–65.1)	7.6±2.65 (5.0–10.3)	7.1±4.3 (2.8–11.4)	13.4±1.87 (8.5–21.1)	21.0±2.84 (14.1–30.1)	1.20±0.18 (0.68–1.87)

However, once again the values tended to normalize after treatment. The rise of proteins during treatment is attributed to the effect of the insulin administered (see also Protopopov 1946, Protopopov et al. 1939, Polischtchuk 1939).

Tschumburidze (1960) obtained rather different results when treating patients with phenothiazines (aminazin). Patients who showed an improvement in the clinical picture in the first two weeks of treatment showed a fall of previously elevated total protein, by on average 4.5 g. percent. The albumins fell by on average 12.5 percent, globulins (particularly α_1- and α_2-globulins) rose and there was also a slight rise of beta fractions. These shifts persisted for five to eight weeks, and subsequently the total protein concentration became normal. The albumin fraction was elevated and the α_1- and α_2-globulin fractions fell and remained at the upper normal limit.

In cases where there was no improvement of the clinical picture after treatment the protein levels took longer to normalize than in the first group. The same was found by Lapteva (1956), Pogodaev and Galenko (1956), Livschitz and Roitrub (1957), Poroschina et al. (1957) and other authors.

Thus far we have been discussing the results of electrophoretic examinations of serum. However, Podoprigora (1960) studied the polarographic properties of protein fractions and he was able to show that seurm proteins in schizophrenics alter according to the stage of the disease. At the onset of the disease and when the symptoms are most in evidence the albumins are depressed and the globulins elevated. Later the depression of albumins is only slight and beta- and gamma-globulins are elevated.

However, polarographic studies also showed that in schizophrenics in *addition to quantitative changes there are also qualitative changes in serum protein.* Initially there is a rise in the second polarographic wave of albumin, and in a few patients there is also an insignificant rise of activity in the polarographic waves for α-, β-, and γ-globulin fractions. In the middle stage of the disease, the first and second polarographic waves of albumins are reduced and the α-globulin wave is increased more than in the initial stage. In the later stage of the disease the albumin curve is flatter with the second wave very much depressed. The α-globulin curves are often elevated and there are twice as many changes as for albumins. γ-globulins are usually elevated, but only when the α-globulins are elevated.

Similar results were obtained by Gorodkova (1953), Danilenko (1954), Cvetkova (1960), Hramcova (1960), Krasilnikova (1960) and others (see Figure 44).

Cvetkova (1960) has studied protein metabolism in patients with delirium tremens and chronic alcoholism, and her findings correlate with those of Jantz (1956), Ronco (1956) and others. At the onset of delirium the level of albumins was depressed by 2.5 ± 0.5 g. percent. Globulins were slightly elevated, by 1.8 ± 0.2 g. percent. The A/G quotient was correspondingly depressed. The findings only altered slightly in the course of delirium, as shown in Table IX. There was also a slight change in serum proteins in patients with chronic alcoholism.

TABLE IX. Serum protein concentration in patients with delirium tremens and chronic alcoholism. (From Cvetkova, N.B., 1960.)

Sequence of Investigation	*Time of Investigation*	*Albumins in g/%*	*Globulins in g/%*	*A/G-Quotient*
0	Kontrol	4.0±0.1 (4.2–6.5)	1.66±0.20 (1.06–2.3)	2.1±0.12 (1.6–2.6)
I	Between 3 and 6 day of illness	2.49±0.5 (1.38–3.75)	1.82±0.20 (1.16–2.68)	1.40±0.33 (0.90–2.44)
II	Between 7 and 15 day of illness	2.69±0.48 (2.12–4.69)	1.91±0.3 (1.31–3.75)	1.56±0.33 (1.06–2.58)
III	Between 16 and 30 day of illness	3.19±0.36 (2.34–4.00)	2.43±0.30 (1.06–3.68)	1.50±0.15 (1.16–2.09)
Investigations into chronic alcoholic patients		3.19±0.2 (2.60–4.30)	2.72±0.30 (1.41–4.53)	1.34±0.23 (1.00–3.51)

During the period when the psychopathological symptoms were subsiding there was a slight rise of albumins and also of globulins, so that the A/G quotient was unchanged. This *was the difference between results from patients with delirium tremens and alcoholism and those from schizophrenics.*

These results illustrate that there are many fine distinctions between epilepsies and schizophrenias as regards changes in serum proteins. There are also differences between these two groups and patients with delirium tremens or chronic alcoholism. However, there are also similarities. A particularly important fact is that where schizophrenia or epileptic attacks have occurred the protein balance in serum, and hence also in the brain, can normalize. Thus, in a psychomotor epileptic the protein balance in his body can normalize, either as a result of an epileptic attack or by the development of a schizophrenic symptomatology. This applies particularly to those epileptic patients who only have psychomotor attacks, and no major attacks. Since only a major attack is capable of normalizing the protein balance and other biochemical changes in the body, a patient with isolated psychomotor attacks is left with the *choice* of schizophrenic symptoms to *help* him to normalize his protein balance.

Amino Acids and Psychoses

In psychoses, changes of proteins seem to be closely related to changes of amino acids (Albert et al. 1946, 1951, Ewalt and Bruce 1948, Fincle and Reyna 1962, Kanig 1966, 1969, 1971, Kety 1968, Pile 1952, Tower 1955, 1956, 1960, Zabarenko and Chamers 1952, Zimmerman and Burgemeister 1950, 1951, 1959, Zimmerman et al. 1947).

In schizophrenias and other psychoses (involutional, asthenic, puerperal, psychopathic and manic-depressive), Schesterikova et al. (1960) found certain elevations of amino acids in blood; this result was significant in schizophrenics who were resistant to treatment. It is interesting to note that the serum level of amino acids is also elevated in other therapy-resistant psychoses (Table X).

The serum amino acids do not respond in this way following a test administration of proteins. At best there is elevation of serum amino acids three hours after the administration (Michnev 1950, Schesterikova et al. 1960).

Following administration of 10 g. aminoacetic acid, in the majority of patients there was a rise in the blood amino acid curve about three hours after administration. If insulin is given, the amino acid concentration in blood falls because insulin promotes protein synthesis (Lotspeich 1949).

After administration of comatose doses of insulin, there were marked falls of amino acids in blood after one, two, three and four and one-half hours in 22 of 27 patients. These falls were similar in patients who were therapy-resistant to insulin and in those who responded to insulin therapy, except that they occurred faster in the first group, with very little relation to the dose of insulin.

Test administration of amino acetic acid to healthy people results in increased urinary excretion of amino acids. However, most of the amino acids are metabolized by the liver, and this results in an increase of ammonia and urea excretion in the urine (Belova 1955, Lapteva 1956). Schesterikova et al. (1960) found aminoaciduria in schizophrenics following administration of amino acetic acid and there was under-production of ammonia. The curve altered in relation to the change in resistance to insulin.

TABLE X. Amino acid concentration in the serum of schizophrenic patients and patients with other mental disorders (mg%) (Schesterikova et al., 1960).

Diagnosis	*Therapy (Insulin shocks)*	*Number of Patients*	*Results*	
			Means	*Variations*
Schizophrenia	Resistent	30	7.64±0.36	3.7—12.5
Schizophrenia	Therapy successful	11	6.90±0.14	4.8—10.0
Other Psychoses	Resistent	14	7.10±0.58	3.55—10.9
Other Psychoses	Therapy successful	6	7.06±0.22	5.70—8.5

In polarographic studies of serum amino acids, Krasnova (1960) found no definite differences between schizophrenics and healthy subjects. However, in epileptics (who were studied in parallel to the schizophrenics) the polarographic wave was flattened, i.e. the concentration of amino acids was reduced. Mison-Crighel et al. (1955) were also able to demonstrate flattening of the polarographic curve for cerebrospinal fluid, as compared with healthy subjects. Pogodaev (1956) also found that the polarographic curve for serum was flattened in schizophrenics.

When assessing these results it must be emphasized that the height of the polarographic waves depends on the content of sulph-hydryls (- SH -) and disulphide groups (- SS -) in the test fluid. Thus, there may be some disparity in the results for amino acids (cystine, cyteine), since sulphhydryl and disulphide groups from proteins are also determined. Proteins containing sulphur may therefore affect the results for amino acids containing sulphur (Balle-Helaers 1955, Brdička 1933, Hasselbach and Schwab 1955, Mitev and Harisonova 1958, Petrasch and Wilschanski 1954, Turek and Cizinsky 1955).

Now, turning to the problem of amino acids in psychoses it is again possible that we are dealing with an epileptic equivalent here. Where there is a fall of amino acids in serum and cerebrospinal fluid of an epileptic, there is the possibility that these may be compensated for by development of a psychotic symptomatology.

Endogenous Amines

We have already alluded to the role of *Adrenaline* in psychoses, and *serotonin* was also mentioned in this connection. Endogenous amines probably have an important part to play in psychoses as well as in epilepsy. Unfortunately, their role here is not thoroughly understood. According to Wolfsohn (1960), the activity of *cholinesterase* was substantially reduced in schizophrenics. During the treatment, the group which responded well to therapy showed a tendency for cholinesterase activity to rise or to normalize, whereas there were no changes in the group of patients resistant to therapy.

While studying the activity of *acetylcholine* in peripheral blood, the author found a paradoxical reaction which was particularly marked in the therapy-resistant group. When acetylcholine activity normalized there was also normalization of the concentration and activity of cholinesterase.

Alpern (1948), and Teleschevskaya and Plotitcher (1949) also found a low level of cholinesterase activity and acetylcholine deficiency in blood of schizophrenics. The latter authors point out that inadequate neurohumoral compensation has an unfavorable effect on the prognosis, i.e. where the ratio of cholinesterase to acetylcholine is disturbed, and vice versa.

There was a rise of cholinesterase activity in the cerebrospinal fluid of schizophrenic patients (Birkhäuser 1941, Pope et al. 1952). The other endogenous amines will be discussed in Chapter VI. Figure 46 illustrates the variations of endogenous amines in brain and blood.

Coppen (1968) has reviewed endogenous and other amines in psychotic states, and he also gives the appropriate literature references on this subject.

Dysrhythmias in the EEG of deeper cerebral structures following administration of acetylcholine into the septum pellucidum and neighboring areas (Health and Guerrero-Figueroa 1965) has already been discussed. Gamma-aminobutyric acid (GABA) has also been studied. The authors conclude that both epilepsy and schizophrenia may show similar or identical symptoms, but pathogenetically they are different diseases. There is also the problem of the extent to which metabolic equilibrium can be achieved in a psychomotor epileptic by development of schizophrenic symptomatology. There is no definite evidence for this, but we believe that the possibility certainly exists.

Ammonia and Other Protein Products

As we pointed out in our discussion earlier, the *ammonia concentration in brain, blood and urine* may be elevated for various reasons (Krainski 1896, Pavlov and Nenski 1951, Protopopov 1946, Slutchevski 1944).

Various noxae are capable of producing a rise of ammonia in *nerve tissue* (Butt 1953, Pravditchneminski 1933, 1958, Tashiro 1922, Winterstein and Hirschberg 1925). Stimulating the nervous system by electroshock, hypoxia, and producing conditioned and non-conditioned reflexes also leads to an increase in the ammonia concentration in nerve tissue (Benitez et al. 1954, Budanova 1950, 1957, Richter and Dawson 1948, Torda 1953, Vladimirova 1938, 1954).

Examinations of blood serum of psychotic and epileptic patients were carried out by many authors (Borsunova 1952, Ferdman 1950, Klein 1957, Leschtchinski 1938, Markova 1944, Rasin 1955, Skuin 1956, Vrba 1956, 1957, Wolfsohn 1960). From their results, all these authors come to the conclusion that the ammonia concentration in blood is *elevated* in both schizophrenics and epileptics. The concentrations vary considerably, so that the mean value is often meaningless or not significant.

Wolfsohn (1960) studied non-protein nitrogen (non-protein N) in the blood of schizophrenic patients and demonstrated that in these patients the concentrations may alter in relation to the clinical picture and the course of clinical symptomatology. In patients who responded well to treatment he did not find any elevation of the levels of non-protein N in blood, whereas in patients who were resistant to therapy the concentration of this substance in blood, was elevated (Table XI). However, in the course of treatment the non-protein N in blood fell in both groups, and the reduction was statistically significant ($p < 0.05$) in the therapy-resistant group. The fall of non-protein N was not significant in the non-resistant group since the concentration had not been as high as in the therapy-resistant group before therapy.

The author carried out further studies of *total nitrogen* in serum and he also differentiated between urea nitrogen and amino acid nitrogen.

Urea nitrogen in serum was substantially elevated before treatment in schizophrenics (Table XVI) and in the course of treatment it fell by 35.2 percent of the initial value in the group which responded well to therapy ($p < 0.01$). In the group which did not respond well to treatment, the values showed considerable variation before treatment. After treatment there were fewer variations and deviations from the mean. However, the mean value remained the same.

The serum concentration of amino acid nitrogen (Table XI) varied before treatment in schizophrenics. In patients who responded well to treatment the concentration of amino acid nitrogen was 2 mg. percent lower than that of healthy subjects. On the other hand, there was a high concentration in patients who did not respond well to therapy ($p < 0.01$). In the course of treatment, the amino nitrogen concentration rose by 106 percent compared with the initial value in the first group ($p < 0.05$), whereas in the second group the amino nitrogen in blood serum was 28.2 percent lower ($p < 0.05$). Wolfsohn believes that this change in concentration of amino nitrogen can be used as an indication of the prognosis.

By examining the *aromatic compounds in blood,* Sorokina (1960) was able to demonstrate that there is a substantial rise of these substances in catatonic patients. This author also found that the processes of detoxification were impaired, and this was reflected by the urinary findings. The author does not consider that these results are very specific, although they could certainly have a part to play in catatonia. This was reported in the introduction to this section.

We have already discussed the results of Tolkatchevskaja and Wunder (1960). Their investigations revealed some measure of parallelity between epilepsy and schizophrenia, and we should like to mention this here. Lando and Krupenina (1962) compared nitrogen values from schizophrenics and epileptics and found certain similarities and also certain discrepancies in the results.

The *urinary* concentration of by-products of protein degradation in schizophrenics has been studied by many authors (Aschkenasy-Lelu 1952, Azima 1952, Kridzanovskaya 1954, Munkvad 1950, Shevko 1958, Skuin 1956, 1960).

Shevko (1960) carried out 725 examinations on 335 patients. 280 of these patients were schizophrenics and 35 of them had other symptoms:

TABLE XI. Concentration of ammonium fractions in the blood of schizophrenics who had been treated with or without success (mg%). (From Wolfson, N.M., 1960.)

Parameter	Therapy: Successful			Therapy: Resistent		
	Before	*During*	*Difference*	*Before*	*During*	*Difference*
Total nitrogen	23.3±2.3 (17—34)	21.1±2.2 (15—28)	—2.1 ±3.2	28.3±2.6 (17—48)	19.9±2.6 (14—28)	—8.4 ±3.7
Urea nitrogen	18.2±1.2 (14—22)	11.8±1.6 (11—18)	—6.4 ±2.6	16.1±2.8 (6—36)	15.2±2.1 (8—25)	—0.9 ±3.5
Amino acid nitrogen	4.7±1.6 (2—12)	9.6±1.5 (4—15)	+4.9 ±2.2	12.2±1.7 (4—20)	8.8±1.1 (1—10)	—3.4 ±2.0

alternating psychoses, asthenic depressive states, reactive psychoses, neuroses. Twenty practically healthy people were used for comparison. Of the schizophrenic patients, 147 had paranoid-hallucinatory symptoms, 42 catatonic symptoms, 51 symptoms of nervous excitement, 14 were hypochondriacs, 14 hebephrenics, six had schizophrenia simplex and six had schizophrenia with mental deficiency. The examinations comprised: volume of urine, specific gravity, total nitrogen, urea nitrogen, ammonia nitrogen, amino acid nitrogen (amino nitrogen) and oxidizing reactions. The results were as follows:

In catatonic patients total urinary nitrogen was depressed in 51 ± 5 percent of cases, and in paranoid patients it was depressed in 30 ± 8 percent of cases. Total nitrogen in the urine was more often depressed in acute catatonic patients than in chronic cases. This finding correlates with the results of Gjessing (1935, 1953), Protopopov (1956), Protopopov et al. (1939).

Normalization of urinary nitrogen varies in the different forms of schizophrenia. Normalization is more common and more complete during the recovery phase in patients with paranoid forms of schizophrenia than in catatonic patients. In the latter, total urinary nitrogen is depressed even after recovery or after therapeutic measures have been instituted, irrespective of whether or not these measures are successful. In the other forms of schizophrenia listed above, urinary nitrogen normalizes in the course of recovery or treatment.

In contrast to these results, in 50 percent of cases urinary amino nitrogen was elevated, and the ratio of amino acid nitrogen to total nitrogen was increased. After treatment there is normalization or a tendency to normalize.

Although we are not yet certain as to the role of ammonia and nitrogen in schizophrenia and epilepsy, it is certainly significant that these substances alter before, during and after the disease. It can be seen from our discusion that the findings in these two diseases have very many points in common.

If we go along with Krainski (1896), Slutchevski (1944), Selbach (1965), Selbach et al. (1965) and other authors, in describing an epileptic attack as a *protective mechanism,* then by this we imply that the metabolic processes normalize in the course of an attack and thereafter. The epileptic with psychomotor epilepsy without grand mal may perhaps *choose* a schizophrenic symptomatology because his psychomotor attacks will not correct his metabolic defects. It is the paranoid-hallucinatory form of schizophrenia (rather than the catatonic form) which resembles psychomotor epilepsy. This may explain why epileptics develop paranoid-hallucinatory symptoms more often than the catatonic psychotic form (see Chapter I).

Table XII shows the variations of serum and urinary nitrogen in patients with delirium tremens and chronic alcoholism. As can be seen from

TABLE XII. Concentration of nitrogen in serum and urine in patients with delirium tremens and chronic alcoholism. (From Cvetkova, N.B., 1960.)

Sequence of Investigations	*Group*	*Blood* Total nitrogen mg%	*Blood* Nitrogen of Urea mg%	*Diuresis in ml*	*Urine* Total nitrogen in mg%	*Roben's Quotient*
0	Control	30±1 (22–40)	27±2 (21–44)	1550-2000	11.5+0.2 (9.5–16.0)	83±2 (79–86)
I	Between 3 and 6 day of illness	37±5 (23–26)	26±3 (14–48)	1340	8.4±0.8 (3.5–13.0)	76±2 (66–84)
II	Between 7 and 15 day of illness	25±0.8 (21–26)	28±2 (15–41)	1650	8,8±1.7 (5.1–15.4)	87±2 (80–94)
III	Between 16 and 30 day of illness	27±1.5 (22–28)	25±3 (16–46)	1750	10.2±1.0 (5.5–13.0)	82±4 (70–98)
IV	Chronic state	25±1 (23–28)	25±3 (15–16)	1800	10.2±0.9 (6.0–16.0)	84±2 (77–98)

this table, there are both similarities and differences in the findings from these patients and in the results obtained in schizophrenias and epilepsies.

Other authors, including Cvetkova (1960), Ignatova (1960) and Troyanova (1960) have also examined this problem.

Examination of sulphur in serum (calculated as SO_4) produced some interesting results. The sulphur concentration in blood was depressed before treatment in both groups of patients (Table XIII.) The value for serum sulphur before treatment did not reach the lower normal limit of 3.0 to 5.5 mg. percent in any of the patients. The mean was 1.5 mg. percent lower than in healthy subjects.

In all patients who responded well to therapy, the serum level of sulphur was 81 percent higher after treatment ($p < 0.05$). In some patients the serum sulphur after treatment was rather higher than in healthy people. The reverse was true in patients who did not respond to therapy and the sulphur concentration fell a further 23 percent below the initial value. However, if these patients in the second group were given a different type of treatment which had a good effect, there was then a rise in the blood sulphur concentration after therapy.

The serum concentration of *organically bound sulphur ions* (organic compounds not contained in proteins) was 2 to 4 mg. percent in healthy test subjects. In schizophrenics who responded well to therapy, the serum level of organic sulphur was only 0.5 mg. percent. In cases with a poor prognosis it was higher, i.e. 1.08 mg. percent. The difference between these two values is statistically significant ($p < 0.05$).

TABLE XIII. Concentration of organic (non-protein) and inorganic sulphur in the blood of schizophrenics who had been treated with or without success (mg%). (From the author of Table XI.)

Parameter	*Therapy*					
	Successful			*Resistent*		
	Before	*During*	*Difference*	*Before*	*During*	*Difference*
Total	1.50±0.23	2.72±0.56	±1.22	1.81±0.29	1.39±0.20	—0.42
Sulphur	(0.1—2.8)	(0.3—6.3)	±0.61	(0.2—4.8)	(0.2—3.8)	±0.35
Organic	0.50±0.12	1.56±0.34	+1.06	1.08±0.17	0.49±0.12	—0.59
sulphur	(0.01—1.6)	(0.1—4.4)	±0.36	(0.1—2.9)	(0.1—2.6)	±0.21
Inorganic	0.63±0.11	1.08±0.24	+0.45	0.84±0.14	0.83±0.60	—0.01
sulphur	(0.1—1.6)	(0.2—3.3)	±0.26	(0.1—2.9)	(0.2—2.1	±0.61

In the course of effective therapy (first group), the serum concentration of organic sulphur rose to 1.56 mg. percent (i.e. a rise of 212%) (see Table XIII). This means that in some cases the sulphur concentration was higher than in healthy subjects ($p < 0.02$). In the group which was resistant to therapy, the blood sulphur concentration fell by 54.6 percent (from 1.08 mg.% to 0.49 mg.%) ($p < 0.05$). Once again, as with nitrogen, in the first group there was a rise and in the second a fall in the blood level of organic sulphur ($p < 0.02$).

Before treatment, the concentration of *inorganic sulphur in serum* (normally 1.5 to 2.0 mg.%) fell in both groups, although to a greater extent in the first group. In this group the serum level of inorganic sulphur rose by 71.4 percent of the initial value in the course of treatment. However, in the second group there was no change in the blood level sulphur during treatment, although in a few cases the level of inorganic sulphur fell.

The results described above illustrate that psychoses and epilepsies do not simply involve metabolic disorders as sequelae of the acute symptomatology. There are also many metabolic anomalies whereby catabolism may stop at certain stages. Whereas total urinary nitrogen and urea nitrogen in urine were depressed, amino acid nitrogen and polypeptide nitrogen were elevated. If the metabolic disorders were simply the result of excitation and other acute symptoms, then there would only have been a rise in the end products of metabolism: however, this was not the case.

Cerebral Lipids

In addition to the metabolic changes described above, there are also changes in lipids (lipoids) in mental patients (Lapteva 1956, Lehmann-Facius 1937, Livschitz and Roitrub 1957, Podorigora 1960, Poroschina et al. 1957). The best parameter to study in schizophrenics is blood *cholesterol.* Generally speaking, serum cholesterol was elevated in these patients. These changes were attributed to disturbances of liver function. It is interesting to note that total cholesterol in involutional psychoses and in schizophrenias in older people is higher than in acute schizophrenias. This makes it difficult to compare these findings with results from epileptics, and so we have not attempted to do this here.

Hormonal Changes

Hormonal changes are known to occur in schizophrenias, but it is difficult to compare the results with those from epileptics.

Enzymes and Vitamins

We have already mentioned the problems associated with enzymes (and vitamins) on several occasions, since it is impossible to avoid mentioning enzymes when discussing the metabolism of other biochemical groups. For this reason, here, we shall simply add a little to what has already been said (see also Kanig 1968, 1971 a, b, c, 1972).

In addition to other investigations which we shall mention later, Lando (1960) studied *hyaluronidase* in the serum of schizophrenics (Table XIV). He based his work on studies by Duran-Reynals (1928, 1929), Chein and Duthie (1939, 1940), Bitchkov (1948), Koschtojanc (1948, 1951), Mogilnicki (1949), Smirnova (1951, 1957), Salesski (1955), Stepanjan and Pertchikova (1956), Stepanjan et al. (1957) and other authors, who have reported on the action of hyaluronidase.

Hyaluronic acid occurs throughout the body and it is an important factor in determining the consistency and permeability of cells. It is broken down by hyaluronidase, and hence, hyaluronidase is also important in the genesis and pathogenesis of psychoses (Lando 1960).

TABLE XIV. Serum hyaluronidase activity in healthy people and patients (schizophrenics). (From Lando, L.I., 1960.)

Diagnosis		*Number of People*	*International Units*						
			0	*2*	*2.5*	*3.3*	*5*	*M±S*	*%*
Healthy people		10	2	4	4	—	—	1.8±0.3	19
Schizophrenia (forms)	paranoid	46	9	8	17	10	2	2.2±0.18	26
	catatonic	30	7	11	9	3	—	1.8±0.2	10
	hallucinatory paranoid	18	4	4	7	2	1	2.0±0.34	16
	Asthenic-hypochondric	11	1	2	6	2	—	2.3±0.25	18
	depressed-paranoid	6	1	2	3	—	—	1.9±0.4	—
	Other forms	5	0	1	2	1	—	2.0±0.5	—
Total		116	20	27	47	19	3	2.1±0.1	19

We should also mention that the properties of hyaluronic acid may change. This applies particularly to its viscosity, which is affected by the specific action of hyaluronidase and also by a non-specific effect of ascorbic acid and some phosphate compounds (Geiman 1951, Matusis and Matusis 1951, Schechonin 1949).

There have recently been reports on the relationships between nerve excitation, nerve conduction and permeability of cellular and intracellular spaces (Koschtojanc 1948, 1951, Lando 1960, Seiler 1966). These authors found that chemical agents involved in the processes of nervous excitation also activate hyaluronidase. Studies on the effects of sympathicotonia and parasympathicotonia on the activity of hyaluronidase revealed that administration of Adrenaline to the rabbit increases hyaluronidase activity and hence it also increases cell permeability. On the other hand, acetylcholine inhibits hyaluronidase activity and reduces membrane permeability (Vrubel 1956). Anaesthesia or local anaesthesia reduces hyaluronidase activity (Belov 1956). Hyaluronidase is activated by light and inhibited by darkness (Gorodinskaja and Hvatova 1951). According to these authors, light may result in fairly pronounced activation of hyaluronidase in epileptics, and this may be associated with an attack.

Lando (1960) examined samples of serum from 116 schizophrenics and most of these patients were also examined in the course of therapy. The patients were between 18 and 56 years old. About 87 percent of the patients were between 20 and 40 years of age and only two were over 50 years old. The patients had various symptomatologies: 46 paranoid, 30 catatonic, 18 hallucinatory, 11 asthenic-hypochondriac, six depressive-paranoid and five had other symptoms. 22 patients were experiencing their first attack, which was acute; the others were relapses, although they were mostly in an acute stage. No medication was given before the investigation. The results are summarized in Table XIV).

In the majority of cases there was only a slight rise of hyaluronidase activity, and so the mean value is not significant. There was a sharper rise of hyaluronidase activity in only 19 percent of cases.

In patients with the paranoid forms of schizophrenia, hyaluronidase activity was increased by 26 percent of the initial value. The increase was only 10 percent of the initial value in catatonic patients, 16 percent in hallucinatory cases and 18 percent in asthenic-hypochondriac forms. As Table XIV shows, the deviation from the mean vary in patients with different forms of the disease.

Hyaluronidase activity deviated further from the mean in patients undergoing a relapse than in patients experiencing their first attack. After treatment, hyaluronidase activity normalized in the majority of cases, particularly where reserpine and chlorpromazine were given.

Arnold and Hofmann (1968) lay particular emphasis on enzymopathies, not only in the actual schizophrenic patient but also in other members of his family.

Here again, there are certain parallels between *enzymopathies* in schizophrenia and epilepsy. It is not possible to assert that schizophrenia and epilepsy are pathogenetically one disease. In this sense they are probably two fundamentally different diseases. However, by *adopting* one or other set of symptoms these patients are able to correct their metabolic disorders, and we regard this as a form of biological regulation which is bound to occur in emergencies, when normalization cannot be achieved in any other way.

Sundry Points

We cannot claim to have dealt with all the problems in our discussion; there is much which we have had to omit. For example, we have not mentioned Hartnup's syndrome (Christian 1968 b), maple syrup disease (Cochrane 1960, Dancis et al. 1960, 1963, Grumbach and Kaplan 1960, McKenzie and Woolf 1959, Menkes et al. 1954, Seiler 1966), several forms of cerebral lipoidosis (Crocker and Mays 1961, Klenk 1934, 1939, 1955, Svennerholm 1962, Svennerholm and Raal 1961), Gierke's disease and other syndromes (Cori and Cori 1952), since they are not really of great importance in the problem under discussion.

CHAPTER VI

EPILEPTOGENIC CHEMICAL SUBSTANCE

SUBSTANCES WHICH HAVE A FACULTATIVE EPILEPTOGENIC ACTION

By *substances which have a facultative epileptogenic action* we mean those chemical compounds which are capable of eliciting an epileptic response or producing an epileptic attack, but only under certain conditions.

The epileptogenic action depends on the dose, previous treatment, any additional medication, the patient's condition, basic disease and many other factors. Under different conditions or when they are used as adjuncts, many of the drugs referred to may actually have an anti-epileptic effect and, in view of this, the substances described cannot simply be lumped together as *convulsants,* and the discussion will make it clear how we arrived at this definition.

To keep within the scope of this monograph, we shall confine ourselves to mentioning the drugs which we think most important.

There are a series of chemical substances which may have a negative effect on the EEG and precipitate specific or suspected convulsion-inducing cerebral activity. Apart from the familiar substance *pentylenetetrazol (Cardiazol®)* and *pyribenzamine* (King and Weeks 1965), there are many other substances which, although they are not used as direct provocative agents, may precipitate an abnormal to pathological epileptic specific cerebral activity (Figure 32). Among other agents there are many psychotropic drugs, which are often indispensible as therapeutic agents, which can induce convulsion-specific elements in the EEG. Among others, the following authors have dealt with this problem: Bente and Itil (1954), Fünfgeld (1956, 1968), Shea (1956), Liberson et al. (1958), Faure et al. (1960), Helmchen and Künkel (1960 to 1967), Jovanovic and Tan-Eli (1970), Kiessling (1964), Monnier and Krupp (1959), Pintilie et al. (1970). While using drugs the following may gradually become apparent: a.) the occurrence of convulsion-specific elements in the EEG without clinical manifestation (Helmchen and Künkel 1960-1967); b.) an increase in the frequency of attacks in epileptics in nearly 50 percent of cases (Ceccarelli and Coen-Giordana 1960); c.) a dangerous accumulation of attacks in over 50 percent of cases (Faure et al. 1960) or d.) there may even be status epilepticus (Bauer 1954, Maucerie and Strauss 1956). Isolated EEG changes of

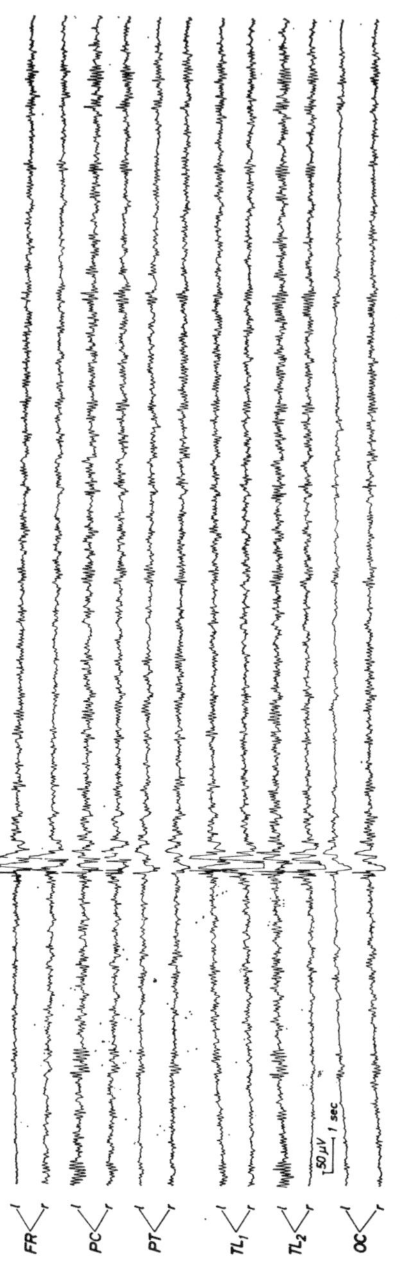

Figure 32. Generalized, short bursts of convulsion potentials in the EEG in the form of spikes, and spikes and waves, in a 14-year-old girl following chlordiazepoxide overdosage (she had taken 30 to 40 tablets with the intention of committing suicide. The exact dose was not known) (our own findings, original).

various grades are relatively common (Haspert 1962, Helmchen and Künkel 1960 to 1967, Jovanovic and Tan-Eli 1968, Klapetek 1963, 1964, Schmalbach 1968).

Analysis of the electroencephalograms revealed the following possibilities:

1.) The cerebral activity only shows *slight activation of the basic alpha wave rhythm,* a suggestion of synchronization of the waves and an insignificant change in the wave frequency. The basic rhythm becomes rather unstable but continues to fluctuate within the normal range of variation (Jovanovic and Sattes 1967, 1970, Jovanovic and Tan-Eli 1970).

2.) In addition to α-waves, *acceleration of between 14 and 30 oscillations per second* (β-waves) appear in the basic rhythm. The accelerated cerebral activity first appears precentrally and frontally, but later it also becomes parietal and occipital, according to the severity of the changes. β-waves are relatively high (40 to 70 microvolts). This form appears under barbiturates (Pieri and Hürlimann 1965), imipramine (Jovanovic and Tan-Eli 1970) or other psychotropic drugs.

3.) *A moderate general change* may be seen as a further stage in the EEG changes under the action of chemical preparations used therapeutically. There is diffuse slowing of the whole basic rhythm as far as the theta wave band, but there are no other characteristic events (Jovanovic and Tan-Eli 1970).

4.) *A moderately severe to severe general change* which may occur is slowing up as far as the δ-wave band with a mixture of slower and faster waves (Helmchen and Künkel 1964 a, b; Boerner, Jovanovic and Henschler 1970). Helmchen and Künkel (1964 b) found that there were general changes in 40 percent of the cases, with a range of variation between 31 and 61 percent, after using psychotropic drugs in psychiatric patients (mainly phenothiazine but also imipramine).

5.) *Basal dysrhythmia* is one of the next changes to occur in the EEG after the action of psychotropic drugs. According to the authors cited above this occurs in 76 percent of the cases, with a range of variation of 55 to 91 percent. In another publication (1964 a), they also found that there was basal dysrhythmia in a very high percentage (96% of female patients). Basal dysrhythmia shows a tendency to localize and this can be regarded as a more severe form of electroencephalographic change after administration of chemical substances.

6.) *Paroxysmal dysrhythmia* is manifest in the form of abrupt, large sharp and slow events which are composed of waves of 1 to 3/sec. These waves project considerably above all other parts of the basic rhythm (Helmchen and Künkel 1961 a, b, 1964a, b, c). In many EEG curves there may also be a tendency to focalize.

7.) *Focal changes* are a further gradual change which occurs after administration of phenothiazines. This usually involves a basal focus. According to many authors, the foci are significantly more frequent in the *left temporal region*. In 1063 EEG tracings, Helmchen and Künkel (1967) found that the foci are not predominate over left temporal region in young people. With increasing age there was an increasing tendency for the foci to dominate the left hemisphere completely. In their publication these authors give an extensive bibliography and a detailed interpretation of this problem. Focal changes may occur as a θ-focus, δ-focus or as focal dysrhythmia. dysrhythmia.

8.) *Suspected convulsion elements in the EEG* with and without general changes, and with and without focal dysrhythmia, are also quite common when using chemical substances (Bente and Itil 1954, Fünfgeld 1968, Helmchen and Künkel 1960 to 1967, Itil 1961, Jovanovic and Tan-Eli 1970).

9.) *A convulsion focus* is also quite often precipitated by using medicaments or other chemical agents, and this may degenerate into a clinical attack (Schmalbach 1968, Fünfgeld 1968). There is a focal phenomenon of slow waves up to the delta band (1 to 3/sec.) and among these sharp and spike events.

10.) It is not uncommon for there to be a generalized sequence of *spikes or spike and wave formations* which do not differ in any respect from the convulsion discharges seen in epileptics. There may also be spikes and waves formations or even *polyspikes and waves elements with diffuse slowing or dysrhythmia*. This is the most severe form of the EEG change and it is often associated with manifestations of clinical epileptic attacks (Fünfgeld 1968, King and Weeks 1965).

As a short supplement to this, we would like to refer to the publications of a few authors. Helmchen and Künkel (1961a) treated 21 female patients with perazine *(Taxilan®)*, in general for 16 (8 to 24) weeks. The average maximum daily dose, which was given for at least one week, was 590 (400 to 1300) mg. Six patients later received additional treatment with imipramine *(Tofranil®)* in doses of 50 to 250 mg. Twenty patients were suffering from schizophrenic or involutional psychoses; one was debilitated. Before treatment, none of the patients showed organic cerebral lesions. After the therapy, only four of 21 patients showed an unchanged EEG. The pneumonencephalographic findings were also given.

In a second publication (1961 b), in 40 female patients with abnormal initial EEG, after treatment with perazine the authors found a change in 24 cases; these changes mainly took the form of paroxysmal dysrhythmia. Focal findings were discussed previously (1961 a).

In a third publication, Helmchen and Künkel (1964 a, b) observed some changes in the EEG after pharmacological therapy in 78 of 96 patients. These changes took the form of basal or paroxysmal dysrhythmia, focal findings or general changes. The next publication is concerned with correlating the findings with the other results (Helmchen and Künkel 1964 c).

In a 54-year-old female patient with severe dementia and cortical atrophy, Fünfgeld (1968) found moderate slowing in the EEG before treatment. The patient was given therapy with promethazine and methylprylon. After anthelminthic treatment with piperazine over a period of one and one-half days with a total dose of 4 g. active substance, there were convulsive attacks with an emphasis on the left side. The EEG revealed convulsion potentials with an emphasis on the right side. After discontinuing the piperazine, the convulsions gradually receded in the course of two days and within two weeks the EEG had reverted to the original picture. The author assumes that additional medication with promethazine may have exerted a synergistic effect and promoted cerebral decompensation. Thus, it is not only children, whose cerebral metabolism is very unstable, who must be excluded from an anthelminthic course of piperazine but, where there are corresponding initial conditions, adults must also be excluded. The author warns against the dangers of combining psychotropic drugs with piperazine.

The illustration of the changes in cerebral activity under the action of drugs must inevitably draw attention to a wide-spread problem. Since (as we shall show later) the chemical substances used *act mainly on the brain stem and in particular on the limbic system,* it is clear that we must focus our attention on the biochemical problems of psychomotor epilepsy.

THE IMIPRAMINE GROUP is an example of drugs, which may have an epileptogenic action under certain circumstances. Since many other conditions have to be fulfilled before they will exert this action, we cannot discuss these drugs in order of activity. Thus for example, although we are beginning with the imipramines, this does not mean that psychotropic drugs from this group have a more powerful epileptogenic activity than the drugs discussed in the next or in the following groups.

During antidepressant treatment with imipramine *(Tofranil,* for formula see Chapter VII) convulsion discharges have been observed in the EEG (Delay et al. 1960, Zappoli 1959). The threshold dose for the attacks is fairly high, being 300 to 400 mg daily (Collier and Martin 1960, v. Ditfurth 1960, Gesenway and Cohen 1960, Hippius and Jantz 1959, Mets 1960, Zappoli 1959). Following an attempted suicide by taking 150 tablets of *Tofranil* the patient finally died with convulsions (Michon et al. 1959). Singh (1960) reported on a woman who had been treated with 15 mg. daily phenelzine *(Nordil®)*; this patient died with sustained convulsions 20 minutes after an intramuscular injection of *Tofranil.* Even patients who were treated with imipramine and survived, suffered from more or less prolonged convulsions (Zappoli 1959).

On the other hand, Jovanovic (1972 a, e), Jovanovic and Sattes (1967, 1970) did not observe any convulsion-specific elements in the EEG when using *chlorimipramine* (3-Chloro-5- (3-dimethylaminopropyl)-10, 11-dihydro-5H-dibenz-hydrochloride, monochlorimipramine, Anafranil®). Continuous EE Gchecks were carried out in 30 of 70 patients and, apart from a slight but not abnormal reduction of frequency and increase in the number of α-waves (signs of emotional tension) and a slight tendency for the waves to synchronize, there were no other abnormalities to suggest the existence of convulsion elements. Thus, chlorination of imipramine seems to reduce its convulsant action, either relatively or absolutely. Indeed, these authors reported that chlorimipramine had a more powerful therapeutic effect and there were no side effects under the therapeutic dose. However, this substance is still relatively new and so it must be studied further.

Monoamino-oxidase inhibitors (MAOI) have recently become the center of scientific interest. There is still controversy on the question of whether MAOI precipitate epileptic attacks or whether they only provoke convulsion specific elements in the EEG. However we have come across a considerable number of published reports of epileptic attacks following administration of MAOI.

At one symposium (Hippius and Jantz 1959) in which 35 specialists in neurology, psychiatry, biochemistry and pharmacology took part, a warning was given on the dangers of using some preparations from the group of MAOI (iproniazid). *Iproniazid* has not achieved as prominent a position as was once expected. After initially good therapeutic results it was found that subsequent use gave rise to many side-effects, including generalized epileptic attacks. The level of catecholamines in the CNS increases, although there is no increase in the sensitivity of the central synapses. If, for therapeutic reasons, iproniazid is given at the same time as imipramine, complications (including seizures) develop much earlier. These authors point out that since imipramine increases the sensitivity of the central synapses (although it does not increase the catecholamine concentration), when combined with iproniazid this may result both in sensitization of the central synapses and an increase in the concentration of catecholamines, thus doubling the danger of convulsions (Körber 1960, Sigg 1959).

Inhibition of *monoamine-oxidase* by MAOI and an increase in the level of endogenous amines may also evoke attacks in other situations. For example, if *reserpine* is given with MAOI preparations this again (as with concomitant use of imipramine) increases the danger to the patient. Reserpine releases these amines from the *stores* where they are normally protected from the action of MAO, and the MAO can then get at them and break them down. If MAO is inhibited by an MAO inhibitor, the concentration of endogenous amines increases and this may lead to a convulsive attack if there is no other defense mechanism available.

In animal experiments, Szimuzu et al. (1964) observed psychomotor excitation states which they interpreted as being due to the increase in the level of amines in the brain following administration of MAOI. These authors consider that serotonin and catechimines are particularly important here. Administration of MAOI (pheniprazine, beta-phenylisopropyl-hydrazine hydrochloride) resulted in a continuous series of slower waves in the electrocorticogram. More rapid, uninterrupted 3 to 5/sec. events occurred over the hippocampus. The authors observed that these changes persisted for several hours without interruption. An arousal effect was also observed during studies on the *cerveau isolé,* but in this case they did not report any increase in predisposition to convulsion. The psychomotor phenomenon and also the EEG changes are seen as a result of the rise of serotonin and, in particular, of catechimine and beta-phenylethylamine.

Detailed surveys of the effects of psychotropic drugs on bioelectric cerebral activity and other neurophysiological and clinical phenomena can be found in Hubach (1963), Müller and Müller (1963), Wandrey and Leutner (1965), Petrilowitsch (1966), Pöldinger 1967), Helmchen (1968). Pöldinger (1967) discusses the problem of incompatibility when using psychotropic drugs. MAOI and thymoleptic agents are extremely incompatible and the author recommends that, after giving MAOI an interval of at least one to two weeks should be allowed to elapse before transferring to a thymoleptic agent. If given in the reverse order, the incompatibility is less marked, but should not be underestimated.

Neuroleptic agents appear to have a more pronounced convulsant action than antidepressants. The following authors in particular have dealt with the problem of activating convulsion-specific elements in the EEG and convulsive attacks in epileptics and in non-epileptics: Friedländer (1959), Frain (1960), Hofmann and Kryspin-Exner (1960), Itil (1961), Lenz (1961), Pauig et al. (1961), Oettinger (1962), Cares (1963), Hubach (1963), Wandrey and Leutner (1965), Haase (1966), Petrilowitsch (1966), and Pöldinger (1967). The last five authors have produced very good reviews.

There are reports of cases where there were no changes whatsoever after receiving neuroleptic agents (chlorpromazine). However, there are only isolated examples (Friedländer 1959). The majority of authors agree that nearly all neuroleptic agents increase the cerebral predisposition to convulsion (in non-epileptic patients) or may have an unfavourable effect in epileptics who experience occasional psychotic episodes.

For example, the action of convulsant drugs is potentiated by chlorpromazine. Sometimes the increased predisposition to convulsion can only be verified with an EEG. Within a few days after oral administration of chlorpromazine in normal doses, convulsion-specific elements or suspected convulsion elements appear in the EEG (Fabisch 1957, Hubach 1963, Jörgensen and Wulff 1958, Turner et al. 1955). As the course of treatment continues there is a definite increase in the number and form of the convulsion elements in the EEG (Bayreuther and Radtke 1958). Intravenous administration of chlorpromazine to both epileptics and non-epileptics quite often elicits convulsion elements in the EEG within a few minutes, and occasionally there are clinical seizures (Fabisch 1957, Shea 1956).

Megaphen (chlorpromazine) is now commonly used as a provocative agent (Christian 1968b, Fünfgeld 1956, Martin et al. 1958, Menšikova et al. 1959, Simons 1959, Stewart 1957). Many other authors have also observed attacks during long-term treatment with phenothiazines (Anton-Stephens 1954, Conrad et al 1956, Fabisch 1957, Jörgensen and Wulff 1958, Lehmann and Hanrahan 1954, Lyberi and Last 1956, Moran and Butler 1956, Năhunek et al. 1959.

Montedoro and Buttighone (1959) were able to demonstrate that the epileptic phenomena are directly related to dose. They found a predominance of nocturnal epileptic attacks in schizophrenic patients when the daily dose of chlorpromazine reached 1200 to 1500 mg. This is a very important point in respect of the problem in hand. In Chapter I we discussed the connection between psychomotor and nocturnal epilepsy. We may again be seeing evidence of this close connection here, and this will be a great help when we come to explaining the mechanism responsible for an attack (Chapter VIII).

Yeager (cited in Hubach 1963) also observed clinical convulsions and convulsion elements in the EEG in 30 patients when the daily dose of chlorpromazine was increased to 1500 mg. The attacks disappeared when he reduced the dose and they reappeared when he prescribed a dose of 1500 mg. several times a day.

According to Sousland and Sigstad (1957), 2 percent of cases become predisposed to attack under clinical treatment with chlorpromazine; this figure is 1.3 percent according to Lomas et al. (1955). Goldman (1956) reports a higher incidence of convulsions (4.2%) in 1250 patients treated with chlorpromazine. If epileptics are given phenothiazines in addition to anticonvulsant therapy, they become more predisposed to develop attacks, (Ceccareli and Coen-Giordana 1961). Grünthal and Walther-Büel (1960) reported a fatality during generalized convulsions following 20 mg. chlorpromazine, within three days of beginning treatment.

Leukotomized patients appear to exhibit particularly poor tolerance to phenothiazines and they are more susceptible than patients who have not been treated surgically. Liddel and Retterslöh (1957) observed convulsions in seven of 21 leukotomized patients under chlorpromazine.

Chlorpromazine preparations taken in attempted suicides also elicit attacks and complications. Jörgensen and Wulff (1958) have reported on a schizophrenic who took 5 g. chlorpromazine in order to commit suicide. This patient suffered a major attack and exhibited convulsion potentials in the EEG; however, he survived. Mauceri and Strauss (1956) observed convulsion potentials in the EEG of a patient who poisoned himself with chlorpromazine in an attempt to commit suicide; the convulsion potentials receded after 12 days.

Other phenothiazine preparations, apart from chlorpromazine (megaphen) are also known to provoke convulsions. Bente and Itil (1960) found convulsion elements in the EEG and clinical epileptic manifestations when using chlorperphenazine (Decetan®), Helmchen and Künkel (1960) found them after using perazine (Taxilan®), Jessel (1961) after prothipendyl (Dominal®) from the series of azaphenothiazine derivatives, Oles (1960) on administration of butyrophenone derivatives (Haloperidol®), and Itil (1961) and Cares (1963) after therapy with thioridazine. The electroencephalographic and clinical symptoms described in these reports differ from one another both quantitatively and qualitatively. However, by and large the overall picture is the same.

The clinical symptoms observed following administration of psychotropic drugs stimulated a wave of experimental work on animals.

Convulsion elements were found in electroencephalograms from experimental animals after administering *Megaphen.*® The form and localization of these convulsion elements resembled spikes and waves in man. These convulsion events were detected in rabbits (Hippius et al. 1955), cats (Ingvar 1957, Steinmann 1954), dogs (Ingvar 1957) and monkeys (Das et al. 1954, Ingvar 1957). Convulsions as well as electroencephalographic symptoms appeared in some animals under megaphen medication.

In order to illustrate just how the predisposition to convulsion changes in relation to the experimental conditions and dose, we shall discuss one or two animal experiments with phenothiazines in greater detail.

In the 1950's and subsequently, experiments were carried out with *aminazin* (chlorpromazine). Cao Sajo-Din (1958) studied the effect of aminazin on the course of an epileptic attack in rats and guinea pigs. In the rat, administration of aminazin in doses of 5, 8 and 10 mg/kg. produced a change in the attack one and one-half to two hours after administration. Aminazin suppressed the clonic phase and the phases following this, but in intensified the tonic phase. Similar changes were also found in the guinea pig three to four hours after administration (10 mg/kg.).

Pogodaev (1964) used different doses of aminazin (3, 4, 5 and 10 mg/kg.) in the rat to study the course of an attack. Within 20 minutes epileptic attacks were induced using an electric current. The experiments were also carried out on control animals under similar conditions.

In general, compared with the corresponding features in control animals the intensity and duration of the phases of the epileptic attack were reduced after each of the doses of aminazin used. The exceptions here were tonic phase and coma phase which are *prolonged* by aminazin (Figure 33). The form of the initial phase (onset of the attack) depends to a large extent on the current strength used and the length of time it is applied. The author attempts to explain the prolongation of the tonic and coma phases by arguing that aminazin reduces the convulsion threshold. Since the same current was used in both groups (test and control group) the current strength in the test animals after the convulsion threshold had been reduced, must have been supraliminal. On the other hand, the current strength in the control animals was at the threshold. A supraliminal current strength has the effect of altering the attack. According to the author, apart from reducing the convulsion threshold, the pharmacological effect of aminazin is also due to the effect on the tonic phase itself. The tonic phase (which is longer than that in control animals) is induced by the clonisms. These clonisms differ from the clonic phase in control animals in that they are shorter and less intense, they do not involve all the muscles at the same time, and they are not fully coordinated. The animals seem to want to escape. The clonic phase is plastic, slower and not so dramatic as in the control animals; it develops much more slowly involving first one and then another group of muscles. This also makes it difficult to assess how long it takes.

Aminazin affects the locomotor phase. Twitching in individual groups of muscles in the hind limbs is more irregular than in control animals.

The postparoxysmal phase (coma) is much longer and deeper than in control animals. The duration and depth of the coma becomes more profound as the dose of aminazin is increased (Figure 33). The animals do not respond to stimuli, and there is a change in the phase of rigidity. This is viscous and can be distinguished from other phases much more easily than in conrtol animals.

It was also possible to see the pharmacological effect of aminazin where there were repeated attacks. After more than two attacks have been in-

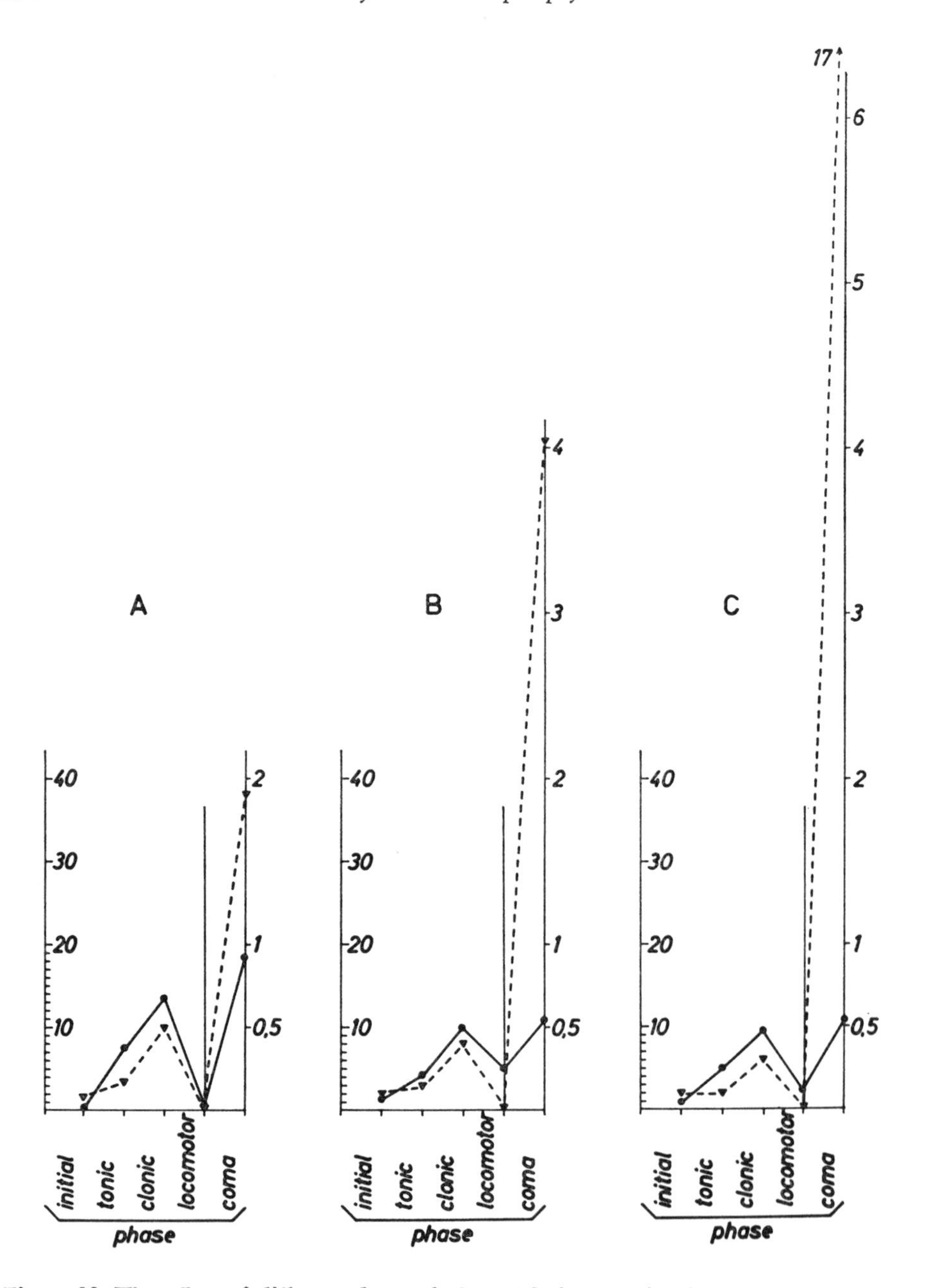

Figure 33. The effect of different doses of phenothiazines (aminazin) on the course and duration of epileptic attacks triggered electrically, in rats. 1 = ●——● control animals; 2 = ▶----◀ test animals. A = aminazin in a dose of 3 mg/kg; B = aminazin in a dose of 4 mg/kg; C = aminazin in a dose of 10 mg/kg. (From Pogodaev, K.I., 1964.)

duced, there is no clonic phase. The initial phase passes rapidly into the tonic phase and the animals assume an *intrauterine* position (embryonic position) with the flexor muscles more stimulated than the extensors, and the locomotor phase and phase of rigidity last longer. The author concludes from the results that aminazin increases an animal's resistance to repeated attacks. Following subcutaneous (s.c.) administration of 3 to 10 mg/kg. aminazin to rats, he observed that the treated rats showed double the resistance to repeated attacks compared with control animals.

Whereas the test animals died after 50 attacks, control animals died after 25 convulsive episodes. The author interprets this as being the result of desynchronization of the attack following aminazin. The brain discharges rapidly in the control animals but later in the test animals since failure of the different phases of the attack to coordinate means that first one and then the other cerebral formation is affected and the brain does not all become exhausted at once, as it does in the control animals.

Pogodaev (1964) also used different doses of the preparation and various provocative agents to study the effect of aminazin on the *convulsion threshold.*

With an *electric current,* a dose of 0.5 mg/kg. s.c. aminazin increases the cerebral predisposition to convulsion and, logically, this means that the convulsion threshold is reduced. The predisposition to convulsions was increased in 70 percent of the experiments. Increasing the dose one hundredfold (50 mg/kg.) also reduced the threshold. A further increase in the dose of aminazin up to the lethal dose (i.e. up to 80 to 90 mg/kg.) again increased the predisposition to paroxysms. For example, whereas convulsions only occurred in 40 percent of experiments under a dose of 50 mg/kg., attacks were induced in 84 to 100 percent of cases after increasing the dose to 80 to 90 mg/kg.

Without aminazin, *Cardiazol* elicited attacks in 72 percent of cases. Following additional administration of 0.5 mg/kg. aminazin, attacks occurred in 100 percent of cases. Predisposition to convulsion is reduced when higher doses of aminazin are used: with 1 mg/kg. attacks occur in 90 percent of the animals, with 2 mg/kg. in 83 percent, with 3 mg/kg. in 80 percent, with 5 mg/kg. in 78 percent and with 10 mg/kg. in 68 percent of cases. Thus, there are fewer attacks following administration of 10 mg/kg. aminazin than when no aminazin is given. With even higher dosages of aminazin the convulsion threshold to *Cardiazol* continues to increase: with 30 mg/kg. attacks were recorded in 60 percent, under 50 mg/kg. in 43 percent, under 55 mg/kg. in 60 percent and under 70 mg/kg. only in 40 percent of the experiments. On the other hand, with a lethal dose of 80 to 90 mg/kg. attacks occur in 80 to 90 percent of the experiments as against 72 percent in control animals. Thus, depending on the dose, aminazin can increase or reduce the convulsion threshold or increase or reduce the cerebral predisposition to convulsion. From this example we can see how chemical substances can have a facultative epileptogenic action, *i.e. they have a convulsant effect on one occasion and an anticonvulsant effect on another.*

In contrast to these effects which have been reported with chlorpromazine and the other phenothiazine preparations mentioned, Kiessling (1964) did not observe any increase in the incidence of attacks when using fluphenazine *(Lyogen®)* in 50 epileptic patients who were kept under observation, some of whom were chronic cases. In 36 of 50 patients for whom EEG checks had been carried out over several years, the author failed to find any changes under treatment with fluphenazine. Kiessling discusses the reports of other authors who have warned against using psychotropic drugs in epileptics, and he concludes that there were no EEG changes in his patients, even in those who were monitored over a fairly long period, when the EEG recordings were compared with those taken before treatment. In order to be certain, he administered the preparation intravenously to 20 patients: 16 epileptics were given 5 mg., one patient 8 mg. and three others 2 to 3 mg. over a period of one and one-half to two minutes. Some of the patients developed other neurological symptoms (extrapyramidal symptoms, visual spasm, spasmodic torticollis, oral movements), but there were no epileptic attacks or changes in the EEG. The author points out that there was no *dangerous* build-up of attacks, although in our opinion this does not necessarily mean that fluphenazine is less *dangerous* as a provoker of attacks. Kiessling also did not observe any build up of attacks when using phenothiazines, although this has been reported by many authors (including some of those referred to above) (see also Ebert and Hess 1965).

Rauwolfia alkaloids also increase the cerebral predisposition to convulsion (Lemere 1956). This fact has already been mentioned above. Barsa and Kline (1955) report generalized attacks in 1.5 percent of psychotic patients under *reserpine* therapy. In epileptics who were given reserpine in addition to anticonvulsant therapy there was an increase in the number of attacks, in particular of minor attacks (65% increase) but of major attacks as well (33% increase) (Zimmermann and Burgemeister 1955). Dazzi and Lagaresi (1956) have reported seeing several patients who developed a petit mal status following *Serpasil®*. Convulsion potentials in the EEG lasting for hours have often been recorded following injection of reserpine (Lien 1960). According to Sterc (1959), the predisposition to convulsion may last for a considerable time after the medication is discontinued. Hospitals have reported fatalities and complications where concomitant neuroleptic and electroshock treatment has been employed (Hubach 1963). According to Leusen (1960), in animals *reserpine* lowers the convulsion threshold for caffeine, pentylenetetrazole, picrotoxin and nicotine and reduces the anticonvulsant action of diphenylhydantoin, mephenesin (see also Chen et al. 1954, Kronenberg 1958, Prokop et al. 1959). In the mouse, 0.19 ml. 0.5 percent Cardiazol solution following reserpine teatment is enough to elicit extension spasms compared with a dose of 0.35 ml. without pretreatment with reserpine (Kobinger 1958). Monnier and Krupp (1959), Monnier (1969) and others observed spontaneous spasms particularly in the hippocampus, under treatment with reserpine.

As the convulsion threshold is lowered by psychotropic drugs, there is a fourfold rise in the mortality rate among rats following shock treatment. This was found in animal experiments by Wortz et al. (1957).

EPILEPTOGENIC SUBSTANCES IN THE NARROWER SENSE

There is no sharply defined borderline between these chemical compounds and the drugs discussed above. Very often it is not possible to tell where the action of *facultative epileptogenic substances* ends and the action of *epileptogenic substances in the narrower sense* begins. The mechanisms of action of epileptogenic noxae vary considerably (see Chapters VIII and IX). We have already mentioned a whole range of these substances in the course of this monograph (see Chapters IV and V). We should add that *many epileptogenic chemical agents are used in hospitals as provocative agents or in animal experiments to induce convulsions.*

In addition to the conventional provocative agents referred to in Chapters IV and V we should mention here a paper which we have not discussed before.

Christian and Hallen (1957) used Aneuxol®, Pyramidon® *(aminophenazone)* to induce attacks and their results are quite interesting. They noticed that patients treated with a Pyramidon preparation exhibited particular clinical symptoms and experienced unpleasant subjective sensations. These authors repeatedly observed the symptoms when treating patients with rheumatic diseases; these symptoms were distinguishable from many side-effects of other preparations.

To examine these effects in more detail, Christian and Hallen observed 15 non-epileptics under slow intravenous i.v. injection of Aneuxol (1 cm^3 per minute) in a dose of 3 to 5 $cm.^3$ The test subjects described the effect of the preparation as an indefinite *funny* or *rather peculiar* feeling; others were vaguely able to localize these sensations and pointed to their stomach or, more rarely, to their head: they said they had a strange feeling in the head; something was coming up from the stomach, *rather like nausea;* something felt *different* in the head *like being in a mist, like being dazed.* If the injection was continued, the sensations changed or became more distinct, and there were other symptoms. "The vague feeling coming up from the stomach turned into a wave of coldness or warmth, rather like retching or a feeling of constriction in the chest; there was sometimes a soft noise in the head; tongue and oral mucosa could feel sticky or furry". These authors also made a note of comments on the odor or taste. Odor and taste could not be defined exactly and sometimes the patients could not distinguish between them. The patients also described sensations which indicated a change in their perception of the surroundings: to many of them the people and objects around them seemed different in an indescribable way; others saw everything at a distance "like looking through the wrong end of a telescope"; one patient saw everything as distorted and sloping and to another patient familiar objects and people seemed strange. The patients spontaneously stressed the particular and strange quality of their perceptions or sensations by exclaiming how *weird, peculiar* or *funny* they were, and they could only approximately compare them to everyday experiences. The sensations were often described as *unpleasant* and the authors think that this was the result of an indefinite feeling of anxiety which often accompanied the whole condition.

These sensations were accompanied by physical changes: increased sweating and salivation, dilatation of the pupils, increased pulse and breathing rate and elevated blood pressure. All the symptoms receded after at the most two minutes. The authors compare the patients statements with the aura which is often observed in epileptics. Had the symptoms been more intense they would have been the same as or similar to the symptoms of psychomotor epilepsy or of oral petit mal (see Chapter I).

These manifestations were interpreted by the investigators as being the result of the specific action of a slow intravenous injection of Aneuxol on the psychomotor episode. In most cases the injection was also followed by a brief period of clouding of consciousness, swallowing and movements and smacking of the lips and licking the lips with the tongue. It was these symptoms in particular which led the authors to assume that the preparation has a specific effect on psychomotor epilepsy. There were also specific changes in the EEG in five of 15 patients; these were in the form of spike and wave complexes which also showed a lateral emphasis.

To confirm this, Christian and Hallen administered the preparation by slow i.v. injection to 25 epileptic patients with psychomotor epilepsy. The symptoms mentioned above and the psychomotor symptoms described in Chapter I were then observed in all of the patients. More violent attacks were recorded in eight patients. In nearly every case the bioelectrical activity in the EEG correlated with that seen in psychomotor epilepsy, with convulsion elements localized over the temporal lobe.

To discover whether this preparation is a general provocative agent in epileptics, i.e. whether or not it is specific to the psychomotor form, these authors injected the drug into epileptics with grand mal and with pyknolepsy and absences. Surprisingly enough, following the injection there were no epileptic symptoms in either of these groups and no electroencephalographic correlates. This indicates that the Pyramidon preparation has a specific action in provoking psychomotor epilepsy and that care should be exercised when prescribing it for patients with rheumatic and other similar diseases.

CHAPTER VII

ANTIEPILEPTIC CHEMICAL SUBSTANCES

SUBSTANCES WHICH HAVE A FACULTATIVE ANTIEPILEPTIC PHARMACOLOGICAL ACTION

WE CAN DRAW AN ANALOGY HERE with the definition, given in Chapter VI, of substances which have a facultative epileptogenic action, i.e. the following chemical agents discussed which are used as drugs in medicine may, under certain conditions, have an anticonvulsant effect and suppress other epileptic or epileptoid phenomena. However, where the conditions are different they may have an epileptogenic effect. The dose of the preparation and the constitution of the patient are particularly important factors here.

To begin with, we would like to mention one or two *amphetamines.* In recent years the central effects of stimulant drugs have been studied by a number of authors (Ekiert 1963, Fleckenstein 1950, 1955, Jung 1963, Rothballer 1957). Since experimental investigations and clinical studies have often produced contradictory results, in the last thirty years many chemical substances with different actions have been tried out.

In man, Grüttner and Bonaklo (1940) observed a fairly pronounced subjective effect and a slight increase in the amplitude of the EEG waves after administrating *methamphetamine* and Greville and Heppenstall (1952) found a less pronounced effect following *amphetamine.*

However, prior to this, using a technique for automatic frequency analysis Gibbs and Maltey (1943) had demonstrated that cerebral activity is slightly accelerated following amphetamine. Pflanz and Schrader (1956) were unable to detect any significant change in the percentage of α-waves, the mean wave frequency and the level of amplitude of the EEG waves following administration of Ritalin®, whereas 2-phenyl-methyl-tetrahydro-1,4-oxazine.HCl and methamphetamine produced a significant increase in the percentage of α-waves and in the level of amplitude of the EEG waves. Radtke (1960) observed that a slow basic rhythm in the EEG was accelerated and the state of dysrhythmia and enlarged amplitude was mitigated following oral administration of *4-phenyl-2-imino-4-oxo-oxazolidine (Tradon®).* In addition to accelerating and activating the basic EEG rhythm, all these investigations *temporarily suppressed convulsion elements in the pathological electroencephalogram of the epileptic patient.* However, the problem here is that all these authors observed the spikes and waves as a very characteristic manifestation in the EEG of an epileptic and they were not really concerned with the spikes which occur locally over the temporal regions of the brain in psychomotor epilepsy. Since initially, the convulsion elements in psychomotor epilepsy differ fundamentally from the spikes and waves which emanate from centrencephalic cerebral structures, it must also be assumed that the various chemical agents used will differ somewhat as regards their effect.

We (Jovanović 1965, 1966 a, b) set out to examine the effects of amphetamines on the EEG of epileptic with spontaneous attacks or with attacks induced by other provocative agents.

In one paper (1965) we reported on the suppression of convulsion potentials in the EEG in patients suffering specifically from psychomotor epilepsy. Among 224 test subjects, 134 had another disease and a normal EEG, while there were 90 patients in the epileptic group. Following oral, subcutaneous and intravenous administration of 2 to 4 mg. *2-diethylamino-5-phenyl-oxazolinone-(4)*, generalized spikes or spikes and waves localized over the temporal lobes were suppressed, temporal foci were suppressed and the general delta-theta dysrhythmia in the EEG improved.

Our second paper (1966 a) dealt with the effect of this substance on the EEG of epileptics alone. 137 patients were used in this study. 19 of these patients had pure, isolated psychomotor attacks and 32 had combined psychomotor and generalized attacks: 51 persons altogether.

In isolated psychomotor epilepsy, the percentage of α-wave (wave index) was significantly increased by the preparation in ten cases, while the θ-wave-index was significantly reduced in 15 cases and convulsion elements were suppressed in 11 of 19 cases. The spikes, sharp waves and biphasic events which appeared over the temporal regions of the brain before treatment were definitely suppressed by the drug. The reduction of the θ-wave index indicates that the abnormally slow basic rhythm in these patients is speeded up and normalized.

In cases where psychomotor epilepsy co-existed with major seizures, following intravenous administration of 4 mg. 2-diethylamino-5-phenyl-oxazolinone-(4) the α-wave index was increased in 13 of 32 cases, and it was reduced (blockade) in 19 cases. The θ-wave index was reduced in eight cases. Convulsion elements were suppressed in two out of four cases. In general, as with isolated psychomotor epilepsy, the slowed EEG rhythms were suppressed and the convulsion potentials reduced.

However, these results only apply to one or two parenteral doses, since the experiment was not continued. Also, the effect wore off within six hours and hence, pathological elements reappeared in the EEGs of these patients. Oral clinical treatment suppressed the predisposition to attacks for a short time (six months to a year). Later on, the attacks recurred as before.

We carried out experiments on individual patients (Jovanovic 1966 a) in order to study the effect of this substance on attacks induced by provocative agents:

In the first test we treated a 48-year-old patient who had been suffering from major and psychomotor attacks for 18 years. During the Second World War, he had sustained concussion of the brain, but no other head injuries. Air encephalography and cerebral arteriography gave no evidence of any local lesion. Before treatment the EEG was characterized by large generalized spikes which were most prominent temporally, and spikes with subsequent slower waves. Intravenous injection of 1.0 ml. pentylenetetrazol precipitated a generalized epileptic attack. One minute after the onset of the attack we administered 2 mg. 2-diethylamino-5-phenyl-oxazolinone-(4) i.v. The EEG became completely normal in about 60 seconds, the basic rhythm normalized and the spikes occurring during the attack disappeared. The spike formations which were observed in the EEG before the attack were not visible at all one hour after the attack and they were much less prominent than before after a further five and one-half hours.

In view of the fact that this patient was particularly predisposed to convulsions and that he had a very low convulsion threshold, we set out to see whether the amphetamine we were using would induce an attack in this patient; so next day we have him 2 mg. 2-diethylamino-5-phenyl-oxazolinone-(4) intravenously and waited for a response. Within the next five or ten minutes the cerebral activity normalized completely. The temporal spikes in the EEG disappeared and only began to reappear to any significant extent six hours later. This amphetamine did not induce an attack, it actually suppressed one, as the EEG normalization showed.

For the second test we examined a 21-year-old woman with centrencephalic epilepsy. Her EEG in the waking state showed generalized formations of spikes, general dysrhythmia and slowing. The cause of her condition was unknown. On one day we gave the patient 2 mg. 2-diethylamino-5-phenyl-oxazolinone-(4) by intravenous injection. The next five to ten minutes brought an improvement; the basic θ-wave rhythm was reduced and the basic α-wave rhythm increased. The number of convulsion potentials was also significantly reduced. On the following day we administered the same substance 40 seconds after the onset of a generalized attack induced by pentylenetetrazole. The generalized attack was halted and the EEG normalized. The effect of the amphetamine as measured by the EEG lasted for five and one-half to six hours.

The third test involved a 28-year-old patient who had been suffering from *dreamy state* psychomotor attacks for three years. Just before this test the man had been found in his nightshirt in a roadside ditch. Apparently his attack had occurred while he was asleep and he walked in his sleep, ending up in the ditch and had not been able to climb out again. He was still in a dreamy condition when he arrived at our hospital. The EEG revealed a fairly pronounced α-wave rhythm with generalized spikes which were prominent temporally, and spikes followed by δ-waves. At a few points there were generalized and paroxysmal bursts of sharp waves for four to seven seconds.

Following intravenous administration of 4 mg. of the test amphetamine, the bursts of sharp waves disappeared within five minutes. An hour later there were no more convulsion elements, even during a trial period of hyperventilation. The convulsion elements did not reappear for over an hour and even then they occurred far less frequently than before the injection. After five more hours the convulsion elements appeared to be exactly as they had been before therapy and we were unable to detect any other differences.

In the fourth test we treated a 23-year-old patient who had been suffering from diffuse epilepsy with generalized and psychomotor attacks for six years. His EEG showed almost classic right temporal and temporo-frontal spikes which closely followed one another; these did not change under trial hyperventilation. Four minutes after intravenous administration of the test amphetamine, these temporal and fronto-temporal spikes were no longer visible. At first the convulsion potentials became less common, then they diminished in size and became more ill-defined and deformed and by the fifth minute there was a continuous α-wave rhythm in the patient's EEG. Instead of convulsion elements there were groups of spindle-shaped α-waves. One hour after injection the convulsion elements reappeared in the EEG, but they continued to be significantly less prominent than before therapy for a further five hours. Six hours after injection the EEG convulsion potentials were the same as before administrating the amphetamine.

To summarize it can be concluded from these results that *2-diethylamino-5-phenyl-oxazolinone-(4) suppresses spontaneous convulsion potentials, and suppresses convulsion elements and attacks induced by other agents, but only for the period in which it has an active effect on the EEG, i.e. for five to six hours.* This substance has not really proved of great value as an anti-epileptic agent since if it is given for several weeks its anti-epileptic action gradually declines.

In a third report we described (Jovanovic 1966 b) the effect of this preparation on the EEGs of 578 test subjects, 160 of whom were healthy individuals. Here, 168 patients had epilepsy, 22 isolated psychomotor attacks and 51 combined major and psychomotor attacks. Convulsion elements were suppressed in 50 to 60 percent of the EEGs. However, these convulsion elements reappeared as before, after five to six hours. Here again we tried to treat the patients with the amphetamine, but after six months it became clear that the experiment had failed. The action of 2-diethylamino-5-phenyl-oxazolinone-(4) was considered to be due to its ability to reduce cerebral predisposition to convulsion. This substance is an *oxazolidine,* and oxazolidines are known to have anti-epileptic properties. On the other hand, this chemical compound is an *amphetamine* which, according to the authors mentioned above, also *(but only temporarily)* suppresses or reduces increased predisposition to convulsions.

Other or similar amphetamines have also been studied by animal experiment (Berlucci 1955, Bochnik and Spigelberg 1957, Bradley and Elkes 1949, Bradley and Key 1958, Colombati and Canestrari 1956, Grundfest 1959, Marchini 1957, Purpura 1957, Purpura et al. 1956 to 1959, Toman and Davis 1949, Ziem et al. 1970). Nearly all these authors report that the basic EEG rhythm is activated following administration of methamphetamine, amphetamine or 2-phenyl-3-methyl-tetrahydro-1,4-oxazine.HCl. Using these substances it was possible to mprove or normalize the pathological or slightly abnormal cerebral activity induced by other drugs. EEG convulsion elements were also temporarily suppressed in animals. However, since this experimental technique involves producing a state of acute intoxication or artificially inducing convulsion elements in the EEG for a short period of time, we do not consider these EEG phenomena can readily be applied to the EEG seen in psychomotor epilepsy in man, although it is possible to draw certain analogies.

Phenamine (amphetamine) is a substance which, according to Pogodaev (1964), has the characteristics of *Adrenaline* and *ephedrine* both as regards chemical constitution and for the point of view of its effects in the body. The special properties of phenamine are that it has a better effect on excitation of the CNS, particularly on the cortex, than either of the other two substances (Arbusov 1944, 1950, Gubar 1944, Kuznecov 1945, 1947). Faddeev's studies on white rats (1951) showed that the effect depended on the dose of the preparation (on the cortex and on the subcortex) and on the initial functional condition of the CNS, particularly of the cortex. An effective dose gives rise to a sequence of different effects which occur one after the other and which mainly involve higher nervous functions. The author noticed that the changes may be of either type.

According to Faddeev (1951), the optimum dose of the preparation in the rat is 0.6 mg/kg. as a single dose. This intensifies both nervous processes —excitation and inhibition—in the cortex and also in the adjacent subcortical structures and this effect is manifest as a shortening of the latent period of conditioned reflexes, the animal runs faster to the food trough, some non-conditioned reflexes are accentuated and the animal becomes generally more lively. In most cases a mean dose of 1 to 2 mg/kg. phenamine had a three-phase action on the CNS: 1.) *the first phase* was similar to the action of the optimum dose and was characterized by shortening of the latent period of conditioned reflexes; 2) *in the second phase* there was a phasic effect on the instincts of self-preservation or sexual drive, and the animals refused to eat, and 3.) *the third and last phase,* which was associated with the elimination of the basic constituents of phenamine, was characterized by an increase of cortical activity and gradual normalization of activity in the proximal subcortex (here formations rostral to the diencephalon).

The author found that when exerting its maximum effect, a higher dose (2.4 mg/kg.) and the medium dose (1.2 mg/kg.) of phenamine inhibit the suppressant mechanism in the cortical centers. Even higher doses (6.0 mg/kg.) eliminate conditioned responses and the instincts of self-preservation and sexual drive. A dose of 60 mg/kg. may kill the animal. After a brief period of recovery of cortical excitation, Faddeev (1951) found that suppression returned and was maintained in both the cortical structures and the structures near the cortex. The effect of the preparation on the brain stem has not yet been studied in detail.

After these general remarks on phenamine we would like to mention Pogodaev's studies (1964) on the effect of this substance on epileptic attacks in animals. Pogodaev used various dosages of this preparation in rats.

The experiments were carried out in three series. The rats weighed between 150 and 200 gr. Phenamine was administered subcutaneously in all cases (aqueous solution), the concentration varying depending on the desired dose (0.6 mg/kg., 1.2 mg/kg., 2.4 mg/kg. etc.). The epileptic attacks were induced with 80 to 120 V electric current, with a burst of 0.5 sec. The results are very interesting.

EXPERIMENTS WITH LOW DOSES *(0.6* MG/KG.*)* OF PHENAMINE: Two groups of experiments were set up in this series. The first group was used to study the effects of low doses on the course of an *isolated epileptic attack* and the second to test the effect of phenamine on *repeated attacks* which were induced one after another until the animal died.

In the first group, ten minutes after administration of phenamine the tonic phase was reduced from 8.2 to 4.2 seconds ($p < 0.05$) and the clonic phase from 22.4 to 10.2 seconds ($p < 0.05$). On the other hand, the locomotor phase was longer and more intense; it increased from 12 to 32.4 seconds and the initial phase from 3.8 to 7.2 seconds. The overall duration of the attack was not affected. These results indicate that the preparation has a favorable effect, since the generalized phase of an epileptic attack are substantially curtailed and the less dangerous or inhibition phases are prolonged.

About 30 minutes after injection of phenamine, the initial values gradually return but they do not normalize completely. This dosage did not alter the convulsion threshold (85 to 88 Volts).

Experiments involving many repeated attacks (second group) also showed that the epileptic phases differ from those in control animals. If the attacks are induced in quick succession in control animals, the initial tonic and clonic phases are soon curtailed. The locomotor phase is also curtailed so that the overall duration of an attack becomes shorter and shorter after each repeat attack. The control animals die after ten to 15 attacks.

However, the prevailing picture is quite different in the phenamine experiments. The animals did not die until 29 to 35 attacks had been induced, and the convulsions after repeated attacks were more constant than in the control animals: after nine to 12 attacks they were the same, then after a further four to five attacks the phases became slightly shorter and after this they remained constant until the end of the experiment. Initial and locomotor phases disappeared.

EXPERIMENTS WITH MEDIUM DOSES *(1.2* MG/KG.*)* OF PHENAMINE*:* Two groups were again used in this series of experiments. The changes which occurred with a *single attack* (first group) were the same as those occurring after low doses, but the results were more significant (i.e. a higher level of statistical significance). For example, the initial phases were two to two and one-half times longer ($p < 0.01$) 10, 30 and 150 minutes after the injection. The tonic and clonic phases were substantially shorter ten minutes after the injection (as with the low doses) and also 30 and 150 minutes after injection. The locomotor phase was substantially longer, much more so after 150 minutes than after 10 or 30 minutes. The phase of rigidity was curtailed more than after low doses of the preparation. As after low doses the convulsion threshold was unchanged. The overall duration of an attack was the same.

When *the attacks were repeated* (second group) the animals were still alive after as many as 55 attacks induced in succession, i.e. the life expectancy of these rats was increased one and one-half to two times compared with the situation after giving the low doses and it was four to five times longer than that of animals which had not been treated with phenamine. The overall duration of the attacks was substantially reduced after ten attacks and this continued until the 15th attack when they began to get longer again. The clonic phase became prolonged after 23 to 25 attacks and then gradually began to get shorter, depending on the constitution of the particular animal. After the 44th attack, all that remained was the clonic phase and this persisted until the animal died.

THE FAIRLY HIGH DOSAGE OF PHENAMINE *(2.4* MG/KG.*)* AND THE LETHAL DOSE *(60* MG/KG.*)*: Three groups were set up here. The attacks were induced at different times after the injection.

The fairly high dosage (2.4 mg/kg.) produced the type of experimental result after four minutes which was seen ten minutes after administration of the low and medium doses. The effect of the fairly high dose persisted for 120 and 150 minutes, and also for four days. *The difference compared with previous experiments was that the convulsion threshold was very much higher three to four minutes after injection of 2.4 mg/kg. phenamine.* After 30 to 60 minutes it was one and one-half times higher and it remained so until 120 to 150 minutes after the injection. The convulsion threshold did not become normal again for two days.

With the lethal dose (60 mg/kg.) the author found that the convulsion threshold increased within three to four and 30 minutes after the injection. In these groups the duration of the attacks also changed four minutes after the injection. After administering lethal doses, after 10 and 30 minutes the course of the attack was the same as that recorded after fairly high doses (2.4 mg/kg.). However, there are certain differences between these findings and those following 2.4 mg/kg., as follows: 1.) the animals died after only 24 to 30 attacks, 2.) the attacks are substantially reduced both as regards duration and intensity, 3.) the attacks are more uniform and oligosymptomatic than under fairly high doses, 4.) the clonic phase appears from the 16th attack on. Lethal doses (60 mg./kg.) produce results similar to those obtained with attacks which are frequently repeated under fairly high doses (2.4 mg/kg.).

Analysis of the results from all three services of experiments, and employing four different dosages (low, medium, fairly high and lethal) reveals some interesting points. Doses of 0.6 mg/kg., 1.2 mg/kg., 2.4 mg/kg. and 60 mg/kg. prolong the initial phase and the locomotor phenomena, but reduce the tonic and, in particular, the clonic phase. Parallel to this, the phase of rigidity is also curtailed (see Chapter V) and in rare cases it may disappear altogether.

The changes which occur in the clinical picture of an attack depend on the dose and the changes increase with the dose of phenamine. Under the experimental conditions used by Pogodaev (1964), fairly low and medium doses do not substantially alter the course of an attack. According to this author, under fairly high and lethal doses the convulsion threshold is increased in the cortex and, in particular, this increase becomes more pronounced in the deeper structures.

According to Pogodaev (1964), attenuation of the phase of rigidity and prolongation of the locomotor phase can be interpreted as the effect of phenamine in intensifying the inhibitory functions in the deeper cerebral structures. It is possible that the locomotor phase is intensified as the higher nervous centers relinquish their control over the function of the spinal cord.

We know that when used in optimum doses phenamine reduces fatigue and drowsiness and increases the capacity for work; it increases muscular strength and reduces rigidity and tremor. It is capable of increasing both the duration and intensity of motor activity (Pogodaev 1954, Sereiski 1943). According to these authors, this is due to the fact that following phenamine mobilization and tonicity of the organism are improved, and resistance is increased. The effect of phenamine on the CNS is seen mainly as the result of its effect in promoting oxidation processes in the brain, promoting protein metabolism and increasing cerebral blood flow (Palladin et al. 1957, Sereiski 1943). In this way, phenamine increases resistance to anoxia which may result from a temporary reduction of oxidation processes in the brain. The increase in the convulsion threshold in the brain and the greater resistance to attacks under low and medium doses of phenamine is sen by Pogodaev (1964) as being due to the effect of this substance in improving the metabolic processes, and this results in integration of the defence mechanisms and mobilization of the reserves in the CNS and hence, this gives better protection to the body. All parts of the brain work together here (cortex, subcortex, brain stem, cerebellum).

Pogodaev (1964) compares the results he obtained by inducing seizures in rats with the findings reported in the literature on the effect of phenamine on the higher nervous functions under physiological conditions (see Faddeev 1951).

Nicotinic acid and a xanthine substance in combination suppress convulsions (Jovanović 1970 c, d, 1972 b, c). This applies particularly if they are used before one embarks on a procedure which is likely to induce convulsions.

In view of the immense importance of this question, we would like to discuss in detail the results obtained using the substances mentioned.

Here we shall be describing our own experiments carried out with the preparation manufactured from two chemical agents: *L-hexyl-3,7-dimethylxanthine (SK-7) and nicotinic acid (200 mg or 50 mg per dose, respectively)* (see formula). The preparation is marketed under the name *Cosaldon®*.

This trial was instigated by, on the one hand, the existence of many results regarding the vasoactive effect of the two chemical substances combined in one preparation and, on the other hand, results regarding ischaemia of the brain in epileptic attacks.

Structural formula :

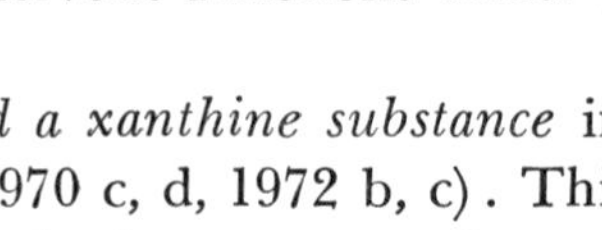

1-Hexyl-3,7-dimethylxanthine (SK 7)

Structural formula :

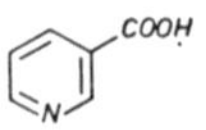

Nicotinic acid

The properties of nicotinic acid, particularly its vasoactive effects, have been described in the literature many times. These properties are illustrated in Chapters III and V.

There have been several publications on the action of SK-7 in animal experiments (Betz and Rodenhäuser 1962, Ueki 1962; Ramos et al. 1963, Neubauer 1965, Rodenhäuser 1963). These experiments revealed an increase of blood flow, dilatation of the vessels, and increased filling of the arterioles and venules in the region of the central nervous system (CNS) and fundus of the eye.

Cosaldon promotes the passage of glucose and phosphate across the blood-brain barrier (Quadbeck 1962). In man, this preparation has been used to good effect in the initial or advanced stages of disorders due to cerebral sclerosis (Felstein 1963, Leube 1959, Meyer 1957, Schenck 1957, Schmidt 1960, Sperling 1960, Vita 1967, Waldron 1963). Moreover, after this medication there was a favorable effect even in severe cases of reduced mental efficiency due to arteriosclerotic brain diseases (Bjurwill 1963, Rerse 1956, Paffrath 1959, Paquay 1962). These findings also stimulated the use of Cosaldon as an adjuvant to electroshock therapy, since it is known that the mental efficiency is transiently impaired after the electro-convulsive procedure. Cosaldon has also proved effective in other diseases of the CNS, such as in the Parkinson syndrome (Ehlers 1961, Mustard 1964), in schizophrenia and epilepsy (Hackstock and Bielinski 1961), and also in peripheral blood flow disorders (Ehlers 1961, Paulusch 1960) which may also be precipitated by electroshock treatment (v. Baeyer 1951).

After administering this preparation, one also found that there was a tendency for the human electroencephalogram to normalize (Paquay 1962, Philippopoulou 1963). *This fact led us to use the EEG as an objective indicator for recording changes in the CNS in patients after electroshock treatment.*

Our tests were carried out in three stages.

In the first stage our group of 60 patients to be studied was divided into two groups so that the indication fo electroshock treatment was the same for all the patients.

Group I (comparison group): 30 patients were treated by electroshock *without* Cosaldon therapy. The age of this group was between 20 and 62 years, the mean age being 43.2 years.

Group II (test group): 30 female patients with the same age range (23 to 63 years). The mean age was 43.4 years. In addition to the electroshock therapy, this group was also treated *with* Cosaldon. The patients were not specially selected.

As a rule, the test group of 30 patients received one tablet Cosaldon three times daily *for one week before the beginning* of electroshock treatment. Treatment was continued during the course of electroshock therapy and for several weeks after it had ended.

In special cases, the preparation was prescribed at the beginning of electroshock treatment (three cases). In two cases, the treatment was instituted three days after convulsive therapy. Electrical induction of the convulsion was carried out in the same way in both groups.

After premedication with 0.5 to 0.4 g. Hexobarbital and 0.9 ml. suxamethonium, the convulsion was induced with a current of 550 to 650 ma. with a Standard Neuroton.

Electroencephalographic investigations were carried out before, during and after the treatment. The EEG was recorded on admission to hospital. After the patients had received Cosaldon for one week, an additional EEG check was carried out on the day before the first electroshock. There was an EEG check once again after the end of electro-convulsive therapy. This check was made as soon as the patients had recovered consciousness from the anaesthetic after the final electroconvulsion. Further EEG checks were carried out at ten-day intervals for up to six months and longer.

For assessing the effect of electroshock on the cerebral activity, the initial EEG and the final EEG after electroshock were compared and evaluated in detail. During the convulsion, the duration of the convulsion, the respiratory arrest after the convulsion and the duration of cyanosis were also timed.

On average, eight to ten electro-convulsions were induced. We only used the *block,* with three electroconvulsions induced on three consecutive days, in exceptional cases.

The data from the electro-convulsion and also the EEGs were statistically evaluated electronically by computer. In both groups of patients the branch leads from the left temporo-occipital regions were used for determining the wave frequency, amplitude and the α-wave indices in the EEG.

This gave the following results:

Group I—Comparison Group

Duration of convulsive therapy with the electric current. The results are summarized in Table XV. The time taken to induce the convulsion was 2.96 (s ± 0.21) to 4.47 (s ± 0.47) seconds. The duration of convulsive shock therapy was only less than three seconds in one case. In all the other cases it was only possible to trigger a therapeutic convulsion with a duration of longer than three seconds. The mean duration for all patients was 3.52 (s ± 0.58) seconds.

Duration of electro-convulsion. With a passage of current lasting 3.52 seconds, on average, this triggered convulsions which lasted between 21.33 (s ± 5.77) and 29.33 (s ± 1.15) seconds. In no case did the electroshock last for less than 20 seconds. The mean duration of the convulsion was

TABLE XV. Statistical evaluation of the results of the parameters studied in 30 patients with manic depression under electroshock treatment without additional prophylactic drug treatment (our own observations).

Patient's Number	*Duration in seconds of* Electric current			Electric convulsions			Respiratory arrest		
	ε	$\bar{X}$	*s*	ε	$\bar{X}$	*s*	ε	$\bar{X}$	*s*
1	39.1	3.26	0.56	320.0	26.67	4.03	335.0	27.92	4.23
2	28.7	3.59	0.61	199.0	24.87	5.28	197.0	24.62	6.63
3	45.7	4.15	1.19	296.0	26.91	9.09	288.0	26.18	7.29
4	29.9	3.74	0.20	208.0	26.00	8.55	197.0	24.62	6.63
5	21.7	3.62	0.37	140.0	23.33	5.89	156.0	26.00	7.07
6	21.2	3.03	0.18	156.0	22.29	6.05	179.0	25.57	6.55
7	33.9	3.39	0.45	266.0	26.60	7.31	270.0	27.00	7.67
8	25.8	3.23	0.49	186.0	23.25	6.23	180.0	22.50	6.61
9	33.1	3.68	0.48	214.0	23.78	6.04	217.0	24.11	6.35
10	30.5	3.81	0.24	188.0	23.50	6.93	197.0	24.62	6.63
11	26.4	3.77	0.71	170.0	24.29	5.94	195.0	27.86	2.48
12	35.5	3.55	0.37	236.0	23.60	9.18	229.0	22.90	6.12
13	23.7	2.96	0.21	220.0	27.50	7.98	199.0	24.87	8.77
14	22.1	3.16	0.24	176.0	25.14	5.27	180.0	25.71	6.50
15	27.9	3.49	0.27	186.0	23.25	5.65	217.0	27.12	7.57
16	21.8	3.69	0.38	152.0	25.33	5.75	124.0	20.67	4.37
17	22.9	3.27	0.18	168.0	24.00	6.32	182.0	26.00	6.45
18	24.5	3.50	0.41	180.0	25.71	9.20	185.0	26.43	7.85
19	27.0	3.38	0.37	216.0	27.00	8.28	210.0	26.25	5.65
20	17.7	3.54	0.09	138.0	27.60	6.58	110.0	22.00	4.18
21	25.6	3.20	0.22	208.0	26.00	8.14	205.0	25.62	6.30
22	9.7	3.23	0.25	86.0	28.67	1.15	87.0	29.00	8.54
23	20.9	4.13	0.65	120.0	24.00	6.48	121.0	24.20	3.90
24	11.4	3.80	0.70	88.0	29.33	12.06	69.0	23.00	5.00
25	23.7	3.39	0.13	195.0	27.86	8.25	169.0	24.14	3.72
26	24.4	3.05	0.09	197.0	24.62	6.99	205.0	25.62	6.07
27	19.7	3.94	0.83	122.0	24.40	5.90	117.0	23.40	5.55
28	26.7	3.81	0.70	200.0	28.57	7.09	176.0	25.14	3.93
29	26.2	3.74	0.78	164.0	23.43	5.86	179.0	25.57	5.97
30	13.4	3.55	0.37	236.0	23.60	9.18	229.0	22.90	6.12
Total:	760.8	3.52	0.58	5459.0	25.27	6.77	5444.0	25.20	6.07

25.27 (s ± 6.77) seconds. There was a relatively large deviation from the mean value in only one case (No. 24, Table XV).

Duration of respiratory arrest and cyanosis following the electro-convulsion differed substantially from the value obtained from the test group. In group I (see Table XV) the respiratory arrest lasted between 22.50 (s ± 6.61) and 29.00 (s ± 8.54) seconds. The mean duration of respiratory arrest and cyanosis after the end of electro-convulsion was 25.00 (s ± 6.07) seconds. *Thus, in the comparison group, the convulsion and the respiratory arrest with cyanosis last for the same length of time.*

Electroencephalographic checks (Table XVI) revealed that there were considerable disturbances of bioelectric cerebral activity not just in isolated cases, but in all the patients but one.

The *frequency* shifted out of the normal α-wave rhythm into θ- and δ-wave regions. The EEG results are shown in Table XVI. This shows that there is considerable scatter of the frequency.

The *amplitude* rose above the normal level and showed wide scatter after only two or three electroconvulsive treatments. The EEG curves showed maximal slowing and were very active in respect of amplitude, so that the electroencephalographs after electro-convulsion were not comparable with those obtained before treatment (Figure 34).

The *α-wave percentage* became very much smaller after the treatment since the EEG waves then came in the regions of the theta and delta wave band. From a value of over 90 cm/metre it was possible to observe a fall in the indices of the α-waves to ten or even to zero (Table XVI).

The *appearance of new elements in the EEG* which had not been recognized before treatment; in addition to the θ- and δ-waves which were present as an expression of slowing and non-specific alteration of the EEG picture, this is *characteristic by the occurrence of suspected convulsive frequencies and of convulsive events.*

In one case (a 34-year-old female patient) we were able to detect generalized polyspike wave formations in the EEG (Figure 35). These were not concentrated on one particular side, they persisted for over three months and, clinically, bilateral symmetrical clonic muscular contractions occurred as a correlate.

In two further cases, after eight electro-convulsive treatments, the EEG showed generalized spike-wave element although it was not possible to record any clinical symptoms of an epileptic event. *In nine cases* there were generalized, very high and slow sharp waves with an emphasis on the left side in the EEG, although there were no corresponding clinical symptoms.

With one exception, all the EEGs showed generalized slow sharp waves with an emphasis on the left side and, from time to time, these occurred in the region of the δ-wave band. The maximum waves (slow δ-waves of 0.8 to 1.2 cycles) were mainly recorded in the frontal and frontotemporal areas, and they were certainly more concentrated on the left than on the right side.

It is interesting that, relatively speaking, the EEG changes do not remain normal for very long even if other vasoactive or anabolic therapy is used subsequently. Over periods of three, or even six months, it is only possible to achieve fairly slow and (between checks in some cases) insignificant regression of the electroencephalographic changes, and in some urgent cases these changes may prove to be a contraindication for further electro-

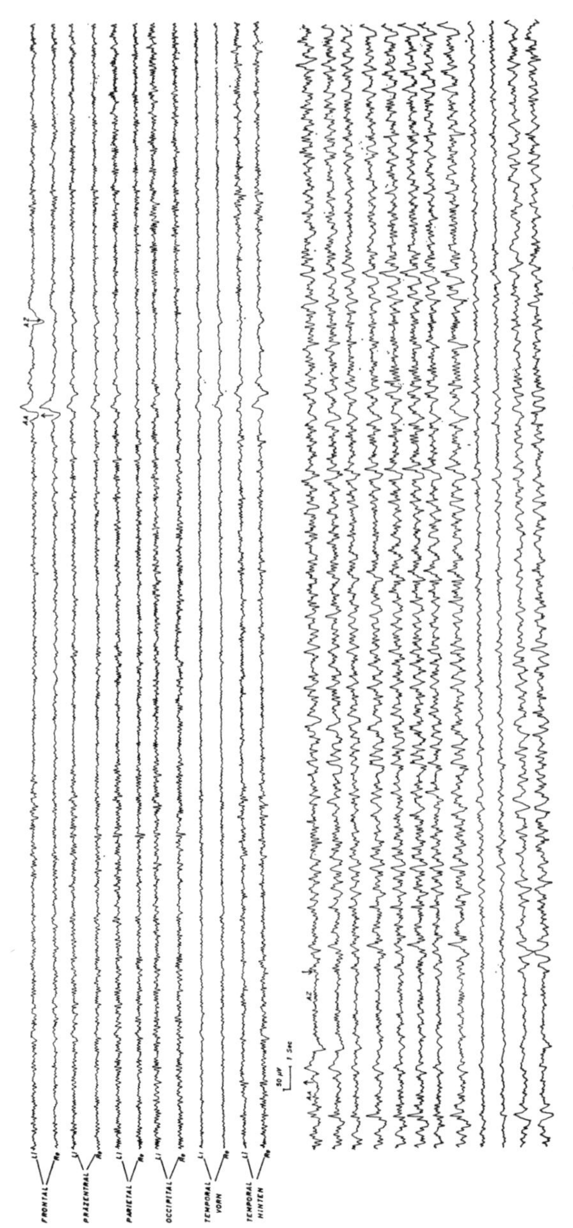

Figure 34. Changes of bioelectrical cerebral activity before (a) and after (b) four electroshock treatments in an adult female patient with manic depressive symptoms. There is evidence of a serious general change in the EEG which can become even more serious after fairly prolonged electroshock therapy (cp. Figure 36) (our own results, original).

Table XVI. Changes in the frequency, amplitude and alpha-wave portions in the EEG of 30 patients with manic depression under electroshock treatment without additional prophylactic drug treatment (our own observations).

	Electric Shocks					
Patient's	*Frequency/per sec*		*Amplitude*		*α-Wave-Percentage*	
Number	*before*	*after*	*before*	*after*	*before*	*after*
1	8	6	70-90	100-140	85	30
2	9	6	80-100	100-160	96	25
3	8	3	80-100	100-170	70	1
4	10	6	70- 80	100-180	65	3
5	11	10	50- 70	100-120	64	55
6	12	10	50- 80	60-100	43	30
7	10	3	50- 70	60-140	30	1
8	10	2	50- 68	60-180	36	1
9	11	3	50- 68	100-200	66	3
10	10	2	52- 68	100-140	67	4
11	8	4	54- 68	140-160	60	10
12	9	3	64-100	60-100	90	15
13	10	6	60- 80	70-140	95	30
14	11	6	70-100	70-140	99	25
15	8	2	70-100	70-160	76	8
16	9	4	60- 70	80-180	80	10
17	9	3	60- 80	80-180	67	10
18	9	2	70- 90	100-240	63	1
19	10	3	40-100	60-280	43	5
20	8	4	60- 80	40-240	32	10
21	9	6	60- 90	60-140	40	12
22	8.5	8	90-100	60-200	44	16
23	10	10	90-100	40-240	46	43
24	11	10	80-100	60-230	66	42
25	10	8	70- 90	70-250	68	68
26	10	7	50- 70	60-140	40	32
27	8	4	50- 70	60-130	90	18
28	9	8	50- 80	50-140	80	16
29	8	3	60- 90	60-130	57	2
30	9	2	60-100	200-240	87	3
M	9.4	5.13	73.70	128.0	65.5	16.83
S	±1.13	±2.71	±11.75	±31.07	±19.48	±15.14
P	<0.01		<0.01		<0.01	

shock treatment (where there is a new endogenous and acute manic depressive phase).

In all cases in the comparison group, there was first a recession of suspected convulsive events and convulsion elements (as the specific changes) and, rather later, there was recession of the maximally slowed EEG curves (as an expression of the general and non-specific changes).

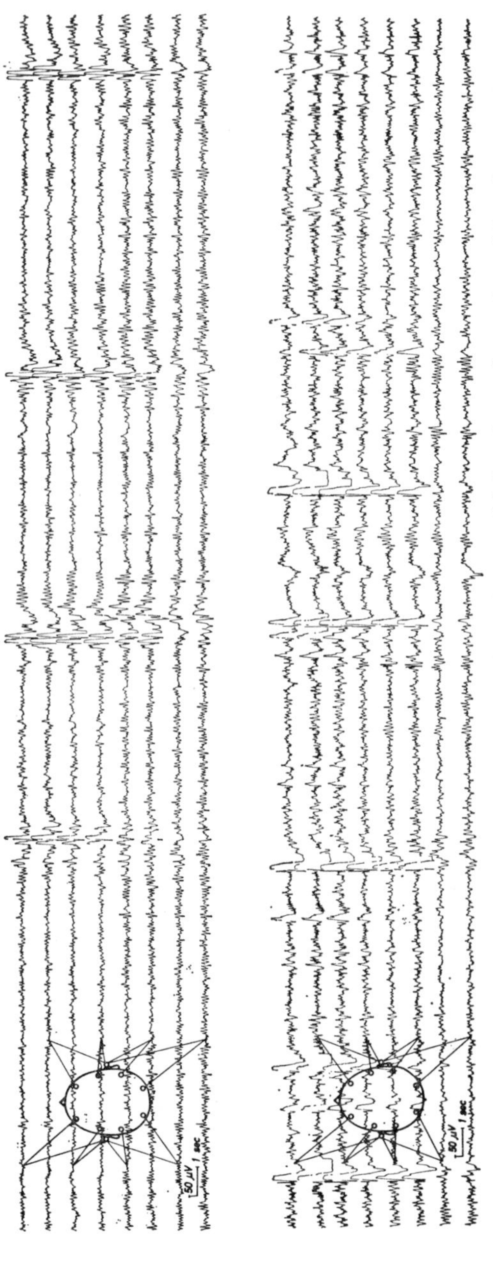

Figure 35. Bioelectrical cerebral activity in a 46-year-old female patient after eight electroshock treatments, with no concomitant drug treatment. There is evedienec of periodic, generalized spike and wave complexes with a general EEG change (our own results, original).

Group II—Test Group

In this group which received additional Cosaldon treatment, following the electro-convulsive treatment, there were significant differences compared with the comparison group with regard to: 1.) the duration of convulsive shock therapy up to the beginning of convulsion; 2.) the duration of respiratory arrest after the electro-convulsion had ended; 3.) the presence and duration of cyanosis and, 4.) the changes in the electroencephalographic picture.

The results in the test group are shown in (Table XVII).

The mean duration of convulsion shock therapy up to induction of the electro-convulsion in group II was 2.57 (s ± 0.39) seconds. To trigger a convulsion of the same duration in the comparison group, on average, the current had to be passed for *one second longer* (3.52 ± 0.58 seconds). In one case the period was 3.09 (s ± 0.60) seconds. In all the other 29 cases these values were less than three seconds. This was very much in contrast to the results obtained from the comparison group.

The duration of the convulsion in the test group was, on average, 24.66 (s ± 6.14) seconds and this is not significantly different from the duration in the comparison group ($p < 0.10$).

The duration of respiratory arrest and cyanosis after the convulsion has ended is very much shorter in the test group treated with Cosaldon and, in all cases, it differs from the corresponding values measured for the comparison group. While in the comparison group the duration of the convulsion and the duration of respiratory arrest after the convulsion with the development of cyanosis were very much the same, in the test group the duration of respiratory arrest after the end of the convulsion was noticeably curtailed. On average, the respiratory arrest in the test group, reckoned from the last twitch up to the first intake of breath, was only 3.48 (± 2.82) seconds. The standard deviation is large since, in many cases, there was no respiratory arrest at all after the end of the convulsions, while in a few patients it lasted for up to ten seconds.

It is characteristic that in over 75 percent of the patients who received additional Cosaldon treatment, it was not possible to observe any cyanosis at all, even when the respiratory arrest lasted for a few seconds. The faces of the patients were pink-red and they usually began to breathe immediately after the last convulsive twitch. Artificial respiration was not necessary in any case.

We consider that the significant curtailment of the duration of cyanosis and of respiratory arrest after the end of the convulsion compared with the comparison group, is the most important result of our experiments with Cosaldon in electro-convulsive treatment.

The electroencephalogram (Table XVIII) was used as an objective

Table XVII. Statistical evaluation of the parameters observed in 30 patients with manic depression under electroshock treatment and additional oral treatment with Cosaldon® (nicotinic acid and a xanthine compound, see text) (our own observations).

Patient's Number	*Duration in seconds of* *Electric current* ε	$\bar{X}$	*s*	*Electric Convulsions* ε	$\bar{X}$	*s*	*Respiratory arrest* ε	$\bar{X}$	*s*
1	6.9	2.30	0.10	86.0	28.67	1.13	7.0	2.33	2.52
2	20.1	2.23	0.27	215.0	23.89	4.43	28.0	3.11	3.62
3	8.2	2.73	0.12	72.0	24.00	7.21	10.0	3.33	3.06
4	23.6	2.36	0.08	242.0	24.20	5.85	39.0	3.90	2.92
5	15.8	2.63	0.34	150.0	25.00	6.29	31.0	5.17	2.99
6	19.7	2.46	0.31	208.0	26.00	8.94	31.0	3.87	2.95
7	14.4	2.40	0.26	140.0	23.33	5.89	17.0	2.83	2.56
8	13.8	2.30	0.32	130.0	21.67	5.83	17.0	2.83	2.56
9	14.4	2.40	0.28	129.0	21.50	4.46	13.0	2.17	2.71
10	28.0	2.80	0.36	242.0	24.20	8.19	39.0	3.90	2.92
11	27.8	3.09	0.60	236.0	26.22	8.39	37.0	4.11	2.85
12	20.1	2.51	0.36	198.0	24.75	5.65	34.0	4.25	2.87
13	16.8	2.80	0.62	162.0	27.00	9.36	29.0	4.83	2.71
14	13.0	2.60	0.24	120.0	24.00	5.66	21.0	4.20	2.49
15	7.3	2.43	0.32	76.0	25.33	6.43	8.0	2.67	3.06
16	13.1	2.62	0.40	122.0	24.40	5.90	10.0	2.00	2.43
17	15.7	2.62	0.31	140.0	23.33	5.89	25.0	4.17	2.99
18	20.8	2.60	0.39	186.0	23.25	5.65	26.0	3.25	3.15
19	13.7	2.74	0.49	122.0	24.40	5.90	13.0	2.60	2.79
20	6.7	2.23	0.06	84.0	28.00	0.00	4.0	1.33	1.15
21	23.3	2.59	0.26	206.0	22.89	5.84	26.0	2.89	2.80
22	7.5	2.50	0.61	86.0	28.67	1.15	8.0	2.67	3.06
23	17.5	2.92	0.20	167.0	27.83	5.95	21.0	3.50	3.33
24	8.0	2.67	0.29	86.0	28.67	1.15	19.0	6.33	1.53
25	14.1	2.82	0.28	120.0	24.00	6.48	18.0	3.60	3.58
26	18.0	2.25	0.21	186.0	23.25	5.65	23.0	2.87	2.53
27	7.6	2.53	0.31	63.0	21.00	2.65	10.0	3.33	3.06
28	15.9	2.65	0.26	164.0	27.33	8.91	29.0	4.83	2.71
29	15.5	2.58	0.47	152.0	25.33	5.75	13.0	2.17	2.71
30	8.3	2.77	0.25	74.0	24.67	7.57	6.0	2.00	2.00
Total:	455.6	2.57	0.39	4364.0	24.66	6.14	616.0	3.84	2.81

Comparison		*Table 18*	*Table 16*	*Probabilty (p)*
Electric current	ε	455.60	760.80	<0.01
	$\bar{X}$	2.57	3.52	
	s	0.39	0.58	
Electric convulsions	ε	4364.00	5459.00	No differences
	$\bar{X}$	24.66	25.27	
	s	6.14	6.77	
Respiratory arrest	ε	616.00	5444.00	<0.01
	$\bar{X}$	3.48	25.20	
	s	2.81	6.07	

Table XVIII. Changes in the frequency, amplitude and alpha-wave portions in the EEG of 30 patients with manic depression under electroshock treatment and additional therapy with Cosaldon® (nicotinic acid and a xanthine compound, see text) (our own observations).

	E E G-W a v e s a n d E l c t r i c S h o c k s					
Patient's	*Frequency/per sec*		*Amplitude*		*α-Wave-Percentage*	
Number	*before*	*after*	*before*	*after*	*before*	*after*
1	8	8	70-90	90-100	86	80
2	10	9	68-100	90-100	96	86
3	10	9	60-70	70-80	78	96
4	9	9	50-60	60- 80	60	59
5	8	8	80-88	80-90	53	39
6	7	7.6	70-90	90-100	36	38
7	8	7.8	50-70	60-80	66	68
8	9	8	60-80	70-80	78	68
9	10	9	50-90	70-100	76	66
10	10	9	60-90	90-100	65	79
11	9	9	70-90	90-100	76	89
12	9	8	60-100	100-120	73	68
13	9	8	50-110	100-120	65	69
14	9	8	60-100	70-110	40	89
15	8	9	90-100	90-120	99	78
16	7	6	70-90	90-100	100	68
17	8	7	60-70	70-100	30	48
18	6	6	60-70	90-100	100	66
19	8	7	40-80	60-90	96	76
20	9	8	60-90	90-100	46	75
21	10	9	60-80	80-100	36	60
22	11	9	60-80	80-110	63	66
23	12	10	40-80	80-120	74	70
24	10	10	60-100	70-100	56	23
25	9	8	70-90	70-90	56	11
26	8	3	60-70	60-80	57	10
27	7	2	60-80	80-100	39	20
28	8	7	63-100	80-110	86	50
29	9	8	60-90	80-110	95	65
30	10	8	65-90	90-110	98	50
M	8.78	7.80	73.97	89.67	69.23	61.73
S	±1.28	±1.75	±9.20	±10.98	±21.43	±22.66
P	>0.05		>0.05		>0.05	

method for detecting changes in the bioelectrical cerebral activity. There was noticeable difference between recordings taken from the comparison group and those from the test group (cf Figures 34, 35 and 36). In only one case were we able to observe maximum slowing of the basic EEG rhythm up to the δ-wave band.

Even after treatment with electro-convulsion repeated ten times, the *frequency* was in the range of the α-wave rhythm.

The *amplitude of the waves* did not increase significantly after the convulsion treatment, but it remained within the range of normal amplitude fluctuation. Thus, the standard deviations are very much smaller than those for the amplitudes recorded after treating the comparison group.

Here, by way of exception, it was possible to see isolated waves projecting from the α- or even from the θ-wave band, in the basic rhythm. As a rule, such events did not occur. In the test group and also in the comparison group, the localization of individual EEG waves projecting from the basic rhythm is recorded over the frontal and frontotemporal cerebral regions and with greater emphasis on the left side.

The *α-wave index* (percentage) in the EEG was not substantially reduced in the test group treated with Cosaldon, following electro-convulsion treatment. Since the EEG did not slow significantly after the treatment mentioned, the α-wave index measured initially remained essentially unchanged. This is in contrast to the results obtained from the group of patients who did not receive additional treatment with Cosaldon.

It was only possible to record *fresh elements in the EEG* in exceptional cases, and these were non-specific. *In no case in the test group were there suspected convulsion or convulsion-like events or convulsion elements such as are seen in the untreated comparison group. There was no clinical symptomatology of an epileptic episode in the test group.*

As a result of the electro-convulsive treatment, there was mainly activation of the α-wave rhythm, activation of the α-waves which existed before treatment and an occasional slight slowing over the frontal to the anterior temporal cerebral regions. This slowing was concentrated over the *left temporal regions* of the brain.

Our results confirm electroencephalographically (by objectivizing the altered bioelectrical cerebral activity) the neuropathological findings on the changes in the brain following convulsions of various etiologies. This applies to patients who did not receive Cosaldon treatment in addition to the electro-convulsions.

Now, how can the action of Cosaldon in preventing the undesirable bioelectrical and clinical manifestations of electro-convulsion be explained?

In our opinion, the major contribution of Cosaldon is its chemo- and haemodynamic effects. During electro-convulsions, among other things there is spasm of the cerebral vessels during passage of the current through the brain, and then there is respiratory arrest with cyanosis.

The spastic changes result in anoxia or hypoxia of the local cerebral tissue and this damages the membranes of the nerve cells. This damage causes changes in the bioelectrical cerebral activity and this is manifest in the EEG as severe general changes.

The immediate reaction in the vessels not only causes a change in the local cerebral tissue but it also has an effect on the vessels themselves, so

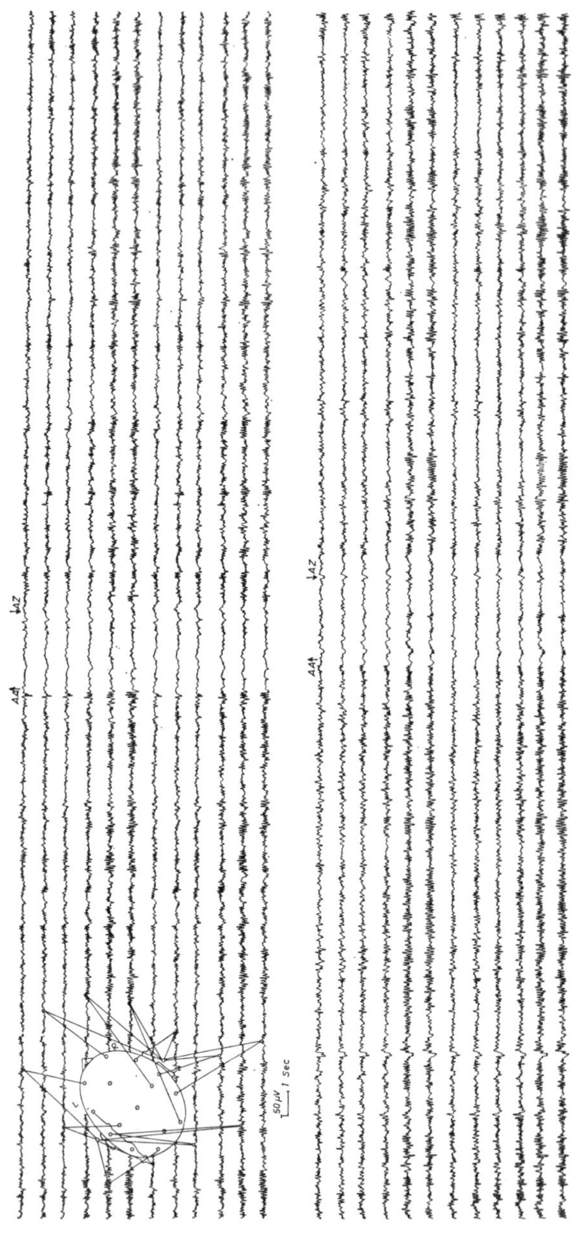

Figure 36. Bioelectrical cerebral activity before (a) and after (b) ten electroshock treatments in a 56-year-old female patient who had also been given oral prophylactic treatment with nicotinic acid and xanthine. As compared with Figure 34, it can be seen that these two drugs, which were combined in one preparation, had a prophylactic effect since there was very little change in the EEG after the electroshock treatment (our own results, original).

that there is a change in the permeability of the blood-brain barrier and this then causes further cerebral lesions. Since it is known that electro-convulsions must be repeated several times before psychotic symptoms disappear, this causes more and more fresh changes in the cerebral vessels and it leads to further changes in the permeability or lesion of the nerve cell membrane (Alexander and Löwenbach 1944, Quandt and Sommer 1966, 1969; Scholz 1951).

By dilating the cerebral vessels, the xanthine substance in Cosaldon increases blood flow and this results in improved blood supply to cerebral tissue (Betz and Rosenhäuser 1962, Quadbeck 1962, Ramos et al. 1963, Ueki 1962).

Probably, during *electro-convulsive therapy* there is no spasm of the cerebral vessels under the action of Cosaldon and thus there is no anoxia of the brain. Accordingly, temporary damage due to the action of the electrical energy is avoided. Again as a result of the improved blood flow through the brain due to Cosaldon, there is no longer any major changes of bioelectrical cerebral activity at the nerve cell membranes. Thus, the EEG no longer reveals the pronounced changes which are seen in the untreated group of patients, and the specific manifestations indicating an increased readiness of the brain to produce convulsions, are no longer observed. Further, it may be assumed that the prophylactic action of Cosaldon is sustained after the direct effect of the electrical energy during the convulsion. This means that there are no changes of permeability and also that there is no anoxia of the cerebral tissue.

The curtailment of respiratory arrest *after the convulsion* is of decisive importance in the action of Cosaldon. According to Scholz (1951, 1959), where there are convulsions there is anoxia of the cerebral tissue. This anoxia occurs both during the convulsion and also later, as a result of the respiratory arrest (and the defective O_2 saturation of the blood), as cyanosis. Cyanosis is certainly a very visible indicator of central anoxia and this is no longer seen, or is hardly apparent, after additional treatment with Cosaldon. Thus, Cosaldon not only improves the circulation and thus provides more favorable conditions for nutrition in the brain during the convulsion, but it also has an effect after the convulsion. The significance of glucose uptake for cerebral nutrition has recently been re-emphasized by Gottstein (1967). We discussed this question in Chapter V. It is understandable that variable cerebral damage during electro-convulsion mainly occurs after the convulsion has ended since it is then that the cyanosis is most pronounced. In the comparison group (without additional Cosaldon treatment) the convulsion lasted for about 25 seconds. In addition to this, there was a further approx. 26-second period of respiratory arrest after the electro-convulsion. Thus, the brain was without normal blood circulation and nutrition for *a whole minute.* When the treatment is repeated eight to ten times, the effects of this therapy can be appreciated.

In the patients treated with Cosaldon, the entire convulsion also lasted for about 25 seconds. However, on average the respiratory arrest only lasted for three to four seconds. It is clear from these figures that the brains of these patients can only be without normal biological blood circulation for *half a minute.* Thus, in contrast to the comparison group, the disturbance of the physiological processes is reduced by more than half by Cosaldon. It can be concluded from this that the effect is twofold: *on the one hand, during the passage of the electric current and during the convulsion it prevents changes in the blood vessels, provides better circulation in the brain and thus prevents cerebral anoxia; on the other hand, it shortens the period of respiratory arrest after the convulsion and hence shortens the total period in which the electro-convulsion has a profound effect on the brain; this means that there is never, or hardly ever, any cyanosis.* This explains the decisive effect that Cosaldon has on the nutritive processes in the brain both during and after the electro-convulsion, since it maintains the supply to the brain cells at a normal level.

In the second stage of the experiment, which involved two groups each of 30 patients (a total of 120 patients in the two stages), the results from the first stage were confirmed. Thus, we did not carry out a fresh statistical assessment (see also Jovanović 1970c, d).

However, in the course of time two further patients developed clinical epileptic attacks so that out of a total of 60 patients who did not receive additional Cosaldon therapy there were three clinical and electro-encephalographic epileptic attacks and in nine it was possible to observe electroencephalographic convulsion-specific elements. In the other group of 60 patients who received Cosaldon orally during the course of electroshock, there were neither clinical nor electroencephalographic signs of increased predisposition of the brain to convulsion. (Jovanović 1970c).

In the third stage of the experiment, we examined nicotinic acid and SK-7 in separate ways. We found that the effects of these two substances differed from (Jovanović 1970 d, 1972 b, c).

In conclusion it should be pointed out that there are many other substances which occur naturally in the body or which can be administered artificially, which may have a facultative anticonvulsant or anti-epileptic action. We have not been able to go into detail on these, but many were discussed in Chapter V.

ANTIEPILEPTIC AGENTS FROM THE THERAPEUTIC POINT OF VIEW

DIBENZAZEPINES *(DIBENZOAZEPINES, CARBAMAZEPINES).* Here we should like to discuss a fairly new substance which has aroused great interest among research workers and physicians in recent years (see also Chapter IX).

Carbamazepine (Tegretol®, Tegretal®, see formula) is produced by the chemical combination of two psychotropic drugs, the antidepressant *iminodibenzyl* (imipramine, *Tofranil®*, see formula) and *imidostilbene* (opipramol, *Insidon,* see formula).

Structural formula: **5-carbamyl-5H-dibenzo(b,f)-azepine, carbamazepine, Tegretol, Tegretal)**

C=C
H H
N
C=O
NH_2

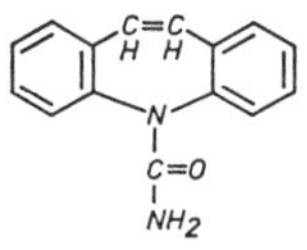

Structural formula: **5-(3-dimethylamino-propyl)-10,11-dihydro-5H-dibenz (b,f)-azepine (imipramine, Tofranil)**

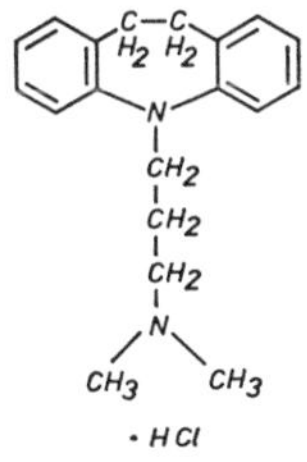

C—C
H_2 H_2
N
CH_2
CH_2
CH_2
N
CH_3 CH_3
· HCl

Imipramin

Structural formula: **imidostilbene (opipramol, Insidon)**

C=C
H H
N
CH_2
CH_2
CH_2
N
N
CH_2
H_2C—OH
· 2 HCl

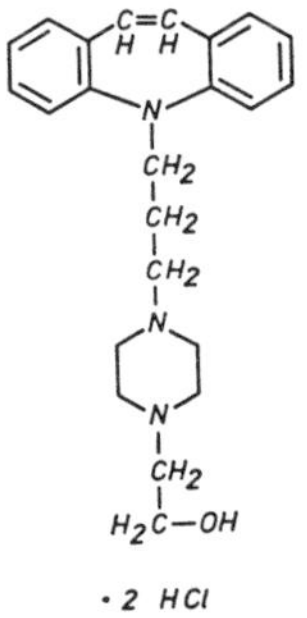

Opipramol

In Chapter VI we dealt with imipramine as a potential epileptogenic substance. However, here it appears—combined with a substance from the same chemical group—as an *anticonvulsant with a psychotropic action.* The action of the combination is quite different from the actions of the two components alone, and as this combination occupies a special position among both psychotropic drugs and anti-epileptic agents we would like to examine it more closely. We shall also be most interested in this substance when we come to discuss the various mechanisms of action of drugs in epileptics (Chapter IX).

Theobald and Kunz (1963) were among the first authors to experiment with this substance. They found that its properties resemble those of phenobarbitone when used in rats where the convulsions are induced by electroshock. However, its anticonvulsant action is quite different from that of *diphenylhydantoin.* An oral dose of about 20 mg/kg. diphenylhydantoin gives partial protection against convulsion, and it is not possible to protect the animal completely from a convulsive attack with any dosage below 400 mg/kg. *With carbamazepine, convulsions are partially inhibited with a dose of about 5 mg/kg. while 18 mg/kg. gives total protection against 80 Volts, and 107 mg/kg. total protection against 100 volts.*

Further investigation indicated that carbamazepine has a mild sedative and tranquillizing effect. On the other hand, these preliminary experiments did not reveal any analgesic or anti-emetic action.

The oral LD_{50} in mouse is 3750 mg/kg. and in rat it is 4025 mg/kg.

Following the preliminary experimental investigations, the drug was examined clinically. Lorgé (1963) observed the effects of Tegretol in a total of 154 patients with epileptic attacks, over a period of three and one-half years. Treatment could not be continued right up to the end of this period in 22 cases and so 132 patients remained for final assessment. 68 of these were male and 64 female. At the beginning of treatment the youngest was one year and four months old and the oldest 72 years old. Most patients were between 10 and 20 and 29 years of age. More than half had been suffering from epilepsy for 10 to 20 years and the remainder had had epilepsy for more or less time than this. Most patients had a mixed form of epilepsy (52 cases), 32 had grand mal, 24 had epilepsy with oligophrenia and 11 cases had temporal lobe epilepsy. The rest were suffering from other forms of epilepsy. There were co-existing psychopathological symptoms in 101 patients.

In most cases treatment lasted for three to six months or two to three years, and the dose varied between 200 and 800 mg. daily.

Under this regimen Lorgé found that there was complete freedom from attacks in 32 cases, the attacks were reduced by 75 percent in 29 cases and by 50 percent in 18 cases, and in eight the effect was doubtful. The psychotropic effect was described as *very good* in five out of 101 cases, as *good* in 10 and as *fair* in 15 cases. There was no substantial change in 18 patients and in 10 the preparation had to be discontinued prematurely because of side-effects.

Before treatment, convulsion elements were present in the EEG in nearly every case. Following treatment with Tegretol, convulsion potenials increased in 13 cases, there was no change in 29 cases and there was a decline of convulsion-specific events in 23 cases. In some of these 23 patients the changes in the cortical EEG disappeared completely. In eight cases there was an increase of cerebral dysrhythmia, in eight other cases it declined, and it remained the same in the rest of the patients. Tegretol proved to be effective in nearly all forms of epilepsy, particularly in *psychomotor epilepsy*. However, the preparation did not have any effect on pure petit mal seizures. The author regarded this new anti-epileptic agent with its concurrent psychotropic effects as an important advance in the treatment of epilepsy.

Following Lorge's first report (1963), Jongsmann (1964) examined and treated 70 epileptics with Tegretal. 43 of these patients had grand mal, three petit mal and 24 psychomotor attacks. The preparation proved to have an anticonvulsant effect, particularly in grand mal. There were very good results in 23 of the 43 cases with grand mal and equally good results in *psychomotor epilepsy* (10 of 24 cases become free from attacks). The author stressed the unusually good psychotropic effect in these forms of epilepsy.

Jacobs (1964) then tested the medicament in 80 children and adolescents. There was an improvement from the point of view of incidence and intensity of attacks in 63 patients with grand mal, psychomotor and combined attacks. The author recommends Tegretal for treatment of hospitalized patients and also for treatment of ambulant patients, since there do not appear to be any side-effects. Much better results can be expected in ambulant patients than in epileptics who have been in hospital for years on end. Very good results were obtained in the 18 children and adolescents (ambulant patients).

Horyd and Patelska (1965) have dealt with the problem of treating epilepsy (including treatment with Tegretal) in great detail. They observed 50 of their own patients, and they also include a discussion on the literature which had appeared on this subject up to that time.

In the same year, Dreyer (1965) treated an imposing number of patients with Tegretal: 416 epileptics (203 men, 156 women and 57 children). Dreyer instituted the therapy himself in 401 cases and continued it for months; for the purposes of this report, a special examination of 120 cases was carried out. 21 of these 120 cases were from the group with *essential* epilepsy, 70 had symptomatic epilepsy and 29 had epilepsy of unknown origin. There was a confirmed familial predisposition in 15 cases. The average age was 29.9 years, the youngest was 14 and the oldest 56 years old. The average duration of the disease was 14.2 years, the longest 48 and the shortest two years. All patients were hospitalized.

Most patients had either isolated (27 cases) or combined psychomotor epilepsy (74 patients), and only a few of the patients had other forms of epilepsy.

The results were promising. Freedom from attacks was achieved in 33 of 120 epileptics, the attacks were reduced by 75 percent in 10 cases and by 50 percent in 16 cases. In 60 patients (i.e. in 50% of cases) he found no change and the clinical picture deteriorated in one case. However, the author points out that his patients had been to many hospitals before they were referred to the institution and hence, there were special problems with this therapy. The best results were achieved in cases of grand mal combined with psychomotor attacks (38 of 74 cases) and where there were isolated psychomotor attacks (14 of 27 cases). The favorable psychotropic effect approximately paralleled these results.

Bioelectrical cerebral activity was unchanged in 50 patients, improved in 33 patients and it deteriorated in 23 cases; the EEG findings could not be assessed in 14 cases. In 15 cases the bioelectrical cerebral activity did not correlate with the clinical result.

At the end of his discussion, Dreyer adds that the substance carbamazepine is an anti-epileptic agent and not a psychotropic drug or a neuroleptic agent. He says that further studies are needed to discover the extent of its dual mechanism of action, i.e. its anticonvulsant and psychotropic properties.

Braunhofer (1965) treated 193 epileptics with carbamazepine for 25 months and he found a considerable number of patients were freed from attacks (143 cases). There was a substantial reduction in the number of attacks in a further 33 cases. According to Braunhofer, the action of this preparation differs from that of other anti-epileptic agents. Tegretal does not cause central sedation and it does not tend to accumulate as compared with barbiturates and hydantoins. Even with prolonged use and higher dosages atactic disorders do not develop. On the other hand, there is a thymoleptic component of action which is of particular advantage to patients who are at work. There is no need to combine Tegretal with other anti-epileptic agents or psychostimulants. There are comparatively few side-effects: slight fatigue, feeling of dizziness and more rarely nausea and transient fusion disorders with double vision, only occur during the first few days.

All forms of attack responded in the same way and Braunhofer concludes from this that Tegretal is a broad spectrum anti-epileptic agent.

Lasich (1966) reported on seven patients and one patient with trigeminal neuralgia who were successfully treated with Tegretal. Haneke (1966) used this preparation in children. He studied 92 children and adolescents in whom psychomotor epilepsy was the most common disorder.

There were very good therapeutic results and comparatively few side-effects. Of 54 patients with psychomotor epilepsy (isolated or combined with grand mal) only eight remained resistant to therapy (approximately 15% of cases). Haneke does not consider that Tegretal is superior to other conventional anti-epileptic agents for treating other forms of epilepsy.

Following Tegretal treatment, the electroencephalographic pictures corresponded to the reconstituted clinical picture.

Livingston et al. (1967) observed 87 patients under therapy with carbamazepine. 63 of 87 patients had isolated psychomotor attacks or psychomotor attacks combined with other forms of seizure. All patients had previously been treated with one or more conventional anticonvulsants without success. The author points out the very good and good results, and only a few side-effects (mainly diplopia).

In one of his most recent papers, Vasconcelos (1967) reports on 250 cases treated with Tegretal. However, results from only 125 cases were used since the author was not able to examine the rest personally. There were 79 men and 46 women, the youngest being nine years old at the beginning of therapy and the oldest 74 years of age. All patients had been suffering from attacks for at least five years, and most of the group were chronic cases. Therapy lasted for between one and 36 months; it was less than a year in most patients. The results are similar to those obtained by the other authors referred to. Visconcelos compared his results with those of the other authors and he includes a number of summary tables.

Out of a total of 432 cases with grand mal which the author had assembled from the literature, 181 patients (41%) were completely freed from attacks under therapy with Tegretal. The incidence of attacks was reduced by at least 50 percent in a further 127 cases.

The following obtained for psychomotor epilepsy: out of a total of 240 patients, 74 (30%) became completely free from attacks and the incidence of attacks improved by at least 50 percent in a further 83.

Comparing these results with the therapeutic results with other anticonvulsants, there is no advantage in treatment with Tegretal. However, Tegretal is superior from the point of view of side-effects. One woman treated by Hansek and Sartorius took 20 gr. Tegretal in an attempt to commit suicide. After a phase of acute poisoning, there were no further harmful effects.

Leder and Timäus-Wolf (1967) and Knauel and Grüter (1967) studied the psychotropic action of Tegretal. Both groups of authors were able to demonstrate that the substance has a pronounced psychotropic effect.

Leder and Timäus-Wolf examined 30 patients and Knauel and Grüter 191 cases. The remarkable feature of these results is that Tegretal was *astonishingly effective even in apparently severe cases of dementia.* Thus, the term *dementia* can no longer be considered clinically valid as a description of a state of mental deficiency.

In his most recent paper, Leder (1968) has reviewed the results of treatment with Tegretol from all the literature that has been published throughout the world, with particular regard to the problem of the preparation's psychotropic effect. He also includes the results of his own objective studies using various psychological tests in 50 patients (mainly with psychomotor epilepsy).

The results gleaned from the literature appear to him to support the hypothesis that Tegretol improves the pathological behavior of epileptics, particularly the *enechetic* personality. The clinical finding improved in one third of his patients following a three-month course of treatment with Tegretol. Corresponding comparative figures from the literature examined by Leder indicate 30 to 59 percent. Delving deeper, it was not possible to establish for certain the extent to which Tegretol differs from the placebo in its effect on the condition of his patients. Leder does in fact say that some of his patients reported some improvement in their condition even after the placebo, although such improvements could not be demonstrated objectively.

However, in four of the ten diagnostic tests selected, differences were confirmed at the 5 percent level of significance. The patients treated with Tegretol considered themselves to be more vital and to be fresher (list of qualities), in the ideation stress test (test d_2 after Brickenkamp) their performance improved quite considerably, there were fewer complaints of somatic symptoms under Tegretol (list of symptoms) and the m-reaction in the Szondi test did not occur so frequently.

According to Leder (1968), in nocturnal epileptics who have undergone an *enechetic* change Tegretol stimulates self-restraint of action and the range of the intentional arc, encourages openness in relations with other people and elevates the patient's mood. The symptoms of an attack in themselves often become less severe. The patients completely lose their hypochondriac self-consciousness.

Each day brings more reports on the anticonvulsant and psychotropic activity of carbamazepine. So much literature has been published on this subject in recent years that we shall have to confine ourselves to the most important reports (Dalby 1971, 1972; Elian 1972; Espinosa 1972; Fumi 1972; Krüger 1972; Mamoli 1972; Meijer 1971; Pryse-Phillips and Jeavons 1970; Scheffner and Schiefer 1972; Singhal et al. 1972; Vaneva and Achikova 1971).

Now we shall briefly discuss our own results which have not yet been published (see also Jovanović 1972a, d). From evening to the next morning we continuously monitored the patients' electroencephalograms and in addition to leads for the cortical EEG we included electrooculogram, respiragram, ECG, electromyogram and measurements of the galvanic skin reflexes, and in this way, among other drugs, we also tested Tegretol. Up to the time that we compiled this report, we have studied 30 patients with psychomotor epilepsy (16 isolated and 14 combined) each on two nights before administrating the preparation and on three nights following therapy with Tegretol. The first night monitored immediately followed a one-day course of treatment, the second followed a three-month course of treatment and the third followed a six-month course of treatment.

The dose varied between two and four tablets daily or 400 to 800 mg. Sixteen patients were given Tegretal alone (isolated psychomotor epilepsy) and 14 (combined psychomotor epilepsy) were given the preparation combined with 250 to 500 mg. Mylepsinum.

The course of sleep, attacks and attack equivalents *before* treatment corresponded to the features described in Chapter I, but here we are mainly concerned with the phenomena occurring *after* treatment.

After a one-day course of treatment sleep is deepened and it may be disturbed. Otherwise the seizure phenomena still did not normalize. *After a three-month course of treatment* there were significant changes.

The patients now took longer to get to sleep than before therapy, indicating that this phase of sleep was normalized. The process of falling asleep was the same as that of 20 healthy test subjects used for comparison.

The first sleep period (*sleep period,* see Jovanovic 1969 b) was more superficial, the deeper stages of sleep were shorter and the superficial stages longer. This meant that sleep, which had been altogether too deep before, had become normal. The second sleep period was also more superficial and shorter so that it now resembled that of healthy test subjects. The third sleep period was much the same. However, before treatment it had been very much the same as that of healthy subjects. There was little change in the fourth and fifth sleep periods since, before treatment, they had been much the same as in healthy subjects.

Considering sleep from the point of view of its different stages, these tended to become more normal, and this paralleled the change in the sleep periods.

The patient's cortical motoricity was more active as he fell asleep and during sleep. Motoricity had been depressed previously and thus it was normalized by the medicament. This motor activity was manifest as normal sleep movements and not as convulsive twitching, which may increase after administering certain drugs and which is not a positive sign of the medicament's efficacy. After three months, the patient's sleep situation resembled that of a healthy person.

After this three month course of treatment the dream phases were longer. Before treatment the dream phases in psychomotor epileptics had been shorter than in healthy persons. The dream content (in patients awakened during the dream phases and questioned in the morning) was richer and the content was acceptable to the patient. Before treatment the dream content had been poor and memories of it were confused.

There was a significant rise in respiration and heart rate. Activity of the sweat glands was reduced after treatment, i.e. the patients did no sweat so much during sleep.

Convulsion elements in the EEG were clearly reduced in number and intensity after three months' treatment. On average, there was a 75 percent reduction over the whole night and the convulsion elements which remained during sleep were distributed in a different way than before therapy.

Before treatment there was actually a very high percentage of convulsion elements during the first hour of sleep (36.6% where the total in one night is taken as = 100%). This figure was reduced to 6 percent after treatment. The percentage of convulsion elements was also significantly reduced in the second hour of sleep. The fall in the percentage during the third hour of sleep was also significant, although it was also significantly different from the percentage in the second hour of sleep, i.e. the fall in the percentage of convulsion elements in the third hour of sleep is less than in the second hour.

The fall in the percentage of convulsion elements in the fourth hour of sleep was not significant, but there was a clear tendency to normalize. In the fifth hour of sleep there was again a slight reduction of convulsion elements in the EEG under the action of Tegretal. In the sixth hour of sleep the number of convulsion elements was not definitely reduced. From the sixth hour (seventh and eighth hours) there was very little effect on convulsion elements in the sleeping EEG.

If we now consider the percentage distribution of convulsion elements in the EEG (which have been reduced by 75%) throughout the hours of sleep during the night and compare this with the corresponding percentage distribution before treatment we find that the picture is reversed: *before treatment there was an accumulation of convulsion elements in the sleep of patients with EEG psychomotor epilepsy in the evening, and after treatment there is an accumulation in the morning,* i.e. the effect of the preparation wears off as the night progresses, so that we need to consider the possibility of producing a sustained action preparation. However, there is still an absolute effect on the convulsion elements in the morning after six hours of sleep ($p < 0.05$).

Fewer attacks arise out of sleep after a three-month course of treatment

($p < 0.01$). However, 14 of the 30 patients had also been treated with Mylepsinum and this combination reduced the number of attacks arising out of sleep by in all, 89 percent Somnambulism ceased after this treatment. When symptoms of an attack did occur, they were confined to smacking of lips, sucking or licking, with the corresponding correlatives in the EEG, but these attacks did not last for longer than 12 seconds. The patients did not wake up or attempt to get out of bed as they had done before therapy (see Chapter II). In the morning the patients seemed to have slept well; they were not tired, but they were wide awake, responsive and very active.

The daytime EEGs were definitely altered by Tegretol. The dysrhythmia which may have been seen in the first few days disappeared after eight to ten days. Pathological elements in the EEG and the basic rhythm both showed a significant tendency to normalize ($p < 0.05$).

No fresh pathological elements appeared in the EEG after three-months' treatment, and there were no foci or other changes which may have indi-

Daytime attacks were reduced by about 75 percent by Tegretol alone or combined with Mylepsinum. No more prolonged twilight states were recorded although these had occurred before treatment. Any psychomotor attacks experienced by the patients resembled brief absences, like an interruption of thought processes or a condition like dizziness. However, this dizziness could not be related objectively to genuine vertigo, nor was it a side-effect of the preparation.

After six months' treatment, sleep, which had already improved, only altered slightly. The process of falling asleep was a little longer than after three months' therapy and the deeper stages of sleep were rather more brief ($p > 0.05$). Although sleep resembled that of a healthy person. Cortical motoricity was even more active than after three months' treatment, but still within normal limits.

The distribution of deep sleep throughout the night was the same as that of healthy subjects and this was not concentrated mainly in the first two-thirds of the night as was the case before treatment. The period of wakefulness, which before treatment occurred mainly in the morning, was then distributed over all three thirds of the night and the period was no longer than in healthy persons. Waking in the night was also like that of healthy people.

Autonomically (as measured by respiratory rate, cardiac action and galvanic skin reflexes) the patients were now just the same as healthy subjects.

The dream phases were also normal after six months. The content of the dreams was rather richer than after three months' treatment but still normal and not unpleasant for the patient. On a percentage basis, the convulsion elements in the sleeping EEG were the same as that after three months' treatment. However, there was a significant fall in the number of convulsion elements after six months as compared with after three months ($p < 0.05$).

The number of clinical attacks showed a marked decline, and after six months very few attacks were recorded during sleep. Isolated, transient episodes of motor twitching occurred but these did not make the patient wake up, or precipitate changes in the EEG.

There was a further significant fall in the number of daytime attacks ($p < 0.05$).

We have kept these cases under observation as ambulant patients over the last three years and the number of manifest attacks has not increased again during this observation period. All but six patients are at work.

On the basis of all these results, we can regard carbamazepine (Tegretal) as a good anti-epileptic agent and psychotropic drug. These studies also demonstrate that Tegretal occupies a special position as a therapeutic agent, and this is not due simply to its chemical composition. (see also Jovanović 1970g).

We did not find that there were any side-effects during our observation period. However, from the very outset, i.e. before stabilization, we attempted to find an optimum dosage, and this was checked by continuous monitoring on a polygraph over 12 hours, so that there was no question of overdosage.

Maxion (1968, 1971) has studied the sleep patterns in patients treated with Tegretal. Quick comparison of his results reveals differences, but only at first sight. His patients slept deeper after administration of Tegretal, i.e. their sleep was not more superficial as in the case of our patients. However, this discrepancy can be explained by the differences in the patients selected. We selected patients with psychomotor epilepsy which had preexisted for from three to eight years. Some of Maxion's patients had psychomotor epilepsy, but his group also included some cases with other diseases. The age distribution among Maxion's patients was also different from ours. Our patients were between 20 and 40 years old. He studied 25 men between 10 (i.e. children) and 60 years old (elderly, and far above the age in our group). Only six of his patients had psychomotor epilepsy, 15 had generalized attacks and four were suffering from other complaints. Of the five women examined whose ages ranged from 16 to 49 years (again the range is greater than in our patients) only two were suffering from psychomotor epilepsy.

As we demonstrated in Chapters I and II, epileptics from other groups (centrencephalic epilepsy) may also exhibit sleep disturbances and experience superficial sleep, and medicaments will have a different effect on sleep here, as compared with deep-sleeping subjects.

On the other hand, we have also observed that to a certain extent the sleep of patients who have only been taking Tegretal for one day is deepened. However, this effect of deepening the sleep recedes after prolonged treatment. Maxion (1968) only gave Tegretal for one day and observed the sleep during the following night. He attributes the resultant deepening of sleep to a *euhypnic* property of the preparation.

Maxion (1968) observed that paradoxical sleep was shorter after one day's treatment with Tegretal. We did not find that it was shortened, in fact the reverse was the case. This phenomenon must be a result of the heterogeneity in Maxion's collection of patients. Disturbed sleep also leads to shortening of paradoxical sleep. If orthodox sleep (Jouvet 1969, 1972; Monnier 1969, Jovanovic 1970 a, 1971 a, 1972 a) is deepened, paradoxical sleep disturbances disappear. However, there is another reason for curtailment of paradoxical sleep, for when deeper stages of sleep predominate there is little time left for paradoxical sleep.

However, our results correlate with those of Maxion as regards motoricity during sleep for he too reports vigorous motoricity during sleep, and this becomes more marked in the morning. Both authors found that the incidence of attacks was reduced in epileptics.

We should not conclude our discussion on Tegretal without mentioning one further point. Patients with psychomotor epilepsy do not only exhibit deep sleep; their sleep is also superficial on the night of an attack and possibly for one or two nights beforehand (see Chapter II). These attacks, which aggravate the disorder, disappear following administration of Tegretal and this promotes the deepening of sleep. However, this is probably not due to a *euhypnic* action of Tegretal, as was assumed by Maxion (1968, 1971), but is the result of eliminating these sleep disturbances.

However, to conclude, it can be assumed that *Tegretal promotes sleep where sleep is disturbed and inhibits sleep where it is very deep.* This is the desired effect, and it is rare to come across drugs which are capable of exerting a dual action, the nature of the action being *determined* by the *substrate* (in this case by the nature of the sleep disturbance).

We shall deal with the neurophysiological action of Tegretal on the bioelectrical cerebral potentials in various formations and nuclei in the brain, in Chapter IX.

BENZODIAZEPINES have become increasingly important in recent years for antiepileptic and psychotropic treatment of epilepsy. It is not easy to compare their status with that of carbamazepine; in fact, there are indications and situations where benzodiazepines are the only drugs which can help. Some benzodiazepine derivatives have proved to be very effective particularly where the condition is acute, such as in status epilepticus or in severe forms of epilepsy in children where all the conventional antiepileptic agents have failed. We shall now mention the most important benzodiazepines.

In recent years *chlordiazepoxide* (Librium®) has found increasing use in the treatment of epilepsies. According to Lowell and Randall (1960), Librium has a more powerful anticovulsant effect than hydantoins or barbiturates on convulsions induced by pentylenetetrazole and electroshock in the mouse. Clinical experience has also shown that chlordiazepoxide has at least the same effect, and it may actually be superior to diphenylhydantoin and Luminal (Kaim and Rosenstein 1960, Keith and Ardoline 1960, Rosenstein 1960, Voelkel 1960, Hollister (cit. in Hubach 1963) administered 100 to 600 mg. Librium daily to 30 patients for many months.

When side-effects were seen in 11 patients the preparation was abruptly discontinued. Two of these 11 patients experienced major attacks during the treatment-free period. However, it must be emphasized that a high dose was used. During withdrawal of barbiturates and alcohol, Tauber (1960) gave patients Librium and he found that the convulsions were milder. Other authors have also dealt with this question (Bowes 1960, Breitner 1960, Caliezi 1962, Clark 1961, Cohen et al. 1961, Farb 1960, Voelkel 1960). Trolle (1965) has reported good results from using Librium in epilepsy. Focal attacks showed good improvement, and the preparation had a very good effect in psychomotor epilepsy. 35 patients were treated.

Broser's recommendations (1966) for treating personality change, depressive states and similar psychical abnormalities include the use of *7-chloro-2-methylamino-5-phenyl-3H-1,4-benzodiazepine-4-oxide* (Librium). However, he does not recommend this drug for use in severe psychotic conditions in epileptics, although we have found Librium to be effective in these cases also.

Diazepam (Valium®) has proved to be a better and more powerful anticonvulsant than chlordiazepoxide. In recent years, several authors have reported very good results in combatting status epilepticus and *psychomotor attack status.* Severe twilight states with complete loss of consciousness and disorientation also respond extremely well to Valium. Trolle (1965) treated 50 epileptics with diazepam. Twenty of these were male and 30 female; 44 were adult and six children. Twelve patients were only troubled by one type of attack, 24 had two types and 14 had a combination of several forms of attack. 35 patients had grand mal, 30 psychomotor attacks, 12 focal attacks, 13 petit mal and 12 other uncharacteristic attacks. In the course of treatment, 45 patients were also given other preparations: five received diazepam alone. Freedom from attacks was achieved with this preparation in five patients with psychomotor attacks, in one with petit mal and in one with combined major and minor attacks. A 90 percent reduction in the number of attacks was achieved in one case with psychomotor epilepsy, in six cases with focal attacks and in two cases with petit mal. The attacks were reduced by from 50 to 90 percent in eight patients with psychomotor epilepsy and in two with focal epilepsy. A favorable, but transient effect was reported in 19 cases with psychomotor epilepsy, four with focal epilepsy, five with petit mal and one with combined major and minor attacks. No more than a slight improvement or less than a 50 percent reduction in the attacks was recorded in 10 patients with psychomotor epilepsy, one with focal epilepsy two with petit mal and eight with other attacks. The clinical picture did not deteriorate in any case and there was no response in 11 cases. The dose varied between 30 and 40 mg daily.

Piqué and Herking (1965) achieved very good results in acute and dangerous epileptic conditions. Diazepam was administered intravenously to five of eight cases in status epilepticus. The status was terminated and the patients recovered consciousness. The clinical picture was very much improved in three other patients. These authors also reported the effect of diazepam on 51 EEG's. All electroencephalograms normalized very well. These authors present and discuss an extensive bibliography on the subject of diazepam and Librium, and many other authors mention Valium as an anti-epileptic agent (Tchacaloff 1965, Weinmann 1966).

Recently the amount of literature on diazepam has increased considerably (Angst 1968, Bamberger and Matthes 1966, Bettis et al. 1968, Elian 1969, Gänshirt 1967 a, b. Gastaut et al. 1971, Isler and Dumermuth 1968, Ketz 1967, Müller et al. 1966, Mumenthaler 1967, Parsonage and Norris 1967, Penin 1967, Prior et al. 1972, Roth 1968, Santamouris and Heye 1966, Tassinari et al. 1972, Weinmann 1966).

Diazepam has proved of particular value in *status epilepticus,* particularly in patients who have failed to respond to any other anticonvulsant or psychotropic drugs.

Bamberger and Matthes (1966) treated 30 children with status epilepticus. The mean dose of the preparation was 4 mg. by slow intravenous injection. In seven cases a satisfactory response was achieved with a dose of only 2 mg. i.v. The highest continuous injection of Valium was 14 mg. in one patient. The EEG was monitored in all cases during the injection and improvement in the clinical picture and disappearance of convulsion potentials in the EEG were taken to be the most reliable signs of an improvement in the condition. 10 of the 30 cases were grand mal patients in status epilepticus at the beginning of treatment. Following administration of 1.5 mg. (maximum 10 mg.) Valium, the tonic-clonic spasms ceased with five minutes in every patient. In three cases convulsions recurred 15 to 40 minutes after the end of injection. In one case a repeat injection of Valium terminated the status again, whereas another patient had to be transferred to other preparations and the last of the three patients could not be saved. One injection was sufficient to terminate a prolonged *hemi-grand mal status* in two of four patients, while the injection had to be repeated in the other two patients before they responded. This drug was used in three infants with confirmed *propulsive petit mal status,* and this inhibited this serious clinical picture for 40 to 50 minutes in two cases. The hypsarrhythmia in the EEG also subsided temporarily. In the third case there was simply a reduction in the convulsion potentials. Six cases in a *myoclonic-astatic petit mal status* were also treated, and in all cases the status was immediately terminated, but four cases then relapsed after 20 to 50 minutes. Three of them then responded to a further injection. Good results were also obtained in the remainder of cases with *absence status.* 16 of 30 cases in status epilepticus responded to a single injection. 14 cases relapsed after some minutes, but a repeat injection brought lasting relief to six of these 14 cases.

According to these authors, the principal advantage of Valium is its lack of hypnotic effect and the fact that it is well tolerated even by infants. However, it has the disadvantage that it only has a relatively short duration of action.

Müller et al. (1966) used diazepam to treat 12 cases with status epilepticus. Nine cases were in convulsive and three in a non-convulsive state. One of these patients, who was admitted to a hospital in a hopeless condition with convulsive status epilepticus, only showed a partial response, but in all other cases the result was described as good to excellent. Compared with treatment with barbiturates, there was a rapid onset of action, less impairment of consciousness and less respiratory and circulatory depression.

Müller et al. recommend 10 mg. i.v. followed by an infusion of 30 mg. in 300 ml. 5 percent glucose over five hours as a suitable dosage for adults. Santamouris and Heye (1966) have also reported termination of *status pycnolapticus* with 10 mg i.v.

Parsonage and Norris (1967) also used diazepam in nine cases of convulsive status epilepticus. The condition was brought under control immediately after the injection in seven patients, while an infusion had to be set up for the other two cases. Ketz (1967) has published a survey on this problem.

In five cases we achieved rapid normalization of convulsions, the psychotic state and cerebral activity, using diazepam. These results have not yet been published. We shall now describe two of these five cases, because they seem to us to be extraordinarily impressive.

Case 8

One afternoon a man about 30 years old, athletic constitution and 168 cm. tall appeared in our Out Patients' Department. He was not able to answer any questions, and could not even give his name, and it was impossible to find out what we wanted and why he has come to us. No one was with him. He was restless and walked up and down the room. He showed no motor symptoms of psychomotor epilepsy, but he was sweating profusely. However, he allowed us to examine him. We immediately took an EEG. This revealed very slow cerebral activity and now and again convulsion elements appeared. While the EEG was being monitored, 10 mg. diazepam was injected i.v. in 10 minutes. The entire picture changed during the injection.

PSYCHICALLY: In the first minute of injection there was no improvement. In the second minute he raised himself on the examination couch and began to make orderly movements. In the third minute he made a further series of coordinated movements. In the fourth minute he was able to tell us his name. It was H.M. In the fifth minute he replied to our question of how old he was: 30 years. In the same minute he told us that he was a trained engineer. In the sixth minute he told us that he was married and had two children. Between the seventh and tenth minutes he was able to give us a short case history without any important errors. We learned that he experienced twilight attacks and twilight states and was being treated at our hospital. We were able to check from his case history that what he had told us under continuous injection of Valium, was correct.

EEG: In the first minute there was slight synchronization, but no improvement. In the second to third minute the basic rhythm speeded up and theta waves of 4 to 7/sec. were recorded; these had not been present before injection. In the fifth minute the EEG rhythm was still in the theta wave-band. However, there was further acceleration of the electroencephalogram. Between the fifth and tenth minutes after starting the injection, cerebral activity returned to 7 to 8/sec. with a high amplitude, but without any delta waves. Within half an hour of continuous monitoring of cerebral activity, it had returned to within normal limits.

At the end the patient was completely normal both psychically and as regards his motor system and he was able to leave hospital that day unaccompanied. We had obviously terminated a twilight state very near to a status, and this did not recur during the days which followed.

Case 9

One afternoon the doctor on duty in our Out Patients' Department received a telephone call from a man asking for help because he was experiencing an attack and he had lost his way. In reply to the doctor, the man told him that he was alone in a telephone box in the town. His voice broke off suddenly and the doctor called to him loudly telling him to come to the hospital, but he did not turn up. The next day a colleague brought him into the EEG department; he had found the man outside the hospital, completely disorientated and confused. The patient was not able to tell us anything, his name or the name of the doctor he was speaking to even though he knew the doctor. An EEG was taken immediately. Cerebral activity showed large, irregular polyspikes and waves with isolated sharp waves (see Chapter II). The electroencephalogram was very much slower and characterized by large slow delta waves. Earlier EEG curves for this patient had shown many more spikes and waves, but there was not much slowing of the basic rhythm. One injection of 10 mg. Valium in 10 minutes transformed the picture in the same way as in Case 8.

The patient was able to say where he was and to converse normally. On the previous day he had drifted off into a twilight state and did not know what had happened since then. He was a philosophy student and had learned about epileptic attacks from some educational literature he had read. His attacks covered the entire spectrum of epilepsy, except BNS spasms, and hardly a day went by without him experiencing some kind of attack.

The electroencephalogram improved with the clinical condition. However, the condition did not normalize since the patient's EEG persistently showed irregular synchronous and generalized spikes and waves even when he was not experiencing clinical attacks—i.e. in the interval.

On the basis of these results, we would point out the following in respect of diazepam: *it has an extraordinarily rapid onset of action, but the action wears off equally rapidly.* Status epilepticus may recur within the hour and be arrested again with the same drug. Generally speaking the effect is even more short-lived in children. Recently, these characteristics have been emphasized again and again by research workers, but we are still not sure of the mechanism responsible for these actions (see Chapter IX).

Nitrazepam (Mogadon®, Mogadan®) is the third substance from the benzodiazepin group which has an anti-epileptic action (see Chapter IX). However, its action is slightly different from that of Librium and very different from that of Valium, although the substances are similar chemically.

Nitrazepam has not proved of value in status epilepticus. However, promising results have been obtained in a severe—perhaps the most severe—form of epilepsy, Blitz-nodding-salaam spasms (BNS spasms). This is a relatively new agent and it is not yet possible to say whether these good preliminary results will be confirmed by further trials.

Weinmann (1966) treated 15 children with propulsive petit mal (BNS spasms) and he found a very good improvement both in the clinical picture and in the EEG. His publication is illustrated with EEG curves which show an astonishing degree of normalization only 10 days after beginning administration of Mogadan. After 10 days' treatment, severe dysrhythmia with generalized and diffusely scattered spikes and sharp waves (which Gastaut calls hypsarrhythmia) no longer appear in the EEG.

We have performed experiments in reverse (Jovanovic 1969 b) to see whether convulsion elements appear in healthy subjects (20 test subjects between 20 and 40 years of age) when nitrazepam (Mogadan) is given to them in the evening. Polygraphic recordings were taken continuously in the following 10 to 12 hours throughout the night's sleep and during the waking period in the evening and morning. No elements which could be interpreted as epileptic appear in the EEG, although before treatment there were variations between the patients as regards cerebral activity and the autonomic system at different levels of sleep and during the waking period. We do not know what effect the preparation has in toxic doses in man. We used single doses of 10 to 20 mg.

Preparations from the meprobamate group impair the level of consciousness slightly, they are fairly powerful muscle relaxants and they are also anticonvulsant agents. They act both centrally and peripherally (Henry et al. 1957, Unna 1957). However, the anticonvulsant action is demonstrated most clearly in petit mal and in BNS–spasms already mentioned (Geratz 1959, Nissen 1970, Perlstein 1956, Quilliam 1957).

This preparation induces interesting withdrawal phenomena, including *twilight states* (Barsa and Kline 1956, Bokonjic and Trojaborg 1960, Essig and Aibslie 1957, Haizlip and Ewing 1958, Hubach 1963, Kalinowsky 1958, Lemere 1956, Tucker and Wilensky 1957).

Although meprobamate is not a powerful anti-epileptic agent and is seldom used as such in general practice, attacks with convulsion potentials in the EEG occur immediately after discontinuing the preparation. Essig (1958) observed convulsions in dogs following withdrawal of meprobamate. Hollister and Glazener (1960) observed the same in man and Hubach (1963) has discussed in detail the withdrawal symptoms of many preparations including meprobamate.

ALDEHYDE PREPARATIONS used to be commonly used but nowadays they are only given on rare occasions to treat serious and acute conditions. Prolonged administration does not improve an epileptic condition, indeed the condition may actually deteriorate (Hubach 1963). Use of *paraldehyde* cannot be avoided in some cases and it is quite often employed in status epilepticus. However, it is no longer used as an anti-epileptic in the strict sense of the word.

BROMIDES are one of the oldest types of anti-epileptic preparation and at one time they were used in nearly all forms of epilepsy. Bromine can still be found in some modern preparations, but it is often left out because of its side-effects. Bromide poisoning (Ammann 1916), clouding of consciousness (De Boor 1956), coma (Geiger 1955), brominism due to chronic use, tremor, ataxia, speech disorders, addiction, delirium and other signs of intoxication and unpleasant effects were quite common when bromine preparations were in common use (Casamajor 1911, Curran 1938, Diethelm 1930, Geiger 1955, Holmden 1890, Kolle 1955, Levin 1960, Meggendorfer 1928, Möllenhof 1928, Schabelitz 1915).

BARBITURATES (see also Chapter IX) have long been in use as anticonvulsants. Luminal and Prominal are often used indiscriminately to treat any form of epilepsy, even though their antiepileptic effect is limited to certain forms. They are most effective in centrencephalic epilepsy, but less effective in the temporocephalic group of epilepsies, including psychomotor epilepsy (see Chapters III and IV.)

Since the effects of barbiturates are well known, we shall confine ourselves to a brief discussion on a new substance which has recently aroused some interest.

This is a chemical combination of phenyl-ethyl-barbituric acid and a mild stimulant. The chemical name of the compound is *L-1-cyclohexyl-2-methylamino-propane (CHP)-5-phenyl-5-ethylbarbiturate* (see structural formula). This compound is marketed under the name *Maliasin®*.

Structural formula: **L-1-cyclohexyl-2-methylamino-propane (CHP)-5-phenyl-5-ethylbarbiturate (Maliasin)**

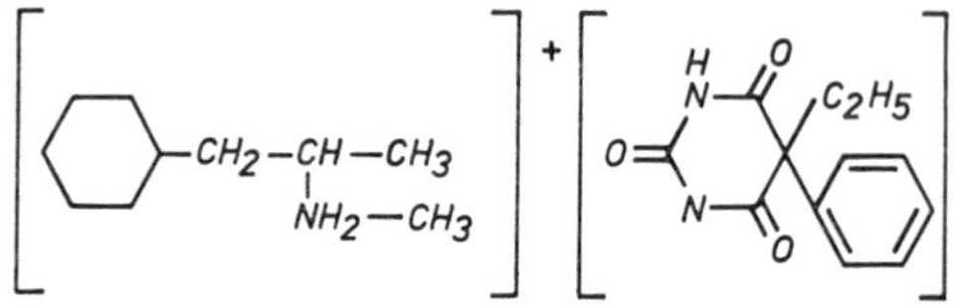

From the therapeutic point of view, this compound has proved particularly valuable in the centrencephalic forms of epilepsy, particularly in matutinal epilepsy. Good results have also been reported in petit mal (Becker 1968, Canger and Wahl 1968, Christian 1961, Faerø et al 1972, Haas 1963, Hallen 1953, Jovanovic 1966 d, 1967 b, 1968 c, Krüger and Schwartz 1965, Penin 1964). Canger and Wahl (1968) reported on the results of treating 298 epileptics over a period of four years. Many of the patients could not be used for evaluating the results, so that the authors were only able to assess the results in 110 patients.

The preparation was effective in cases of grand mal. However, according to Canger and Wahl, this drug does not seem to have a specific action in one of the forms of epilepsy, as was suggested by the authors referred to above. Canger and Wahl only report a marginally better action in matutinal epilepsy and there was no significant effect in the psychomotor form of epilepsy.

However, we (Jovanović 1970 b, 1972 a) found that this drug had a certain amount of activity in our cases of psychomotor epilepsy, particularly in patients who frequently suffer psychomotor episodes during the night, causing them to get out of bed—*somnambulistic form of epilepsy* (see Chapter II). In these forms of epilepsy a sleep disorder may develop unexpectedly and it is not easy to treat.

Hydantoin preparations have recently become a very important form of treatment in epilepsy, although here again they cannot be prescribed indiscriminately without taking into account the type of epilepsy involved. For example, matutinal epilepsy and petit mal do not respond very well to hydantoins and it is beter to revert to barbiturate in these cases. In our experience, *Maliasin*—a combination of barbituric acid with it hypnotic action and CHP which has a stimulant effect—is the drug of choice in these forms of epilepsy (Jovanovic 1968 c). Nocturnal epilepsy and psychomotor forms respond better to the hydantoins, but here again there are limitations.

Merrit and Putnam (1938) first discovered the anticonvulsant action of *diphenylhydantoin.* While examining a series of test substances they noticed that diphenylhydantoin was particularly active. Knoefel (1940) succeeded in increasing the *convulsion threshold of the cerebral cortex* in the cat by 50 percent and this significantly suppressed convulsions which originated in the cerebral cortex. He used a dose of 5 mg/kg. diphenylhydantoin. Diphenylhydantoin does not prevent cocaine or strychnine convulsions. Thus, these experiments show that deeper structures of the brain are not greatly affected.

Since then, a great deal of literature on diphenylhydantoin has been published (Kimball 1939, Kröber 1950, v. Lehoczky and Dubos 1941, Mezei 1941, Robinson et al. 1941, Ross and Jackson 1940, Weinland 1950, Winemiller 1941, Zanello 1940). Merrit and Putnam (1938) treated 350 epileptics with diphenylhydantoin and they found that there was a sharp fall in the number of major attacks. The authors stress the fact that unlike bromide preparations and barbiturates, diphenylhydantoin does not cause any side-effects. They state that the activity of diphenylhydantoin does not decline, even after two year's therapy.

According to initial observations by Frankel (1940) and Robinson (1942) diphenylhydantoin has a favorable effect on an epileptic's personality and improves his vitality. These preliminary results were later supplemented and corrected.

Lennox (1947) recommends diphenylhydantoin for use in grand mal and focal attacks. He regards this preparation as the drug of choice in focal attacks, whereas it has to be combined with barbiturates in grand mal.

Janz (1950) initially treated 85 epileptics with diphenylhydantoin. This substance was strictly successful in 54 patients. About half of the patients had previously been under treatment for years with other drugs, without success. The results from 16 patients could not be included in the evaluation because these patients did not follow the doctor's instructions.

Rommelspacher (1950) treated 20 patients with diphenylhydantoin (Zentropil®) and found that the preparation was effective in all forms of epilepsy, particularly twilight attacks and emergency conditions. However, he used too few patients for statistical evaluation of the results.

Weinland (1950) prescribed diphenylhydantoin for 712 of 1,294 hospitalized epileptics. He demonstrated that the preparation has a very favorable effect in major attacks and very few patients failed to respond to treatment. Ziehen (1950) also found that there was a good effect in grand mal and he reports that the preparation is more powerful than other anticonvulsants in suppressing the tonic phase of an attack, and this may actually disappear completely. He suggests that diphenylhydantoin reduces convulsive activity at every level in the CNS. However, this hypothesis has not been completely confirmed.

Kröber (1951) recommends diphenylhydantoin for use in grand mal and psychomotor epilepsy. Stauder (1951) refers to all the literature on the preparation available up to then, and he draws attention to the fact that it is better tolerated than other drugs. However, our own practical experience has shown that side-effects are not all that uncommon.

Schleissing (1951) and Bittner (1953) have discussed the problems of diphenylhydantoin therapy, and they consider that this preparation is very suitable for treating grand mal, and it is also recommended for use in pregnant women with epilepsy. Bittner (1953) reports his results in individual patients.

Dreyer (1953) has had a considerable amount of experience in this field and he believes that diphenylhydantoin can be used to advantage in grand mal forms of different aetiologies, but it is of little or no use in petit mal.

When treating 38 chronic epileptics, Lustig and May (1955) found that there was a definite reduction in the incidence of attacks following diphenylhydantoin alone or in combination with barbiturates (Zentronal®). Szobar and Frater (1955) were able to relieve their patients of attacks even in musicogenic epilepsy (one case).

Vollmering (1955) considers this preparation to be a highly active antiepileptic agent and that it is superior to other anticonvulsants in many respects; however, there is emphasis on the motor component of the attack here. The mechanism of action has still not been elucidated (see Chapter IX).

Ziehen (1955), Brauknecht (1956) and Zeuner (1959) have reported on their results using diphenylhydantoin, although unfortunately these are not suitable for statistical evaluation. Zeuner describes his results obtained in individual patients.

Geese (1961) reports good results with diphenylhydantoin combined with barbiturates in five cases. All his patients were able to go back to work after treatment.

Janz (1962) reports on the problems of treating a large number of epileptics who were applying for annuities. He also provides statistical data on his good results in an even larger number of other epileptics under diphenylhydantoin treatment.

Ulrich (1962) and Stucke (1964) have reported the results of treating various forms of epilepsy with diphenylhydantoin and and they also mention some side-effects.

According to Ulrich (1962) and many of the authors mentioned above, common side-effects of diphenylhydantoin treatment are gastric disorders, nausea, eosinophilia, and more rarely allergic reactions, rise of temperature and glandular swelling, dizziness, ataxia, cerebellar gait, reactions in bone marrow such as agranulocytosis, panmyelopathy, thrombopenia, and (harmless) gingivitis.

These authors, state that the dose of diphenylhydantoins is generally between 300 and 400 mg/kg. and more rarely up to 500 mg/kg.

We should now like to take this opportunity to point out a connection between epilepsy and trigeminal neuralgia. Hydantoin preparations have proved valuable in both diseases (Dam Mogens 1970, Danielson et al. 1971, Frid et al. 1972, Gabka 1961, Jensen 1954, 1955, 1956, Joss 1957, Fulian and Halperin 1972, Krings 1955, Pincus et al. 1970, Popp 1954, Seliger 1956, Sorrell et al. 1971, Sperling and Stender 1955, Stille 1960) and carbamazepine preparations are also used in both diseases. The two diseases exhibit a similar dysrhythmic EEG over the cortex and they are both by nature paroxysmal. These diseases also resemble one another in many other respects. The mechanisms of action of the diphenylhydantoins is interesting here (see Chapter IX).

Now we should like to give a brief survey of our own experience in using diphenylhydantoin (Zentropil®).

Following administration of diphenylhydantoin, we observed the clinical picture, the effect on convulsion elements in the EEG particularly in the sleeping EEG, the effect on the sleep pattern, and effect on dream phases and the psychical response during the waking hours.

In one report (1967b) we discussed the sleep pattern in epileptics before and after treatment, and we included all forms of epilepsy. As we have already pointed out in Chapter II and above, patients with nocturnal and psychomotor epilepsy sleep deeply, fall asleep rapidly and they have a sleep excess and attacks and convulsion elements in the EEG arise out of sleep.

Following administration of Zentropil to nocturnal and psychomotor epileptics the period of falling asleep (normally short) is delayed and prolonged, and the patients have enough time to adapt to the trophotropic situation (Monnier 1969). As time goes on sleep becomes more superficial and the patient's cortical motoricity becomes more lively; the number of attacks is reduced and convulsion elements are rarer, or they disappear altogether.

However, in this report we emphasized that administration of hydantoins over a period of time results in such a superficial pattern of sleep that, rather than an excess of sleep, the patient may acquire a sleep deficit. We suggested that in these patients hydantoins alone should only be prescribed at the beginning of treatment. After a couple of weeks, and at the latest after three months, therapy should be combined with a hypnotic preparation.

Later trials (Jovanovic 1968 c) confirmed our initial results and also provided some additional information. Up to then, we had examined 129 epileptics. Twenty-eight patients were suffering from nocturnal epilepsy combined or not combined with psychomotor attacks; 37 patients were suffering from diffuse epilepsy combined or not combined with psychomotor episodes, and 14 patients had pure psychomotor epilpesy. The remaining patients had other forms of epilepsy.

Nocturnal studies during sleep by EEG and other polygraphic monitoring were carried out after *three* and *nine* months. *In nocturnal epileptics three months' treatment* with 100 to 400 mg. *Zentropil* daily lengthened the period of falling asleep and increased motor disturbances on falling asleep, which sometimes disturbed the sleep. Fewer convulsion potentials were observed in the EEG on falling asleep, as compared with the period before treatment. The sleep was more superficial than before, but it was still within the normal limits. Significantly fewer attacks arising out of sleep were observed as compared with the situation before treatment.

At *the nine-month check,* there were more twitchings and other motor disturbances than after three months and the sleep was more restless and longer. Patients who had a sleep surplus before treatment now showed a sleep deficit. However, there were fewer convulsion elements in the EEG than before treatment. There were more motor disturbances during dreams than before therapy and more was remembered about the dreams.

There were no more major nocturnal attacks after nine months' treatment, and minor and psychomotor attacks were significantly reduced. Concomitant therapy with a hypnotic (Maliasin® or Mylepsinum®,) improved the sleep and potentiated the favorable effect on attacks, attack equivalents and convulsion potentials in the EEG.

As in nocturnal epilepsy, in diffuse epilepsies with and without psychomotor attacks, after three and nine months it was found that the process of falling asleep was delayed, sleep was more superficial, there was an increase of motor disturbances (unpredictable motor twitching and movements), convulsion elements in the EEG were reduced and there were fewer clinical attacks during sleep or while the patient was awake. The results were much better if hypnotic agents were given in addition to Zentropil. Sleep was not then disturbed by a great deal of motoricity and there were significantly fewer convulsion potentials and attacks than with Zentropil alone.

Diphenylhydantoin had the same effect in psychomotor epilepsy as it did in nocturnal epilepsy.

Our experience to date, some of which has been published (Jovanovic 1969 c), confirms these results.

These findings indicate that hydantoin preparations are particularly effective in suppressing the motor components of an attack particularly during the waking hours. Here again within a short time other drugs have to be given as adjuncts since the motor disturbances increase. This is most clearly seen during sleep.

This means that therapy with diphenylhydantoin alone is not quite sufficient for treatment of psychomotor epilepsy and that this form of epilepsy demands several types of combination since the focus is not in the neocortex (see Chapters II and III), which is the principal site of action of these preparations (see Chapter IX).

A PYRIMIDINE DERIVATIVE, *5-phenyl-5-ethyl-hexahydropyrimidine* (Mylepsinum®) is sometimes considered to be a member of the acetylurea group of anticonvulsants (Dreyer 1964). However, it is of special interest among anti-epileptic agents which are effective in psychomotor epilepsy. The structural formula bears some resemblance to barbituric acid (see formula) so that many authors have explained the action of this preparation as being due to its being metabolized to phenobarbitone in the body (Butler and Waddell 1956, Plaa et al. 1958).

Structural formula: **5-phenyl-5-ethyl-hexahydropyrimidine (Mylepsinum®) (Mysoline)**

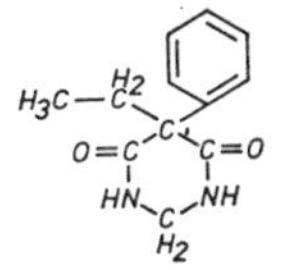

H_3C-CH_2 / $O=C$, C, $C=O$ / HN, NH / CH_2

As we shall report later, many of the properties of Mylepsinum differ completely from those of phenobarbitone and Frey and Hahn (1960) have confirmed that *primidone* (Mylepsinum) has, per se, an anticonvulsant effect and that this is not, or not always due to its being converted into phenobarbitone.

The properties of Mylepsinum were first examined by Bogue and Carrington (1953) and Goodman et al. (1953). These authors found that it has a more powerful anticonvulsant effect than hydantoins or phenobarbitone against electrically induced convulsions. It also has a pronounced anticonvulsant effect following pentylentetrazole convulsions.

Grand mal and psychomotor epilepsy respond the best to this medicament (Booker et al. 1970, Cartellieri 1956, Dreyer 1956, 1964, Haneke 1965, Matthes 1967, Wenzel 1958). Janz (1962) carried out a statistical analysis and he found that out of 3350 patients with epileptic symptoms, there were good results with Mylepsinum in 72 percent with nocturnal epilepsy, in 65 percent with matutinal epilepsy and in 55 percent with diffuse epilepsy. 81 percent of patients with petit mal were freed from attacks (impulsive petit mal) and 40 percent of cases with psychomotor epilepsy responded similarly. Other forms of petit mal did not respond so well to Mylepsinum.

The side-effects reported are usually harmless symptoms such as a feeling of intoxication and dizziness. Drowsiness is also quite common, but this recedes after eight days (Dreyer 1964). Thus, a low initial dose is recommended (Dreyer 1964, Janz 1962 a, b). In very rare cases, megaloblastic anemia may also develop following prolonged treatment. Occasionally more rapid frequencies from the β-wave region are observed in the EEG (Dreyer 1956). However, as the incidence of attacks is reduced, the dysrhythmia is improved or normalized, and the convulsion potentials disappear (Wenzel 1958). With regard to side-effects, primidone is often recommended since it causes fewer side-effects than other anticonvulsants (Dreyer 1964, Lempp 1954). A 28-year- old patient of ours took 78 tablets (in an attempted suicide) and survived. However, she passed through two phases of unconsciousness.

The *first phase* occurred about one to one-and-a-half hours after the tablets were taken. The patient regained consciousness six hours after treatment.

Shortly after the woman had regained consciousness and the symptoms of poisoning had abated, the *second phase* of unconsciousness developed. This lasted until almost 24 hours after she had taken the tablets. These two phases of unconsciousness must be due to primidone being converted into phenobarbitone. The first phase is probably the result of the action of primidone itself. Following the recovery and when the primidone had been metabolized, there must have been a large quantity of phenobarbitone and this resulted in the protracted second phase of unconsciousness.

We have also collected together our own results from treating epileptics with Mylepsinum and the results of our studies using polygraphic monitoring (as described above,—Jovanovic 1967 b, 1968 c, 1970 g, 1972 a) and we shall report on these briefly.

Administration of 750 to 1000 mg. Mylepsinum daily to 53 epileptics with major attacks and psychomotor episodes produced a substantial improvement or normalized all the epileptic manifestations which had been present before treatment. For example, after *three* and *nine* months there was a distinct tendency for total, relative and actual sleep to become normal (Jovanovic 1970 g, 1972 a). The superficial stages of sleep were shorter and the deeper stages longer, as in healthy people. The latent period before falling asleep which was long before therapy, was shortened and normalized after treatment with Mylepsinum. Sleep became normally distributed over each third of the night or there was a tendency for it to normalize in this way.

Convulsion potentials disappeared from the EEG or were significantly reduced by the preparation. In 30 of 53 cases, Mylepsium alone was capable of suppressing all the epileptic phenomena. In the remaining 23 cases, additional therapy with diphenylhydantoin was attempted. Mylepsinum treatment did not have to be discontinued in any case.

In a further 48 cases of combined or isolated psychomotor attacks, Mylepsinum and hydantoins were combined since (as has already been reported) hydantoins alone may have an adverse effect on the patient's sleep and later also on the general condition of the epileptic. Supplementary administration of primidone normalized the sleep pattern and significantly reduced the convulsive attacks or convulsion elements in the EEG. Where these phenomena had already been partially suppressed by diphenylhydantoin, the picture was normalized by concomitant use of Mylepsinum.

We have reported (Jovanovic 1970 g), that sleep becomes disturbed in all forms of epilepsy immediately before, or a few days before an attack, and sleep is disturbed during the night in which the attacks occur. In these cases, we would recommend the use of Mylepsinum in addition to hydantoins and other stimulant anti-epileptic agents, since disturbances of sleep tend to provide an attack.

EFFECTS APPEARING AFTER THE WITHDRAWAL OF ANTIEPILEPTICS

It is known that seizures and twilight states often occur after discontinuing an anti-epileptic agent and there is no need for us to stress the importance of this point here. The mechanism by which an attack is precipitated following withdrawal of the anti-epileptic agent is important. This is known as *post-inhibitory rebound.* We should again emphasize that even *anticonvulsant agents may have a convulsant effect if they are abruptly withdrawn.*

It is worth mentioning in this connection that phenamine and other fast-acting and potent drugs have a short duration of action. This also applies in the same or a similar way to other substances including endogenous amines, other neuromodulators, *diazepam* and *cocaine,* which all have a rapid and favorable effect on epileptic manifestations. However, after peak activity has been reached, there is a rebound phenomenon so that the danger is then greater than it was before giving the drug.

CHAPTER VIII

A NEUROPHYSIOLOGICAL AND BIOCHEMICAL MODEL OF EPILEPTIC MANIFESTATIONS

OUR MODEL OF epileptic and epileptiform manifestations is based on results of clinical (see Chapter I), electroencephalographic (see Chapter II), neuro-anatomical (see Chapter III), experimental neurophysiological (see Chapter IV), and neurobiochemical investigations (see Chapter V), which correlate well with one another. This evidence was supplemented by the findings described in Chapters VI and VII.

We realise that much of this chapter will, to a certain extent, be rather speculative. The use of models is fraught with limitations since they are seldom completely reliable and faithful representations of the actual truth. However, there are occasions when they have to be used since they offer the only possible way of solving a particular problem.

There are a number of mechanisms which may be involved in producing epileptic manifestations.

Firstly, an epileptic episode may be due to a *failure of the blocking* mechanisms in the CNS (failure or inadequacy of inhibitory processes or mechanisms). This can be considered to be the mechanism in many cases (see also Chapter IV) and is discussed further.

The second possibility is an *increase in predisposition to convulsion* (increased neuronal excitability, increased excitation). In these cases some other form of epileptic manifestation often occurs first (i.e. an isolated attack of psychomotor epilepsy is relatively rare here) and so we have dealt with this although we have not discussed this at such length as the mechanism described under previously.

Finally, there is the third possible mechanism which, along with the other two possible mechanisms, may have some part to play, i.e. the *combination* of impaired inhibitory ability and increased excitability in the brain. We shall briefly mention this third possible mechanism at the end of this chapter.

Although we have dealt in some detail with the whole of this problem in previous chapters, before we can construct our model we still need to discuss briefly and *systematically* the *sites* at which disinhibition may occur.

The abolition of inhibitory mechanisms or the occurrence of disinhibition may occur at tvarious places in the CNS (see Chapters II to V) and various mechanisms may be responsible. Here we shall just mention one or two.

1.) Disinhibition occurs at the site of origin of epileptic excitations which, in psychomotor epilepsy, is in the *formations of the Ammon's horn,* so that the excitation is not properly blocked at its site of origin, i.e. in the convulsion focus. *Epileptic discharges* then develop.

2.) Disinhibition occurs a little farther away from the convulsion focus, i.e. further away from the site of origin of the excitations. The interneuron does not inhibit the excitations properly and more impulses are propagated.

3.) Disinhibition occurs at the site of origin and also in the interneurons so that epileptic impulses transmitted from the site of origin are not even inhibited in these neurons. This type of disinhibition occurring at *two* sites is a rather more serious disorder than disinhibition occurring at a single site.

4.) Disinhibition may occur at a third site (the neocortex) during the spread of excitations. In this case, more impulses are transmitted to the periphery via the efferent projections.

5.) There may be a failure of *first, second and third phase* inhibition (from the site of origin to the neocortex) . Here there is a very much greater danger than when disinhibition occurs at one or two sites.

6.) The structures of the lower brain stem do not exert any inhibition.

7.) Failure of the inhibitory mechanisms at the site of origin, in the interneuron, in the neocortex and in the brain stem caudal to the diencephalon.

Similar sites and combinations also occur in the case of increased excitation or where there is interaction of disinhibition and increased excitation.

As we have seen in Chapters IV, V and VII and as will be discussed in Chapter IX, in the last resort, the neuronal transmitters (neurohormones, endogenous amines) play the most important part in the mechanisms responsible for an epileptic attack and attack equivalents. In order to avoid repetition, here we shall simply discuss the effect these neuronal transmitters have in the model of epileptic manifestations. To simplify matters, we are assuming that acetylcholine and/or serotonin are mainly responsible for triggering epileptic impulses in the Ammon's horn formations and the other structures of the limbic system *(acetylcholine/serotonin excitation).* The triggering agent in the thalamus-hypothalamus and the remaining medial structures rostral to the mesencephalon would then be acetylcholine and/or noradrenaline or *acetylcholine/noradrenaline excitation.* Noradrenaline and/or acetylcholine would be responsible in the neocortex or *noradrenaline/acetylcholine impulse generator* and in the brain stem (caudal to the diencephalon) epileptic discharges are mainly produced by serotonin and/or noradrenaline or *serotonin/noradrenaline impulse generator.*

All these neuronal transmitters are discussed later. The part played by the neurohormones mentioned will not be particularly emphasized in the other sections of this chapter, however it is presupposed and should be borne in mind.

A MODEL OF EPILEPTIC MANIFESTATIONS IN CENTRENCEPHALIC TYPES OF EPILEPSY (FIGURE 37)

We must first deal briefly with the problem of the model of the mechanisms responsible for producing an attack in centrencephalic types of epilepsy, since this model is simpler and will help the reader to understand the more complicated model of epileptic manifestations in psychomotor epilepsy (temporocephalic types of epilepsy). However, we must first mention a few events which occur under normal physiological conditions.

Pattern of the Discharges (Excitations, Impulses) Under Normal Physiological Conditions

For reasons of simplicity, we shall assume that the site of excitation is right in the thalamus (it can also be in other adjacent and rather more distant centrencephalic formations). We shall now consider the course this excitation takes on its way to the periphery.

In order to reach the periphery, discharges triggered in the thalamus have to traverse many barriers (bars, relays, synapse groups). We (Jovanović 1968 a) now describe this unknown number of barriers as y. For practical reasons, we shall use a scheme of four groups (y_1, y_2, y_3, y_4) since these can be analysed. These barriers (sum of barriers), which have intentionally been very much simplified, are actually four groups of systematically arranged and extraordinarily complicated functional circuits in the CNS (v. Holst and Mittelstaedt 1950, Jovanović 1968 a, McCulloch 1951, v. Uexküll 1928).

These four barriers can be considered systematically as follows (see Jovanović 1968 f):

THE FIRST BARRIER (y_1) is the site of occurrence of the bioelectrical events which occur after an impulse is triggered, in our case corresponding to the structures of the thalamus.

THE SECOND BARRIER (y_2) would then be the neocortex of the brain. If the excitations break through the first barrier, there is then a rather larger and more complicated functional circuit between the site of occurrence (thalamus) and neocortex. According to our theory, the second barrier also includes projections of the thalamus into the neocortex, since the first barrier was limited to the nuclei of the thalamus and intrathalamic projections.

THE THIRD BARRIER (y_3) occurs in a functional circuit between the neocortex and reticular formation caudal to the diencephalon, and in the reticular formation itself. If the impulses pass through the second barrier in the neocortex, the excitations will be partially or completely suppressed in the formatio reticularis mesencephali et pontis (= RF).

THE FOURTH BARRIER *(y_4)* is centered in the spinal cord (Renshaw 1940, 1941).

To put this in more concrete terms and to simplify the model, let us assume that in the thalamus or adjacent centrencephalic structures $96x$ ($= A_o$) impulses pass from the presynaptic membrane into the postsynaptic functional structures (we have chosen the figure 96 because it is readily divisible; it is also possible to use an algebraic term "*x*", but this would involve frequent use of less practical fractions). Normally, stimuli at synaptic membranes can be classified as *excitatory postsynaptic potentials (EPSP) and inhibitory postsynaptic potentials (IPSP)* (see Chapters III and IV) and fairly powerful excitatory impulses are necessary to produce explosive discharges or *spikes.* For the above-mentioned reasons, the impulses take a physiological course; *activation and blocking* (inhibition).

To simplify matters further, we can assume that each barrier *halves* the impulses. In this case the $96x$ impulses, a figure which we selected at random, will be reduced to half ($A_0/2 = 96x/2 = 48x = A_1$) at the *site of origin (y_1).* The 48x impulses will be halved again in the *neocortex* (y_2). This leaves $24x$ ($A_0/4 = A_1/2 = 96x/4 = 48x/2 = 24x = A_2$) for further propagation. These impulses pass from the neocortex to the caudal brain stem where they reach the *reticular formation (y_3),* where they are again reduced by half ($A_0/8 = A_1/4 = A_2/ = 96x/8 = 48x/4 = 24x/2 = 12x = A_3$). This leaves $12x$ excitatory impulses for transmission to the *spinal cord.* Here we have the fourth barrier *(y_4)* at which, if the impulses are too powerful, they are again halved by a feedback mechanism ($A_o/16 = A_1/8 = A_2/4 = A_3/2 = 96x/16 = 48x/4 = 24x/4 = 12x/2 = 6x = A_4$). Thus, only $1/16$ of the original $A_0 = 96x$ excitatory impulses arising in the thalamus (y_1) actually reach the periphery, i.e. only $6x$ impulses. These are translated into mechanical movement by the effector muscle which carries out the command and hence, has an effect on the environment, which may have been the original source of the stimulus. The synergy of the musculature means that only one group of muscles will function while the antagonists will be inhibited. We have called this the *law of successive inhibition* (Jovanović 1968 a).

The Course of Excitation in the Case of an Epileptic Reaction

If we now consider the effect of excitation in an epileptic and compare this with what we have assumed to be the normal physiological excitatory process described above, we come to the following conclusions.

The provoking factors in the centrencephalic types of epilepsy (matu-

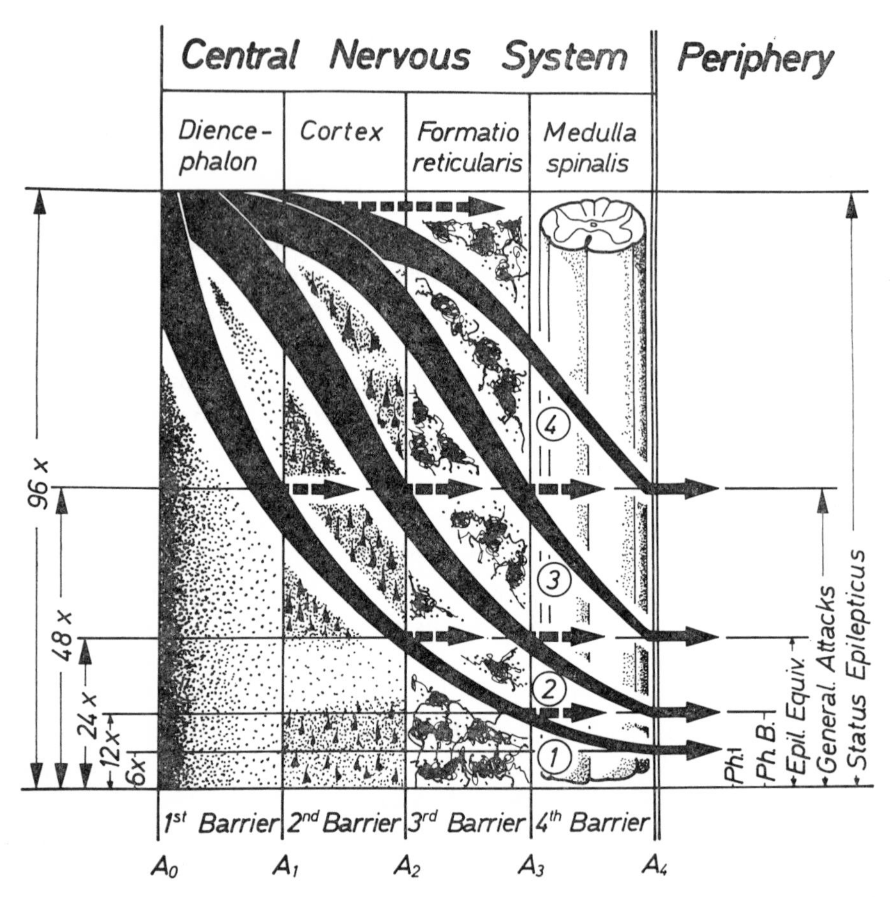

Figure 37. Model of an epileptic attack in centrencephalic forms of epilepsy. Ph = physiological responses at the periphery; Ph.B = possible physiological (i.e. non-pathological) range of peripheral reactions; Epil.Equiv. = epileptic equivalents manifest at the periphery; General Attacks = generalized attacks at the periphery. (See text for further explanation. Our own diagram).

tinal epilepsy of the grand mal and petit mal type) *differ from those in the temporocephalic types of epilepsy (psychomotor epilepsy). In centrencephalic epilepsies, attacks can be precipitated both from the periphery (exogenous) and also from the focus itself or from other structures in the CNS (endogenous)* (see Chapter III). Once the excitation has been triggered the picture does not remain physiological. Because the membrane potential is depressed (partial depolarization, as described in Chapters III, IV and V) even at rest, the IPSP are not capable of suppressing the impulses in the convulsion focus. A state of relative *hyperexcitation or epileptic excitation* develops. If the inhibitory mechanisms are defective at the site of origin (thalamus = y_1), epileptic stimuli build up (Baumgartner 1967, Blasius 1962, Henatsch 1962, Jung and Tönnies 1950) and are transmitted *in unison* (Nigro 1964, 1965). The $96x = A_0$ impulses are not halved at the first barrier (y_1), i.e. reduced to $48x$, but more are transmitted. Now if we assume, for the sake of simplicity, that all $96x$ impulses are transmitted, the demands made of the second barrier would then be at least double those normally found in healthy people.

While the epileptic stimuli are at the site of origin (y_1) the patient may be agitated, more emotionally unstable and he may complain of subjective symptoms, show external signs of unrest and suffer from brief episodes of absence. The electroencephalogram may show a brief period of desynchronization over the convexity, which may be followed by synchronization of the waves with mild to fairly marked dysrhythmia.

There are at least *two* possibilities at the second barrier (neocortex).

First, if the neocortex is still functioning reasonably well, it may be capable of reducing the $96x$ impulses by half. The inhibitory effect in this barrier (y_2) may occur in two ways: by interactions via the thalamo-cortical, non-specific projection system (see Chapters III, IV and IX), and by inhibitory, synaptic elements in the neocortex itself. So the $96x/2 = 48x$ impulses would be transmitted caudally and reach the third barrier (y_3).

Clinically, the effect on the neocortex of double the number of impulses is manifest in the form of absences and *electroencephalographically* as spike-and-wave complexes. If the number of impulses is halved in the neocortex (y_2) and halved again at each of the next two barriers (y_3 and y_4), then double the number of impulses, i.e. $12x$ impulses instead of $6x$ impulses, will reach the periphery. Working on the basis of our model in Figure 37, these impulses will not be capable of eliciting epileptic manifestations, but the patient may show increased psychomotor activity.

Now, if after a certain time and depending on a number of factors (see Chapter III) the neocortex (y_2) is also damaged by this doubled *bombardment* (ictally-induced lesions), it will then be even less capable of inhibiting the epileptic discharges (which are doubled) which reach it from the convulsion focus (y_1). Attack equivalents will then develop. These equivalents may be manifest *clinically* as jerking of the head, forward jerking of the trunk (propulsive petit mal, Janz and Mathes 1955, Janz 1968 b), backward jerking of the trunk (retropulsive petit mal, Janz 1968 b) or jerky tossing movements of the upper arms, head and trunk (impulsive petit mal, Janz and Christian 1957). *Electroencephalographic recordings* show spikes and waves, polyspikes and waves, diffuse dysrhythmia with spikes and other convulsion elements over the neocortex.

Under normal conditions, $24x$ impulses would reach the third barrier

(y_3). In our case, if the neocortex is not damaged, 48x impulses would reach the third barrier, or if the cortex is damaged the full 96x impulses will arrive; this means that they cannot be reduced to their physiological level at the fourth barrier (y_4), so that at the periphery we now have 24x instead of 6x impulses. This would still not produce a generalized seizure, but would lead to isolated epileptic equivalents.

The inhibitory power of the third barrier (y_3) has often been considered when examining the mechanisms responsible for producing an attack. Dell et al. (1961) (see also Chapters III and IV) assume that there is a physiological interaction between the lower part of the reticular formation and the neocortex. The reticular formation (y_3) could exert a certain inhibitory effect on the neocortex (y_2) and could in this way suppress the convulsion elements. Nigro (1964, 1965), Catania and Nigro (1964) and Ardizzone et al. (1965) took a look at the mechanisms responsible for producing an attack from a neurocybernetic point of view, and they considered the reticular formation to be of primary importance. Based on experimental results, in 1965 Nigro stated: "Via corticoreticular pathways, convulsive activity in the cortex affects, in particular, the reticular system and activates it. The reticular system then suppresses the convulsive condition in the cortex by transmitting an appropriate excitatory pattern to the cortex via reticulocortical pathways. The condition of predisposition to epilepsy is due to a disorder of the corticoreticular pathways which prevents information about the convulsive state of the cortex reaching the reticular system. This failure in the controlling mechanism allows a diffuse spread of cortical activity over the whole of the cortex." According to Lindsley et al. (1960) and many other authors (see Chapter IV), collateral branches reach the reticular formation of the pons and medulla oblongata from both afferent and also efferent specific pathways. These are capable of suppressing and reducing to a physiological level stimuli which reach the CNS from the outside and also efferent impulses produced by higher cerebral formations, which are travelling caudally. In this way the reticular formation is capable of controlling impulses both from the periphery and also from the cortex. It follows from what has been said that the reticular formation can also exert its blocking effects in two ways: by interaction between itself and the cortex, and by inhibiting the impulses in its own synaptic elements. Here again, there may be several possibilities.

If the neocortex (y_2) exerts an inhibitory effect on the discharges (which are doubled, 96x instead of 48x) which are being transmitted from the thalamus (convulsion focus), then these will be halved. In turn, the reticular formation will then receive double the number of discharges (48x instead of 24x) and, by the law of successive inhibition, these 48x impulses will be reduced to 24x. The fourth barrier (y_4) again halves the number, leaving $12x$ impulses and, in this case, there will be no peripheral manifestations of attacks or their equivalents.

The doubling of the demand made on the neocortex (y_2) and lack of proper treatment has involved the neocortex itself in this condition and, instead of reducing the number of impulses by half, it allows all the impulses to reach the reticular formation. Now, instead of the normal number of $96x/4 = 24x$ or $48x$ in the case of centrencephalic epileptics without cortical damage, in this case the reticular formation will receive the full salvo of $96x$ impulses and if the reticular formation is still capable of halving these it will send $48x$ instead of $12x$ to the fourth barrier (y_4) where they will be reduced to $24x$ impulses. Assuming that these $24x$ simultaneous impulses are not capable of triggering a classic generalized seizure, the patient will show a few attack equivalents such as jerky twitches, uncoordinated movements, tossing movements of the trunk or extremities and possibly an akinetic seizure or similar symptoms.

However, there may also be clinical and electroencephalographic evidence of the event as a result of hyperexcitation and stimulation of the reticular formation. *Clinically* there may be brief disturbances of consciousness, obnubilation, agitation, psychomotor unrest and excessive emotionalism. The *electroencephalogram* reveals a short or fairly long period in which the waves are flattened, there may be acceleration of the basic rhythm, the convulsion elements which would otherwise be present are blocked or there may be flat dysrhythmia.

In time, the third barrier (y_3) will also be unable to reduce the $96x$ impulses it receives and the full quota of $96x$ impulses will then reach the spinal cord. Even if the fourth barrier (y_4) halves this number, there will still be a generalized attack.

The RF and also the interaction between RF and the neocortex can be enhanced or blocked by certain pharmacologically active compounds, and these compounds are capable of producing specific effects (Werner 1958). Catania and Nigro (1964) succeeded in blocking corticoreticular pathways using *trimetadione.* According to the authors, this abolished the controlling effect of the reticular formation on the neocortex and produced convulsions. In our opinion, chemical and pharmacological effects on the RF and its connections with the cortex and other higher cerebral structures are of great importance in the treatment of epilepsy, since epileptic impulses can be blocked or promoted by using appropriate medicaments (see Chapters VI, VII, and IX).

With the first generalized attack we are faced with another aspect of this problem, i.e. *facilitation,* which can also be produced by chemical substances. Facilitation cannot be incorporated into the model in Figure 37.

Facilitation creates conditions which favor development of major seizures and these seizures damage structures of the brain (see Chapter III), and so a vicious circle develops.

However, the synaptic or direct (see Chapter IV) blocking of hyperexcitation (epileptic impulses) does not end completely after the reticular formation. Whether all $96x$, half of this number $= 48x$, or only $24x$ impulses descend from the convulsion focus to the anterior horn cells (y_4), if they are still above the normal physiological level they will be suppressed. The Renshaw cells (Renshaw 1940, 1941) are in the immediate vicinity of the actual motor neuron and its synergists and they form blocking synapses with these. Collaterals run backwards to these cells (= biocybernetic feedback) from the efferent neurites in front of the anterior horn (Bleichert 1962, Henatsch 1962, Renshaw 1940, 1941). This feedback mechanism prevents excessive contraction of the effector muscle and so these cells are bound to have some effect in the mechanism responsible for producing an attack. Although these devices cannot always prevent a generalized seizure, according to our model they can mitigate such a seizure. In the fourth barrier (y_4) there are even more possibilities than in previous barriers.

In $24x$ impulses $= 96x/4$ pass through the first three barriers and are reduced to $96x/8 = 12x$ at this fourth barrier, then there will not be an attack or an equivalent.

If the epileptic excitations from the site of origin (y_1 = convulsion focus) are not halved in the neocortex (y_2), $96x/2 = 48x$ impulses will arrive at the fourth barrier. This will mean that two barriers (y_1 and y_2) in the brain have failed. In this case these $48x$ impulses will be reduced to $24x$ in the fourth barrier (y_4). According to our model, a generalized attack is not possible here but there will be epileptic equivalents with motor disturbances.

If barriers y_1, y_2 and y_3 in the brain fail, the fourth barrier will receive all 96x impulses and even if these are halved at y_4 there can still be a generalized attack.

In the course of time, the fourth barrier (y_4) will also be damaged and it will no longer be capable of reducing the $96x$ impulses, so they will all reach the periphery.

In theory, our model shows that if status epilepticus is bound to develop (Figure 37); there are other factors which are also responsible for this.

According to our model, in centrencephalic types of epilepsy a generalized attack can only be prevented *if the impulses are properly blocked in the CNS at at least two barriers, i.e. the epileptic impulses are reduced by half at each barrier.* Disorders in the functional circuits (Blasius 1962, Bleichert 1962, Eccles 1953, 1957, 1964, Eccles and Lundberg 1958, Eccles et al, 1964, Grundfest et al. 1938, Henatsch 1962, Jovanović 1968 a, f, Lorente De Nó 1938, 1939, 1943, McCulloch 1951, Raines and Standaert 1969, Renshaw

1940, 1941, Selbach 1938, Selbach and Selbach 1950, v. Uexküll 1928) play an important part here.

A MODEL OF EPILEPTIC MANIFESTATIONS IN PSYCHOMOTOR EPILEPSY (TEMPOROCEPHALIC TYPES OF EPILEPSY, TEMPORAL LOBE EPILEPSY (FIGURE 38)

As can be seen from previous chapters, the biochemical and neurophysiological problem in psychomotor epilepsy or in the temporal lobe type of epilepy is rather more complicated than in the centrencephalic type of epilepsy discussed above. In temporal lobe epilepsies the site of occurrence in the brain of epileptic discharges is *asymmetric* (see Chapters II and III). Over and above this asymmetry, the problem is further complicated by the functional-anatomical and topographical heterogeneity of the focus (see Chapter III). In order to produce a model in this case, we shall assume that the convulsion focus or site of occurrence (y_1) of the epileptic discharges is confined exclusively to the *Ammon's horn.* This focus is in front of a complete blocking system—axial cerebral structures such as subcortical ganglia, thalamus, mesencephalon, rhombencephalon, pons, medulla oblongata—so that here, instead of four groups of barriers there are at least five. This increase in the number of barriers means that, mathematically, there is a definite multiplication of the epileptic manifestation and also of the blocking processes.

The Course of Excitation from the Ammon's Horn to the Periphery in Normal (Physiological) Cases

On the basis of the facts we have already described, there are the following possibilities:

THE FIRST BARRIER (y_1) is in the Ammon's horn which is the site of origin of the bioelectrical impulse.

THE SECOND BARRIER (y_2) occurs in the block of diencephalic structures (to simplify matters: thalamus). To this we must add efferent projections of the Ammon's horn (y_1) up to the second barrier, so that the first barrier only includes nuclei of the Ammon's horn and intrahippocampal projections. Connected in series between the two barriers is the interneuron (Blasius 1962, Eccles 1953, 1957, Eccles et al. 1941, McCulloch 1951) which will have the effect of reversing the excessive number of activating impulses it receives and which acts like a functional *current reverser* in that it forms inhibitory synapses at its efferent endings (see also Chapter IV).

THE THIRD BARRIER (y_3) in this case is the neocortex which receives epileptic stimuli via the thalamic barrier.

THE FOURTH BARRIER (y_4) is in the reticular formation caudal to the diencephalon, and

THE FIFTH BARRIER (y_5) is to be found in the spinal cord where, in centrencephalic types of epilepsy, the fourth is found.

In order to elicit peripheral effects similar to those which occur following transmission of impulses from centrencephalic structures, stimuli from the first barrier (from the Ammon's horn) must be at least *double* those from the thalamus, and so, instead of $96x$, $2 \times 96x$ impulses $(2 \times 96x = 192x = A_0)$ must be generated at the site of origin.

Assuming that the $192x$ impulses (A_0) are normally halved at the site of origin (y_1), under physiological conditions the resultant number of impulses will be $(A_0/2 = 192x/2 = 96x = A_1)$ and these $96x$ impulses will be transmitted to the second barrier $(y_2 =$ thalamus). The blocking effect on these impulses will halve the number $(A_0/4 = A_1/2 = 192x/4 = 96x/2 = 48x = A_2)$ and so $48x$ stimuli will be propagated to the neocortex (y_3) where they will again be halved $(A_0/8 = A_1/4 = A_2/2 = 192x/8 = 96x/4 = 48x/2 = 24x = A_3)$. These $24x$ impulses (A_3) will be transmitted into the fourth barrier (y_4) in the reticular formation caudal to the diencephalon. This will halve the $24x$ impulses $(A_0/16 = A_1/8 = A_2/4 = A_3/2 = 192x/16 = 96x/8 = 48x/4 = 24x/2 = 12x = A_4)$. According to the rule of successive inhibition, the 12x impulses reaching the spinal cord will be reduced to the physiological number (see Figure 38), i.e. $A_0/32 = A_1/16 = A_2/8 = A_3/4 = A_4/2 = 192x/32 = 96x/16 = 48x/8 = 24x/4 = 12x/2 = 6x = A_5$. This means that A_5 would then be 1/32 of the initial impulse (A_0). If, as in the case of the centrencephalic structures, only $96x$ impulses were produced in the Ammon's horn (A_1), only $3x$ $(A_5/2)$ would reach the periphery and, as we have seen above, this impulse level would not elicit a physiological effect. It is on this that we have based our assumption that double the number of excitatory impulses must be produced in the limbic system to elicit a peripheral physiological action or reaction.

The Course of Excitation from the Ammon's Horn to the Periphery in Psychomotor Epilepsy

Having described the normal physiological situation, we shall now go on from the problem of centrencephalic epilepsy to the problem of epileptic stimuli in *psychomotor epilepsy. In this case, an attack and other attack equivalents are virtually bound to be produced by the convulsion focus and peripheral provocation similar to that which occurs in the centrencephalic type of epilepsy is less common* (see Chapter I).

In line with our hypothesis, the processes of the *first barrier* (y_1) may occur as follows: if for any pathophysiological reason (biochemical changes, see Chapters III, IV, V and IX) 192x excitatory impulses (A_0) are triggered in the convulsion focus, the affected synapses may partly or completely fail to assume their inhibitory role. The impulses build up and spread un-

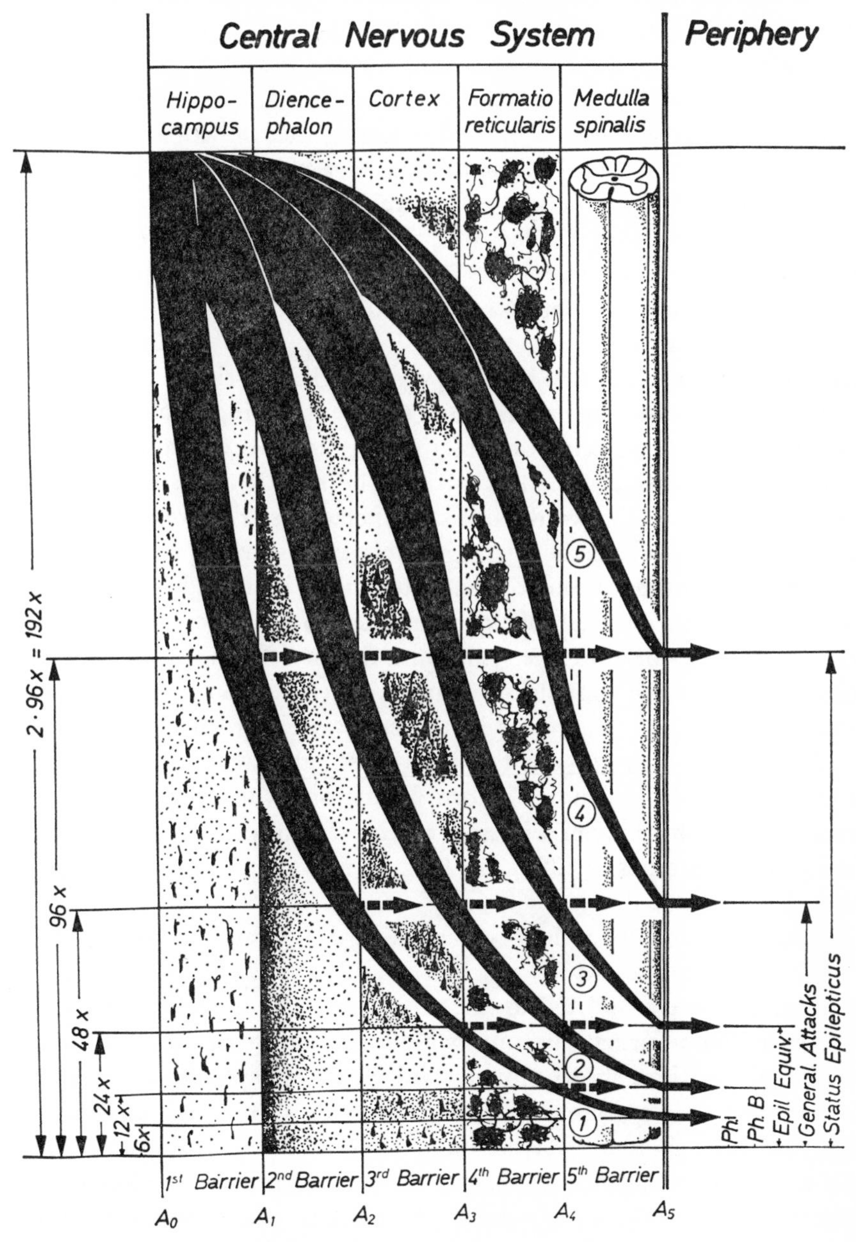

Figure 38. Model of an epileptic attack in temporocephalic forms of epilepsy. See text and Figure 37 for further explanation (our own diagram).

checked. As this type of epileptic excitation spreads in the temporal lobe and towards the diencephalon and reticular formation caudal to the thalamus, the patient develops *clinical* and *electroencephalographic* symptoms which are familiar in psychomotor episodes. Even at this stage there may be external evidence of many of the phenomena mentioned in Chapter I, although the epileptic impulses themselves have not been transmitted to the periphery. In this case, *active* peripheral symptoms such as those which occur with a convulsion are less in evidence and the main emphasis is on symptoms which occur *due to a "deblocking"* of psychomotor functions (isolated psychomotor epilepsy). The patient becomes fairly or extremely restless and suffers from very brief or longer periods of disorientation. If there are changes in the first barrier (y_1) or if this barrier is not functioning properly, the patient may experience a transient feeling of mental obnubilation, changes or a narrowing of consciousness, loss of consciousness, acoustic, olfactory and/or gustatory hallucinations, he may become aggressive, make defensive movements, have dreamlike experiences *(déjà vu, vecu* etc.), his activity may stop altogether without motor disturbances, there may be masticatory and other automatisms, hysterical or hysteroid behavior, he may become stuporous or catatonic or even develop a psychotic reaction and there may be aura or aura-like symptoms, depending on the histological and functional site of the convulsion focus. Abnormal events, which have been described in Chapter II, appear in the cortical electroencephalogram.

The second barrier (y_2) in the centrencephalic structures includes efferent projections of the Ammon's horn formations which extend as far as the diencephalon. This barrier will now receive a total of $192x$ impulses instead of the normal number of $192x/2 = 96x$. Here we have at least two possibilities.

First, if the second barrier (y_2) is capable of halving the doubled number of excitatory impulses which reach it $(A_0/2 = 192x/2 = 96x)$, then $96x$ impulses will be transmitted to the neocortex (y_3). As the stimuli spread in the diencephalic formations and where excitation of these structures is doubled, the patient shows clinical and electroencephalographic symptoms which combine with those developing following stimulation of limbic structures. *Clinically* there may be mental changes including increased emotional instability, excessive emotionalism, increased aggressiveness, longer periods of consciousness changes and similar phenomena (these symptoms still come under the heading of isolated psychomotor epilepsy).

The *electroencephalogram* reveals local changes over temporal regions of the brain and also other, more diffuse phenomena which complicate the overall bioelectrical picture.

The second possibility is that the $192x$ impulses (A_0) transmitted from the Ammon's horn to the thalamus are not reduced by half. They will then be passed on to the neocortex which, instead of $48x$ impulses under normal conditions or $96x$ impulses where the second barrier is functioning properly, will receive the full salvo of $192x$ excitatory impulses. This will result in a generalizing of epileptic stimuli all over the brain and produce manifest clinical and electroencephalographic phenomena.

Clinically, instead of a brief period of disorientation, there will be total amnesia, the patients will experience a fairly short or longer period of absence and they may run away, become rather aggressive and fail to understand the situation, there may be various other psychotic symptoms, tonic deviations of the head and trunk or general tonic muscular changes. Masticatory automatisms and other fairly marked psychomotor disturbances are quite common. The symptomatology varies a lot and tends to change because at one moment the limbic system may be dominant and the next moment dominant factors may be the centrencephalic structures or structures of the neocortex (isolated or semi-generalized psychomotor epilepsy).

The cortical EEG may show isolated spikes, high sharp waves, biphasic or triphasic events, sharp waves in a positive direction, general slowing and hypersynchronization. For short periods there may also be fairly pronounced slowing down to the δ-wave band during which the patient may show psychomotor symptoms.

The third barrier (y_3) is more or less (ir) regularly bombarded with an excess number of epileptic stimuli. Here there are at least *three* possibilities.

In the first case the neocortex (y_3) has only received $96x$ epileptic impulses. Here there is only a *deblocking* at the site of origin of the convulsion elements, i.e. in the first barrier (y_1), which in this case is in the Ammon's horn. We have already described the symptoms above (isolated psychomotor epilepsy).

In the second case the neocortex receives $192x$ impulses or, in other words, the second barrier has failed. We have already described the symptoms which will occur here. If the neocortex is capable of reducing the number of impulses by half, then the fourth barrier (y_4) will receive $96x$ impulses. If these are reduced by half in the fourth and also in the fifth barriers ($48x$, $24x$), then a generalized attack may be prevented. However, a peripheral, *active* motor component may be combined with *passive* psychomotor phenomena which occur as a result of *deblocking* in the brain.

In the third case the neocortex is no longer capable of halving the $192x$ impulses. This will occur sooner or later when the brain has been damaged by epileptic manifestations and excessive amounts of strain imposed upon it. $192x$ impulses will now reach the fourth barrier and if they are reduced by half at the fourth and the fifth barriers, $48x$ impulses (A_2) will reach the periphery. Returning again to our model, this level of impulses is capable of producing a generalized attack (combined psychomotor epilepsy)

(Figure 38). The first seizure causes facilitation which then promotes the development of further attacks, and so a vicious circle develops.

The fourth barrier (y_4 = reticular formation caudal to the diencephalon) may affect the situation in various ways. There are *four* possibilities here.

Half the epileptic stimuli from the limbic system are transmitted to the neocortex ($192x/2 = 96x$). After this number is halved, $48x$ are transmitted to the reticular formation which is left with double the normal number of impulses to halve. This means that attacks and equivalents can be prevented.

In the second case the neocortex (y_3) has received the full quota of $192x$ epileptic stimuli from the Ammon's horn, indicating that the second barrier in the thalamus has failed. The neocortex then reduces this number by half so that $96x$ impulses reach the retitcular formation. The reduction in the number of impulses here in the fourth barrier prevents a generalized attack from developing since the stimuli are further reduced to $24x$ (A_3) in the spinal cord (y_5). However, psychomotor attacks with active peripheral motor components are not inhibited.

In the third case the neocortex, having been damaged, is not capable of halving the $192x$ impulses (A_0) which reach it and so the reticular formation receives the full salvo of $192x$ impulses. Having halved these, they are transmitted to the fifth barrier where they are again halved, so the periphery receives $48x$ excitatory impulses, which are capable of precipitating a generalized attack (combined psychomotor epilepsy).

In the course of time, the reticular formation also loses its ability to halve the $192x$ impulses and so the full quota of $192x$ impulses is transmitted to the fifth barrier and in theory this could produce status epilepticus. Other factors will be discussed later.

At the fifth barrier a number of situations can determine the clinical picture.

If all but the site of origin (y_1) reduce the epileptic stimuli by half, i.e. the impulses are halved at each of the other barriers (y_2, y_3, y_4), instead of the normal $12x$ the fifth barrier (y_5) will now receive $24x$ discharges. If this number is now halved again there will be no attack and no epileptic equivalents.

The second barrier has been bombarded for a fairly long period by epileptic discharges and it is now no longer capable of halving these discharges but it transmits the full number ($192x$) to the third barrier. If these are now halved at each of the following barriers, instead of the normal $6x$ or $12x$ in the case of first barrier failure, $24x$ impulses (A_3) will now reach the periphery. This number of impulses will be capable of producing epileptic equivalents, but not a generalized attack.

Here the third barrier is also damaged so that the $192x$ impulses are passed on in full to the fourth barrier. They are halved to $96x$ by the fourth barrier and transmitted on to the fifth. Even if these are reduced to $48x$ impulses here, a generalized attack will still occur.

In the fourth case the $192x$ impulses are not even blocked at the fourth barrier. Where the disease has been fairly long-standing, the reticular formation (y_4) will have been damaged to such an extent that it is no longer capable of halving this level of hyperexcitation, so thte ffull quota of $192x$ impulses will be transmitted to the fifth barrier (y_5), halved and then passed on to the periphery. Here a generalized attack may be followed by a number of attacks until status epilepticus develops.

In the fifth case the epileptic stimuli pass unimpeded or virtually unimpeded through all the barriers. They are not halved at the site of origin in the Ammon's horn nor in the diencephalon, nor in the neocortex, nor in the reticular formation, so that all $192x$ impulses reach the periphery without being blocked. Our model indicates that this can be fatal (in acute poisoning with convulsant poisons, nerve gases etc.).

Mechanisms Responsible for Producing Status Epilepticus in Patients with Psychomotor Epilepsy

We have already mentioned several times a fairly straightforward way in which status epilepticus can be produced in patients with *psychomotor epilepsy with generalized attacks (combined psychomotor form)* (see Chapter I). However, this mechanism is probably less common than the one which we shall now describe. In status epilepticus there tend to be several successive attacks interspersed with phases of exhaustion during which the patient loses consciousness, and it is less characteristic for all the stimuli to reach the periphery from the brain at once in status epilepticus. This would produce a prolonged attack with no remissions. In our opinion, one of the possible mechanisms responsible for producing status epilepticus with repeated attacks could be as follows.

If the $192x$ (A_0) stimuli are not reduced to half in the Ammon's horn (y_1), then all $192x$ will reach the second barrier by an axo-neuronal pathway or via artificial synapses. The second barrier, i.e. the diencephalon, becomes *hyper*excited and it does not only conduct this hyperexcitation to the neocortex, but it also sends a reverse wave of excitation (reverse stimuli) back to the first barrier (y_1), i.e. back to the limbic system. As we have shown in Chapters III, IV and IX, stimuli can easily reach thalamic, hypothalamic and adjacent structures via a few afferent projections, the old cortex and nuclei of the limbic system (amygdala). In this way, formations in the brain which have already undergone pathological change can be restimulated and a pathological functional circuit formed so that fresh stimuli are constantly leaving the limbic system *(y_1)* and travelling to the periphery. The first series of impulses causes a generalized attack and fresh epileptic impulses descend from the convulsion focus *to elicit a second attack.*

Some of the epileptic stimuli return from the second barrier *(y_2)* to restimulate the first (the Ammon's horn) while more of them continue on into the neocortex. This third barrier then continues to transmit stimuli down to the brain stem. In this situation, the first barrier in the Ammon's horn may be restimulated by impulses returning from the neocortex and so *three series* of epileptic impulses may reach the periphery: *the first series* passes directly from the limbic system via the second, third, fourth and fifth barriers to the periphery where it elicits a generalized attack; *the second series* returns from the thalamus and restimulates the Ammon's horn to produce epileptic stimuli; *the third series,* which is transmitted to the neocortex via the thalamus, stimulates the convulsion focus for a third time and again produces epileptic impulses. In this case, *three generalized attacks* will occur in succession and the patient will not have time to recover consciousness completely after each attack and subsequent phase of exhaustion.

Also, up until they reach the mesencephalon, the impulses may act in reverse and restimulate the Ammon's horn formations, i.e. the convulsion focus *(y_1)*. In this case the first barrier will be stimulated *four times: firstly* by a metabolic defect (see Chapters V and IX) ; *secondly* by a throw-back from the second barrier (from the thalamus) ; a *third time* by a throw-back via the neocortex and thalamus, and a *fourth time* by a throw-back via the thalamus, neocortex and mesencephalon. Consequently there will be *four generalized seizures* in succession and the overall effect may be regarded as status epilepticus.

There is a fourth possibility for reverse stimulation from the reticular formation of the pons and medulla oblongata *(y_4)*. When the first series of impulses reaches the second barrier in the thalamus, stimuli are conducted backwards from the thalamus to the convulsion focus. When the impulses reach the neocortex stimuli are again conducted backwards via the thalamus and other projections to the convulsion focus (Ammon's horn) . A third series of stimuli travel in reverse from the mesencephalon to the Ammon's horn. If the first series of stimuli reach the pontine and medullary reticular formation, they will stimulate the serotonergic (in the raphe system) and noradrenergic neurons (which are somewhat to the side of the median line) (Jouvet 1969 a, 1972) . The release of serotonin and noradrenaline produces a new series of epileptic impulses in the Ammon's horn. In this case *five generalized attacks* may occur in succession, and the patient remains unconscious between each attack. *This cycle may be repeated directly or indirectly several times.*

Another possible mechanism responsible for producing status epilepticus is the effect of stimuli produced by Ammon's horn formations. Let us say, for example, that the convulsion focus is in the *left* Ammon's horn. The epileptic impulses will travel from here to the thalamus and they will also be transmitted to the Ammon's horn in the *right* cerebral hemisphere. These epileptic impulses will then be capable of producing the same or similar types of stimuli and reverse stimuli from the right Ammon's horn so that there may be several generalized attacks following one after the other. In this case, some other blocking mechanism or fatiguing of the convulsion focus may be the only way of altering this process or inhibiting the seizures.

Mechanisms Responsible for Producing a Psychomotor Status

In isolated psychomotor epilepsy (see Chapter I) there can only be psychomotor attacks, i.e. there are no generalized seizures. In this case the process is, in principle, the same as that in status epilepticus with generalized seizures, with the one difference that, here, the impulses *circulate in the brain* but do not reach the periphery. The peripheral phenomenology is of a different type (see Chapter I) since the peripheral musculature of the body is not involved as a result of stimulation of the precentral region of the neocortex. Masticatory and other symptoms occur as a result of a deblocking, i.e. inadequate psychomotor blocking from the limbic system. This type of status is rather rare since, without generalized seizures, *psychotic episodes* or other psychic manifestations are more common. The organism needs to discharge but this cannot be completely achieved by means of a status of psychomotor attacks.

Mechanisms Responsible for Producing Psychotic Manifestations Without Visible Symptoms of Epilepsy

The powerful blocking system in the medial (axial) line (midline) of the brain stem from the lower reticular formation upwards to the subcortica ganglia, also plays an important part here. The medial blocking system can conduct stimuli but, as already described, it can also exert a *powerful blocking action.* During random psychomotor attacks which afflict these patients from time to time, this blocking system may be so powerfully stimulated that every neuronal stimulus emanating from the asymmetric formations of the brain and reaching this block is totally blocked and eliminated. In this case the stimuli are not suppressed at source and they live on in the convulsion focus, but they can only spread as far as the thalamus and cannot reach the periphery. Consequently the organism and brain cannot be bioelectrically discharged. If they are not completely blocked in the diencephalon, stimuli may spread to other formations in the brain and they will circulate in the brain without being able to reach the periphery.

Psychotic episodes with a variable symptomatology (see Chapters I and II) occur as an *alternative* to epileptic manifestations.

Now, what are the neurophysiological possibilities here? No doubt there is a plethora of mechanisms responsible for producing the psychotic manifestation in patients with psychomotor epilepsy and we cannot list all of these here.

The epileptic stimuli *circulate in the limbic system* (y_1) and the route to the thalamus and neocortex is blocked so that they cannot get as far as the thalamic structures. *In this case only the functional-anatomical formations of the limbic system itself would be stimulated.* There are several possibilities here:

a.) If the predominent effect is to stimulate *activating synapses* in the Ammon's horn with release of acetylcholine and serotonin, then the patient will tend to develop a more *illusory-hallucinatory psychosis.*

b.) If the main effect is to stimulate *inhibitory synapses* of the limbic system, then there will be psychomotor retardation, taming, inactivity, blocking of motor activity, obnubilation, anxiety and emotional depression. A *catatonic-stuporous psychosis* will develop.

c.) If more powerful stimuli are produced so that the activating synapses become fatigued, then the inhibitory system will become functionally dominant and the *psychosis will be of a more catatonic type.*

d.) If the convulsion focus (y_1) is bombarded by even more powerful epileptic stimuli, the inhibitory synapses may also become fatigued. This will produce more marked *catatonia,* more marked *stupor* or a *catatonic-stuporous condition.*

Epileptic impulses reach the *second barrier* (y_2); the thalamus and other neighboring subcortical structures are already involved. The patient may then show symptoms produced by the convulsion focus and also symptoms produced by a disturbance of diencephalic function (y_2). Various formations in the thalamic structures may also be affected.

a.) If all medial structures of the thalamus with activating projections to the neocortex are stimulated (Monnier 1962, 1969), then the patient will develop *agitated, aggressive, paranoid or paranoid-hallucinatory psychotic symptoms.* The cortical EEG will not become completely normal; waves continue to be slow and do not extend into the α-wave rhythm. However, the convulsion potentials are suppressed, diffuse dysrhythmias disappear and focal changes are also suppressed.

b.) However, if inhibitory structures and their projections (Demsey and Morison 1942, Moruzzi 1972) are stimulated, then there will be psychomotor and bioelectrical blocking. The symptomatology here will be mainly *depressive, depressive-stuporous* with *catatonic, catatonic-*

cataleptic psychotic symptoms due to the irritation of the limbic system. The cortical EEG will then show diffuse slowing, possibly with slight or fairly marked synchronization of the waves, a basal dysrhythmia (see Chapter II) or a general change with periodic bursts of hypersynchronous waves.

c.) If the activating formations are stimulated until they are fatigued, then the inhibitory formations may become dominant. In this case, the patients become very inhibited with a fairly marked *stuporous, stuporous-catatonic* or *catatonic-cataleptic* clinical picture such as that which occurs during stimulation of inhibitory structures. There are fairly pronounced changes in the cortical EEG or maximum slowing of the waves.

d.) On the other hand, if the inhibitory structures are suppressed until they become fatigued, the patient will present with a picture of *acute agitation, aggressiveness* or *paranoid* symptoms with a tendency for the cortical EEG to normalize. However, this will not be forced normalization in the EEG (a term used by Landoldt, see Chapters I and II) but a tendency for the slowed basic rhythm in the EEG to accelerate.

In all these cases the clinical picture is variable; most of the patients show an *organic-type psychosis* with a number of uncharacteristic symptoms, so this is rarely mistaken for an endogenous psychosis.

If the epileptic stimuli reach the third barrier (y_3 = neocortex, the clinical picture becomes even more complicated. Affective and psychomotor symptoms combine with hallucinatory and thought disturbances. The EEG tends to normalize, but this is still not a psychosis with forced normalization (see Chapters I and II).

If the *fourth barrier* (mesencephalon, pons, medulla oblongata = y_4) is also involved, the psychosis may develop in several ways.

a.) Excitation of the activating structures of Moruzzi and Mogoun (1949) with activation of higher formations and of the cortex produces a *paranoid, paranoid-hallucinatory* or *agitated psychotic form* with forced normalization in the cortical EEG (see Chapters I and II). With forced normalization there is the development of a psychotic picture which is very like or practically the same as a schizophrenic-type endogenous psychosis (see Chapter I). It is often difficult to make a diagnosis in these cases, and diagnosis can be greatly facilitated by study of the patient's case history.

b.) If the activating structures of the reticular formation (Moruzzi and Magoun 1949) are excited to such an extent that their function is blocked, then the clinical picture may take an *inhibited, catatonic-*

stuporous or *catatonic form* since the inhibitory neurons become functionally dominant (see Chapter I).

c.) Where the inhibitory formations are stimulated (Magoun and Rhines 1946), here again, *inhibition will dominate the clinical picture* but the symptoms will be rather different because the activating structures will still be fully functional and may change everything.

d.) If the inhibitory structures of the reticular formation of Magoun and Rhines (1946) are so powerfully inhibited that their function is paralyzed, then the activating projections become dominant. In this case there may also be a *schizophrenic-type psychotic symptomatology with forced normalization in the cortical EEG* after Landolt (see Chapter I).

e.) In most cases simultaneous stimulation of activating (Moruzzi and Magoun 1949) and inhibitory (Magoun and Rhines 1946) structures of the reticular formation caudal to the diencephalon produces an *agitated* or *excited agitated* form or, more rarely, an inhibited psychotic form.

f.) Both formations (activating and inhibitory) are so powerfully blocked that they become virtually non-functional (see Chapter III) and then *various forms* of psychotic symptomatology may develop. In these cases the phenomena are mainly produced by the limbic and/or diencephalic systems. The cortical EEG will show slowed cerebral activity and there may even be convulsion potentials in spite of the psychotic symptoms. This is probably a psychosis without forced normalization in the EEG after Landolt (see Chapter I).

Chronic mental changes in patients with psychomotor epilepsy occur as a result of changes in the vicinity of the convulsion focus. These symptoms are to be regarded as a result of functional elimination or extirpation of these anatomical-functional regions, and they have not been taken into account above (see Chapters I and III).

MECHANISMS RESPONSIBLE FOR PRODUCING OTHER CLINICAL AND NEUROPHYSIOLOGICAL PHENOMENA

Here we shall discuss a few biochemical and neurophysiological aspects of *abnormal sleep* and of *somnambulistic episodes* in patients whom we have treated ourselves (Jovanović 1970d, 1971a, 1972a).

In order to understand the biochemistry of sleep, of sleep disturbances and of pathological episodes arising out of sleep, we shall have to take another look at the problems of regulation of the sleeping-waking system. In recent years, a vast amount of literature has been published on the reticular formation of the brain stem and on the sleeping-waking system (Baust

1970; Demsey and Morison 1942; Hess 1954; Hopf 1970; Jouvet 1969, 1972, Jovanović 1970 a; Magoun and Rhines 1946; Moruzzi 1972; Moruzzi and Magoun 1949 and Chapter IV) .

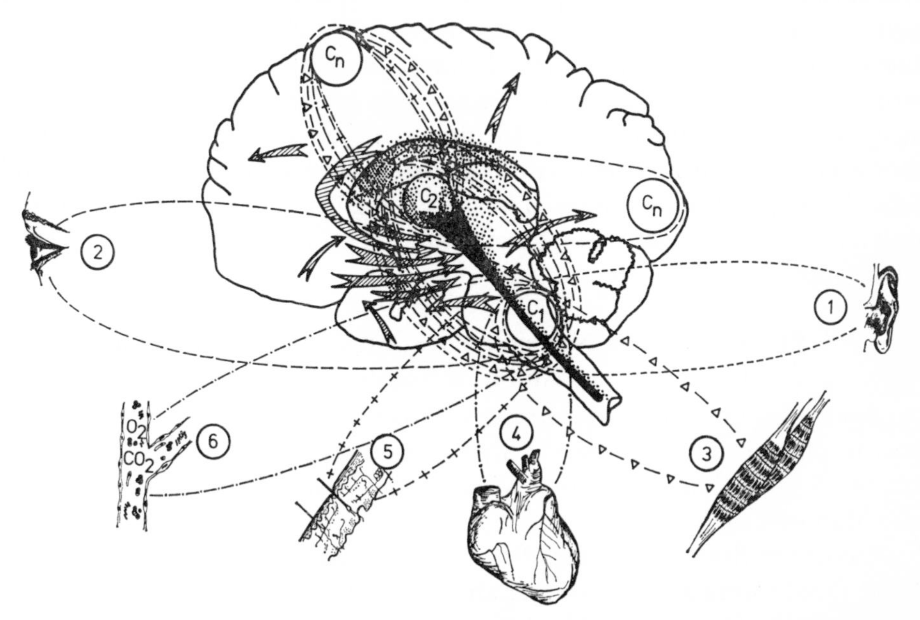

Figure 39. Diagrammatic representation of the extent of the sleep-waking system in the brain and its connections with the interior of the body and the environment via sense and other organs. *Black* = formations which are primarily responsible for the waking state. *Stippled* = cerebral structures which are primarily responisble for regulating sleep. *Hatched arrows* = projections of the sleeping-waking system (activating and suppressing system. (1) = hearing; (2) = light perception; (3) = muscle; (4) = heart and circulation; (5) = tactile perception; (6) = blood with partial 0_2 and CO_2 pressure. C = centers in the brain. The connections shown in the diagram do not necessarily correspond to the actual anatomical course. (From Jovanovic, U.J.: *Nervenarzt, 41*:5-23, 1970a.)

As Figure 39 demonstrates, the *sleeping-waking system extends from the anterior end of the spinal cord as far as the anterior end of the diencephalon including the limbic system and the thalamo-cortical projections.* The formations of the medulla oblongata of the rhombencephalon and midbrain (4th barrier) are mainly responsible for inducing and maintaining the waking state. The formations in the thalamus and hypothalamus (2nd barrier) are mainly responsible for the function of sleep. The limbic system (1st barrier) is a functional unit with the sleeping-waking system of the brain system and together they form a harmonic biocybernetic mechanism. This does not only apply to the sleeping and waking states. This mechanism is also responsible for many other vital functions, and it is connected with the environment via the sense organs. Any change in the environment either has a calming, sedating and hypnotic effect, or an arousing, tonic or agitating effect on the individual. However, it is not only the surroundings which can have these calming, sedating and hypnotic, or arousing, tonic or agitating effects; they can also be induced by changes in the internal homeostasis of the CNS. If there is an active pathological process in the structures of the sleeping-waking system, this can trigger a set of abnormal symptoms. As we have shown in Chapter III, the convulsion foci in psychomotor epilepsy are localized within the structures of the medial temporal lobe, i.e. in the limbic system. Thus, they are in a position to disturb not only the sleep and the waking state, but they can also produce epileptic stimulation.

Biochemical and Neurophysiological Control of Sleep on Non-Ictal Nights

Serotonin (5-hydroxytryptamine = 5-HT) probably has an important part to play in the deep sleep of a patient on a non-ictal night. In the last ten to 15 years, Jouvet (1969 a, b, 1972) has dealt with this problem (see also Matussek 1970).

Using the fluorescence technique of Falk and Hallip, Dahlström and Fuxe (1964) were able to discover and describe two *monoaminergic neuron* systems in the brain stem. The first system of neurons is *catecholaminergic* (most of which are noradrenergic). These neurons show a green fluorescence and they usually lie in 12 groups (A 1 to A 12) in the *lateral part* of the medulla oblongata, of the pons and of the mesencephalon. In addition to this, high concentrations of sympathin have been found in the hypothalamus, infundibulum and area postrema (Monnier 1969). On the other hand, the *serotonergic neurons* which show a yellow fluorescence which is intensified after injection of monoamine oxidase inhibitors (MAOI), occur almost exclusively in nine groups in the nuclei of the raphe system of the brain stem (nuclei raphes rhombencephali). Ends of these neurons have been found in the spinal cord, in the brain stem itself and in the rostral part of the brain as far as the hypothalamus (Jouvet 1969 a, b, 1972; Monnier 1969, Vogt 1954). About six to eight days after destruction of the serotonergic neurons, the serotonin in these endings disappears completely. After ten days there is no more monoamine staining.

As a result of their topography, the serotonergic neurons can be completely destroyed and this means that appropriate experiments can be carried out. The nuclei of the raphe system are actually fairly small and fine. This makes it possible to correlate the extent of the destruction with the resulting duration of sleep and with the quantity of cerebral monoamine which occurs rostral to the lesions.

The following observations have been made *after subtotal (80 to 90%) destruction* of the raphe system (Jouvet 1969 a, b, 1972):

The first effect in the experimental animals (cats) was a condition of permanent wakefulness in the first three to four days. The animals lay on their sides, made continuous running movements, and developed mydriasis. There was usually an increase of heart rate and moderate polypnoea. Throughout the whole period there was rapid and low voltage activity in the EEG. In addition, there were persistent volleys of monophasic spikes in the corpus geniculatum laterale (deep electrode). There was an increase of muscular activity in the region of the neck, and the eyes of the cats followed any moving object. The EEG did not reveal any sleep activity in the first 100 hours. After four days there were a few brief periods of normal sleep (synchronized, slow sleep according to the EEG nomenclature). These periods never lasted for longer than a couple of minutes and only represented 3 to 5 percent of 24 hours (compared with 50 percent in control animals).

Where the raphe system was *partially destroyed* (we are still quoting Jouvet 1969 a, 1972) there were the following results:

In the first few days there was the customary complete loss of sleep. However, sleep returned rapidly on the third day. The correlation between the amount of sleep and the extent of destruction of the raphe system and the cerebral monoamines is highly significant. The reduction in the amount of sleep parallels the selective reduction of serotonin. The noradrenaline was not significantly changed.

These experiments demonstrate that serotonin is an important modulator of sleep and that the slow (synchronized, normal, orthodox, dreamless) *sleep is promoted* (Jouvet 1969 a, b, 1972; Matussek 1970). Since, like every other vital process, sleep is not regulated by one chemical substance but by *a system,* we may assume *that in patients with psychomotor epilepsy (who experience deeper sleep as compared with healthy people) the serotonin system is in a dominant position compared with the other chemical systems (the brain stem).*

There are a few more points which should be mentioned about this hypothesis. Jouvet (1969 a, 1972) enlarged on this further in his summary publication: serotonin cannot traverse the blood-brain barrier. If an increase of cerebral serotonin is required, a precursor, *5-hydroxy-tryptophane (5-HTP),* must be injected or the deoxidative deamination of serotonin can be inhibited by administration of MAOI (see also Berlucchi 1970).

In the cat, injection of 30 to 50 mg/kg. 5-HTP induces a condition resembling slow sleep and this then persists unbroken for about five to six hours (Green and Sawyer 1964, Kramer and Seifter 1966). During this period there have been no instances of paradoxical sleep (paradoxical sleep in animals corresponds to dream sleeping in humans, see Baust 1970 and Hartmann 1968). We have pointed out that sleep with dreaming in patients with psychomotor epilepsy is substantially shorter than in healthy people. This clinical finding correlates with the results of experimental investigations by the authors mentioned.

Gangloff and Monnier (1957) and Monnier (1960, 1969) were able to induce incipient sleep symptoms by direct injection of serotonin. Subsequently, a state of mixed arousal and relaxation developed and the behavior of the animals became passive (Monnier 1960) due to activation of the hippocampus and reduction of thalamic suppression.

However, if the cerebral serotonin and noradrenaline are reduced by injection of *reserpine* (0.5 mg/kg.) both the slow and also the paradoxical sleep very soon disappear and incessant bursts of discharges of ponto-geniculo-occipital spikes (deep electrode) occur together with a rapid cortical EEG and the muscular activity is also increased. Intravenous injection of 50 mg/kg. 5-HTP six hours after administration of reserpine leads to immediate recurrence of slow sleep, whereupon the bursts of spikes from the corpus geniculatum laterale disappear. About five to six hours after the injection of 5-HTP there is a return to the condition seen after administration of reserpine (Berlucchi 1970, Delorme et al. 1965, Gangloff and Monnier 1957, Matsumo and Jouvet 1964).

Injection of MAOI (iproniazid, phenylisopropylhydrazinenialamide, see also Chapter VI) leads to an *increase of slow sleep* in the cat. The most active substance is *nialamide.* After one injection of 10 mg/kg., slow waves occur in the EEG for almost 80% of the time (over a period of three to four days). *The increase of the slow (i.e. deep) sleep during this period is accompanied by complete disappearance of paradoxical sleep in the animals* (Jouvet 1965). In Chapter VI we have discussed the MAOI as convulsion-provoking agents. Thus, substances which under certain circumstances can deepen sleep, can also induce convulsion elements in the EEG. In our case this is the MAOI. The tremendously deep sleep with marked curtailment of dreaming in patients with psychomotor epilepsy correlates with these findings. It can be assumed that in these patients there is either a primary increase of serotonin in the structures of the limbic system (1st barrier) and of the brain stem (4th barrier) which elicits convulsions, or that monoamine oxidase is inhibited so that there is a secondary effect involved in increasing the serotonin concentration.

We have already considered (Jovanovic 1967 d, e) psychomotor epilepsy to be, neurophysiologically, a temporocephalic or a rhomboencephalocortical form of epilepsy (see also Table I and Chapter I). This hypothesis fits very well with Jouvet's findings (which we are now discussing) on the role of serotonin in sleep. *Biochemically, this form may be considered as serotogenic epilepsy.* However, we have no direct evidence that serotonin induces sleep and the convulsion elements in psychomotor epilepsy. The results quoted here were only obtained from animal experiments. There are also many findings, which are discussed in Chapters VI and VII, to support the hypothesis of *serotonin or acetylcholine epilepsy.* Now we should like to cite a few more results of other authors with regard to the serotonin hypothesis.

According to Koe and Weisman (1966), it may be possible to reduce the serotonin by inhibiting its synthesis at the tryptophane-hydroxylase stage by injection of *P. chlorophenylalanine.* It is also possible to reduce cerebral serotonin by injection of P. chloroamphetamine (Pletscher et al. 1963).

Delorme et al. (1966) have carried out experiments in cats and rats using *P. chlorophenylalanine.* A single injection of 400 mg/kg. or two injections of 200 mg/kg. completely inhibited sleep in these experimental animals. There is first a latent period of 24 to 30 hours during which sleep is normal. After this period there is a parallel reduction both of deep and also of paradoxical sleep, and after 72 hours the effects of the waking state are seen. Sleep gradually returns again after 80 hours. The amount of sleep becomes normal again about eight to ten days after the injection. If 5-HTP (40 to 50 mg/kg.) is injected during the permanent waking state (i.e. at least 60 hours after the injection of p. chlorophenylalanine), there is an almost immediate return to slow sleep and five hours after this there is paradoxical sleep.

Delorme et al. (1966, see also Jouvet 1969 a, b, 1972) carried out a further experiment with *P. chloroamphetamine.* Injection of 15 to 30 mg/kg. selectively reduces the level of serotonin while noradrenaline and other catecholamines remained unaffected by this dose. Almost immediately, this substance leads to a condition of total sleeplessness accompanied by a permanent state of wakefulness with motor unrest, and this is maintained for about 16 to 18 hours. Subsequently, there is gradual recovery and a return to sleep.

Like serotonin, *noradrenaline* must also have a considerable part to play in the sleep of patients with psychomotor epilepsy (and thus also with the type of sleep seen in grand mal). Using a dose of 150 to 300 mg/kg. of *α-methyl-para-tyrosine,* a drug which inhibits the synthesis of noradrenaline, Delorme (1966) was able to inhibit paradoxical sleep in experimental animals for a period of six to eight hours. Slow sleep was not changed. *Alpha-methyl-meta-tyrosine* (100 to 200 mg/kg.) or *α-methyl-dopa* (100 to 200 mg/kg.) specifically inhibit paradoxical sleep for a period of 12 to 18 hours (Berlucchi 1970, Matussek 1970, Peyrethon et al. 1967).

Injection of dihydroxyphenylalanine (DOPA) in a dose of 50 mg/kg. produces definite prolongation of the waking state and reduces sleep (Delorme et al. 1966). On the other hand, injection of *dihydroxyphenylserine,* which is a direct precursor of noradrenaline (Blaschko et al. 1950), produces an increase of slow and of paradoxical sleep in the rat (Harlicek 1967). *All these experiments indicate that noradrenaline is an important chemical substance which promotes paradoxical sleep.* However, substances which promote paradoxical sleep at the same time inhibit deep and slow sleep in proportion. Thus, in patients with psychomotor epilepsy, the effect of noradrenaline must be a secondary factor, and so the serotonin system (serotonergic system, serotonergic mechanism) is dominant. Accordingly, all other substances which inhibit the noradrenaline system and promote the serotonin system, promote deep sleep, and vice versa.

We must now say a few words about the predisposition to attacks and the condition of deep sleep. In Chapter II we have already mentioned that the period taken for patients with psychomotor epilepsy to fall asleep is shorter and thus they fall asleep more quickly than healthy subjects. In the same Chapter we have reported that, just at the moment of falling asleep, the convulsion potentials show a rapid numerical increase and they become much more distinct. The deeper the subject sleeps, the more convulsion potentials are recorded in the EEG.

In an earlier report (Jovanovic 1968 a) it has already been noted that generalized attacks of nocturnal epilepsy also arise at the moment of falling asleep, as the sleep deepens, and out of deep sleep. *This gives us our working hypothesis: all mechanisms which promote the serotonin system increase the predisposition to attacks.*

There is evidence in other publications (Jovanovic 1966 d, e, 1967 e, 1968, c, d, 1970 a, 1972 a) *that no, or practically no, convulsive symptoms are recorded in paradoxical sleep while there is dream activity.* Even in cases where the cerebral predisposition to convulsion is considerably increased (Jovanovic 1968 c, 1970 g) or where there is a catatonic condition in which the EEG in the waking state is normal and the sleeping EEG during deep sleep is extremely pathological, during paradoxical sleep (dreaming sleep) there are no clinically manifest epileptic reactions or convulsion potentials observed in the electroencephalogram. *Dreaming, or more precisely, paradoxical sleep with dream activity, appears to offer patients with epilepsy of any type benevolent protection against ubiquitous attacks during sleep.*

This gives us an additional working hypothesis: *Any mechanism which inhibits the adrenaline-noradrenaline system in the brain stem promotes the predisposition to attacks, and vice versa.*

Biochemical and Neurophysiological Control of Sleep During Ictal Nights

The sleep disturbance in psychomotor epilepsy differs basically from other forms of sleep disorders since, among other things, it is associated with attacks occurring during sleep. Thus, we are faced with two problems: the first is the significance of the sleep abnormalities and the second is the attacks during this abnormal form of sleep. Since, as yet, these two problems have not been explained biochemically, we are faced with a very difficult task. There are several hypotheses which can be put forward.

First, if one assumes that the sleep disturbances in these patients are caused by inadequate synthesis or release of serotonin, then an arousal reaction with prolongation of paradoxical sleep must be expected. In addition, there should also be a reduction of the cerebral predisposition to convulsion. Neither of these in fact occur. The sleep is disturbed, but the patients do not remain awake as a neurotic would, but they are drowsy and they fall into light sleep, although they are not capable of deep sleep. The paradoxical sleep is disturbed almost completely (Jovanović 1967 d, 1968 a, d, 1970, 1972 a, e).

Second, if one assumes that there is an increased concentration of serotonin, there would be deep sleep and curtailment of paradoxical sleep. However, we only observe such activity in the non-ictal nights and so this hypothesis must be rejected.

Third, as yet we have not dealt with a third modulator, the *cholinergic system*. There is no accepted view on the action of *acetylcholine* in the sleeping and waking states.

In animal experiments it is possible to elicit an arousal reaction following administration of acetylcholine, but the animal does not behave as if it were awake. Electrical stimulation of the mesencephalic structures (4th barrier) causes a five to six-fold increase in the concentration of acetylcholine in the ipsilateral cortex (Kanai and Szerb 1965). According to Monnier (1969), cholinesterase inhibitors (see Chapter IX) are also capable of inducing an arousal reaction in the EEG over the upper reticular formation (mesencephalon and thalamus). This arousal reaction can be abolished by *atropine* and other parasympathicomimetic agents (amyzil, banactyzine, methylamizil, diphemin: Bradley and Key 1958, Ilyutschenok 1962, 1968, 1965, Monnier 1969, Monnier and Romanovski 1962, Rozanova 1964).

On the other hand, several authors have found that acetylcholine activates sleep. Bowers, Hartman and Freedman (1966) recorded an increase in the amount of cortical acetylcholine during sleep. Hernandez Peón (1965 a, b) induced sleep activity by application of acetylcholine crystals along the line of the hypothalamus-thalamus (2nd barrier) and rhinencephalon (1st barrier), which has been exactly defined anatomically. According to

Yamaguchi et al. (1963), acetylcholine produces drowsiness with a synchronized EEG and it potentiates the effect of low frequency electrical stimulation (i.e. the *recruiting* response) (Monnier 1962) when it is applied locally into the intralaminar thalamus. Administration of acetylcholine in a dose of 20 mg/kg. to the bulbar, pontine and mesencephalic reticular formation has also produced sleep in the cat. This sleep is accompanied by salivation and vomiting (Cordeau et al. 1963).

It can be seen from these results that the part played by acetylcholine in normal sleep has still not been explained. It is possible that this substance contributes to the disturbances of sleep in the epileptic. According to Monnier (1960), activation of the adrenergic system together with the cholinergic mechanism causes definite desynchronization of the EEG over the motor and sensory cortex and, at the same time, it causes synchronization of the waves over the hippocampus and thalamus in the form of a medium-frequency theta rhythm. In psychomotor epilepsy occurring during sleep we see neither persistent desynchronization over the motor and sensory cortex nor constant medium-frequency theta waves over the hippocampus. Thus the hypothesis cannot be vindicated on the basis of this mechanism alone.

Fourth, the sleep disturbances arise due to primary elevation of Adrenaline and noradrenaline levels. In this case we ought again to observe an arousal reaction and also prolongation of the paradoxical sleep. Both systems, noradrenaline and paradoxical sleep, would then have the effect of suppressing convulsions, and the attack would be inhibited. Thus, this hypothesis is also invalid.

Fifth, if one assumes that there is a primary defect in synthesis in the adrenaline-noradrenaline system, there would be deepening of the sleep with a relative elevation of the serotonin level and also an increased predisposition to convulsion. The increase of predisposition to convulsion is in fact seen in these nights, but the deep sleep is not seen.

Sixth, according to Monnier, serotinin and LSD which is chemically related to it, produce stimulation of the rhinencephalon (palaeocortex) similar to that produced by convulsant agents (picrotoxin) (see also Matussek 1970).

Having established this we have reached a point where we can produce a plausible explanation of the *sleep disturbances and the attacks* which arise out of sleep in psychomotor epilepsy. In these cases there must be several mechanisms involved.

Initially, stimulation from the convulsion focus (1st barrier) probably causes an increase in the concentration of serotonin and acetylcholine. This prevents paradoxical sleep and wakefulness and promotes deep sleep. The patients are drowsy and tend to fall asleep, but deep sleep is prevented by additional mechanisms. There is probably a compensatory release of adrenaline-noradrenaline and this results in a counter-regulatory reaction. As Selbach (1953, 1965) suggests, in epileptics there is a primitive metabolic disturbance so that the process of counter-regulation is not simply a smooth adjustment. Thus, there are crises ranging from extreme vagotonia to extreme sympatheticotonia, or vice versa. The attack balances out these extreme situations. After the attack a certain stability is restored until an extreme situation again develops in the body as a result of the primitive metabolism.

We can detect the compensatory release of Adrenaline shortly before an attack during sleep. There is a critical desynchronization in the EEG (see Figure 12 and 18) and this lasts for a few seconds. After this, there is gradual synchronization which may be a function of the elevated concentration of serotonin. This process culminates in an attack and after this the sleep is more peaceful than before.

Many other factors also have a part to play in this mechanism (see also Chapters III, V, and IX).

Biochemical Basis and Neurophysiological Control of Somnambulistic Episodes

As with the disturbed sleep in epileptics on the ictal nights, the biochemical mechanism responsible for somnambulistic episodes is complicated by an increased cerebral predisposition to convulsions. However, simple somnambulistic episodes in sleep-walkers cannot be explained biochemically.

Somnambulism is explained as partial activation of the reticular system of the brain stem (Jung 1963, Bauer 1965). However, what causes this activation?

When dealing with this problem, it is necessary to analyse the regulatory system again (see also Figure 39). Here we should mention just a few points. It is known that sleep occurs in two important phases: one is *orthodox* (normal, synchronized, dreamless) *sleep,* the other is *paradoxical* (desynchronized, dream-, D-state) *sleep.* These two components can each be further subdivided into two, one part being the *tonic,* the other part being the *phasic* component. Both the tonic and the phasic components can be further broken down into *psychic, autonomic and motor components.* Dissociation of the motor and psychic components is particularly well known in sleep-walkers *sui generis.* In psychomotor epilepsy the attacks are an additional component (Jovanovic 1970 b, Jung 1963, 1965).

According to Monnier (1969) *it is possible to classify waking activity into elementary arousal reactions, affective, impulsive reactions and higher psychomotor activities.*

MASSIVE AROUSAL REACTION. This is induced by the ascending reticular formation of the brain stem (4th barrier), mainly by the caudal part. We have already discussed the fact *that in this area, laterally there are more catecholaminergic (noradrenergic) neurons and medially there are serotonergic neurons.*

THE MESENCEPHALIC STAGE (4th barrier) of the arousal reaction is characterized by rapid desynchronized activity in the cortex and, in the rabbit, by synchronized θ-activity in the hippocampus and thalamus. At this stage there is still marked concentration of *serotonergic neurons or their endings.* The *cholinergic system* has also been detected in the mesencephalon (Bradley and Key 1958, Monnier 1960, 1969, Monnier and Tissot 1958).

THE DIENCEPHALIC STAGE (2nd barrier) organizes, according to Monnier (1969), the instinctive reactions in the posterio-ventral hypothalamus, particularly in the dynamogenic field of Hess (1943). Here, the function of the improved state of wakefulness and readiness is to further the selfpreservation of the individual and it is a defence against the hostile environment. According to Mac Lean (1949 to 1958), the limbic system (1st barrier) also has this function. The *cholinergic mechanism* is mainly localized at this stage (1st and 2nd barriers).

THE RHINENCEPHALIC STAGE (1st barrier) of the arousal reaction is characterized by more active behavior (Hassler 1964 a, b, Mac Lean 1957, Monnier 1969) and also by activity directed to preservation of the individual and the species (Mac Lean 1957, 1958). As mentioned above, *serotonin* is localized in this region with *acetylcholine* in the cortical structures.

From all that has been said it seems likely that somnambulistic psychomotor episodes are triggered from the reticular formation, i.e. from the fourth barrier. However, if the fourth barrier is directly stimulated by the convulsion focus (1st barrier), then a generalized seizure will occur even before the patient wakes up. However, if firstly the second (thalamus and adjacent structures) and then the third (neocortex) is stimulated from the fourth barrier, then the patient will show *increased motor activity.* He will get up, wander about for a time like a somnambulist and then he will develop psychomotor symptoms triggered from the rhinencephalon (as in isolated psychomotor epilepsy, see Chapter I), since the excitatory impulses will have eventually spread even to these out-of-the-way cerebral formations.

MECHANISMS RESPONSIBLE FOR PRODUCING EPILEPTIC MANIFESTATIONS WHERE THERE IS INCREASED NEURONAL EXCITATION (INCREASED CEREBRAL PREDISPOSITION TO CONVULSION)

We just discussed the model of epileptic phenomena where there was *inadequate blocking or the blocking mechanism was itself blocked (deblocking).* In this section we should like to deal with the problem of epileptic attacks where there is *an increased level of excitation* (increased cerebral predisposition to convulsion) due to an activation of stimuli. Under these conditions epileptic seizures may occur even when the body or brain of the subject is healthy, and these seizures are frequently fatal. Chemical and pharmacological drugs are usually responsible for this and, in this respect, nerve gases and fluorinated insecticides (see Chapters III, V, VI and IX) are particularly dangerous.

If we attempt to adapt our model in Figure 38, we find that there may be several possibilities, not all of which will produce a seizure or death.

If the level of excitation in the convulsion focus (first barrier = Ammon's horn = y_1) is *doubled,* then these stimuli can follow the same route as the epileptic stimuli in cases where there is inadequate blocking (see above). This increased (doubled) level of epileptic impulses (i.e. $384x$) cannot be suppressed in the convulsion focus, and so all $384x$ impulses are transmitted to the second barrier (thalamus = y_2). If they are halved at y_2, $192x$ excitatory impulses will reach the neocortex. The neocortex then halves this number and the remaining impulses are passed on down to the fourth barrier (y_4 = reticular formation). They are again halved in the fourth barrier (to $48x$) and halved again in the fifth (y_5). The remaining $24x$ are not capable of eliciting a generalized attack but there will be *epileptic equivalents* with motor components. *Hence, double the number of epileptic impulses is not a potentially fatal number.* However, if there is no convulsion focus in the brain (as in healthy people) then there will be no epileptic symptoms; that is to say, when the blocking mechanism is still completely intact, on the basis of our model, a larger number of impulses are necessary before the creature's life is threatened.

Now let us examine an example of *four* times the number of stimuli affecting a convulsion focus. These $768x$ impulses build up in the convulsion focus and are conducted to the second barrier, where the number of epileptic stimuli is halved. The neocortex receives $384x$ impulses which it then halves again, passing on $192x$ impulses to the fourth barrier. The process is repeated and the spinal cord, the fifth barrier, then receives 96x impulses. Even if this number is halved to $48x$, here, on the basis of our model, this number is still capable of eliciting a generalized attack. However, the epileptic will still not lapse into status epilepticus unless there are additional factors at work.

In a healthy brain the 768*x* impulses would also be halved at the site of origin, 24*x* excitatory impulses would arrive at the periphery and so, in this case, four times the number of stimuli would not produce a generalized attack. *Thus, in healthy people, a discharge of four times the number of impulses in the Ammon's horn will not produce a potentially dangerous peripheral symptomatology.*

If we assume that *eight times* the number of epileptic impulses are generated in the convulsion focus and that these are not blocked, 1536*x* impulses will reach the second barrier (y_2). Here they will be reduced to 768*x*, in the third barrier to 248*x*, in the fourth to 192*x* and in the fifth to 96*x* impulses and, in an epileptic, these 96*x* impulses would be capable of producing status epilepticus without the aid of additional factors.

In a healthy person with no convulsion focus in the limbic system the total number of 1536*x* impulses would be halved at the site of origin. 48*x* impulses would arrive at the periphery and these would be capable of producing a generalized attack but there would be no status epilepticus. *In a healthy brain (all the blocking mechanisms intact) eight times the number of impulses will not produce a potentially dangerous situation.* The generalized attack may remain isolated as long as it is not complicated by other factors. However, if there are any other detrimental factors to be taken into account, every affect, be it exogenous or endogenous, can act as an epileptic stressor.

A *sixteen-fold* increase in the number of impulses building up in the limbic system cannot be blocked in epileptics and 3072*x* impulses will be conducted to the second barrier (thalamus y_2). Even if this quantity is halved at each successive barrier, 192*x* impulses will still reach the periphery. Thus, a sixteen-fold increase in the number of impulses generated could be fatal in an epileptic. In a healthy person, 96*x* impulses would reach the periphery and this number would be capable of producing status epilepticus. *However, since a status epilepticus would still be controllable, even a sixteen-fold increase in the cerebral predisposition to convulsion would still not present a very great danger to the healthy brain as long as there were no complicating factors. The individual is in much less danger when the blocking mechanism is fully functional as compared with the situation which would obtain were this blocking mechanism impaired or eliminated.*

If *32 times* the number of excitatory impulses built up, as we have shown in Figure 38, even a healthy person's life would be threatened. *In these circumstances, the individual would not survive even if the blocking mechan-*

isms were fully intact. With a build-up of 6144*x* impulses at the site of origin, without blocking, 192*x* would reach the periphery and these would be fatal even if the patient were given appropriate treatment. Thus, we must not underestimate the danger of, e.g., nerve gases, fluorinated insecticides, ABC warfare etc.

MECHANISMS RESPONSIBLE FOR PRODUCING EPILEPTIC MANIFESTATIONS WHERE INHIBITORY AND EXCITATORY MECHANISMS IN THE BRAIN ARE DISTURBED

There is a very much greater risk of attacks and also a danger of death where deblocking is combined with an increased level of excitation in the brain. We have seen above that a build-up of even double the number of stimuli (384*x* impulses instead of 192*x*) can produce epileptic manifestations if the blocking mechanisms fail at only one place. If there is deblocking at two barriers, then a two-fold increase in the cerebral predisposition to convulsion may produce a generalized seizure. If there is deblocking at three barriers, then a two-fold increase in the cerebral predisposition to convulsion may produce status epilepticus, and if four barriers are disrupted the outcome may be fatal. Thus, when the whole brain is affected, as can occur during short-term administration of, or poisoning with epileptogenic agents (see Chapter VI), then even a two-fold increase in the cerebral predisposition to convulsion may be fatal.

It is clear from what has been said *that the brain possesses a vast range of powerful blocking mechanisms, and profound, potentially fatal functional disorders do not develop unless the whole brain is affected. The existence of a convulsion focus must certainly be regarded as serious since epilepsy cannot occur unless there is one. However, in many dangerous situations a convulsion focus can develop extremely quickly since the brain always has a latent predisposition to convulsion.*

CHAPTER IX

SUPPLEMENTARY REMARKS ABOUT THE PROBLEM OF THE MECHANISMS OF ACTION OF CHEMICAL COMPOUNDS

One or two remarks about the effects of chemical compounds on cerebral metabolism were made in Chapters III, V, VI, VII and VIII in connection with psychomotor epilepsy. However, in each of these chapters we discussed the matter from some other point of view. We would now like to deal with this problem by summarizing and *supplementing* this material within the context of the task in hand. Here we shall discuss both epileptogenic noxae and possible pharmacological treatment. The results here are still incomplete and they are often contradictory. We have deliberately left many of the interpretations of other authors without adding our own comments. The problems are illustrated by examples from recent research work.

As far as we know from studies on the mechanisms of action of chemical compounds on the human CNS (Adler 1969, Bente and Brodey 1964; Boerner et al. 1970; Coper and Selbach 1970, Eccles, 1953, 1957, 1964; Grundfest 1959; Himwich and Schadé 1965; Hodgkin and Keynes 1955; Jovanović 1965, 1966 a, b; Jovanović et al. 1970; Jung 1958; Maynert 1969; Millichap 1969; Müller and Müller 1972; Müller et al. 1972; Pogodaev 1964; Purpura 1969; Swinyard 1969; Woodbury 1969; Woodbury and Kemp 1970, and many other authors) there are the following possibilities: a.) The effect on cerebral metabolism is mediated via an effect on the enzymic processes; b.) This results in depolarization or hyperpolarization of the nerve cell membrane; and finally c.) Effects on the cerebral bioelectrical potentials.

ENZYME-MEDIATED MECHANISMS OF ACTION OF CHEMICAL COMPOUNDS ON CEREBRAL METABOLISM

Possible mechanisms here are: a.) Effect on the electrolytes or electrolyte-activated enzymes; b.) Effects on oxygen, carbon dioxide, pH and oxidizing processes; c.) Effect on carbohydrates; d.) the problem of protein metabolism in the brain; e.) Energy changes. Nucleotides and nucleic acids under the action of chemical compounds; f.) Amino acids and chemical compounds which affect their metabolism; g.) Concentration and activity of neuromodulators (endogenous amines and other neurohormones) ; h.) Chemicals with a pharmacological action, and cerebral lipids; i.) Other problems regarding enzymes, vitamins and hormones when using pharmacological agents.

Impairment of Electrolytes by Centrally-Acting Drugs

According to Squires (1965) and other earlier authors, *chlorpromazine* affects the interactions of K^+, Na^+, Mg^{++}, ATP and ATP-ase. Chlorpromazine may impair the harmonic effect of the electrolytes. This action has been described by the Hill equation. Certain changes in the electrolytes (indirect conclusions following administration of aminazine and Tofranil) have also been observed by Levtova (1966).

Davis and Brody (1966) studied a number of psychopharmacological agents from the point of view of their effect on ATP-ase (which is activated by Na^+ and K^+) in the brain, including *promazine.HCl, propiomicine.HCl, promethazine.HCl, chlorpromazine.HCl, prochlorperazine edispylate, trifluoperazine dihydrochloride, thoridazine.HCl, mepazine.HCl, perphenazine, triflupromazine, fluphenazine dihydrochloride, imipramine* and *sulfoxide derivative* of *promazine, chlorpromazine* and *trifluoperazine.* They found that all the phenothiazines used inhibited enzyme activity in concentrations of 1×10^{-4} M. In concentrations of up to $5 \times 10^{\infty 4}$ M, D-amphetamine, strychnine, GABA and phenobarbitone had no effect on Na^+- and K^+- stimulated ATP-ase activity. In concentrations of 1×10^{-4} M, promazine sulfoxide, chlorpromazine sulfoxide and trifluoperazine sulfoxide sometimes had no inhibitory effects on the activity of Na^+- and K^+- activated ATP-ase, whereas, in the same concentrations, the parent compounds of these agents inhibited the activity of this enzyme in 6 percent, 38 percent and 98 percent.

Green (1967) also tackled this problem, but by another method, and obtained similar results. Kraus and Simane (1967) studied Mg^{++}- activated ATP-ase under the effect of perathiepin [10-(4-methylpiperazino)-10,11-dihydro-dibenz-(d,f)-thiepin] (a thymoleptic agent) in comparison with chlorpromazine. Both drugs inhibited the activity of Mg^{++}- stimulated ATP-ase. Perathiepin also inhibited the activity of 2,4-dinitrophenol-stimulated ATP-ase. In concentrations of 0.2 — 0.5 mM, both drugs inhibited Na^+- and K^+- activated ATP-ase, which is one of the components of the sodium pump (see Figure 16). Chlorpromazine inhibited this activity by 100 percent, perathiepin by 90 percent. Thus, both of these drugs are similar in their effects on the enzymes under study.

According to the results of studies by Woodbury and Kemp (1970), *diphenylhydantoins* reduce both the total and the calculated sodium ion concentration in the cortex of normal rats, but potassium ion concentrations remain unchanged. The substances act to prevent induced reduction of sodium ion concentration and increased potassium ion concentration in rat brain.

Oxygen, Carbon Dioxide, pH and Oxidizing Processes

In common with a number of authors, Pogodaev (1964) worked with *aminazine*. He found that, 20 minutes after injection of doses of 10 mg/kg or more, there is a toxic suppression of respiratory processes in brain homogenates from rats. After using *Luminal* (40 min incubation), there was a substantial reduction of O_2 consumption compared with control animals. This reduction was 33 percent in the cortex, 28 percent in the subcortex, 30 percent in the brain stem and 22 percent in the cerebellum. Additional administration of vitamins B_1, B_2 and B_6 to the preparations described had a favorable effect on the results. Addition of the vitamins to the Amytal-sodium mixture increased O_2 consumption and respiratory processes in the brain (compared with the results with Amytal-sodium without vitamins). If *nicotinic acid* was also added, respiratory activity was enhanced even more. This reduced the toxicity of Amytal-sodium (as regards nicotinic acid and epilepsy, see also Chapters V, VII and Pogodaev and Krasnova 1955).

Dimitrov and Kolotilova (1967) obtained some interesting results in their studies on the action of *chlorpromazine* on respiration and oxidative phosphorylation in mitochondria of the cerebral hemispheres of the rat. Both respiration and oxidative phosphorylation were inhibited by using various concentrations of chlorpromazine and by administering the substrates glutamate and α-ketoglutarate. This inhibition was related to the drug concentration and the effect was more pronounced on the glutamate. Where there was no ATP in the non-phosphorylating milieu, there was no inhibition of the respiratory rate with glutamate. The respiratory processes were actually accelerated with α-ketoglutarate. These results indicated that chlorpromazine acts by disrupting oxidative phosphorylation and it was noticed that there was no enlargement of the mitochondria.

Tursky et al. (1965) studied the metabolic effects of *imipramine* and *prothiaden* compared with those of chlorpromazine, in sections of rat cortex. These authors found that, in relatively high concentrations, imipramine and chlorpromazine inhibited O_2 consumption in the mitochondria. Prothiaden produced effects similar to those of imipramine. As the concentrations of imipramine and prothiaden were reduced, the inhibitory effect on O_2 consumption also declined. All concentrations of imipramine, prothiaden and chlorpromazine used significantly reduced the penetration of free L-phenylalanine into the sections. With high concentrations of imipramine and prothiaden there was an increased level of transformation of L-phenylalanine into proteins. With lower concentrations there was again a reduction of this transformation compared with the situation with high concentrations. With a further reduction of concentrations (down to 10^{-4} M) transformation was the same as in the controls. 5×10^{-3} M chlorpromazine had no effect on the transformation of L-phenylalanine into proteins.

Pogodaev (1964) found that there were substantial differences in oxygen consumption in rat brains compared with controls, following pretreatment with *phenamine*. Four minutes after injection there was a 47 percent increase in O_2 consumption in the cortex of the test animals. The animals which were decapitated after 30 minutes showed a further increase of 22 percent. The picture was somewhat different in the brain stem. In the test 30 minutes after injection, there was an increase of 42 percent compared with the controls and of 22 percent compared with the test 4 minutes after injection.

The findings revealed contrary pictures: in the neocortex there was a fairly sharp increase of O_2 consumption immediately after injection and this then declined with time. On the other hand, there was only a slight rise in the brain stem immediately after injection, but this then increased considerably with time. Immediately after injection and later, there was only a slight rise in the subcortex after phenamine (17% after 4 minutes; 20% after 30 minutes). Pogodaev and Mechmedova (1957) also dealt with this problem and obtained similar or the same results.

The effect of antiepileptic agents has been discussed in previous chapters.

The Effect of (Psychopharmacological) Drugs on Carbohydrates

In the course of his studies, Gey (1965) found that *chlorpromazine, reserpine* and *phenobarbitone* have a certain inhibitory effect on glycolysis. The changes of cerebral carbohydrate metabolism was studied by measuring the concentrations of glucose, glucose-6-phosphate, fructose-6-phosphate, fructose-1,6-diphosphate, dihydroxy-acetone-phosphate, adenosine-5′-triphosphate and inorganic phosphate in the brain and blood of rats which had been pretreated with chlorpromazine (25 mg/kg), reserpine (2 mg/kg) or phenobarbitone (100 mg/kg). The intracellular levels were determined from the total levels in brain and blood. By this procedure, it was found that there was a reduction of glucose-6-phosphate and fructose-6-phosphate in the brain at the time of maximum depression of motor activity in the experimental animals. There were no conspicuous changes of other phosphorylated metabolites and inorganic phosphate. There were no significant changes in the glucose metabolites under study, in blood. After the time of peak tranquilization of the experimental animals, reserpine and phenobarbitone increased the concentration of glycogen. The author concluded that the reduction of hexose-phosphates in the brain indicates that the sedation action of psychopharmacological drugs is due to an inhibitory effect on glycolysis in the CNS. This inhibition of glycolysis may be due to inhibition of glucose phosphorylation.

The effect of chlorpromazine on glucose and nucleotide metabolism in the brain of mice has also been studied by Chowdhury et al. (1968) and other authors. Chlorpromazine reduced protein and lipid synthesis. Glucose and glucose phosphate were increased. *In vitro,* chlorpormazine promoted oxidative phosphorylation with an increase of high-energy phosphates. This explained the reduction of protein and lipid synthesis. The concentrations of AMP, ADP and ATP were not changed by chlorpromazine, whereas the *in vivo* activity of ATP-ase was inhibited. Thus, these metabolic changes are also due to other mechanisms apart from the change of high-energy structures.

Protein Metabolism in the Brain, Drugs and Epilepsy

According to Pogodaev (1964), *aminazine* altered the activity of proteinases in cerebral tissue (doses: 2, 5, 7 and 10 mg/kg s.c.). Twenty minutes after injection, the 40 rats showed a reduction of free ammonia concentration in all areas of the brain studied (Figure 40). The pharmacological effect also increased as the dose of aminazine was raised: *inhibitory bioelectrical and metabolic processes dominated in the brain.* The best results were seen in the cortex and subcortex. For example, a dose of 2 mg/kg aminazine reduced the concentration of ammonia in the cortex by 50 percent and by only 36 percent in the brain stem. A dose of 10 mg/kg reduced the ammonia concentration in the cortex by 67 percent and by 55 percent in the brain stem, compared with the controls.

Gosh (1967) studied the effects of drugs on cerebral riboproteins in rats. The drugs used included *chlorpromazine, strychnine, prochlorperazine, chlordiazepoxide* and *picrotoxin.* The results showed that these compounds produce more or less marked disorganization of ribonucleoproteins and change the RNA structure (as regards RNA, see also Chapter III).

The fluorometric studies of Teller et al. (1968) revealed that chlorpromazine and *thioproperazine* are bound to subcellular organelles. This binding occurs in several stages. Thus, for example, the binding of thioproperazine to the mitochondria of cerebral neurons altered the particle structure and permitted secondary binding of chlorpromazine and thioproperazine. The authors suggest that the structural changes, which can be produced in subcellular particles by phenothiazine concentrations of less than 10^{-6} M, may explain some of the *in vivo* actions of these and other drugs.

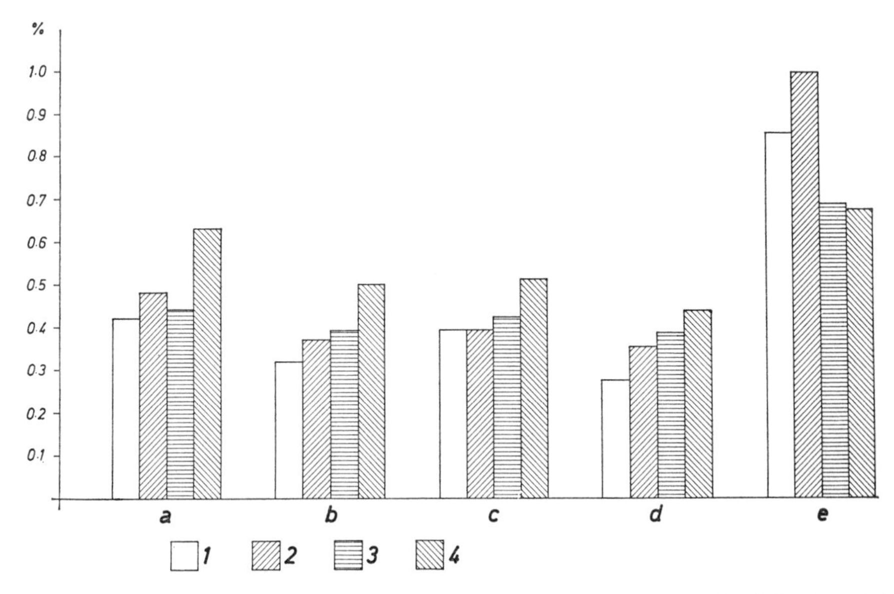

Figure 40. Free ammonia concentration in different parts of rat brain following injection of different doses of phenothiazine (aminazin) (in mg% of fresh cerebral tissue). a = aminazin in a dose of 2 mg/kg; b = aminazin in a dose of 5 mg/kg; c = aminazin in a dose of 7 mg/kg; d = aminazin in a dose of 10 mg/kg; and e = control animals (normal saline solution). 1 = cortex; 2 = subcortex; 3 = brain stem; 4 = cerebellum. (From Pogodaev, K.I., 1964.)

Pogodaev (1964) obtained some very important results by studying the effects of drugs on proteolytic enzymes of cerebral tissue in epileptic rats. After *phenamine,* the activity of proteolytic enzymes changes during autolysis of the cerebral homogenates. The concentration of ammonia in the cortex increased by 22 percent only four minutes after the injection. After 30 minutes it fell by 36 percent. So, at this stage, it was 20 percent lower than in control animals. The subcortex provided similar findings: the ammonia concentration rose by 36 percent four minutes after injection, but had fallen by 37 percent, 30 minutes after injection so that, compared with the control animals, there was a reduction of 16 percent. The findings in the brain stem were quite the reverse: four minutes after injection the proteolytic enzyme activity had only increased by 4 percent but it had increased by a further 23 percent after 30 minutes so that, at this stage, the ammonia concentration in the brain stem was 27 percent higher than in the control animals. The author concluded that the activity of proteinase after phenamine undergoes different changes under electrical stimulation of convulsions in different areas of the brain and at different times. In the cortex and subcortex, the activity of these enzymes increases immediately after the injection and later falls to below the level in the control animals. On the other hand, there is a steady increase in the brain stem.

After autolysis of the brain homogenates, the activity of proteolytic enzymes in the cortex increased by 26 percent in animals decapitated four minutes after injection of phenamine. It fell by 44 percent in animals decapitated after 30 minutes. Corresponding findings in the subcortex were as follows: increased by 36 percent and reduced by 31 percent. Four minutes after the injection, the activity of proteinases in the brain stem was 12 percent lower. After 30 minutes it increased by 54 percent so that this activity was then 34 percent higher than in control animals. The dose of phenamine was 1.2 mg/kg. Working in Pogodaev's laboratory, Mechmedova (cited from Pogodaev 1964) obtained similar findings with doses of 2.4 mg/kg in the two to three minutes after injection. From this Pogodaev (and Mechmedova) concluded that, *in the doses used here, phenamine activates metabolic processes of proteins in the brain and thus causes neuronal excitation.* This excitation begins in the cortex and is then transmitted to the subcortical ganglia; this can be seen from the activity of proteinases (and respiratory processes) four minutes after injection. About 30 minutes after injection an inhibitory process assumes dominance in the cortex and subcortex, whereas the excitatory process is dominant in the brain stem. In this test preparation, excitations begin in the cortex and, as time goes on, wander into the deeper cerebral structures.

These results correlate with those of Faddeev (1951), which he obtained from studying conditioned reflexes under the action of phenamine. Other authors have also demonstrated the wandering of excitation from the cortex to the subcortex and brain stem (see Chapters III and IV) in other test preparations. As far as epilepsy is concerned, the precondition is that the focus is in the cortex itself. However, if it is in deeper formations of the brain (as may be the case in psychomotor epilepsy) the excitation arises from this convulsion focus (see Chapter III), wanders into the cortex and only then does it return to deeper cerebral structures, whence it passes into the periphery (see also Chapters IV and VIII).

Pogodaev (1964) carried out a series of experiments in which he studied the activity of proteinases in rats during the autolysis of brain homogenates of the cerebral hemispheres and cerebellum after giving other chemical compounds. The experimental animals were first treated for 15 days with *Amytal-sodium* or a mixture of *Luminal* and *strychnine.* After this treatment, proteinase activity was lower than in control animals. After Amytal-sodium it was 14 percent lower in the cerebral hemispheres and 36 percent lower in the cerebellum; after the mixture of Luminal and strychnine it was 14 percent lower than in control animals in the cerebral hemispheres and 10 percent lower in the cerebellum. As a result of the suppression of proteolytic enzymes, production of ammonia was reduced by five or 20 percent in the hemispheres and thirty or 40 percent in the cerebellum. This suppression of ammonia production in the cerebellum was up to 41 percent lower than the level in control animals after Amytal-sodium and up to 34 percent lower with Luminal-strychnine.

In a second series of experiments, test and control animals were treated for up to two and one-half months with the drugs mentioned. Proteolytic activity in brain homogenates was reduced by 40 percent in the test animals after both groups of compounds. Proteolytic activity following use of tridione (77 mg/kg Trimetin) responded in approximately the same way as with the first two groups of compounds. There were no definite changes with a mixture of Trimetin and strychnine. However, the group of test animals was too small to calculate the significance level.

Other antiepileptic agents such as *diphenylhydantoins* have an effect on proteolytic enzymes similar to that of Amytal-sodium (Woodbury and Kemp 1970).

Energy Changes. Nucleotides and Nucleic Acids Under the Action of Other Chemical Compounds

Decsi and Méhes (1958) assumed that, compared with the effects of pure *sedatives,* the mechanisms of action when using *neuroleptic* and *ataractic* agents must be more complicated. According to Sutherland and Rall (1960), adrenaline and glucagon stimulate synthesis of AMP and its breakdown is inhibited by *glucagon* and *caffeine.* Moreover, via a kinase system and with the help of ATP, cyclic AMP activates the phosphorylase necessary for degradation of glycogen. Lewis and van Petten (1963) examined the effects of a number of compounds including *imipramine* and MAOI on the adenine nucleotides in rat brain and they found that there was a rise in the ATP/ADP quotient. It was concluded that there is a connection with the antidepressant action here.

Kaul et al. (1965) made a specific study of adenine nucleotides (and phosphocreatine and inorganic phosphorus compounds) in the whole brain and in the hypothalamus of rats, under the action of *chlorpromazine.* Chlorpromazine was administered i.p. in doses of 20, 25 and 50 mg/kg (or triflupromazine 20 mg/kg). After three hours there was a significant reduction in the concentration of ATP in the whole brain, and there was a significant elevation after six hours. In the hypothalamus ATP was elevated after 1.5 and six hours, but was depressed after three hours. There were more marked variations of ATP in the whole brain with 25 mg/kg than after 50 mg/kg. With a dose of 25 mg/kg, ADP was elevated after 1.5 hours and reduced after six hours. After 50 mg/kg there was no significant change of ADP at these times. However, both doses increased the level of ADP after 0.5 and three hours. Hypothalamic ADP was elevated after three hours and reduced after six hours under the action of 25 mg/kg and 50 mg/kg chlorpromazine. The total increase of adenine nucleotides (ATP, ADP, AMP) in the whole brain was the same as the controls. However, in the hypothalamus the total quantity of adenine nucleotides was elevated after 1.5 hours with 25 mg/kg and depressed after three hours with 50 mg/kg chlorpromazine. See also Davis and Brody (1966) as regards these findings.

Studies on adenine-containing nucleotides under the action of drugs and in psychoses have revealed many important changes. Frohmann et al. (1967) have discovered characteristic changes of adenosine phosphate metabolism in the blood of schizophrenic patients after high-dosed insulin treatment; we mentioned this in Chapter V from another point of view. The disruptive factor is to be found in plasma. Hofmann and Arnold (1967) discovered by a succinate loading test that the disruptive factor is in the erythrocytes, i.e. in their membrane. Other authors (Biesold et al. 1965) did not find any changes of adenosine phosphate in the blood of schizophrenic patients without using the succinate loading test.

Hofmann and Arnold (1967) failed to find any changes of adenosine phosphate metabolism in manic-depressive patients. ATP and its degrading enzyme ATP-ase definitely play a decisive role in maintaining normal membrane function (Kanig 1969), in our particular case the function of the nerve cell membrane. If this function is disrupted, enzymes may leave the nerve cell (Amelung 1964); this has already been demonstrated by a number of authors (Bengzon et al. 1966; Hippius et al. 1964). The demonstrable *in vitro* and *in vivo* effects of psychopharmacological drugs on adenosine phosphates are *due to inhibition of ATP synthesis partly as a result of disruption of oxidative phosphorylation, and also due to inhibition of ATP-ase* (Kanig 1966, 1969).

The *in vivo* investigations of Kanig (1963, 1965, 1966, 1967, 1969, 1971 b) on rats with *butyrylperazine* revealed that the balance between these two active components results in a higher concentration of ATP in the brain compared with that in controls. Neuroleptic agents can be regarded as having an economizing effect on metabolism (Coper 1971, Kanig 1969, 1970, 1971 a, b, c, 1972; Quadbeck 1966). Kanig (1969) found that, compared with barbiturates, there was an additional effect in that the amount of 3-adenosine phosphate was increased. The author did not state whether this effect was due to reduced incorporation of adenosine phosphates into nucleic acids. Administration of the psychotonic magnesium pemoline has been shown to increase the nucleic acid content (Plotnikoff 1966). It was thus concluded that psychopharmacological agents act on nucleic acid synthesis.

NAD has already been discussed in Chapters III and V. Here we would like to make one or two brief additions to what was said. Lewis and Pollock (1965) observed the effects of D-amphetamine sulfate (2.5, 5 and 10 mg/kg) and chlorpromazine.HCl (15 or 30 mg/kg) on oxidized NAD and reduced $NADH_2$ in the brain of rats. They found that D-amphetamine sulfate (10 mg/kg) causes a significant fall of NAD content but there was no significant change in the concentration of $NADH_2$. As a rule, amphetamine alone and other stimulants increase the concentration of ATP in the brain. Since, in the experiment of Lewis and Pollock just discussed, amphetamine and chlorpromazine did not cause a significant increase of ATP, it was concluded that additional chlorpromazine causes a reduction in the cerebral concentration of ATP. For this reason, in this type of test, the otherwise comparable relationships between the concentrations of ATP and NAD are not valid.

Walaas and Walaas (1965) found that large quantities of NAD inhibit the oxidation of catecholamines to aminochromes. The authors assume that this type of oxidation reaction also occurs with copper-containing enzymes in the synapses of the brain. If this hypothesis was to be confirmed, then the combination of neuroleptic agents and high doses of nicotinamide would be the treatment of choice for psychoses, especially schizophrenia (Kanig 1969, 1970, 1971 a, b, c, 1972; Kanig and Oesterle 1971). In the case of epilepsy, the triggering of seizures could be prevented by administering high NAD doses (or nicotinamide) in addition to neuroleptic agents or antidepressants in the case of a psychotic condition. In these cases it would be possible to control the psychotic symptomatology in epilepsy without running the risk of triggering an epileptic seizure. Further research work needs to be done to confirm this hypothesis.

After special preparation, Hoffer (1966) achieved a dramatic improvement in schizophrenia with NAD. There was no success in chronic schizophrenia with NAD without this preparation (see in Kanig 1969). Nicotinamide produces a temporary increase in concentration of NAD in the brain. Pretreatment with chlorpromazine or reserpine prolongs this rise (Burton et al. 1960; Coper 1963, 1971, Coper and Selbach 1970, Coper et al. 1972). It was thus concluded that nicotinamide or nicotinic acid would be of some help in schizophrenia since this compound provides structural units for producing NAD. Since the work of Hoffer (1967), these compounds have been used in high doses in schizophrenia. The effect of nicotinamide and nicotinic acid in epilepsy has been discussed in Chapters V and VII. All these results indicate that NAD will influence metabolism of the central neurons in schizophrenia and epilepsy.

The phenothiazines antagonize flavine nucleotides such as flavine mononucleotide (FMN) and flavine adenine dinucleotide (FAD), particularly

(FAD) (Kanig 1963, 1966, 1969, 1970, 1971 a, b, c, 1972). Competitive suppression of flavoproteins has been suggested (see also Chapters III and V). Lasslo and Mayer (1951) found that phenothiazines inhibit D-amino acid oxidase, which also contains FAD as the coenzyme. Gabay and Harris (1966) actually attempted to find a correlation between the intensity of this inhibition and clinical activity. According to a number of authors (Nagatsu et al. 1967; Yagi et al. 1960), to a certain extent FAD is capable of abolishing the effect produced by chlorpromazine. It is therefore assumed that small quantities are capable of penetrating into the brain. As regards extrapyramidal symptoms and phenothiazines, it should also be mentioned that the central ganglia are rich in riboflavines (Kanig 1966, 1969, 1970, 1972; Leemann and Pichler 1941).

Compared with the picture in other organs, in the brain there are high concentrations of the next group of nucleotides, the guanine nucleotides such as guanine triphosphate (GTP), guanine diphosphate (GDP) and guanine monophosphate (GMP). These compounds are involved in the production of energy-rich compounds in the citric acid cycle, and in protein metabolism (Kanig 1969). Butyrylperazine and reserpine increase the sum of guanosine phosphates in rat brain (Kanig 1967, 1969, 1972).

It was also thought likely that chlorpromazine has an effect on cytosine nucleotides (Ansell et al. 1964).

Antiepileptic agents such as *diphenylhydantoin* and others affect the metabolism of nucleotides and nucleic acids (see Woodbury and Kemp 1970).

Amino Acids and Chemical Compounds Which Affect Their Metabolism

By treating rats with 77 mg/kg *cystine,* Pogodaev (1964) found a 51 percent increase in the levels of this compound in the brain in test animals compared with the results from controls. As a rule, levels of cystine and cysteine fall with repeated epileptic attacks. Lajtha and Todh (1965) studied the effects of a number of neuroleptic agents on the uptake and output of cerebral amino acids *in vitro* and *in vivo* in mice. Most of the drugs reduce amino acid metabolism in the brain, but a number of different mechanisms were recognized here. Reserpine and phenobarbitone inhibited the *in vitro* uptake of L-lysine and cycloleucine in brain sections. However, this type of change was not found with pentylenetetrazole. Low concentrations of chlorpromazine tended to enhance the uptake of these amino acids but this was reduced with higher concentrations. Cocaine abolished the inhibitory effect of protoveratine on cerebral amino acid uptake, but not after prior administration of oubain or chlorpromazine.

Pentylenetetrazole and phenobarbitone did not produce any *in vivo* changes. Under conditions of hypothermia, to a large extent phenobarbitone was capable of reducing the uptake of lysine. Chlorpromazine reduced the cerebral uptake of lysine, whether it was given by i.p. or i.c. injection. I.p. injection of reserpine also inhibited the uptake of lysine. However, with i.c. injection a tendency to promote uptake of this amino acid was found. The uptake of cycloleucine *in vivo* responded in the same way as that of lysine.The *in vivo* output of cycloleucine by the brain declined with reserpine and chlorpromazine. However, with phenobarbitone this only occurred under hypothermic conditions.

Singh and Malhotra (1967) observed the effect of chlorpromazine on GABA, aspartic acid, glutamic acid/glutamine, cystine/cystathionine, alanine, serine and glycine in the frontal lobes, amygdala, mesencephalon, hippocampus, hypothalamus and cerebellum of apes. The chlorpromazine dose was 10 mg/kg i.v. After administration of chlorpromazine there was a reduction in the concentrations of GABA and cystine/cystathionine in all regions of the brain. The concentration of alanine fell in all observed cerebral regions except the mesencephalon. There was an increase of aspartic acid levels in the mesencephalon, hypothalamus and cerebellum and a reduction in the other areas of the brain. The levels of glutamic acid/glutamine increased in the frontal lobe, mesencephalon and cerebellum and fell in the other cerebral regions. The level of serine was only depressed in the frontal lobe and amygdala, and it increased in other regions of the brain apart from the hypothalamus where there was no change. The glycine concentration increased in the frontal lobe, amygdala and mesencephalon, but it was depressed in the remaining three regions.

As mentioned in Chapters III and VI, a number of *antiepileptic agents* also have an effect on amino acid metabolism (see also Toman 1949; Woodbury and Kempf 1970).

Concentration and Activity of Neuromodulators

The most important factor in the effect of drugs on the CNS is the change of concentration and activity of neuromodulators (neurohormones). A number of mechanisms must be involved here and some of these are shown in Figure 41 (see also Hassler et al. 1971; Matussek 1964, 1966, 1970).

One or two of the mechanisms involve alterations in the production and degradation of endogenous amines and other neuromodulators. In their studies on the effects of chlorpromazine in intact white rats, Gey and Pletscher (1964) discovered a number of changes which cannot be caused by hypothermia. This was demonstrated by two experiments. First they injected the animals with chlorpromazine (20 mg/kg) i.p. 30 minutes before an s.c. injection of DL-2- ^{14}C-DOPA (20 mg/kg). About 60 minutes after the last injection, the radioactivity levels in the fractions of amino acids, monoamines and phenolcarboxylic acids were determined. The results that showed that chlorpromazine increased the blood levels and reduced urinary levels of these three ^{14}C-labelled fractions. This was plain where there was hypothermia.

In the second experiment, chlorpromazine was given to a group of animals with hypothermia and another group of normothermic animals. Here there was an increase of radioactivity in the brain of the experimental animals, both in the hypothermic and in the normothermic animals. This was mainly due to an increase in the concentration of ^{14}C-phenolcarboxylic acids. At the same time there was also an absolute increase of ^{14}C-noradrenaline. In another experiment the rats were pretreated with an MAOI (iproniazid) and this reduced the chlorpromazine-induced increase of radioactivity of ^{14}C-phenolcarboxylic acids.

Among other things, Anden (1966) discovered that administration of haloperidol, chlorpromazine and reserpine blocked the transformation of dopamine and its transport across the blood-brain barrier. Various authors including Ingenito and Bonncastle (1967) studied the interrelationships between temperature regulation and changes in the concentration of cerebral monoamines. α-Methyl-m-tyrosine, 4-chloro-N-methyl-amphetamine and 5-hydroxy-DL-tryptophan affected the levels of cerebral monoamines without influencing temperature regulation. Resperine had similar effects. Chlorpromazine, dinitrophenol and DOPA did not affect the levels of 5-HT and noradrenaline, but they did influence regulation of body temperature. In rats, the authors did not find any direct relationship between regulation of body temperature and the concentrations of 5-HT and noradrenaline in the whole brain.

Among other authors, Bird et al. (1967) used an indirect method to examine the effect of phenothiazines on production of monamines in the brain. They examined the manganese and dopamine concentration in the basal ganglia of the brain of primates. After a three-day and three-month course of phenothiazines, in apes they found a significant increase in the manganese concentration in the caudatum and putamen, but not in the other basal nuclei studied. After the three-day experiment, there was a significant increase of dopamine, and in a one-month experiment this returned to the control levels. The authors concluded from this that phenothiazines exert their extrapyramidal effects by altering the concentrations of manganese and dopamine, i.e. by impairing production of noradrenaline in the brain.

Guldberg and Yates (1968) studied the effect of chlorpromazine on cerebral catecholamine metabolism in dogs. Various regions of the brain were observed. Certain changes appeared in the caudate nucleus two hours after administering the preparation. After 5 mg/kg chlorpromazine, the concentration of dopamine remained unchanged, but it declined after a dose of 15 mg/kg. The concentrations of homovanillic acid (HVA) and 3, 4-dihydrophenylacetic acid were increased with 5 mg/kg but they remained unchanged with a dose of 15 mg/kg. Both doses of chlorpromazine reduced the concentrations of methoxydopamine. Similar changes in the level of dopamine and its metabolites were seen in the globus pallidus. Both doses of chlorpromazine increased the concentration of noradrenaline in regions of the brain which contained more noradrenaline than dopamine (hypothalamus, thalamus, mesencephalon, cerebellum). However, in general there was no significant change in the concentration of dopamine and its metabolites. These authors found that the chief effect was stimulation of catecholamine synthesis. However, the results cannot be explained simply on the basis of catecholamine synthesis. It has been assumed that chlorpromazine exerts several effects on the cerebral amines and this will be dealt with again later.

ANOTHER MECHANISM CAN LEAD TO A REDUCTION IN THE CONCENTRATION OF NEUROMODULATORS AT THE RECEPTORS. This is *blockade of the release of monoamines* from the presynaptic regions of the neurons, i.e. from the stores. Dresse (1966) studied the effect of 15 neuroleptic agents (butyrophenones and phenothiazines) on the variation of cerebral noradrenaline content and on the activity of experimental animals (rats) in autostimulation tests. The most important neuroleptic agents used were fluphenazine, thioperazine, haloperidol and triperidol. The drugs were injected s.c. two hours from the administration of tranylcypramine (1.25 mg/kg). Higher doses of neuroleptic agents reduced or completely suppressed the increase of extracellular noradrenaline. Doses which were necessary for this suppressant action varied according to the drug used. A selective effect of neuroleptics on specific cerebral structures was also found.

In studies on the effects of neuroleptic agents on the activity of catecholaminergic neurons, Haessle et al. (1967) used haloperidol, chlorpromazine and the methyl ester of DL-α-methyltyrosine hydrochloride (H 44/68) on rat brain. Haloperidol alone resulted in a weaker intensity of fluorescence (fluorometric method) of the noradrenergic nerve endings than H 44/68 alone. With dopaminergic nerve endings the fluorescene was the same after treatment with H 44/68 as after treatment with H 44/68 and haloperidol.H 44/68 and haloperidol together caused an increased loss of noradrenaline but not of dopamine. Similar results were observed after treatment with H 44/68 and chlorpromazine. Chlorpromazine alone produced a significant reduction of the dopamine level. There was no significant reduction of fluorescence activity of catecholaminergic nerve endings after clorpromazine alone, compared with control animals. Repeated injection of haloperidol and chlorpromazine resulted in a depletion of endogenous amines at the noradrenergic and dopaminergic nerve endings.

BLOCKADE OF INTRACELLULAR ENZYMES MAY RESULT IN AN INCREASE OF MONOAMINES. Naturally enough, in this case the increase will first occur inside the cells. Later there will also be an increase in the subsynaptic concentration of noradrenaline. This also applies to serotonin (Hippius and Jantz 1959; Matussek 1964, 1969, 1970; Ross 1965; Shimuzu et al. 1964). This is particularly marked by blockade of MAO by MAO inhibitors (MAOI) so that monoamine which returns into the nerve cells after the end of stimulation, cannot be broken down. This results in excessive intra- and extra-cellular levels of monoamine, which can cause psychomotor excitation in experimental animals and in psychotic patients, or trigger epileptic manifestations in epileptic patients. A number of antidepressant agents (see Chapter VI) are known to be monoaminoxidase inhibitors.

THE RELEASE OF MONOAMINES FROM THE STORES is an important feature in the mechanisms of action of psychopharmacological agents. The use of rauwolfia preparations has led to our understanding this. Among other authors, Ross (1965) observed the effects of reserpine, chlorpromazine and haloperidol on the concentration of 5-HT, dopamine and their metabolites in the CNS. He established that reserpine causes a release of 5-HT and dopamine from their stores. Minimum values were reached one hour after administration of reserpine and recovery took a week (see also Chapter VIII). Since there is no concurrent inhibition of MAO, the destruction of these neuromodulators results in an increase in the levels of their metabolic products in the brain. Destruction can also be brought about by catecholamine-O-methyltransferse (which again is not inhibited in this case) which is a more extracellular enzyme. Experiments with chlorpromazine and haloperidol have shown that there is an increase in the concentration of degradation products of 5-HT and dopamine in the brain; for example, there is an increase in the levels of homovanillic acid. The mechanism of action of these latter two compounds has not yet been definitely explained.

Many other authors have also found changes in the cerebral metabolism of dopamine in the brain stem due to monoamine-releasing psychopharmacological agents. Pletscher and Prada (1966) observed a significant and dose-related increase of HVA in the cerebellum of rats with 2-hydroxy-2-ethyl-3-isobutyl-9, 10-dimethoxy-1,2,3,4,6,7-hexahydro-11-bH-benzo-(a)-quinolizine (Ro 4-1284, Hoffmann la Roche) and chlorpromazine (here, both compounds were regarded as fast-reacting monoamine releasers).

Ro 4-1284 produced a definite increase in the concentration of 5-hydroxyindoleacetic acid and a reduction in the concentration of 5-HT and dopamine. Thus, Ro 4-1284 appears to exhibit similar effects to those of reserpine. According to these latter authors, other psychotropic compounds such as tranquilizers (meprobamate, chlordiazepoxide), hypnotics (phenobarbitone) and thymoleptic agents (imipramine, amitryptiline) do not affect the concentration of HVA or 5-HT or their metabolism in the brain stem.

Vysotskaya and Shugina (1967) studied the catecholamine content in the brain stem of white rats and the sedative effect of neuroleptic agents (aminazine, chlorpromazine) and tranquilizers (reserpine, meprobamate) and found that the sedative effect of various tranquilizers is accompanied by variable changes in the catecholamine content in the brain stem. Thus, reserpine, trypthiazine and, to a certain extent, also meprobamate tended to reduce adrenaline and noradrenaline in the brain stem. Chlorpromazine and mepazine did not alter the monoamine content. According to Sulser and Dingel (1968), reserpine caused a dramatic increase of total radioactivity in experimental animals pretreated with desipramine. The results reflect the *in vivo*, desipramine-induced inhibition of the amine transport mechanisms. In order to demonstrate this, the authors used ^{3}H-noradrenaline which was injected into the lateral ventricle of rat brain. There was then continuous release, re-uptake and metabolism of the catecholamine. Reserpine was administered (5 mg/kg i.p.) one hour after beginning the perfusion of ^{3}H-noradrenaline into the anterior hypothalamus. In the next two hours there was an increase in the total radioactivity released into the perfusate.

In their experiments, Vysotskaya et al. (1968) concentrated on the action of reserpine, trifluoperazine, amphetamine and pipradol on the free, active but unstable noradrenaline (NA) in the brain of rats and compared the results with the effects on behavior in experimental animals. The results showed that trifluoperazine had a tranquilizing effect if the total NA content of the brain stem was reduced. The rats' behavior became normal before the normal level of NA was restored. Other rats were given reserpine for seven weeks (0.2 mg/kg daily). The behavior of the experimental animals returned to normal one day after the last injection in spite of the marked reduction of NA content in the brain stem. In these animals, trifluoperazine and reserpine produced tranquilization which correlated on a time basis with changes of NA content. Amphetamine (2.5 mg/kg) and pipradol (12.5 mg/kg) increased motor activity in these reserpine-treated rats. Tranquilization which then followed was accompanied by a fall of NA levels in the brain stem. Motor activity increased again as the NA level increased.

Blockade of the return of monoamines into the neurons after they have been released from the presynaptic regions by a nerve impulse again results in an increase in the concentration of these substances at the receptor and hence, leads to increased bioelectrical and psychomotor excitation

(Matussek 1964, 1969). This is the particular mechanism of action of antidepressants (and, according to a number of findings, of neuroleptic agents as well).

In studies on chlorpromazine- or haloperidol-induced catalepsy in mice and rats, Maj and Przegalski (1967) obtained a result which indicated an increase of cerebral noradrenaline. In addition to the specific effects of DOPA, MAOI and O-methyltransferase inhibitors on psychopharmacological-drug-induced catalepsy in experimental animals, the authors observed the action of α-β-hydroxylase inhibitor (disulfiram). Mice were injected with nialamide 18 hours, chlorpromazine 3.5 hours and haloperidol 1.5 hours s.c., disulfiram two hours and DL-DOPA 0.5 hours i.p. before the test. The catalepsy was determined at intervals. The rats were given reserpine 3.5 hours, chlorpromazine and haloperidol one hour, disulfiram two hours and DL-DOPA immediately before the test. DOPA and nialamide did not control the reserpine-, chlorpromazine- or haloperidol-induced catalepsy in disulfiram-treated mice.

In rats, DOPA and nialamide reduced the cataleptic effect of haloperidol, whereas the results with chlorpromazine were not significant. The anticataleptic effect in disulfiram-treated experimental animals was not observed. These results appear to confirm that the anticataleptic effect of DOPA and nialamide may be due to an increase of cerebral noradrenaline, but that it has nothing to do with the dopamine level. Schanberg et al. (1967) also dealt with the problem of changes of noradrenaline concentration in the brain. To do this, ^{3}H-noradrenaline (NA) was injected i.c. Imipramine, desmethylimipramine, chlorpromazine and lithium chloride were injected i.p. before and after this injection. The rats were sacrificed at different times and their brains with the spinal cord homogenized and examined in the usual way. The homogenate was examined for total radioactivity, radioactive NA and radioactive acids. The pretreatment with imipramine and desmethylimipramine revealed that these two drugs reduce the ^{3}H-NA and increase the ^{3}H-normetanephrine concentration. Chlorpromazine reduced the ^{3}H-NA concentration but did not affect the ^{3}H-normetanephrine. Lithium chloride had no effect on ^{3}H-NA but reduced ^{3}H-deaminated catechol metabolites. It was concluded from these results that *antidepressants cause a useful increase of noradrenaline for the central receptors.* Lithium chloride may exert an opposite effect.

EVEN MORE PRONOUNCED EFFECTS ARE OBSERVED BY BLOCKING THE RETURN OF NEUROMODULATORS FROM THE SUBSYNAPTIC GAP (see Chapter IV, Figures 27 and 41) *and the release of these substances from the stores.* In particular, this is the mechanism of action of neurostimulants and thymoleptic agents (de Boor 1956; Dengler et al. 1961; Fleck 1925; Herting et al. 1961; Matussek 1964).

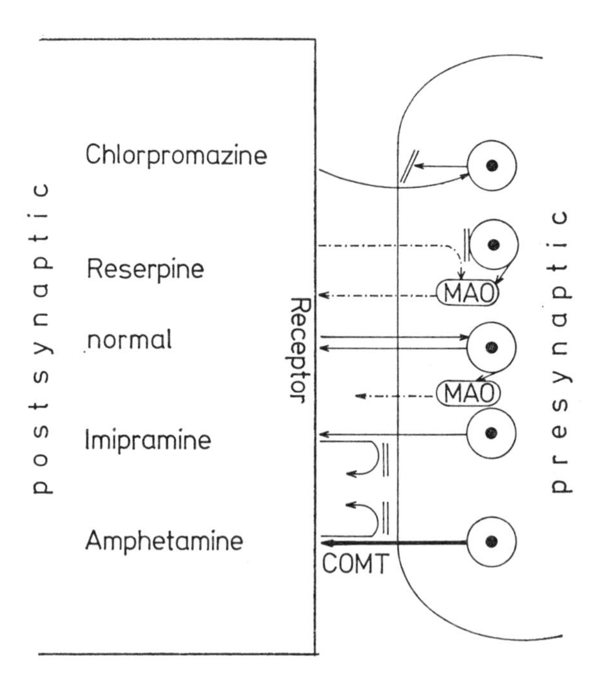

Figure 41. Effect of various centrally acting chemical compounds on the concentration and activity of neuromodulators at the nerve cell membrane (synapses) and within the cells. There is particular emphasis on noradrenaline metabolism which is used as an example for the other neuromodulators. MAO = monoamine-oxidase; COMT = catecholamine-O-methyl-transferase; ⊙ = noradrenaline storage granules; = = inhibition of the return and outflow of noradrenaline at the neuronal membrane. Arrows show the strength and direction of flow of noradrenaline under various conditions. (Based on Axelrod, J., 1966. From Matussek, N.: in *Molekular-Biologie.* p. 254, UMSCHAU-Verlag, Frankfurt/Main, 1969.)

While studying the mechanism of action of drugs on affective diseases and noradrenaline metabolism in rat brain, Schildkraut et al. (1967) came across an interesting result. Cocaine (5.15 or 30 mg/kg)inhibited ^{3}H-NA uptake by the neurons. The level of ^{3}H-noradrenaline rose and that of deaminated catecholamine metabolites fell. These effects were dose-related. Pretreatment with imipramine and desmethylimipramine (25 mg/kg) impeded ^{3}H-NA uptake and resulted in an increase in the level of ^{3}H-NA. Chlorpromazine had a similar effect on the ^{3}H-NA level and a reduced effect on the ^{3}H-normetanephrine level. Electroshock following i.c. pretreatment with ^{3}H-NA reduced the level of ^{3}H-NA in the brain compared with that in control animals, although there were no longer any visible differences three minutes after the electroshock. Experimental animals given i.c. injection of ^{3}H-NA followed by 50 mg/kg lithium chloride showed higher concentrations of ^{3}H-catecholamines, but lower concenrtations with ^{3}H-normetanephrine, compared with the controls. It is concluded that there is a fairly consistent connection between the known clinical effects of drugs and their effects on the concentration and activity of monoamines in rats. *According to the authors, stimulants like cocaine, amphetamine etc. and antidepressants can increase the levels of NA at the receptors in the brain,* while lithium, which is used in agitated psychomotor states, is capable of reducing the level of NA at these receptors. Sharman (1967) was also able to confirm this finding in another way, by studying the effect of various psychopharmacological agents on the production and removal of homovanillic acid (see also Matussek 1964, 1969; Simpson et al. 1967). Sharman (1967) regarded the action of reserpine and amphetamine as being a result of the effect on noradrenaline, serotonin and dopamine.

Sulser and Dingel (1968) showed that chlorpromazine is a central adrenergic blocker and that catecholamine-O-methyltransferase (COMT) is capable of inactivating the free noradrenaline which interacts with the adrenergic receptors. ^{3}H-α-amphetamine (3 mg/kg i.p. 4.23 c/mmol) had a marked psychomotor stimulant effect in rats. Pretreatment with desipramine (1.25 to 10 mg/kg i.p.) potentiated and prolonged this effect. Low doses of chlorpromazine (1.25 to 2.5 mg/kg) also intensified the central effect of amphetamine, which, however, is blocked by higher doses (10 to 20 mg/kg). This example again illustrates the *facultative* epileptogenic effort of chemical compounds (see Chapter VI): a lower dose of chlorpromazine does not have the same effect as a higher dose; this was also mentioned in the chapter just referred to. A lower dose of amphetamine may exert an antiepileptic effect, a higher dose may have an epileptogenic action (see also Chapter VII).

Jonas and Scheel-Krueger (1969) demonstrated that amphetamine-induced stereotyped behavior in animals correlates with the increase in concentration of O-methylated dopamine. The effect of amphetamine on the cerebral concentration of dopamine and noradrenaline and their O-methylated metabolites such as 3-methoxytyramine and normetanephrine has been observed in reserpinized rats. Amphetamine with reserpine produced marked central excitation. This excitation is followed 60 to 90 minutes later by a phase of characteristic stereotyped behavior in which the animals snuffle, lick and gnaw. Rats which have been treated with reserpine (7.5 mg/kg), nialamide (500 mg/kg) and amphetamine (10 mg/kg) always showed this behavior. However, experimental animals which have been treated with reserpine (7.5 mg/kg), perphenazine (5 mg/kg), nialamide (Niamid 200-500 mg/kg) and D-amphetamine sulfate (10 mg/kg) behaved in a quite different way.

In rats pretreated with nialamide, amphetamine increased the accumulation of O-methylated metabolites; corresponding findings were obtained with normetanephrine and 3-methoxytyramine. However, there was a difference between the dopamine metabolites and noradrenaline metabolites in rats which had been given reserpine, nialamide and amphetamine; there was a significant reduction in the concentrations of noradrenaline, normetanephrine and dopamine, but a significant increase in the level of 3-methoxytyramine. The amphetamine-induced accumulation of 3-methoxytyramine in rats pretreated with reserpine is not affected by the neuroleptic drug perphenazine. Perphenazine opposed the hypothermic effect of amphetamine without there being any influence on the accumulation of 3-methoxytyramine. Thus, all these results indicate that where there is a reversal of reserpine-induced tranquilization and catalepsy by amphetamine into pronounced central excitation with stereotyped behavior, there is increased transformation of dopamine.

THE COMBINATION OF BLOCKADE OF THE INTRACELLULAR ENZYMES WITH A RAPID RELEASE OF MONOAMINES from their stores can also result in an increase in the concentration of these agents at the receptors. This situation can occur, for example, if a monamine releaser like reserpine and a monoamine oxidase inhibitor like iproniazid are administered in combination. This can produce severe excitation in experimental animals, delirious states and other excitation states in patients with psychotic symptoms or convulsive seizures in epileptics (see Chapter VI).

ANOTHER COMBINATION OF DRUGS CAN BLOCK THE RETURN OF MONOAMINES FROM THE SYNAPTIC GAP AND ALSO BLOCK MAO. Sensitization of the central synapses by using imipramines was discussed in Chapter VI. Here, we have suggested that this sensitization occurs such that imipramines block the return of monoamines (noradrenaline) from the synaptic gap into the neurons. Simultaneous admininstration of MAOI as antidepressants results in an accumulation of monoamines even in the nerve cells. This concentration causes monoamines to leave the cells and pass into the synaptic gap which is already *saturated* with monoamines. Again in this case there are either excitation states (psychoses) or increased excitation (epilepsy).

THE NEXT POSSIBLE COMBINATION OF DRUGS can increase the intracellular concentration of monoamines and subsequently increase the extracellular concentration. As we have described above, phenothiazines (chlorpromazine) prevent noradrenaline from leaving the nerve cells. According to the authors cited above and other authors, this results in psychomotor tranquilization. If additional MAOI are given, there is a considerable increase in the concentration of monoamines in the neurons. The result is that these neuromodulators leave the intracellular space and there is an increase in the concentration of these agents at the postsynaptic receptor. The effect of neuroleptic agents can be more or less abolished.

However, restlessness and other delirious states which are observed in patients are also known to occur after other drug combinations. We can imagine that a combination of monoamine releaser (reserpine), MAOI (iproniazid) and a drug which blocks the return of monoamines from the synaptic gap (Tofranil), can cause profound restlessness with signs of delirium. The psychiatrist will come across these types of conditions fairly frequently if the drugs are combined in this way. Epileptic reactions are common here (see Chapter VI).

In rare cases we come across a multiple combination of psychotropic compounds. For example, if a combination of reserpine (monoamine releaser), iproniazid (MAOI), imipramine (blocker of the return transport of monoamines) and amphetamine (blocker of the return transport and monoamine releaser) are used, the bioelectrical and clinical consequences may be incalculable. We shall not describe any more potential combinations of drugs here since, in practice, they are less common than those described above.

We must not forget neuroreceptor blockade. In this case the concentration of neuromodulators may be normal, but the substrate is blocked. Here are a few examples.

While studying the effects of various psychotropic compounds on the concentration of homovanillic acid (HVA) and 5-hydroxyindoleacetic acid (HIAA) in the brain stem of rats, Prada and Pletscher (1966) set out to discover whether the increased production of dopamine is the result of a *feed-back* mechanism which functions during the blockade of dopaminergic receptors. The rats were given neuroleptic agents (chlorpromazine, chlorprothixen, haloperidol), thymoleptic agents (imipramine, amitryptiline), tranquilizers (meprobamate, chlordiazepoxide, diazepam) and hypnotics (phenobarbitone, hexobarbitone) i.p. in doses of 5 to 50 mg/kg.

In some of the experiments, 10 mg/kg chlorpromazine was injected s.c. at different intervals of time after 2.5 mg/kg reserpine i.p. The compounds used produced a marked increase in the concentration of HVA in the brain stem of the experimental animals. In all cases, there was only a slight rise in the level of HIAA, apart from the thymoleptic agents which produced a slight fall. After reserpine had depleted the stores of dopamine, chlorpromazine had little effect on HVA. The authors concluded that there may be some connection between disturbed extrapyramidal function and the increased production of cerebral homovanillic acid since neuroleptic agents cause a major rise of HVA. The role of dopamine in the feed-back mechanism was not fully explained, although the authors suggest that the increased production of dopamine is due to compensatory biosynthesis in the stores since there is *receptor blockade*.

Anden (1968) observed changes of the bioelectrical impulses of central monoaminergic neurons produced by preparations which affect monoamine receptors. The tyrosine-hydroxylase inhibitor, i.e. α-methyltyrosine-methyl ester (H 44/68), and the tryptophan hydroxylase inhibitor, i.e. α-propyldopacetamide (H 22/54), caused a reduction of monoamines in the whole *intact* spinal cord, but only proximal to the lesions in the *severed* spinal cord. Adrenergic α-receptor blocker (phenoxybenzamine) and neuroleptic agents (chlorpromazine and haloperidol) increase the H-44/68-induced noradrenaline depletion in the whole, intact spinal cord, but only proximal to the lesions in the severed spinal cord. In the author's opinion, these three drugs possibly block the NA receptors. LSD delayed the H 22/54-induced loss of serotonin (5-HT) in the spinal cord and brain. LSD may stimulate the spinal serotonin receptors, because there are similar effects with the 5-HT precursor 5-hydroxytryptophan. Atropine also inhibited the H 44/68-induced disappearance of dopamine; its action was blocked by haloperidol. It is suggested that the blockade of monoamine receptors causes an increase in activity due to a feed-back mechanism in the presynaptic neurons. A reverse effect is obtained after stimulation of the receptors mentioned.

Pharmacological Compounds and Cerebral Lipids

The lipids (lipoids) of the brain can also be affected by certain drugs. Imipramine and prothiaden stimulate incorporation of L-phenylalanine into the lipid fraction (into lipoproteins or lipoamino acids). The result of increased incorporation of L-phenylalanine into lipoids in brain sections shows that imipramine and prothiaden can act via a different metabolic pathway on cerebral lipids (Tursky et al. 1966, see also above on the effect of imipramine and prothiaden on L-phenylalanine and oxygen consumption).

Further Problems Regarding Enzymes, Vitamins and Hormones with the Use of Pharmacological Compounds

Studies by Ilyuchenok and Mateeva (1965) on 110 experimental animals (rabbits, cats), and many other authors (Hauschild 1960; Hubach 1963; Roos 1965; Ley 1958; Moeller 1958) have shown that, among other things, *chlorpromazine* is a cholinesterase inhibitor but, in the course of its interaction with anticholinesterase and parasympathicomimetic agents it is capable of exerting a central antispasmodic effect and of blocking central cholinergic structures. This effect is usually unmediated, of short duration and weaker than that of central antispasmodic agents. Ilyuchenok and Mateeva conclude from this that the mechanism of action of chlorpromazine and anticholinesterase is based on the fact that chlorpromazine is involved in the blocking of m-cholinergic systems. E 605 and the fluorinated insecticides, which are known to be convulsant poisons, act by blocking cholinesterase (Hauschild 1960, Ley 1958, Moeller 1958 etc.). The modern gaseous convulsants derived from fluorinated insecticides (Hubach 1963; van Sim 1961) have not lost the effect of the parent compounds (see Chapter V). We still cannot say whether the military nerve gases sunk deep in the Atlantic off the coast of Florida U.S.A. had been made completely harmless.

In passing we should like to mention one more finding. Mishkinsky et el. (1966) found that lactation in rabbits was suppressed by hypothalamic implantation of perphenazine. This was explained as being due to the inhibition of the prolactin inhibitors causing activation of prolactin in the anterior lobe of the pituitary and increased growth of the mammae. However, the direct importance of these results from the point of view of our problem is not absolutely obvious.

MECHANISMS INVOLVING CHANGES AT THE NEURONAL MEMBRANE

Changes of the neuronal membrane have already been discussed in detail in Chapters III, IV and V. There was also some discussion on this subject in Chapters VI and VII. Also, changes in the nerve cell membrane are often very evident from the descriptions in the first section of this chapter. This problem will be mentioned again in the summary and so we do not need to embark on further discussion of this question here.

PROBLEMS OF LOCALIZATION. TARGETS OF ACTION OF DRUGS WITH A CENTRAL EFFECT. CHANGES OF CEREBRAL BIOELECTRICAL ACTIVITY DUE TO CHANGES OF THE SYNAPSES AND NEURONAL RATE OF CONDUCTION IN THE BRAIN

We have already dealt with the problem of localization at a given moment, in sections above. The following section is intended, as far as possible, to fill in any gaps there were in the previous sections.

The sites of action of chemical compounds are best studied by microneurophysiological techniques (microleads to monitor spontaneous potentials or discharges after direct or indirect stimulation). It is not possible to survey all the literature on this subject and here we shall summarize it quite briefly. As was done in Chapter VIII, here again we would first like to consider the processes in the brain at each of the barriers (i.e. from a different standpoint from that used earlier). Here again, we shall have to confine ourselves to a few examples.

The First Barrier (y_1 = Ammon's Horn and Adjacent Rhinencephalic Cerebral Structures) as a Site of Action for Drugs

In part, *neuroleptic agents and antidepressants* exert their effect via the first barrier, where they exhibit their negative rather than their positive action (see Chapter VI). In animal experiments, with medium dosages of *phenothiazines* (chlorpromazine) the amygdaloid nuclear complex is activated first, then the hippocampus and finally the cerebral cortex (Monnier 1969, Monnier and Tissot 1958). This sequence corresponds approximately to the predisposition to convulsion of individual central nervous structures (Jung 1957, 1958) and this sequence also appears in psychomotor epilepsy. With higher dosages rather different mechanisms probably come into play.

On the other hand, *neurostimulants* have rather more effect on the remaining regions of the brain and less effect on the limbic structures.

From the *dibenzoazepine* group (dibenzazepine, carbamazepine Tegretal) should be mentioned (see Chapter VII). From the few reports there are, we should like to deal briefly with the results of Holm et al. (1970). In recent years, these authors have examined a number of drugs including Tegretal. In their electrophysiological experiments on cats they concentrated on three methods: 1.) monitoring the spontaneous cortical EEG; 2.) stimulating bioelectrical arousal reactions and monitoring the potentials, and 3.) measuring the thresholds of subcortical response potentials to single stimuli. The following structures were studied: amygdaloid nucleus and anterior hippocampus (our barrier y_1); pallidum, caudatum, nucleus ventralis anterior thalami and the posterior lateral hypothalamus (in most cases our second barrier = γ_2); reticular formation of the mesencephalon and pons (our barrier four = γ_4). Barrier three (neocortex = γ_3) was only observed in respect of response potentials. The authors themselves regarded the findings in the mesencephalon as doubtful so that here we shall only discuss the reticular formation of pons.

These experiments showed that with high doses of Tegretal (60 and 120 mg/kg) there was slight suppression of α-synchronization of the hippocampus which was produced by stimulating the pons. There was more powerful inhibition of neocortical desynchronization. With medium doses (20 mg/kg), the hippocampal synchronization actually showed a threshold reduction. With response potentials to single stimuli, there were suppressant effects in the hippocampus when the nucleus ventralis anterior thalami was involved at the site of stimulation or (more rarely) at the monitoring site. Tegretal only suppressed the amygdaloid efferents in doses of 120 mg/kg and above. For the most part, there was negative correlation between changes of the reticulo-amygdaloid projections and those of the amygdaloid efferents. The occasional inhibitory effects of low or high concentrations of

Tegretal on response potentials which followed hippocampal, hypothalamic or striopallidal stimulation, appeared to be minimal. The afferent projections to the amygdaloid nucleus (apart from the reticulo and caudato-amygdaloid responses) only responded convincingly to doses of 120 mg/kg and above, with moderate threshold rises. The hippocampal afferents responded quite differently; with single doses of Tegretal their thresholds were in part increased, in part reduced.

Of the *benzodiazepine* group we should mention nitrazepam (Mogadan, Mogadon). According to Holm (1969), doses as low as 3 mg/kg Mogadan produced pronounced rises of threshold in all afferents of the amygdaloid nucleus and very slight rises in the reticular formation of pons. Some of the connections with the limbic system are also suppressed. However, the amygdaloid and hippocampal afferents do not present a consistent picture. According to Holm, the symmetrical inhibitions of the efferents of the amygdaloid nucleus can only be located in the *structures of this nuclear region.* Here suppression of those formations also affect stimuli responses with a longer latency, for instance amygdalo-reticular responses (latency 11.1 msec). However, the asymmetric amplitude losses of limbic afferents still do not prove that Mogadan has any influence on the amygdaloid nucleus or hippocampus. We would be dealing here with reticulo- and thalamo-limbic connections of long latency (8 msec or more) where changes are not due to corresponding de-activation at the stimulus sites, but they could be explained by an impairment of the particular relay regions. Nevertheless, Holm (1969) poses the question as to whether the amygdaloid nucleus and reticular formation of pons are the primary sites of action of Mogadan or whether this compound only has a secondary influence on these areas.

Some information has been obtained by comparing the effects of Mogadan with those of *barbiturates.* After administration of barbiturates, amygdaloid after-discharges showed a threshold rise, their duration was curtailed or, at the very least, their spread was limited (Delgado and Mihailović 1956; Holm 1969; Killam and Killam 1957; Killam et al. 1957; Strobos and Spudis 1960). Low doses of Mogadan are even more effective here (Hernández-Peón and Rojas-Ramirez 1966, Holm 1969, 1970; Lanoir et al. 1965a; Schallek and Kuehn 1965; Schallek et al. 1965 a, b). Morillo (1962) assumed that Mogadan has a direct effect on the amygdaloid nucleus. This interpretation is confirmed by the inhibition of many amygdaloid efferents, which is always found after injection of 3 mg/kg. The response of the afferent projections to the amygdaloid nucleus originating from the nucleus ventralis anterior thalami, has shown losses of amplitude. The remaining amygdaloid afferents were not impaired after 3 mg/kg Mogadan. As Holm (1969) went on to explain, the afferents to the amygdaloid nucleus which were studied were partially inhibitory in character. Without exception they were suppressed by *Nembutal®* (pentobarbitone-sodium). Holm explained the fact that the amygdaloid efferents remain unchanged by the functional heterogeneity of the afferents (see also Chapter III). Results of the after-discharge method indicate that barbiturates have an inhibitory effect on the hippocampus (Aston and Domino 1961; Gangloff and Monnier 1957a, Killam and Killam 1957; Killam et al. 1957; Monnier 1969; Schallek et al. 1965; Strobos and Spudis 1960; Takagi and Ban 1960). With the evoked-potential technique, it was possible to make a functional differentiation between intrahippocampal structures by making a separate assessment of afferents and efferents (Andersen 1966; Green 1964). Holm (1969, 1970) and McKenzie (1964) found that there was marked suppression of afferent projections to the hippocampus following injection of pentobarbitone. Since the thresholds of hippocampal efferents were depressed at the same time, Holm went along with Gangloff and Monnier (1957b) in postulating pharmacological suppression of afferent inhibitory impulses to the hippocampus.

From the point of view of our problem, this postulate is only of importance in that here it involves afferent inhibitory impulses from the reticular formation and from the thalamus to the hippocampus. A dose of 3 mg/kg Mogadan will reduce the stimulus response of projections from the reticular formation of pons to the hippocampus far more than the equivalent change of reticular activity (Holm 1969). As regards this projection, the septum and centrum medianum in particular have been attributed with relay functions (Eidelberg et al. 1959; Green and Arduini 1954). Here again, the corresponding effect only assumes significance as regards our problem when there is a condition of status epilepticus (see Chapter VIII). Now, if we take the efferents with a relatively short latency as our criterion, neither septum (Vieth et al. 1969) nor centrum medianum (Holm 1969) exhibits a correspondingly significant influence with medium or low concentrations of Mogadan. Therefore, according to Holm (1969), the principal effect of Mogadan to be considered is its action on intrahippocampal systems. After low and high doses of Mogadan, the remaining response potentials of the hippocampus behaved in very different and sometimes opposing ways, but it was not possible to attribute responsibility to the sites of stimulus (Holm 1969, 1970). The findings would be partly explained if relay structures of the hippocampal formations themselves and also the generators of the derived potentials were involved to varying extents in creating the responses to stimuli and that they responded differently to Mogadan (Holm 1969; Purpura and Grundfest 1959).

According to Green (1964), many afferent stimuli are transmitted via the granular cells of the gyrus dentatus. After afferent stimulation, Eidelberg (1961) identified independent sources of potential in apical and basal dendritic plexuses of the hippocampus. Mogadan had no effect on the after-discharge threshold of the hippocampus (Holm 1969, 1970; Randall et al. 1965). However, this threshold is of prime importance from the point of view of psychomotor epilepsy (see in Kreindler 1965 and Chapter IV). A dose of 20 mg/kg Mogadan is required to suppress the efferent projections of this nuclear region, but high concentrations have very little more suppressant activity. According to Holm (1969), this could again be interpreted as a relay phenomenon. This effect of Mogadan explains its relatively low activity in acute situations with psychomotor seizures and status epilepticus.

It would appear possible from the few known experimental findings that *chlordiazepoxide* (Librium) and *diazepam* (Valium) also have a positive effect on the first barrier of the model in Figure 38, although all the details of the results have still not been confirmed. According to the results of some observations (see above), diazepam has more effect on the reticulo-hippocampal projections. It has a good, but relatively short-lived effect in controlling status epilepticus in psychomotor epilepsy (see Chapter VII).

Vinylbital (Speda®) is also said to affect the first barrier (Holm 1970, Jovanović 1967 g), but this assumption is more speculative and the details have yet to be confirmed.

The other *antiepileptic agents* mentioned in Chapter VII have hardly any effect on the first barrier in psychomotor epilepsy. At all events there are no definite results here. It is possible that *primidon* (Mylepsinun®) has, among other things, an effect on the limbic region, since its pharmacological activity is comparable to that of barbiturates (see Chapter VI).

According to the results of a number of authors, *succinimides* also affect the hippocampus. Steinmann (1964) carried out experiments on 39 rabbits and 11 cats by giving stimulus tests and triggering psychomotor seizures, and this author found that there was a certain increase in the convulsion threshold in the hippocampus following administration of succinimides. In 25 control tests on rabbits, the convulsion threshold for the hippocampus was 17.04 ± 6.06 volt. After administering a dose of 50 mg/kg ethyl-methyl-succinimide, the hippocampal convulsion threshold rose to 27.3 ± 9.7 volt. Diethyl-succinimide also increased the convulsion threshold to 26.5 ± 9.1 volt, whereas propyl-methyl-succinimide did not have a definite effect until a dose of 100 mg/kg was used, when the convulsion threshold rose to 26.11 ± 8.3 volt.

Experimentally-induced psychomotor seizures were suppressed after administration of succinimides. The EEG recordings returned to normal or showed a tendency to normalize. However, it was only possible to influence psychomotor attacks in cats when they were transient hippocampal seizures (see Chapter I). This author attributed the effect of succinimides to stabilization of hippocampal activity.

The Second Barrier (y_2 = Diencephalon and Adjacent Cerebral Structures Rostral to the Mesencephalon) as a Target of Action for Drugs

Neuroleptic agents and antidepressants also affect the second barrier of our model in Figure 38. However, the effect in these regions is rather weaker than that in the limbic system (Monnier 1969).

Neurostimulants have effects in the thalamus and hypothalamus but they are not of any great importance from the point of view of our problem.

Carbamazepine exhibits activity centered in a complicated spectrum of the thalamic projections. The efferent projections of the nucleus ventralis anterior thalami always respond to 20 mg/kg Tegretal. The suppression of these projections is dose-related. With pontine-triggered response potentials, Holm et al. (1970) found that Tegretal (20 mg/kg) primarily impairs the reticulo-thalamic response. With 60 mg/kg, but only definitely with 120 mg/kg, there was a rise in the threshold of the reticulofugal projections to most of the brain regions which they studied. A notable exception was the reticulo-amygdaloid response which lost amplitude after administration of a low dose of carbamazepine, but which did not respond to a high dose.

The authors concluded that carbamazepine exerts its effect most definitely along the *axis: reticular formation of pons—nonspecific thalamus—neocortex,* and low concentrations mainly suppress thalamic structures. Furthermore, there are dose-related effects on limbic afferents and on amygdaloid and pallidal efferents.

As regards the non-specific thalamus (γ_2) *nitrazepam* is effective in a dose of 0.4 mg/kg. With this dose, the excitability of diffusely projecting thalamic increases with concurrent suppression of the reticularis pontis (Bonnin 1965; Faure et al. 1965; Vincent et al. 1966). However, a dose of 1.5 mg/kg had an inhibitory effect on recruiting waves (Lanoir et al. 1965 a, b). With 1 mg/kg there was a significant increase in the threshold of after-discharges of the nucleus centralis lateralis thalami. With *phenobarbitone* a comparable effect only occurred with a dose of 40 mg/kg (Randall et al. 1965; Schallek et al. 1964). After giving an injection of 3 mg/kg, Holm (1969) only found moderate amplitude losses with response potentials following stimulation of the centrum medianum and of the nucleus ventralis anterior thalami. The results obtained up to now still do not reveal a consistent picture of the effects of Mogadan on specific afferents (Bonnin 1965; Faure et al. 1965; Hernández-Peón and Rojas-Ramirez 1966; Holm 1969, 1970; Lanoir et al. 1965 a, b; Vincent et al. 1966). This was only mentioned for comparison with the effect of diphenylhydantoins. Mogadan does not increase the threshold with provoked after-discharges in the caudatum (γ_2); this has been observed by Randall et al. (1965), and by Schallek and Kuehn (1965). The responses of efferent connections of the caudatum also remain normal under Mogadan, or at most there may be a slight reduction of the threshold (Holm 1969). Mogadan was superior to barbiturate in various tests of Mogadan and phenobarbitone on hypothalamic-induced blood pressure responses (Schallek et al. 1964, 1965 a,b). Mogadan suppresses descending impulses from the amygdaloid nucleus (y_1); hippocampus (y_1) and Septum (y_2) to the hypothalamus (y_2); this involves projections of the amygdala-hypothalamus (Holm 1969). Mogadan reduced or inhibited rage and avoidance responses induced in cats and monkeys by stimulating the posterior hypothalamus and the septum (Hernández-Peón and Rojas-Remirez 1966). These authors postulated this effect of Mogadan on excitatory circuits which include the limbic system. In general Mogadan exhibits a much more potent and more reliable effect on the non-specific thalamus than on structures of the limbic region or caudatum. Effects similar to those with nitrazepam can be expected with other benzodiazepine preparations (see Chapter VII).

In low and medium doses, *barbiturates* enhance the triggering of recruiting responses of the neocortex following stimulation of non-specific thalamic structures (Demsey and Morison 1942; Domino 1962; Hold 1969; Jasper et al. 1955; Jung 1963; Killam and Killam 1957; Monnier 1969; Morison and Demsey 1942). These findings have been attributed to suppression of reticulo-thalamic inhibitory impulses *(release phenomenon)* (Domino 1962; Killam and Killam 1958). Thus, the effect is not only local and not only in the thalamic region. The activity changes in the reticular regions may also be responsible for the occurrence of cortical barbiturate spindles (Domino 1955; Holm 1969; Killam 1962). However, there are also other explanations of these phenomena (Monnier 1962, 1969). Gangloff and Monnier (1957b) have suggested that there is some degree of autonomy in the production of cortical spindles in barbiturate-induced sleep.

Also, according to these authors, the recruiting responses are the result of another mechanism. For example, it was still possible to elicit recruiting potentials even in subjects under deep barbiturate anaesthesia, although the optimum stimulus frequency was lower (Domino 1955; Holm 1969; Jasper et al. 1955). If we leave aside the phenobarbitone findings, which were obtained from rabbits (Gangloff and Monnier 1957b, 1958; Monnier 1969), then we find that the recruiting system is less sensitive to barbiturate than the reticular formation of pons. Also, the thalamic-induced changes of existing cortical potentials respond to barbiturates later than the reticular-induced changes (Arduini 1958; Brookhart et al. 1958). The evoked-potential technique finally demonstrates that specific structures of the non-specific thalamus are actually not affected by relatively high doses of barbiturate. Brazier (1960) found that after administration of 13 to 30 mg/kg Nembutal, a response potential of the centrum medianum to a light stimulus is not impaired.

The pitcure is different with the diffuse thalamic projections, which mediate an *arousal* and represent a special non-specific thalamic system (Monnier et al. 1963). This system was inhibited by barbiturates (Killam and Killam 1958; Killam et al. 1957). Phenobarbitone produces threshold elevations to after-discharges provoked in the caudatum (Gangloff and Monnier 1957 b). Mogadan has no effect on these responses or on responses to stimulation of efferent connections of the caudatum (Randall et al. 1965; Schallek and Kuehn 1965). The hypothalamus is particularly sensitive to barbiturates (Feldman et al. 1959). Holm (1969, 1970) observed that, in contrast to Mogadan (3 mg/kg), Nembutal (15 mg/kg) suppressed ascending connections from the posterior hypothalamus to the amygdaloid nucleus, hippocampus and septum. This fact might play a part in the excitations in status epilepticus, but it is not involved in the primary spread of impulses from limbic structures. Inhibition of the descending impulses has not been observed under the action of Nembutal. Reverse effects were recorded with Mogadan. In this case, Mogadan would suppress the spread of primary epileptic impulses from the Ammon's horn to the hypothalamus.

Diphenylhydantoins have very little influence on the excitability of the diffuse thalamic and thalamo-cortical system and they have little effect on the electrical stimulus threshold or on the excitability of limbic system projections. The responses to stimuli in the cortical part of the hippocampus and limbic system are potentiated by hydantoins. The specific projections are not influenced by diphenylhydantoins (Pampus 1958; Stille 1960). Also, other drugs do not have a definite effect or a consistent effect on specific afferents (Arduini and Arduini 1954; Bremer 1937, 1954; Domino 1962; French et al. 1953; Hernández-Peón 1956, 1965; Hernández-Peón and Scherrer 1955 a, b; Holm 1969, 1970; Holm et al. 1970; Killam and Killam 1957; King et al. 1955, 1957; Naquet and King 1954; Scherrer and Hernández-Peón et al. 1955).

The Neocortex (y_3 = Third Barrier) as a Site of Action for Drugs

Neuroleptic agents and antidepressants only have an indirect effect on the neocortex, via deeper cerebral structures (Monnier 1969).

Neurostimulants favor the neocortex as regards the effects (see Chapter VII). Principal drugs here are adrenaline, noradrenaline, phenamine, amphetamine and other analeptics. From the effect of these compounds on the third barrier, i.e. far from the convulsion focus in psychomotor epilepsy, they can be classified as facultative anti-epileptic agents since their favorable effect is only maintained while the neocortex is activated. The anti-epileptic effect of these preparations declines fairly quickly or after a somewhat longer period.

Carbamazepine only produces a very definite rise in the threshold of the arousal reaction in the cortical EEG after a dose of 120 mg/kg. There is a moderate threshold rise after 60 mg/kg, whereas there is no effect with a dose of 20 mg/kg (Holm et al. 1970). Cortical effects have probably been provoked by an effect on the thalamo-cortical projections.

Nitrazepam influences responses in the cortical EEG by affecting reticular and thalamo-cortical projection systems. It inhibits the potentials which correspond to an *arousal* in the olfactory bulb (Domino 1962; Hernández-Peón and Rojas-Ramirez 1966; Holm 1969, 1970). Reticular-triggered arousal reaction of the neocortex is not impaired after injection of 2 mg/kg (Holm 1969, 1970; Morillo 1962). In various animal species the threshold only begins to rise with doses of 3 to 4 mg/kg (Bonnin 1965; Faure et al. 1965; Gogolak and Pillat 1965; Holm 1969; Lanoir et al. 1965 a; Vincent et al. 1966). The response to arousal stimuli is changed earlier by Mogadan in the hippocampus than in the neocortex, whereas barbiturates have the reverse effect (Gogolak and Pillat 1965). According to Holm (1969), this effect must be due to the fact that Mogadan preferentially causes profound suppression of the reticulofugal projections to the hippocampus or to the septal region.

In spite of the high sensitivity of subcortical structures to *barbiturates* and Mogadan, according to Holm (1969) there is evidence that, in quite low concentrations, these drugs first affect the neocortex (y_3). This was also postulated by Brazier (1954) for barbiturates which, in the initial stage of of their effect, induce cortical *fast activity* (Brazier and Finesinger 1945; Chafetz and Cadilhac 1954; Domino and Ueki 1959; Holm 1969; Lennox 1946; Toman and Davis 1949). Low doses of Mogadan also cause high, rapid and regular cortical rhythms when injected into non-anaesthetized cats (maximum dose 0.5 mg/kg). Similar changes of spontaneous potentials have also been induced by other drugs (Cornu 1965; Jouvet 1969; Jouvet et al. 1965; Lanoir et al. 1965 a, b, 1966; Monnier 1962, 1963, 1969; Oswald et al. 1963; Soulairac et al. 1965; Tissot 1965; Vincent et al. 1966). However, we cannot discuss these in detail here.

Diphenylhydantoins increase the convulsion threshold of the motor cortex (Knoell 1940). After use of diphenylhydantoin, the sensitivity of the motor cortex to convulsant agents is reduced (Stille 1960). The convulsion threshold of the neocortex in cats is increased by 50 percent after 5 mg/kg diphenylhydantoin (see also Chapter VII). This site of action of diphenylhydantoins, which is far removed from the convulsion focus, explains the relatively low activity of these compounds in psychomotor epilepsy, compared to their effect in other forms of epilepsy.

Effects of Drugs on the Fourth Barrier (y_4 = Reticular Formation Caudal to the Diencephalon)

Many experimental results have suggested that *chlorpromazine* and other phenothiazine derivatives have a blocking action on the reticular formation mainly in the mesencephalon (Agsphonov 1956; Anochin 1959; Bente 1956; Bremer 1935; Chartan 1954; Surabaschvili 1961; Waldmann 1958; Woronin et al. 1962). Pogodaev (1964) regards the dose-related action of *aminazine* as the result of a series of effects on the reticular formation and on the cortex. Aminazine exerts its action primarily on the subcortical structures, particularly in the mesencephalon. *Amplification* of the mesencephalic reticular formation leads to tonic excitation of the cortex, and tonic excitation of the cortex prolongs the tonic phase of the attack and curtails the clonic phase. Thus, activation of the reticular formation inhibits the motor cortex region and activates the other regions.

Pogodaev considers that higher doses of the preparation lead to dissociation of the deeper and superficial structures as regards inhibition and excitation. He interprets the formation and prolonging of the locomotor phase as excitation of the deeper cerebral structures (rostral to the mesencephalon) and suppression of the higher formations, following administration of higher doses. This functional dissociation of the deeper and higher cerebral formations leads to uncoordinated inhibition and excitation, so that during an attack there are a series of uncoordinated symptoms. Thus, all the epileptic phases which have their origin in the deeper cerebral structures (i.e. the locomotor phase and phase of rigidity) are prolonged. If the entire brain is inhibited, the experimental animals lapse into the coma phase which is then deeper and longer than it would be if phenothiazines had not been given.

According to Pogodaev, the increase in the convulsion threshold of the brain under higher dosages cannot be interpreted as a favorable effect of aminazine. This increase of the convulsion threshold is attributed to a toxic effect of this substance, and toxicity is certainly not a desirable effect. After a certain period, the toxicity alters the body's resistance to other epileptogenic noxae and under chronic conditions the cerebral predisposition to convulsion is increased and the convulsion threshold reduced. Thus, the situation under chronic conditions and that under short-term experimental conditions are basically different. This indicates that caution should be exercised when interpreting the phenomena seen in short-term animal experiments and then attempting to apply them to man (Abdurachimov et al. 1959; Couvpisier and Fournel 1953; Gallenko et al. 1956; Nevsorova 1961; Sack 1957; Usunov et al. 1957).

Neurostimulants have definite effects on the reticular formation. This can be seen from the experimental results already reported.

We mentioned above how *carbamazepine* affects the fourth barrier (y_4). From the results of Holm et al. (1970), carbamazepine may have more effect on the relay stations responsible for propagating an attack than on the sites of origin (convulsion foci) of specific epileptic discharges (see Chapters VIII and VI). As regards the reticular formation, this effect can be regarded more as suppression of back-excitation of the convulsion focus. Comparatively speaking, there is less inhibitory effect on the primary spread of epileptic excitations. However, in our opinion it is possible that the activating neurons of the reticular formation are suppressed so that the inhibitory neurons become predominant. In this case the original epileptic impulses would also be blocked in the fourth barrier as they descend to the spinal cord.

The effect of *nitrazepam* on the reticular formation has been studied by a number of authors (Bonnin 1965; Faure et al. 1965; Hance 1959; Holm 1969, 1970; Holm and Schaefer 1969; Killam 1957; Killam and Killam 1958; Lanior et al. 1965b; Vincent et al. 1966). These authors generally found that, here, Mogadan has considerably less quantitative effect than barbiturates. Using the *evoked-potential* method it was found that inhibitory effects of Mogadan only occur after high doses. With pontine stimulation, doses of 3 and 80 mg/kg only produced a slight change of mesencephalon-triggered response potentials. Even with 80 mg/kg Mogadan, the efferent projections of the reticularis to other cerebral regions were not so powerfully suppressed as they were after administration of 15 mg/kg Nembutal (Holm 1969). However, it must be stressed that even very low doses of Mogadan (0.4 mg/kg) do have some effect on the reticular formation (Bonnin 1965; Faure et al. 1965; Holm 1969; Vincent et al. 1966).

These experiments again demonstrated that there are promoting and inhibiting relationships between the reticular formation of pons and the amygdaloid nucleus. This fact plays a very important part in the construction of our model of epileptic manifestations (see Chapter VIII). 3 mg/kg Mogadan increases the threshold of the efferent connections of the amygdaloid nucleus, but the response of projections between reticular formation and amygdaloid nucleus remains practically unchanged. This projection is suppressed with 80 mg/kg and hence, there is no more inhibition of the amygdaloid efferents. Thus, we can conclude that high doses of the drug suppress ascending influence of a predominantly inhibitory nature. This would result in an increase of excitability of the amygdaloid nucleus *(release phenomenon)* which would virtually balance the direct effect of Mogadan on this nuclear region. Mogadan either has no effect or does not have a consistent effect on the effects of stimulation recorded in the mesencephalic reticular formation (Holm 1969). The mesencephalic reticular formation responds to Mogadan in the same way as the reticularis pontis (Batini et al. 1958, 1959; Baust 1967; Magnes et al. 1961a, b: Moruzzi 1960, 1972).

In addition to what has been said about the effect of *barbiturates* on the reticular formation, it should be added that these chemical compounds inhibit intrareticular connnections (Hance 1959; Holm 1969; Killam 1957; Killam and Killam 1958). Holm (1969) found that there was a profound effect on mesencephalon-triggered response potentials after 15 mg/kg Nembutal with pontine stimulation. It is surprising that the effects of stimulation recorded in the mesencephalic reticular formation either do not respond at all or do not show a consistent response to Nembutal.

According to Holm (1969), the reticular potentials must be evaluated in a different way when, instead of a subcortical nuclear region, a peripheral nerve or a sense organ is stimulated and the afferent signals are transmitted via collaterals of sensory pathways. Then, for the most part, the long-latency response components appear to be determined by the reticular activity. Thus, the suppressant effect of barbiturate on the reticular formation is manifest as an impressive amplitude reduction of such potentials (see also Arduini and Arduini 1954; Collis and O'Leary 1954; Feldman et al. 1959; French et al. 1953; Killam 1957; Killam and Killam 1958; Kletzkin and Swaun 1959; Longo and Silvestrini 1958). However, this fact is of more importance in centrencephalic forms of epilepsy where the seizures can easily be provoked by external stimulation. On the other hand, exogenous stimuli have very little effect on psychomotor epilepsy (see Chapter I). In addition to the mesencephalic reticular formation, caudal regions of the brain stem also respond to barbiturates (Anokhin 1961; Brazier 1954, 1963; Feldman et al. 1959, 1960; Forbes and Morison 1939; Holm 1969, 1970; Magni et al. 1959; Martini et al. 1958, 1959; Monnier 1962, 1969; Moruzzi 1960; Purpura 1955, 1972).

Hydantoin preparations and other drugs affect the fourth barrier (see Chapter VIII).

Possible Methods of Affecting the Fifth Barrier (y_5)

Neurostimulants, strychnine and similar compounds activate the spinal cord, whereas relaxants such as meprobamate, sedatives and tranquilizers suppress the spinal cord. However, this effect rarely has to be considered in psychomotor epilepsy since, in many cases, the seizures are not transmitted via the fifth barrier.

CHAPTER X

SUMMARY AND FINAL CONCLUSIONS

THERE ARE MANY problems involved in studying *psychomotor epilepsy* and, consequently, there are many factors which have to be taken into account. To facilitate systematization of the material, the cerebral structures involved in the genesis of psychomotor epilepsy are classified into regions. Since results so far indicate that disinhibition of excitation is *primarily* responsible for epileptic discharges and manifestations, here we have termed these cerebral regions *barriers.* Based on the model of epileptic excitations, the first barrier is in the temporal lobe (y_1), the second in the medial structures of the brain (y_2), the third in the neocortical regions (y_3), the fourth in the lower part of the brain stem (y_4) and the fifth (y_5) in the spinal cord.

THE MANY FORMS AND SYMPTOMS OF PSYCHOMOTOR EPILEPSY

Psychomotor epilepsy may develop as a *primary* manifestation, or, *secondarily,* from one of the other forms of epilepsy. It may develop *symptomatically* as a result of some demonstrable noxa, or it may be *essential* (idiopathic), where the cause is unknown. From a phenomenological point of view, psychomotor epilepsy may be *isolated* (mainly the primary form) or the symptoms may occur in conjunction with other epileptic manifestations —*combined* psychomotor epilepsy (mainly the secondary form).

Psychomotor epilepsy can occur at any age and it tends to occur more frequently in its combined form. It is usually combined with nocturnal epilepsy of grand mal type and, more rarely, with matutinal epilepsy of grand mal type. It is hardly ever combined with petit mal epilepsy. However, any form of epilepsy can clear up in time or, alternatively, it can develop into the psychomotor form. Hence, this form is regarded as the common *finale* of all forms of epilepsy.

Because there is such a vast range of symptoms, the *nomenclature* in respect of psychomotor epilepsy is poorly standardized. The literature contains references to autonomic epilepsy, uncinate fits, dreamy state, rhinencephalic epilepsy, twilight attacks, twilight states, psychomotor equivalents, visceral epilepsy, temporal or temporal lobe epilepsy, oral petit mal or oral automatisms. From the clinical point of view the most commonly used term has become *psychomotor epilepsy,* whereas *temporal or temporocephalic epilepsy* are the terms used in neuroanatomy and neurophysiology. Further subclassification and systematization of psychomotor epilepsy into more homogeneous, manifest forms is a problem—again because the symptomatology is so diverse and unpredictable. There have been a number of attempts to do this, in the literature.

It is not always easy to distinguish psychomotor epilepsy from other forms. Epileptics of the temporocephalic type (psychomotor and nocturnal epilepsy) can be distinguished from the group of centrencephalic epileptics (matutinal and petit mal) by their clinical symptoms, bioelectrical cerebral activity, by the localization and type of pathological and neurophysiological convulsion focus, by the course, by their intelligence and character, by their processing of experiences, by the way they overcome conflict, by their perception of time and space, by their social relationships, their physique, autonomic functions, by their predisposition to status epilepticus, by the frequency and nature of seizures and by the multiplicity of epileptic manifestations. All these differences are evidence that psychomotor epilepsy is a *biological* as well as being a clinical phenomenon. Much time and effort is required if the problem as a whole is to be solved.

Isolated psychomotor epilepsy is manifest by *psychic symptoms* (alteration or loss of consciousness without the patient falling, disorientation, visual, acoustic, vestibular, olfacto-gustatory and tactile illusions and/or hallucinations which may or may not be preceded by aura, usually with *déjà vu* and mental diplopia), by *sensations* (olfacto-gustatory, cardiac, respiratory, epigastric, tactile sensations or pain, anorexia, vomiting, diarrhea, constipation), by *motor symptoms* (smacking of lips, similar movements of the mouth, clicking the tongue, grinding of the lower jaw, sipping movements, spitting, coughing, wheezing, talking, coordinated or automatic hand movements, fingering the clothes or bed covers, reaching for objects, wiping, rubbing, knitting, tinkering, stereotyped movements, tonic change of posture and position of the body, movements in circles, complicated and ordered actions, impulsive fugues and similar manifestations) and by *autonomic symptoms* (livid facial coloration, salivation, outbreaks of sweating, singultus, waves of heat in the head, tachycardia, palpitation, allodromy, changes of pulse, discharge of urine, evacuation of faeces, ejaculation). Many symptoms can occur simultaneously or consecutively.

Combined psychomotor epilepsy has an even greater abundance of symptoms. However, the situation may be determined by a generalized or semi-generalized seizure. In the *preparoxysmal* phase there is usually an aura, with a sensation of air rising from the epigastrium into the heart and neck. Optical, acoustic, vestibular, olfacto-gustatory and tactile illusions and/or hallucinations are quite common here. The *paroxysmal* phase is characterized by the familiar tonic-clonic attack. The *postparoxysmal* phase involves the process of reorientation and may now and then take the form of postparoxysmal twilight attacks, a postparoxysmal twilight state or terminal sleep. It is not possible to predict the course and duration of these symptoms.

Psychomotor syndromes take several different forms. *Brief* psychomotor paroxysms show several phases: phase I usually consists of an aura. Phase II is the phase of passivity, phase III is the phase of activity, and IV the reorientation phase. *Longer* psychomotor episodes may vary in length and the symptomatology is very varied. In addition to longer psychomotor episodes, there is also the *psychomotor status,* which is rarer than the *generalized-attack status.* When combined with major attacks, the psychomotor status may be relatively prolonged; lasting for two, three or more days. *Productive psychotic* manifestations are also particularly important. Again, these can vary considerably as regards duration and phenomenology, so we shall first mention *productive psychoses with forced normalization* of bioelectrical cerebral activity (EEG) over the cortex. Normalization of the cortical EEG is associated with the sudden onset of psychotic symptoms. Clinical symptoms may be depressive, paranoid or primarily catatonic. *Productive psychoses without forced normalization of cerebral activity in the cortical EEG* are uncharacteristic, they last longer and they are more like an organic psychosis from the point of view of symptomatology. *Hysterical* reactions have also been described in patients with psychomotor epilepsy.

At the end of the fateful course of psychomotor epilepsy comes a *personality change* in the patient, and this can be associated with various symptoms.

THE MANY FORMS OF BIOELECTRICAL CEREBRAL ACTIVITY IN PSYCHOMOTOR EPILEPSY

Bioelectrical cerebral activity in psychomotor epilepsy is very variable. A number of qualitative and quantitative variations are observed during the *interval* between attacks (interictal EEG).

The cortical EEG is normal when there are convulsion foci in quite deep cerebral structures. Here, the cortical EEG does not correlate with the clinical picture, since the focus cannot be detected over the neocortex.

Where the convulsion focus is in a temporal lobe, the *EEG focus is unilateral, localized strictly over the temporal lobe,* and takes the form of isolated spikes with or without subsequent slower waves.

An EEG focus strictly localized *over both temporal regions* is usually observed in *idiopathic* epilepsies. However, this type of focus is quite often found in symptomatic psychomotor epilepsies as well.

A temporal, unilateral focus which is not strictly temporal, but which extends over the precentral, parietal and occipital regions, is usually found when the anatomical focus is situated in the mediobasal temporal regions of the brain.

A bilateral temporal EEG focus with spikes or sharp waves with or without local dysrhythmia, which may spread some distance, is found when the neuroanatomical focus is situated in the lateral temporal regions and neighbouring cerebral structures are involved or where the disease has persisted for quite some time. This type of focus occurs in the EEG in symptomatic rather than in idiopathic psychomotor epilepsy.

Another form of EEG changes in psychomotor epilepsy is found in patients with combined seizures. In these cases there is *general dysrhythmia,* which cannot be definitely localized, in the cortical EEG.

In fairly acute cases we also find *spikes which closely follow one another* and which occur over all cerebral regions with or without dysrhythmia. In these cases, the neuroanatomical focus is probably localized more in the medial cerebral structures and has not yet affected the neocortex or convexity of the brain.

Spike and wave formations with or without dysrhythmia are rarely seen in psychomotor epilepsy. In these cases the focus is in the limbic system, but it also affects the diencephalic structures.

The EEG *during an attack* (ictal EEG) is different from the EEG in the interval between attacks. Here again, there are several variations depending to a large extent on the nature of the clinical attack.

Normal cerebral activity is rarely found during a psychomotor attack.

About 20 seconds before a psychomotor attack, there is critical flattening of the cortical EEG. Immediately after this, the electroencephalogram becomes larger and larger and sinusoidal waves of 3 to 5/sec. appear. 6 to 8/sec. waves in a generalized form are quite often observed. Just before the active phase of the psychomotor attack the cortical EEG also records muscle potentials as an indication of the tense muscles of the head and face. In the attack itself, generalized sharp waves and spikes which closely follow one another are recorded. These elements gradually disappear after the attack.

In many cases, shortly before the attack an EEG focus develops over one or both temporal regions and gradually spreads over the other regions of the brain. During the attack there is an abrupt change in this cerebral activity, which rapidly becomes generalized over the whole brain. As the attack passes off there is a marked slowing of the cerebral waves.

In some twilight attacks, generalized dysrhythmia is transient and only lasts a few seconds, although it is fairly pronounced. Large, unmasked δ-waves are usually recorded.

On rare occasions it is possible to record an outbreak of spikes and waves over all regions of the brain in psychomotor epilepsy. It is still always possible to define the focus in the EEG in these cases.

Occasionally, spikes which closely follow one another are seen over one or both temporal regions of the brain; these become faster and faster during the attack, and then slower and slower after the attack until they completely disappear.

Cerebral activity may be quite different in combined attacks, depending on the clinical course of the attack and on the type of attacks.

In many cases the *convulsion elements (CE)* in psychomotor epilepsy are quite different *morphologically* and *topographically* from those in other forms of epilepsy (particularly centrencephalic epilepsy).

There may be normalization of the cortical EEG during psychotic episdoes (forced normalization) or it may deteriorate further.

The cortical EEG may normalize in psychomotor epilepsy in the course of a hysterical reaction. As mentioned above, *forced normalization* depends in many instances on the course of the clinical psychotic symptoms.

Great importance is attached to the morphological and topographical properties of the EEG convulsion elements since these can provide evidence as to the type and localization of the convulsion focus and the possibility of a convulsion being triggered and inhibited. The cortical EEG in the interval is a better indicator because cerebral activity changes substantially during an attack and the focus may be obscured.

Polygraphic monitoring during the sleep of patients with psychomotor epilepsy revealed that they fall asleep more rapidly, sleep more deeply, do not wake up so frequently during the night, move about less and that their initial autonomic state is one of vagotonia, in contrast to the corresponding parameters in other forms of epilepsy and in healthy people. Convulsion elements (CE) are more common in the sleep EEG than in the waking state in psychomotor epilepsy. During sleeping and waking, the convulsion elements of patients with psychomotor epilepsy are morphologically and topographically different from CE in other forms of epilepsy. Even during sleep there may be attacks in which the course, type and duration can vary.

Somnambulistic episodes during sleep are particularly interesting in patients with psychomotor epilepsy; these differ in a number of important ways from those of genuine sleepwalkers. Somnambulistic episodes may occur following a generalized attack or in isolation.

THE MANY TYPES OF NEUROANTOMICAL CHANGE IN PSYCHOMOTOR EPILEPSY

It is really very difficult to study the neuroanatomical and histochemical substrate of psychomotor epilepsy. However, a vast number of results have been obtained. Changes have been described in both *symptomatic* and *idiopathic (essential, cryptogenic, epilepsy of unknown origin)* forms of epilepsy.

Symptomatic epilepsy is associated with many neuroanatomical changes. The psychomotor epilepsy form is most commonly found where the neuroanatomical focus is in the temporal lobe. Psychomotor epilepsy has been found in 50 to 60 percent of cases with tumors in this region, whereas it occurs in about 30 percent of cases with extratemporal tumors. Slow-growing tumors (gliomas) cause psychomotor epilepsy in 60 to 70 percent of cases, whereas psychomotor attacks were only found in about 30 to 35 percent of cases with fast-growing glioblastomas. As regards temporal tumors, psychomotor epilepsy is most common when the tumor is in a *temporomedial* position (in 58%). Next come the *temporofrontal* (about 52%) and *temporoparietal* (about 49%) localizations. There were no differences regarding tumor localization in the temporal lobe itself in respect of psychomotor epilepsy combined with major seizures. Focal, non-psychomotor attacks occur most often where the focus is in a temporoparietal position. Other stressors which can induce psychomotor epilepsy include perinatal, traumatic, toxic, infectious, metabolic and many other factors. In very many cases the symptomatology of psychomotor attacks is related to the site of the neuroanatomical changes.

Recently, neuroanatomical, microscopic, histochemical and metabolic changes in the temporal lobe have also been found in psychomotor epilepsy of *unknown origin.* Many authors consider that there is no such thing as epilepsy of *unknown origin* (essential, idiopathic form), since, as examination techniques improve, a neuroanatomical focus is found in all forms. In all, there are no detectable, definite changes in the temporal lobe in only a quarter to a third of cases with epilepsy of *unknown* origin. The main positive findings include atrophy, traumatic lesions, diffuse gliosis and tumors which had remained undiagnosed while the patient was alive. Undiagnosed vascular changes with diffuse gliosis also have quite an important role here. As in symptomatic psychomotor epilepsy, here the site of neuroanatomical changes tends to be temporobasal and temporomedial (hippocampal and perifalciform regions). With the advent of electron microscopy, many more neuroanatomical changes are now found.

Secondary psychomotor epilepsy (symptomatic and idiopathic) may also occur when the neuroanatomical focus is in other regions of the brain. In this case, in time the changes spread from these areas of the brain to the temporal lobe.

There is much discussion in the literature about *Ammon's horn sclerosis* as a possible neuroanatomical cause of psychomotor epilepsy. It is still difficult to distinguish between cause and effect here. Clearly, psychomotor epilepsy (and also other forms of epilepsy) must be the outcome of both *endogenous* (disposition) and *exogenous* (exposure) factors.

Disposition is said to include: 1.) constitution (including cerebral angio- and chemoarchitechtonics) ; 2.) genetic enzyme abnormalities resulting in metabolic defects; 3.) pre-existing cerebral damage; 4.) age; 5.) hereditary lowering of convulsion threshold; and 6.) prevailing psychosomatic state. *Exogenous factors* include, among other things; 1.) encephalopathy; 2.) foetal damage; 3.) perinatal cerebral damage; 4.) inflammatory encephalopathy in infancy; 5.) brain tumors; 6.) cerebral trauma; 7.) damage to the blood-brain barrier; 8.) oxygen, glucose, electrolyte and water utilization disorders; 9.) cerebro-vascular insufficiency; 10.) cerebral atrophy; 11.) infections, and 12.) various kinds of poisoning.

BIOCHEMICAL BASIS OF ISOLATED (PRIMARY) PSYCHOMOTOR EPILEPSY

The many functions and neuroanatomical and histochemical structures of the temporal lobe determine the symptomatology of this form of epilepsy. A number of biochemical changes have been found in this region of the brain.

Again and again, the *electrolytes* have been regarded as the principal agent causing neuronal excitation and hyperexcitation. However, changes of electrolyte balance are nearly always linked with other metabolic phenomena. Increased water retention (for example in inflammation) enhances penetration of sodium ions into the nerve cells, since it increases porousness of the neuronal membrane and strips and aqueous sheath from around the sodium ions. Sodium ions have a smaller crystal radius than potassium ions and therefore penetrate into the nerve cells more easily. Conversely, potassium ions can pass out more easily. *This leads to depolarization of the neurons and hyperexcitation.* Similar changes in sodium-potassium transport are also associated with changes in vitamin metabolism. For example, potassium ions are involved in glucose oxidation, and in the oxidation of pyruvic acid, lactic acid and glutamic acid. Other electrolytes apart from sodium and potassium also play an important part in psychomotor epilepsy, e.g. calcium, magnesium and zinc ions. So it is likely that, where there is a metabolic change, there will eventually be metabolic manifestations in respect of metal ions.

Changes of *water balance* in the temporal lobe cause a shift in the metal ion picture. Water retention leads to psychomotor attacks or to symptomatic deterioration. Conversely, forcible dehydration results in a symptomatic improvement. Water retention also induces indirect symptomatic deterioration, because it causes other metabolic shifts. Water retention is found particularly where there are inflammatory, toxic, traumatic and oncological lesions in the temporal lobe.

Up to now, no definite changes of *oxygen consumption* have been found in the epileptic focus of the temporal lobe. Artificially high levels of oxygen supply to the brain evoke epileptic manifestations which, however, play a more important part in other forms of epilepsy. Forced removal of CO_2 seldom elicits psychomotor manifestations. Here again, other epileptic manifestations are more commonly found. On the other hand, supplying CO_2 to the brain results in a symptomatic improvement or mitigates an attack in psychomotor epilepsy.

Changes of *pH* in the first barrier of our model may lead to a deterioration or an improvement of psychomotor attacks. It is therefore assumed that pH shifts also have a part to play in the genesis of psychomotor epilepsy. Local *alkalosis* in the temporal lobe enhances an attack. *Acidosis* results in an improvement. The factors here are intracellular pH changes.

There is a great deal of evidence to suggest that *glucose metabolism* undergoes a change in epilepsy. Glucose degradation is disrupted at the pyruvic acid stage. Hypoglycaemia causes a deterioration of the symptoms; hyperglycaemia has this effect more rarely.

Changes of *protein metabolism* have also been implicated in psychomotor epilepsy. Election microscopy and histochemical studies using antimetabolites have revealed specific metabolic changes in the Ammon's horn which were linked with psychomotor symptoms. Among other changes, there were marked shifts in protein metabolism which resulted in local changes in the nerve cells. The spatial arrangement and structural organization of organelles in regions h_3 and h_4 of the Ammon's horn were altered here. Where there was profound cell shrinkage and a change in shape and position of the organelles, there was also solidification of the karyoplasm and cytoplasm, dilatation of the ergastoplasmic cisternae, loosening and swelling of the internal structure of the mitochondria with multilamellar deposits in the cells. All these changes were linked, among other things, with disturbances of protein metabolism. There was also loss of ribonucleic acid (RNA) from the nerve-cell nuclei. It is also assumed that many exogenous and endogenous processes can produce similar or the same disorders of protein metabolism leading to the development of epileptic manifestations of a psychomotor type.

Many authors have observed changes in the serum protein picture of patients with psychomotor epilepsy. Their findings include: 1.) a slight elevation of total protein; 2.) a relative reduction of highly dispersed, low-molecular-weight albumins; 3.) an increase of globulins, and 4.) a change of colloidal osmotic pressure. In particular, many authors found an increase of the α-1- (and also α-2) fraction of the globulins. The albumin/

globulin quotient was depressed. The differences are said to be even more pronounced in *idiopathic (essential)* epilepsy than in symptomatic psychomotor forms. In other forms of epilepsy, serum proteins remained unchanged or only changed slightly.

Changes in amino-acid metabolism are reported to have a special part to play in psychomotor epilepsy. It is very often stated that glutamic acid (GA) and gamma-amino-butyric acid (GABA) are mainly responsible here. A shift in the ratio of these two amino acids produces many other changes in metabolism, pH and metal-ion balance, and hence, leads to epileptic manifestations.

According to results reported by many authors, GA has an adrenaline-like *stimulant effect* on the neurons of the central nervous system (CNS). GABA is involved in synaptic transmission (membrane stabiliser) and, as an *inhibitory transmitter,* it retards the conduction of impulses.

After administration of hydrazine derivatives it has been shown that the cerebral concentration of GABA falls at the onset of epileptic attacks. The concentration of other amino acids does not change so much. Other chemical compounds which reduce the GABA concentration in cerebral tissue will also evoke attacks. Since, in many cases, there are possible ways of reducing the GABA concentration in the brain, it is quite often this which predisposes the patient to epileptic attacks. GABA deficiency in the brain can occur due to increased utilization or due to inhibition of GABA synthesis, or due to blockage of the entire system of amino acid and glucose metabolism. It is thought that attacks occur in hypoglycaemic situations because of a disorder of GABA metabolism. Artificial administration of GA into the brain also elicits attacks or their equivalents, depending on the dose used. On the other hand, reactions to administration of aspartic acid are far less pronounced than after GA. No epilepsy-type responses were evoked by administering leucine, methionine, novaline, valine, ATP and pyridoxine or isotonic saline solution. Injection of pyridoxal-5′-phosphate (PAL or PYP) may be accompanied by attacks, but these are mitigated by subsequent intravenous (i.v.) injection of GABA. Intracisternal (i.c.) administration of GABA interrupts or prevents the attacks. These phenomena are due to the synthesis of GABA. Injection of GA and PYP reduces glutamic acid decarboxylase (GAD) activity. This results in a reduction of GABA which in turn causes disinhibition and hyperexcitation. PYP can function as a coenzyme of GAD and also as the coenzyme of gamma-aminobutyric acid transaminase (GABAT). However, it has a greater affinity to GABAT than to GAD, and so an increase in PYP concentration increases transamination of GABA and, to a lesser extent, leads to decarboxylation of GA to GABA. The GABA level in the brain falls and the GA concentration rises. This results in a disruption of neuronal function and evokes epileptic reactions, although at first sight this appears rather illogical.

Endogenous amines have either a direct causal role or they are indirectly implicated in practically every case of psychomotor epilepsy.

A large amount of phenylpyruvic acid is produced during transamination of phenylalanine. This is reported to produce imbecility and epileptic reactions, but not so much the psychomotor form. Psychomotor epilepsy may occur if another form develops into secondary psychomotor epilepsy after some time has elapsed. *Adrenaline* is reported to play a special role in psychomotor epilepsy, since more of it is found in phylogenetically older parts of the brain than in other cerebral regions. Less of the stable (bound) form is found in epilepsy, so in an unstable (bound) form it causes hyperexcitation. The protective mechanism is less in evidence in psychomotor epilepsy than in the healthy brain.

Acetylcholine is also involved in producing psychomotor attacks. Mild electrical or chemical stimulation of the brain leads to substantial release of acetylcholine, which immediately reacts with the receptor protein, producing a change of membrane permeability to ions and finally to depolarization of the nerve-cell membrane. Acetylcholine-glutamate and electrolyte metabolism are substantially changed in the human epileptogenic focus of the temporal lobe. Increased cholinesterase activity has been found in the interval between psychomotor attacks and the acetylcholine-binding capacity is lost. In addition to these two neuromodulators, *serotonin* is reported to play a special role in psychomotor epilepsy, and so this form of epilepsy can be regarded as *serotonergic* or *serotogenic.*

There is general disagreement among authors as to the role of *ammonia* and protein degradation products in psychomotor epilepsy. No definite increase of ammonia in the brain has been reported in the interval between epileptic attacks nor was there definite evidence of elevated blood concentrations; sometimes there was actually a fall in the blood levels. However, there are some urinary findings which could be linked with disordered protein metabolism in epileptics: there is a reduction in the urinary excretion of total nitrogen and excretion of urea nitrogen is often reduced too. On the other hand, excretion of amino acid nitrogen is somewhat elevated and urinary excretion of polypeptide nitrogen is said to be even higher, i.e. urinary excretion of the end product of protein metabolism is depressed, amino acid nitrogen excretion is slightly to sharply increased and polypeptide nitrogen excretion is even higher. The conclusion from this is that protein metabolism is impaired at a polypeptide stage in epileptics. Consequently, the initial ergotropic state is changed into one of trophotropism and this leads to an attack and compensation. The epileptic attack is regarded as an emergency mechanism for normalizing protein metabolism. For this reason, acute and chronic mental manifestations are more frequently encountered in pure psychomotor epilepsy than in other forms of epilepsy, because there is no normalizing tonic-clonic seizure in the pure psychomotor form.

Hormones and *vitamins* have different roles in psychomotor epilepsy. The effect of hormones in this form of epilepsy has not been studied sufficiently but vitamins have been examined more thoroughly. Following on injection of ACTH there was a rise of NH_3 and acetylcholine in the brain which then resulted in an increase of cerebral predisposition to convulsion. The vitamins studied in most detail are *thiamine* (Vitamin B_1), *nicotinamide* and *pyridoxal* (Vitamin B_6) and their role in epilepsy has been established.

Administration of antimetabolites such as *methoxypyridoxine* and *3-acetylpyridine* to rats and mice has been found to cause lesions of the pyramidal cells of h_3 and h_4 of the Ammon's horn. The experimental animals also exhibited behavioral disturbances like or similar to those observed in patients with psychomotor epilepsy. The symptoms develop quite soon after methoxypyridoxine, whereas they take several hours to develop after *6-aminonicotinamide* and 3-acetylpyridine. At the very onset of the symptoms there is increased penetration of sodium ions through the membrane into the neurons. On the other hand, these ions are not properly reabsorbed by the renal cells since these cells are also damaged by the poison. There are many factors other than administration of antimetabolites which can impair the vitamins' function as coenzymes.

Phosphorylation of Vitamin B_6 is catalysed by pyridoxal phosphokinase, which is activated by magnesium ions. Zinc ions can activate the enzyme. There are also other reasons for believing that zinc ions play a major role in forming the focus in psychomotor epilepsy. Fields h_3 and h_4 of the Ammon's horn have a high zinc content. It is assumed that a zinc-containing enzyme such as carboxypeptidase or alcohol dehydrogenase is present in these fields. Damage in h_3 and h_4 probably results in the formation of a chelate from the active form of Vitamin B_6 and metal ions. The resulting coenzyme blockade causes the resting membrane potential of the neurons to drop and triggers convulsive excitation. Since the epileptic focus in psychomotor epilepsy occurs in these very fields, it is also very likely that all pathological manifestations originate from there.

Pyridoxal phosphokinase can also be inhibited by *hydrazides* or *deoxypyridoxal*. *Iproniazid* and *amphetamine* evoke the same disorders. Thiosemicarbazide and thiocarbohydrazide have been shown to have a convulsant effect both *in vitro* and *in vivo*. Hydrazides are said to cause

L-GAD inhibition. In addition to changes in the metabolism and concentration of GABA, this also disrupts the activity of DOPA-decarboxylase, 5-hydroxytryptophane-decarboxylase, diamine-oxidase, histidine-decarboxylase and many other coenzymes. Convulsions following penicillin are also due to pyridoxine deficiency. Lack of pyridoxine can also be caused by overproduction of pyridoxic acid, by excessive pyridoxine utilization and by inadequate supply of this vitamin.

When considering the effect of *enzymes* in psychomotor epilepsy there are a number of other factors which are also important. Using vital staining techniques, cholinesterases have been detected in fields h_1 and h_2 of the Ammon's horn. On the other hand, acid phosphatases tended to be concentrated more around the base of the apical dendrites of h_3 and h_4. Fewer respiratory enzymes (succinodehydrogenases) were found in h_1 and h_2 than in h_3 and in the fascia dentata. The oxidases were distributed in a similar way. This enzyme distribution shows that metabolic changes produced by antimetabolites and other toxic noxae and by tumors and trauma do not have to be identical in all fields of the Ammon's horn and that fields h_3 and h_4 are particularly at risk. Local metabolic changes result in potassium, sodium and chloride retention. This impedes water excretion which, in turn, leads to an accumulation of water within and outside the damaged neurons and this also reduces the resting membrane potential.

BIOCHEMICAL BASIS OF COMBINED PSYCHOMOTOR EPILEPSY

Since this form of epilepsy can develop either from isolated psychomotor epilepsy or from the other forms of epilepsy, its biochemistry is more complicated. When it develops from isolated psychomotor epilepsy the biochemical basis is probably similar to that already described. It often takes a long time for combined psychomotor epilepsy to develop from the isolated form, since the anatomical conditions for this do not correspond. Pathways of propagation are required for epileptic impulses to spread from barrier 1 of our model. However, the temporal lobe is fairly remote and poorly linked (compared with the connections of other cerebral formations) to barrier 2.

Functionally speaking, the temporal lobe is situated on one side of an inhibitory block, a powerful retarding system comprising the diencephalon and adjacent basal cerebral ganglia. There are remarkably few connections between the lateral parts of the temporal lobe and the thalamic nuclei, whereas there are better developed functional connections with the adjacent cortical regions. Medial parts of the temporal lobe have better projections to basal centrencephalic cerebral formations, predominantly to the mesencephalic and rhombocephalic reticular formation. Bilateral connections to the amygdaloid nucleus have also been found. However, these projections *in toto* are insufficient to allow the spread of hyperexcitation in psychomotor epilepsy from the temporal lobe into the other regions of the brain and then to the periphery.

The pathway to the dramatic motor seizure in generalized epilepsy is largely blocked and, consequently, many different types of psychomotor equivalent, even to the extent of pronounced psychotic episodes, occur for quite some time. Other factors have to be present before there is a combined psychomotor attack, i.e. a generalized convulsion with psychomotor symptoms. In other words, here, to a greater or lesser extent, vital histochemical regions of large areas of the brain (or the entire brain) are also damaged. There are also chemical changes which are different in the preconvulsive, convulsive and postconvulsive stages.

Changes in the *blood-brain barrier* play an important role here. These may occur following irradiation, infections, toxoplasmosis, intoxication and poisoning, certain drugs, cerebral tumors, trauma.

The *vascular system* of the brain appears to be unstable just before a generalized attack. Vasodilatation is followed by vasoconstriction with cerebral anoxia. During the attack fairly prolonged vasodilatation occurs; at the end of the attack this reverts to vasoconstriction.

The *electrolytes* are unstable just before an attack. The postsynaptic neurons become more permeable to potassium and sodium ions. This reduces the potential difference across the membrane, increases the intracellular level of sodium ions and reduces intracellular potassium ions. The intracellular level of potassium ions remains abnormal throughout the attack. Many authors have failed to find these changes but the ratio of electrolytes to one another nearly always changed, i.e. there is a change in the relative ratio of electrolytes rather than a change in absolute concentrations.

There is a local and general increase of *water retention* just before a generalized attack, and this causes a change in swelling pressure and further retention of potassium. Many other metabolic changes also occur. After the attack the local situation is reversed. An increase of magnesium ion concentration has been found in various organs after a generalized attack. It is assumed that it is the Mg^{++} ions which carry calcium ions back to the membrane surface after an attack. In this way, both types of ion can inhibit convulsions. Sodium ions are transported out of the nerve cells and potassium ions flow back into the neurons. This corrects the potassium deficiency in the neurons and membrane permeability is stabilized.

The oxidizing activity of cerebral tissue is reported to change before a generalized attack. Firstly, CO_2-sensitivity is reduced and, secondly, there is a relative fall in the production of CO_2. The *all or nothing* laws under crisis conditions result in maximal production of and saturation with this and other activators. With assistance from the tonic attack, the life-saving consequence is a tendency to periodic reorganization of physiological surface activity. Increased oxidation of arterial blood has been found a couple of minutes after the clonic attack. Abortive psychomotor attacks which have a protracted course are not capable of increasing this oxidation rapidly. The attack is prevented by the increased amounts of CO_2 produced during the attack. During an attack oxidizing processes in the brain have a specific anatomical-physiological pathway, from which one can conclude that the impulses originate from the temporal lobe and are conducted to the diencephalon and cortex, and to the periphery.

As a consequence of these chemical changes, there is also a change in the *acid-base balance* shortly before an attack. A state of alkalosis prevails before the attack, acidosis develops during the attack. The acidosis is produced in different parts of the brain at different times. After the attack there is a gradual return to normal pH levels, and alkalosis tends to develop again a few days or weeks later.

Carbohydrates are also important as regards generalized attacks. The cerebral glucose and glycogen concentrations decline once an attack has started and, at the same time, there is increased production of lactic acid and the tissue pH falls. The fall of pH has an anticonvulsant effect. High-energy compounds are utilized right at the beginning of a generalized convulsion, and there is a shift in the phosphocreatine and ATP balance. There is also an increase of inorganic phosphorus in the brain during an attack as a result of the breakdown of phosphoproteins, phosphopeptides, ribonucleic acids and ribonucleides, and phospholipids. The cerebral phosphorus concentration increases up to the clonic phase and is depressed by up to 44% of the initial value at the end of the attack. All these changes are accompanied by corresponding shifts in the carbohydrates.

Protein metabolism is changed before, during and after a combined psychomotor attack. Total proteins in the blood are actually elevated during the interval between attacks and they rise further, just before an attack. The albumin concentration falls further and the α_1-globulin concentration increases further. The albumin/globulin quotient is reduced accordingly. Similar changes have only been found in the brain in the convulsion focus. At the beginning of an attack the α_2-globulin concentration tends to fall and the γ-globulin concentration tends to rise. These biochemical changes and subsequent changes in the form of a shift the opposite way take place faster than the attack itself. The bioelectrical cerebral activity shows similar manifestations, which occur faster than the attack itself. These changes are more pronounced in essential epilepsy than in symptomatic epilepsy.

The *amino-acid* picture alters at the beginning of, during and after a generalized psychomotor attack. At the beginning of an attack, in the cortex of experimental animals it has been found that there was an increase of GA, glutamine and glutathion, whereas GABA remained unchanged. According to results from several other experiments, just before an attack there is also a critical reduction of GABA. Once convulsive activity has started, the cerebral GA concentration falls by 50 percent. The glutamate-GABA system alters during an attack and changes in the cystine and cysteine concentrations have also been found at the beginning of, and during an attack. These two amino acids decline shortly before the attack and during the attack, and the cerebral concentration of inorganic sulphur rises.

A change of *endogenous amines* in the brain is of decisive importance for a generalized attack combined with psychomotor symptoms. These changes have been demonstrated particularly clearly and unequivocally after administration and overdosage of psychotropic drugs, and this can be used as a model.

Firstly, we have to consider a change in the *production and degradation* of endogenous amines. According to results obtained by many authors, phenothiazines impede noradrenaline production. Another process is *blocking the release* of monoamines from the presynaptic regions of the neurons, i.e. from the stores. This causes an increase in the intracellular noradrenaline concentration. Here again, psychotropic drugs (particularly the phenothiazines) have been found to have a blocking effect. *Blockade of intracellular enzymes* first leads to an increase in the intracellular level of neuromodulators. Later the subsynaptic concentration also increases. Monoamine oxidase inhibitors (MAOI) are known to cause an increase in the noradrenaline and serotonin concentration in the subsynaptic regions. After an impulse, the monoamines go back into the neurons and cannot be broken down, and so convulsive discharges may occur. Some other antidepressants also inhibit intracellular monoamine-oxidase.

Increased release of monoamies from the stores is another mechanism which can bring about a change of neuromodulators in the brain. Phenothiazienes and rauwolfia alkaloids have been shown to have this effect. There is yet another mechanism here to be considered. This is *blocking the return* of monoamines into the neurons so that the neurons become hyperexcited. Antidepressants are known to block the return of monoamines from presynaptic regions into the neurons.

Combined blockade of the return of neuromodulators from the subsynaptic gap and increased release of neuromodulators from the stores has an even greater effect. Administration of stimulants, such as cocaine, amphetamine etc., combined with antidepressants or neuroleptic agents has this effect. Another potential combination here is *intracellular enzyme blockade combined with rapid release of monoamines from the stores.* This can occur when a monoamine releaser like reserpine is administered in combination with a monoamine-oxidase inhibitor like iproniazid. Another possible way of increasing the monoamine concentration in the subsynaptic region is by *blocking the return of monoamines from the subsynaptic gap, plus simultaneous blockade of MAO*. An overdose of imipramine can result in very powerful blockade of the return of noradrenaline from the subsynaptic gap into the neurons. Simultaneous administration of MAOI causes a build-up of monoamines, even in the nerve cell. As a result of this build-up, monoamines leave the nerve cell and pass into the subsynaptic gap, which is already *saturated* with monoamines. The consequences are obvious.

Even more complicated mechanisms come into play if the *exit* of monoamine from the neurons is *blocked, MAO is blocked* and the nerve cells *sensitized*. A further increase in monoamines and intensification of their epileptogenic action can be caused by combining *increased release* (following rauwolfia preparations), *inhibition of MAO* (following an overdosage of MAOI) and *blockade of the return* of the monoamines from the subsynaptic gap into the neurons. A number of these mechanisms and mechanism combinations may be involved in causing an epileptic attack and chronic epilepsy.

For a certain period of time, a generalized attack brings about a discharge and metabolic equilibrium, which may be disturbed again during the interval if the causes are not eliminated. However, a generalized attack may also pave the way for subsequent attacks so that the epileptic condition may persist even if the original cause is removed. This *facilitation* can be regarded as a new, detrimental element in psychomotor epilepsy.

As far as *enzymes, hormones and vitamins* are concerned, all that we know so far is that there is an abrupt alteration in the activities which are changed even during an isolated psychomotor attack. Here again, for a short time a generalized attack results in a relative compensating effect, or a tendency to compensate.

THE BIOCHEMICAL BASIS OF STATUS EPILEPTICUS

There are two important factors here. First there is *psychomotor attack status* and secondly a *generalized attack status* (combined primary or secondary epilepsy). In the former case, the most decisive factors are the convulsion focus itself, the functional neuroanatomical structure of the temporal lobe and its lack of connections with other cerebral formations, the fact that the disease has existed for some time and the initial functional condition of the body. Biochemical changes (like those mentioned above) may be more severe. There does not have to be a biochemical defect throughout the whole brain; it may be localized simply in and around the focus. Hyperexcitation does not penetrate from the first barrier into the second. In the latter case, there must be a biochemical change in the brain as a whole such that the brain is no longer capable of correcting this biochemical defect by a single attack.

Biochemical neurophysiology has revealed that neither a psychomotor attack status nor a generalized status are capable of correcting the metabolic defects. This also explains why these conditions are more persistent. In many cases it is necessary to precipitate a generalized attack artificially, and this then overcomes the status epilepticus. This technique is used clinically to treat very persistent and severe status epilepticus.

In a status epilepticus it must also be remembered that there may be two or more convulsion foci in the brain. These are activated at different times so that hyperexcitation from one focus may follow hyperexcitation from another. There may also be retro-excitation, since impulses from the fourth barrier in our model (from the reticular formation of the lower brain stem) may travel towards the temporal lobe instead of to the periphery. This retro-excitation may perhaps explain why not all impulses reach the periphery and abruptly elicit a generalized attack; some impulses return while others are transmitted to the periphery. Returning impulses trigger fresh hyperexcitatory activity from the focus which, in turn, gives rise to fresh epileptic manifestations. This produces a vicious circle which may be difficult to interrupt without treatment. Here, generalized attacks are combined with loss of consciousness, but in many cases, from the tonic-clonic point of view, they are weaker than a single generalized attack which immediately alters the biochemical situation in the brain and body.

BIOCHEMICAL BASIS OF LONGER PSYCHOMOTOR AND PSYCHOTIC MANIFESTATIONS

Whereas biochemical changes in the brain, blood and urine are qualitatively similar in status epilepticus and in a simple epileptic attack, the only difference being a quantitative one in the brain, the biochemical basis of psychotic episodes in psychomotor epilepsy is much more difficult to work out. At first sight, the transition from psychomotor epilepsy to a psychosis can be explained by the fact that the temporal lobe, which contains the epileptic focus, is situated on the one side of a powerful blocking system, i.e. the brain stem and its basal ganglia. This blocking system inhibits the spread of epileptic impulses to the periphery. Thus, it could be assumed that *a psychosis occurs as an alternative to an epileptic attack.* However, we still do not fully understand the potential biochemical factors or the possible mechanisms by which the biochemical defects in the brain could be corrected in a psychotic manifestation which replaces an attack, although there are many possible parallels here.

The *electrolytes* should be mentioned first. Some electrolyte shifts have been found in schizophrenia and in manic depressive disease but, not surprisingly, it was not easy to find a close causal connection between the shifts and these diseases. However, more recently it has been found that there is an immediate improvement if lithium salts are used during the manic phases in manic-depressive psychosis. According to results reported by many authors, lithium affects catecholamine metabolism by binding adrenaline and noradrenaline. Some other authors report that lithium affects the serotonin mechanism and binds serotonin. As a result of the binding of adrenaline, noradrenaline and serotonin, the impulsion is suppressed in manic patients. From this we can conclude that the electrolyte system in mania and psychomotor epilepsy is altered at the same level. If for any reason the psychomotor symptomatology of a patient from the psychomotor group is blocked by the processes described above, a manic symptomatology can develop and act as an alternative. If an overdose of lithium is given to a manic patient, there are manifest epileptic seizures even though, originally, there was no epilepsy. Once an attack occurs, the manic symptoms disappear. Thus, here the attack is acting as an alternative to the psychosis.

Water retention has been found in catatonic and stuporous patients. Water retention was also mentioned above, in connection with epilepsy. Here again the physiology of an epileptic and a psychotic are at the same metabolic-biochemical level and so the transition from one set of symptoms to the other is not altogether illogical. However, changes of body weight are not the same. Catatonic and manic patients lose weight during the acute phase, whereas this does not occur in psychomotor epilepsy. We must therefore exercise caution when drawing comparisons here.

Oxidation processes and pH are important factors when comparing the symptoms in epilepsies and in psychoses and the transition from one set of symptoms to the other. The hypnoid state in schizophrenic patients is interpreted as a function of a blockade of oxidation processes and corresponding changes have been found in the striatum and thalamus. Inhibition of cytochrome C, oxygen consumption and carbonic anhydrase have been reported and catalase activity in the brain was also said to be depressed. Impairment of these metabolic processes with enzymic inhibition leads to metabolic *acidosis* in brain and blood. The acidosis has an adverse effect on the psychotic picture, but it mitigates or stops the epileptic manifestations. This is why epileptic symptoms develop into psychotic symptoms. The epileptic's body attempts to correct the prevailing alkalosis by changing into the psychosis. This also explains why two groups of symptoms (epileptic and psychotic) cannot really be present simultaneously. There are more and more clinical results to indicate that only one of these two groups of symptoms can exist at any one time. As soon as one appears, the other disappears, and vice versa.

There is a parallel situation in psychoses and epilepsies in respect of *carbohydrate metabolism.* Most epileptics tend to be *hypoglycaemic.* The greater the hypoglycaemia, the more severe are the symptoms. On the other hand, catatonic and paranoid-hallucinatory schizophrenics exhibit *hyperglycaemia* during periodic endogenous depression, in the depressive phase. Here, if no epileptic attack can occur, the epileptic system is capable of developing into psychotic symptoms to correct the hypoglycaemia.

There are also parallels between epilepsy and psychosis is respect of *protein metabolism.* In all forms of psychosis there is a slight increase of total proteins, a slight to moderate reduction in the albumin concentration and an increase of globulins in the brain and blood. We mentioned the same or similar changes in epilepsy. The argument that this is simply a sequel is discounted by the fact that these changes are also observed in the interval and *before* the outbreak of acute psychotic or epileptic symptoms. Here again, there are two different diseases at the same metabolic level and hence there can be a transition from one to the other.

As far as *amino acids* are concerned, findings in the brain are not altogether significant. It has been possible to adversely affect the blood picture in schizophrenic patients by administering various amino acids. An increase of spontaneously produced amino acids has also been found in the blood of these patients. There is something of a parallel here in that a reduction in the concentration of corresponding amino acids has been found in the blood of epileptics. The epileptic could correct his blood amino acid deficiency via the transition to psychotic symptoms. However, we must be cautious here since these are not cerebral findings.

The most important *endogenous amines* are *acetylcholine* and *serotonin,* followed by adrenaline and noradrenaline. Increased acetylcholinesterase activity has been found in the cerebrospinal fluid of schizophrenics, and in manics many authors have found elevated levels of adrenaline and noradrenaline in the brain. Thus, once again we find that, postulating our theory with every caution, epilepsy and psychosis are at the same metabolic level. Artificial administration of serotonin precursors into the brains of experimental animals elicited psychotic manifestations. At the same time as these psychotic manifestations there were also dysrhythmic changes in deep EEG leads. These dysrhythmic changes correlated with those of patients with psychomotor epilepsy. Furthermore, by monitoring a deep lead from the brain a few weeks before the onset of psychotic symptoms in schizophrenic patients, it was found that there were dysrhythmic changes in the EEG exactly like those in patients with epilepsy. Also, a few weeks before the onset of an epileptic seizure in patients with psychomotor epilepsy dysrhythmia just like that found in psychosis cases before the onset of psychotic symptoms was found in the same deep cerebral structures (septum, hippocampus). Parallel to these electrophysiological phenomena, there was an increase of catecholamine concentration (primarily serotonin) in these regions of the brain in both disease groups. This is our clearest indication of the interrelationship between psychosis and epilepsy. At any given period of time, the brain can only respond in one way—with epilepsy or psychosis. If epilepsy is blocked, then psychosis develops.

Similar parallels between epilepsy and psychosis can be drawn as a result of studies on hormonal, enzymic and vitamin changes. However, these findings require further verification as there are still many unknown factors here.

All the evidence described above points to *two possible ways* in which epilepsy can change into psychosis or epileptic symptoms into psychotic symptoms (if an epileptic seizure is prevented): 1.) first, the biochemical changes of the two clinical pictures are on the same level and so epileptic symptoms can easily *slide* into psychotic symptoms, and 2.) secondly, metabolic defects can be corrected by the transition from epileptic to psychotic symptoms—for example, alkalosis changes into acidosis.

BIOCHEMICAL BASIS OF CHRONIC MENTAL CHANGES IN PATIENTS WITH PSYCHOMOTOR EPILEPSY

Here we shall be discussing the familiar *personality change,* which is much more pronounced in patients from the psychomotor group than in other forms of epilepsy. Some authors assert that all types of epilepsy must eventually lead to the psychomotor form and it is only then that a personality change occurs. Almost all of the results we have to hand indicate that there are two decisive factors in this process: a.) the functional heterogeneity of the temporal lobe, and b.) repetition of attacks.

Complete removal of the temporal lobe produced mental deficiency with personality changes. Major mental changes have been found following removal of the mediobasal temporal cerebral cortex with parts of the anterior hippocampus and gyrus hippocampi. Unilateral extirpation of these cerebral structures induced isolated or vague mental disorders. Sensory sensations were not so marked as mental disturbances, following removal of individual structures of the temporal lobe. Bilateral resection of the gyrus cinguli tranquilized and subdued the experimental subject. Extirpation of various parts of the septum pellucidum and limbic system disrupted autonomic regulation. All these symptoms were found both in animals (experimentally) and in humans (following neurosurgery in severe cases of psychosis and epilepsy).

It is generally agreed in the literature that repeated seizures damage the brain. Many experiments with repeated attacks have shown that there is a further change in electrolyte metabolism, oxygen metabolism (with a reduction of respiratory activity in cerebral tissue), in the acid-base balance, in protein metabolism (increase of activity and degradation), in amino acid levels (blood level was elevated), in endogenous amines, vitamins and enzymes. These changes start after only the second attack, build up after the tenth or twelfth attack and, after the twentieth attack, they are quite different from those after a single attack. The results from animal experiments correlate with those from human studies.

Somnambulistic episodes are fairly rare in patients with psychomotor epilepsy and are not dealt with here under a separate heading. Serotonin is one of the factors which are held to be responsible for these episodes.

THE PROBLEMS OF TREATING PSYCHOMOTOR EPILEPSY

Of all the adult forms of epilepsy, psychomotor epilepsy responds least well to treatment. Infantile spasms (salaam-nodding spasms in young children) are the only form of epilepsy which is more resistant to treatment. Hence, treatment of psychomotor epilepsy has to be individually adapted for each patient and from syndrome to syndrome.

Only restricted amounts of *analeptic amines* can be given, only during brief psychomotor attacks in combination with antiepileptic agents.

Vasodilator agents can also be used to interrupt an attack, but again in combination with antiepileptic agents.

High doses of *vitamins* of the B complex (particularly Vitamin B_6) should be administered in every case, especially in young people and at the beginning of the disease.

The best antiepileptic agent for treating psychomotor epilepsy has been found to be *carbamazepine* (Tegretal, Tegretol). For combined attacks, a pyridine derivative, 5-phenyl-5-ethylhexahydropyridine (Mylepsinum) is given in most cases. Tegretal and Mylepsinum can be prescribed together and in combination with B vitamins.

Drugs of the *hydantoin group* have proved best for treating status epilepticus. The drug must be given intramuscularly or intravenously; 250 to 500 mg every four hours (according to degree of severity) because it is rather short-acting.

Barbiturates can also be prescribed for patients who do not respond to other drugs. A combination of carbamazepine and barbiturates acts on various regions of the brain, and improves treatment.

Drugs of the *benzodiazepine* group (chordiazepoxide, diazepam, nitrazepam or Librium, Valium, Mogadan or Mogadon) can be prescribed for patients with a protracted psychomotor seizure. Twilight states respond well to diazepam, especially when administered intravenously. The injections should be given quite slowly with EEG monitoring and a watch being kept on the patient's mental state. After half-an-hour, this may bring about a prompt improvement and abolish relatively severe twilight states.

A lumbar puncture must be performed to relieve the cerebrospinal fluid pressure in severe cases of generalized status epilepticus.

Electroshock can be used with caution in a status dominated by unconsciousness with weak tonic-clonic seizures. This will induce tonic-clonic discharges in the body. Here, the seizure, which would otherwise have a detrimental effect, can be exploited for therapeutic purposes.

In psychotic conditions it is necessary to resort to psychiatric techniques. These cases are treated with *antipsychotic* agents, antidepressants and other tranquilizers which otherwise have an epileptic or epileptogenic action. Here again electroshock might sometimes have to be used to abolish the psychotic condition.

Somnambulistic episodes can be effectively treated with barbiturates. In many acute cases, treatment will be pointless unless the aim is to prevent the next attack.

BIBLIOGRAPHY

Abducharimov, A.A., Blankfelt, A.E. and Kovaleva, L.V.: Therapeutical experiments in epilepsy with aminazine and serpasil. (Russ) *Med Zh Uzbekistan, 7*:1921, 1959.

Abood, L.G. and Geiger, A.: Breakdown of proteins and lipids during glucose-free perfusion of the cat brain. *Am J Physiol, 182*:557, 1955.

Adams, C.W.M. and Davison, A.N.: The occurrence of esterfied cholesterol in the developing nervous system. *J Neurochem, 4*:282, 1959.

Adams, J.A., Aird, R.B. and Garoutte, W.: Fluid and electrolyte exchange in the brain in experimental convulsions. *Trans Am Neurol Assoc, 77*:34, 1952.

Adler, M.W.: Laboratory evaluation of antiepileptic drugs. *Epilepsia, 10*:263-280, 1969.

Agaphonov, V.G.: The depressive action of aminazine on the central effect of painful stimuli. *Zh Nevropat Psikhiatr, 56*:94, 1956.

Aird, R.B. and Strait, L.A.: Protective barriers of the central nervous system. *Arch Neurol Psychiatr (Chic), 51*:54, 1944.

Ajmone-Marsan, C. and Stoll, J.: Subcortical connections of the temporal pole in relation to the temporal lobe seizures. *Arch Neurol Psychiatr (Chic), 66*:669, 1951.

Ajmone-Marsan, C., Stoll, J. and Jasper, H.H.: Electrophysiological studies of subcortical connections of the tip of the temporal lobe. *Electroencephalogr Clin Neurophysiol, 2*:356, 1950.

Ajmone-Marsan, C., and Zivin, L.S.: Factors related to the occurrence of typical paroxysmal abnormalities in the EEG records of epileptic patients. *Epilepsia, 11*: 361-381, 1970.

Akimoto, H. and Creutzfeldt, O.: Reaktionen von Neuronen des optischen Cortex nach elektrischer Reizung unspezifischer Thalamuskerne. *Z Neurol, 196*:494, 1958.

Alajouanine, Th., Bertrand, I., Gruner, J. and Nehlil, J.: Corrélations électro-anatomocliniques dans un cas d'épilepsie psychomotorique. *Rev Neurol (Paris), 92*:169, 1955.

Albanese, A.A. and Frankston, J.E.: Difference in metabolism of l- and dl-tryptophane in human. *J Biol Chem, 155*:101, 1944.

Albe-Fessard, D.: Activités de projection et d'association du néocortex cérébral des mammifères. *J Physiol, 49*:521, 1957.

Albert, K., Hoch, P. and Waelsch, H.: A preliminary report on effect of glutamine acid administration in mentally retarded subjects. *J Nerv Ment Dis, 104*:263, 1946.

Albert, K., Hoch, P. and Waelsch, H.: Glutamic acid and mental deficiency. *J Nerv Ment Dis, 114*:471, 1951.

Alexander, L. and Löwenbach, H.: Experimental studies on electrical shock treatment: 1. The intracerebral vascular reaction as an indicator of the path of the current and the threshold of early changes within the brain tissue. *J Neuropath Exp Neurol, 3*: 193, 1944.

Allen, D.W. and Schroeder, W.A.: Comparison of the phenylalanine content of the hemoglobin of normal and phenylketonuric individuals—determination with ion-exchange chromatography. *J Clin Invest, 36*:287, 1957.

Allgén, L.G., Lindberg, U.H. and Ullberg, S.: Tissue distribution, excretion and metabolism of heminevrine. *Nord Psykiatr T, 17*:13, 1963.

Alliez, J.: Epilepsie psychique et lobe temporale. Peut-on envisager une pathologie rhinencéphalique? *Evol Psychiatr* (Paris), 1952.

Alpern, E.B.: Polystotic fibrous dysplasia. *J Pediat, 32:*91, 1948.

Alsen, V.: Anfallsleiden und Psychose. *Nervenarzt, 36:*490, 1965.

Altmann, H.W.: Allgemeine morphologische Pathologie des Cytoplasmas. In *Hb.d.Allgem. Pathologie,* Vol. 2/1, Berlin-Göttingen-Heidelberg, Springer 1955.

Altschule, M.D.: *Bodily Physiology in Mental and Emotional Disorders.* New York, Grune & Stratton, 1953.

Altschule, M.D., Goncz, R.M. and Holliday, P.D.: Carbohydrate metabolism in brain disease, X. Lack of effect of chlorpromazine and reserpine on abnormal carbohydrate metabolism of chronic schizophrenia. *Arch Int Med, 99:*892, 1957.

Amelung, D.: *Fermentdiagnostik interner Erkrankungen.* Stuttgart, Thieme, 1964.

Amico, D.: Sull' esplorazione del sistema reticolo endoteliale in neuropsichiatria. *Neopsichiat, 2:*273, 1936.

Amman, R.: Die Bromvergiftung und ihre Schriftstörungen. *Z ges Neurol Psychiat, 34:* 12, 1916.

Anastasopulos, G.: Hypersexualität, Wesensveränderung, Schlafstörungen und akute Demenz bei einem Tumor des rechten Schläfenlappens. *Psychiat et Neurol, 136:*85, 1958.

Anastasopulos, G. and Routsonis, K.G.: Demenzzustände bei Ammonshornläsionen. Über einen Fall mit einseitiger angiopathischer Läsion. *Dtsch Z Nervenheilkd, 186:* 246, 1964.

Anastasopulos, G. and Routsonis, K.G.: Zur Symptomatologie der Schläfenlappentumoren mit Ammonshornzerstörung. *Nervenarzt, 38:*442, 1967.

Anden, N.E.: Changes in the impulse flow of central monoamine nerves by drugs affecting monoamine receptors. *Acta Pharmacol Toxicol, 25:*5, 1968.

Anden, N.E., Dahlstroem, A., Fuxe, K. and Larsson, K.: Functional role of the nigroneostriatal dopamine neurons. *Acta Pharmacol Toxicol, 24:*263, 1966.

Andersen, P.O.: Correlation of structural design with function in the archicortex. In Eccles, J.C. (Ed.): *Brain and Conscious Experience.* New York, Springer, 1966.

Anderson, E.P., Kalckar, H.M. and Isselbacher, K.J.: Defect in uptake of galactose-1-phosphate into liver nucleotides in congenital galactosemia. *Science, 125:*113, 1957.

Andreev, A.L.: Serial studies on the therapeutic problems in patients with psychic disorders regarding the applied amino acids. Proc. of the conference on the metabolism of maino acids and their application in medicine. (Russ) *MGU.* Moscow, pp. 33-43, 1956.

Andreev, A.L.: The magnesium salt of glutamic acid in the treatment of epilepsy. Proc. on the 40 Anniversary of protein research and the application of amino acids. *Sov Med, 30:*172-188, 1958.

Andy, O.J. and Akert, K.: Electroencephalographic and behavioral changes during seizures induced by stimulation of ammons formation in the cat and monkey. *Electroencephalogr Clin Neurophysiol, 3:*42, 1953.

Andy, O.J. and Akert, K.: Seizure patterns induced by electrical stimulation of hippocampal formation in the cat. *J Neuropathol, 14:*198, 1955.

Angst, J.: Neuere Entwicklung der Pharmako-Psychiatrie. *Praxis, 57:*143, 1968.

Angst, J. and Weiss, P.: Zum Verlauf depressiver Psychosen. Vortrag an der 84. *Wanderversammlung Südwestdeutscher Neurologen und Psychiater.* Unpublished manuscript Baden-Baden, 1968.

Anguiano, G. and McIlwain, H.: Convulsive agents in the phosphates of the brain examined *in vitro. Br J Pharmacol, 6:*444, 1951.

Anokhin, P.K.: Advances in modern neurophysiology and their importance in the problem of higher nervous function. (Russ) *Ves AMN SSSR, 5*:40, 1959.

Anokhin, P.K.: The multiple ascending influences of the subcortical centers on the cerebral cortex. In Brazier, M.A.B. (Ed.): *Brain and Behavior. Amer Inst Biol Sci,* Washington, Vol. VI, pp. 139-170, 1961.

Ansell, G.B. and Marshall, E.F. In Bradley, Flügel, Hoch (Eds.): *Neuro-Psychopharmacology*. Amsterdam, Elsevier 1964, vol 3. pp. 200-202, cit. by Kanig, K.: *Arzneim Forsch, 19*:397, 1969.

Ansell, G.B. and Richter, D.: Evidence for a "neutral proteinase" in brain tissue. *Biochem Biophys Acta, 13*:92, 1954.

Anton-Stephens, D.: Preliminary observations on the psychiatric uses of chlorpromazine (Largactil). *J Ment Sci, 100*:543, 1954.

Appel, K.R., Appel, E. and Maurer, W.: Konzentration und Austauschrate des freien Methionins im Gehirn der Ratte. *Biochem Zschr, 332*:293, 1960.

Arbuzov, S.J.: Parallel action of antiepileptic drugs on some functions of CNS: I. Antagonism of antiepileptic drugs to narcotics. (Russ.) *Farmakol Toksikol, 7*:31, 1944.

Arbuzov, S.J.: *Antinarcotical and Arousal Reaction of Stimulation of the Nervous System.* (Russ) Moscow, Medgiz, 1950.

Ardizzone, C., Calabrese, E., Catania, E., Moralito, S., Nigro, A., Salva, L. and Tripodo, M.: *Boll Soc Ital Biol, 41*:275, 1965; cit. by Nigro, A.: *6th Int. Congr. Electroencephalogr Clin Neurophysiol,* Vienna, p 81, 1965.

Arduini, A.: Enduring potential changes evoked in the cerebral cortex by stimulation of brain stem reticular formation and thalamus. In Jasper, Proctor, Knighton, Noshay a. Costello (Eds.): *Reticular Formation of the Brain.* Henry Ford Hospital Symposion. Little, Brown & Co., Boston, pp. 333-351, 1958.

Arduini, A. and Arduini, M.G.: Effect of drugs and metabolic alterations on brain stem arousal mechanisms. *J Pharmacol, 110*:76, 1954.

Armstrong, M.D. and Robinson, K.S.: Excretion of indole derivatives in phenylketonuria. *Arch Biochem, 52*:287, 1954.

Armstrong, M.D. and Tyler, F.H.: Phenylketonuria: I. Restricted phenylalanine intake in phenylketonuria. *J Clin Invest, 34*:565, 1955.

Arnold, O.H.: Epilepsie. Eine statistische Studie am Material einer Epileptiker-Ambulanz. *Wien Z Nervenheilkd, 2*:359, 1954.

Arnold, O.H. and Hofmann, G.: Diskussion. Biochemische Diagnostik des schizophrenen Formenkreises. *Proc. 4th World Congr. Psychiatr. 1966,* Part 1, Amsterdam, Excerpta Med, p. 533, 1967.

Arseni, S., and Cristesar, A.: Epilepsy due to cerebral cyctiarcosis. *Epilepsia, 13*:253-258, 1972.

Arutunov, D.N.: Soj. Psikhonevrol. 4-5, 1939; cit. by Sorokina, T.T.: Biochemical and experimental studies of catatonic stupor of schizophrenic kind. (Russ) In *Obm. Veshtch, Psikhiat, Zabol.,* Moscow, Medgiz, pp. 77-84, 1960.

Åsander, H.: Ambulatory treatment of alcoholics with heminevrine. *Sven Tandlak Tidskr, 59*:418, 1962.

Aschkenasy-Lelu, P.: Le retentissement de la nutrition sur les phénomènes psychiques. *Encéphale, 41*:45, 1952.

Aston, R. and Domino, E.F.: Differential effects of phenobarbital, pentobarbital and diphenylhydantoin on motor cortical and reticular thresholds in the Rhesus monkey. *Psychopharmacol, 2*:304, 1961.

Atzev, E.: Ognistschina Epilepsia. *Medicina i Fizcultura.* Sofia, Bulg. 1962.

Ausst, E.G., Arana, R., Migliaro, E., Sanda, M.T. and Segundo, J.P.: Changes in the

EEG and in the tendon jerks induced by stimulation of the fornix in man. *EEG Clin Neurophysiol, 6:*653, 1954.

Axelrod, J.: Purification and properties of phenylethanolamine-N-Methyl transferase. I. *J Biol Chem, 237:*1657, 1962.

Azima, H.: Biologie de la schizophrénie. (Revue critique 1944-1952). *Encéphale, 41:*527, 1952.

Baastrup, P.C. and Schou, M.: Lithium as a prophylactic agent. Its effect against recurrent depressions and manic depressive psychoses. *Arch Gen Psychiatr, 16:*162, 1967.

Bach, A.H.: Selected writings. (Russ) *A.N.,* SSSR, 1950.

Bailey, P.: *Die Hirngeschwülste.* Stuttgart, Enke, 1951.

Bailey, P.: Betrachtungen über die chirurgische Behandlung der psychomotorischen Epilepsie. *Zbl Neurochir, 415:*195, 1954.

Bailey, P. and v. Bonin, G.: *The Isocortex of Man.* Urbana, U. of Ill. Pr., 1951.

Bailey, P. and Gibbs, F.A.: The surgical treatment of psychomotor epilepsy. *JAMA, 145:* 365, 1951.

Bain, J.A. and Wiegand, R.G.: *J Pharmacol Exp Ther, 119:*131, 1957; cit. by Kanig, K.: *Die Bedeutung der B-Vitamine für das Nervensystem.* Wiss. Berichte, E. Merck, Darmstadt, 1968.

Bakay, L.: *The Blood Brain Barrier.* Springfield, Thomas, 1956.

Balazs, R. and Lagnado, J. R.: Glycolytic activity associated with rat brain mitochondria. *J Neurochem, 5:*1, 1959.

Baldridge, R.C., Borofsky, L., Baird, H., Reichle, F. and Bullock, D.: Relation of serum phenylalanine levels and ability of phenylketonurics to hydroxylate trytophan. *Proc Soc Exp Biol* (NY), *100:*529, 1959.

Baldwin, M.: Modifications psychiques survenants après lobectomie temporale subtotale. *Neurochirurgie* (Paris), *2:*152, 1956.

Baldwin, M.L., Frost, L. and Wood, C.D.: Investigations of the primate amygdala. Movements of the face and jaws. *Neurology* (Minneap), *1:*586, 1954.

Ball, B.: Encéphale 1886, p. 427; cit. by Hallen, O.: *Dtsch Z Nervenheilkd, 171:*236, 1954.

Balley, B.F.S. and Heald, P.J.: Quantitative estimation of proteins in extracts of cerebral tissue after separation by electrophoresis in starch gel. *J Neurochem, 7:*81, 1961.

Bamberger, P. and Matthes, A.: *Anfälle im Kindesalter.* Basel-New York, Karger, 1959.

Bamberger, P. and Matthes, A.: Eine neue Therapiemöglichkeit des Status epilepticus im Kindesalter mit Valium i.v. *Z Kinderheilkd, 95:*155, 1966.

Banga, J., Ochoa, S. and Peters, R.A.: Pyruvate oxidation in the brain: VII. Dialysable components of the pyruvate oxidation system. *Biochem J, 33:*1980, 1939.

Barbeau, A. and Sourkes, T.L.: Some biochemical aspects of extrapyramidal diseases. *Rev Can Biol, 20:*197, 1962.

Barmina, O.N.: Fermentative reduce of proteins—a link in the regulation of water balance of the nervous system. *Proc Med Inst Gorki, 1:*19, 1957, (Russ).

Barsa, J.A. and Kline, N.S.: Treatment of two hundred disturbed psychotics with reserpine. *JAMA, 158:*110, 1955.

Barsa, J.A. and Kline, N.S.: Use of meprobamate in treatment of psychotic patients. *Am J Psychiatry, 112:*1023, 1956.

Baruk, H.: A propos des facteurs régulateurs de la motilité volontaire. Les fonctions cérébrales psychomotrices au point de vue clinique et expérimental. *Rev Neurol, 38:* 629, 1931.

Batini, C., Magni, F., Palestini, M., Rossi, G.F. and Zanchetti, A.: Neural mechanisms underlying the enduring EEG and behavioral activation in the midpontine pretrigeminal cat. *Arch Ital Biol, 97:*13, 1959.

Batini, C., Moruzzi, G., Palestini, M., Rossi, G.F. and Zanchetti, A.: Persistent patterns of wakefulness in the pretrigeminal midpontine preparation. *Science, 128:*30, 1958.

Bauer, E.O.: Erfahrungen mit der potenzierten Narkose. Stizungsberichte Ges. dtsch. Neurol. u. Psychiat.; ref. *Zbl Ges Neurol Psychiatr, 128:*327, 1954.

Bauer, E.O.: Beitrag zur Adrenalinwirkung bei potenzierter Narkose. *Anaesthesist, 3:* 192, 1954.

Bauer, J.: Schlaflähmung und Schlafwandeln. *Wein Klin Wochenschr, 77:*338, 1965.

Bauer, K.F., Haase, J. and Leonhardt, H.: Über Dosis-Wirkungsbeziehungen bei dem durch Cardiazol induzierten Zusammenbruch der Bluthirnschranke von Geigyblau als Schrankenindikator. *Arch Psychiatr Nervenkr, 195:*199, 1956.

Bauer, K.F. and Leonhardt, H.: Zur Kenntnis der Blut-Hirnschranke. Cardiazol-Schock und Schrankenzusammenbruch. *Arch Psychiatr Nervenkr, 193:*68, 1955.

Bauknecht, R.: Epilepsie und Beruf. *Mat Med Nordm, 8:*369, 1956.

Baumgartner, G.: Zur Pathophysiologie der Epilepsie. *Ther Umsch, 24:*506, 1967.

Baumm, H.: Erfahrungen über Epilepsie bei Hirnverletzten. *Z Ges Neurol Psychiatr, 127:*279, 1930.

Baust, W.: Local blood flow in different regions of the brain stem during natural sleep and arousal. *Electroencephalogr Clin Neurophysiol, 22:*365, 1967.

Baxter, C.F. and Roberts, E.: The γ-aminobutyric acid-α-ketoglutaric acid transaminase of beef brain. *J Biol Chem, 233:*1135, 1958.

Baxter, C.F. and Roberts, E.: Demonstration of thiosemicarbazide-induced convulsions in the rat with elevated brain levels of γ-aminobutyric acid. *Proc Soc Exp Biol Med, 104:*426, 1960.

v. Bayer, W.: *Die moderne psychiatrische Schockbehandlung.* Stuttgart, Thieme, 1951.

Bayreuther, H. and Radtke, H.: Klinische Erfahrungen bei der Reserpinbehandlung schizophrener Psychosen unter besonderer Berücksichtigung der Beziehungen zwischen somatischen Befunden und EEG. *Arch Psychiatr Nervenkr, 198:*158, 1958.

Becker, B.: Erfahrungen mit dem Antiepilepticum Maliasin®. *Med Welt, 19:*577, 1968.

Becker, H. and Quadbeck, G.: Tierexperimentelle Untersuchungen über die Funktionsweise der Blut-Hirnschranke. *Z Naturforsch, 7b:*493, 1952.

Belezki, W.K.: On the pathological anatomy of the nervous system in epilepsy. Collection *Problems of Epilepsy* (Russ). p. 170, 1936.

Belov, V.P.: Results of clinical testing of a new antispasmodic hexamidine. (Russ) *Zh Nevropat Psikhiatr, 56:*828, 1956.

Belova, H.A.: Collection of research reports. Machatchkala 1955; cit. by Schesterikova, P.T. et al.: Some metabolic changes of carbohydrate and nitrogen in psychotic patients, resistent and responding to insulin-therapy. In *Obm. Veshtch. Psikhiat. Zabol.* Moscow, Medgiz, pp. 146-153, 1960.

Benedeto, V., Ferraris, G.M. and Pansa, E.: Applicazioni cliniche della autoistoradiografia tiroidea con I 131. *Minerva Med (Torino), 47:*1976, 1956.

Bengochea, F.G., de la Torre, O., Esquivel, O., Vieta, R. and Fernandez, C.: *Trans Am Neurol Assoc, 79:*176, 1954.

Bengzon, A.H., Hippius, H. and Kanig, K.: Veränderungen einiger Serumfermente während der psychiatrischen Pharmakotherapie. *Dtsch Med J,* 217-223, 1966.

Benitez, D., Pscheid, G.R. and Stone, W.E.: Formation of ammonium ion in the cerebrum in fluoracetate poisoning. *Am J Physiol, 176:*488, 1954.

Bente, D. and Itil, T.M.: Zur Wirkung des Phenothiazinkörpers Megaphen auf das menschliche Hirnstrombild. *Arzneim Forsch, 4:*418, 1954.

Bente, D. and Itil, T.M.: EEG-Veränderungen unter chronischer Medikation von Piperazinyl-Phenotiazin-Derivaten. *Med Exp (Basel), 2:*132, 1960.

Bente, D. and Kluge, E.: Sexuelle Reizzustände im Rahmen des Uncinatus-Syndroms. *Arch Psychiatr Nervenkr, 190:*357, 1953.

Bercel, N.A., Travis, L.E., Olinger, L.B. and Dreikurs, E.: Model psychoses induced by LSD-25 in normals. *Arch Neurol Psychiatr, 75:*588, 1956.

Berendes, N., Anderson, J.M., Ziegler, M.R. and Ruttenberg, D.: The disturbance in tryptophan metabolism in phenylketonuria. *J Dis Child, 96:*430, 1958.

Bergen, J.R., Koella, W.P., Freeman, H. and Hoagland, H.: A human plasma factor inducing behavioral and electrophysiological changes in animals. II Changes induced in animals. *Ann NY Acad Sci, 96:*469, 1962.

Bergener, M.: EEG-changes during treatment of delirium tremens with chlormethiazole. *Acta Psychiatr Scand, 42:*65, 1966.

Bergener, M. and Fritschka, J.: Zur Klinik und Therapie des delirium tremens unter besonderer Berücksichtigung der Chlormethiazolbehandling. *Nervenarzt, 36:*156, 1965.

Berl, S., Purpura, D.P., Girado, M. and Waelsch, H.: Amino acid metabolism in epileptogenic and nonepileptogenic lesions of neocortex (cat). *J Neuro chem, 4:*211, 1959.

Berl, S.,Tagaki, G. and Purpura, D.P.: Metabolism and pharmacological affects of injected amino acids and ammonia on cortical epileptogenic lesions. *J Neurochem, 7:* 198, 1961.

Bernheimer, A.W. and van Heyningen, W.E.: The relation between the tetanus toxin-fixing and influenca virus-inhibiting properties of ganglioside. *J Gen Microbiol, 24:* 121, 1961.

Bernheimer, H., Birkmayer, W. and Hornykiewicz, O.: Homovanillinsäure im Liquor cerebrospinalis: Untersuchungen beim Parkinson-Syndrom und anderen Erkrankungen des ZNS. *Wein Klin Wochenschr, 78:*417, 1966.

Bernheimer, H. and Hornykiewicz, O.: Herabgesetzte Konzentration der Homovanillinsäure im Gehirn von parkinsonkranken Menschen als Ausdruck der Störung des zentralen Dopaminstoffwechsels. *Klin Wochenschr, 43:*711, 1965.

Bertaccini, G.: Effect of convulsant treatment on the 5-hydroxytryptamine content of brain and other tissues of the rat. *J Neurochem, 4:*217, 1959.

Bertler, A., Falck, B., Hillarp, N.A., Rosengren, E. and Torp, A.: Dopamine and chromafin cells. *Acta Physiol Scand, 47:*251, 1959.

Bertler, A. and Rosengren, E.: Distribution of monoamines and enzymes responsible for their formation in brain. *Experientia, 15:*382, 1959.

Bessey, O.A.: Role of vitamins in the metabolism of amino acids. *JAMA, 164:*1224, 1957.

Bessey, O.A., Adam, D.J.D. and Hansen, A.E.: Intake of vitamin B_6 and infantile convulsions. A first approximation of requirements of pyridoxine in infants. *Pediatrics, 20:*33, 1957.

Bessman, S.P. and Baldwin, R.: Imidazole aminoaciduria in cerebromacular degeneration. *Science, 135:*798, 1962.

Bettis, T.A., Kalra, P.L., Cooper, R. and Jeavons, P.M.: Epileptic fits as a probable side-effect of amitriptyline. Report of seven cases. *Lancet, 1:*7539, 390-392, 1968.

Bettzieche, F.: Untersuchungen über den Stoffwechsel bei Schizophrenen. *Z Neurol Psychiatr, 124:*136, 1930.

Betz, E., and Rodenhäuser, J.H.: Gleichzeitige Durchblutungsregistrierung von Gehirn, Aderhaut und Ciliarkörper bei Einwirkung vasoaktiver Substanzen. *Klin Wochenschr, 512:*40, 1962.

Beyer, L. and Jovanović, U.J.: Elektroencephalographische und klinische Korrelate bei

Aufwachepileptikern mit besonderer Berücksichtigung der therapeutischen *Probleme Nervenarzt, 37:*333, 1966.

Bhagat, B. and Lockett, M.F.: The effect of deficiency and small excess of thiamine on the rat phrenic nerve-diagram preparation. *J Pharm Pharmacol, 14:*161, 1962.

Bickel, G., Barazzone, J., Engel, E., Falbriard, A., Greder, G., Rentchnik, P. and Secretan, P.: Les effets seconds des antibiotiques. *Rev Med Suisse Romande, 73:*817, 1953.

Biehl, J.P. and Vilter, R.W.: Effect of isoniacid on pyridoxine metabolism. *JAMA, 156:* 1549, 1954.

Biehl, J.P., Vilter, R.W., Beall, F.C. and Kennedy, C.E.: Effect of isoniazid on vitamin B_6 metabolism; its possible significance in producing isoniazid neuritis. *Proc Soc Exp Biol Med, 85:*389, 1954.

Biesold, D., Weise, K. and Canzler, E.: Untersuchungen über das Verhalten von Phosphorsäureverbindungen im Blut von Schizophrenen. *Psychiatr Neurol Med Psychol,* (Lpz) *17:*232, 1965.

Binswanger, O.: *Die Epilepsie.* Wien, Hölder, 1899.

Bird, E.D., Ellis, W.H. and Anton, A.H.: Effect of phenothiazine on manganese and dopamine concentration in basal ganglia of primates. *Clin Res, 15:*42, 1967.

Birkhäuser, H.: Cholinesterase and Monoaminoxidase im zentralen Nervensystem. *Schweiz Med Wochenschr, 71:*750, 1941.

Bittner, C.: Diphenylhydantoin (Zentropil und Zentronal) in der Epilepsiebehandlung. *Mat Med Nordm, 5:*222, 1953.

Bjurwill, B.: Der Effekt von Cosaldon auf Orientierungund Denkvermögen bei älteren Menschen mit Zerebralsklerose. *Svenska Läkartid,* 3, 1963.

Blashko, H.: The specific action of L-dopadecarboxylase. *J Physiol (Lond), 96:*50, 1939.

Blashko, H.: The activity of L-dopadecarboxylase. *J Phyisol* (Lond), *101:*337, 1942.

Blashko, H., Burn, J.H. and Langemann, H.: The formation of noradrenaline from dihydroxyphenylserine. *Br J Pharm Chemother, 5:*431, 1950.

Blashko, H. and Welch, A.D.: Localisation of bovine adrenaline in cytoplasmic particles of bovine adrenal medulla. *Arch Exp Path Pharmakol,* 219, 17, 1953.

Blasius, W.: Allgemeine Physiologie des Nervensystems. In *Landois-Rosemann: Physiologie des Menschen,* 28th Ed. München, Urban & Schwarzenberg, vol. II, 1962.

Bleichert, A.: Grundlagen biologischer Regelung. *Klin Wochenschr, 40:*497, 1962.

Bleuler, E.: Dementia praecox. In *Hb.d.Psychiatrie,* Spez. Teil, Abt.4, Hälfte 1, Leipzig, Deuticke, 1911.

Bleuler, E.: "Hystero-Epilepsie." *Schweiz Med Wochenschr, 55:*1005, 1925.

Bleuler, M.: Die Psychopathologie des Cushing-Syndroms. In *Endokrinologische Psychiatrie.* Stuttgart, Thieme, 1954.

Bleuler, M.: Endokrinologie und Psychiatrie. *Wein Z Nervenheilkd, 14:*16, 1957.

Blickenstorfer, E.: Zum ätiologischen Problem der Psychosen vom akuten exogenen Reaktionstypus. Lysergsäurediäthylamid, ein psychisch wirksamer toxischer Spurenstoff. *Arch Psychiatr Z Neurol, 118:*226, 1952.

Blochin, H.H.: 1951; cit. by: Tchalissov, M.A.: Carbon. phosphate metabolism and its importance in psychiatry. In *Obm. Veshtch. Psikhiat. Zabol.* Moscow, Medgiz, pp. 14-20, 1960.

Block, W.: Paradoxe Reaktionen im vegetativen Bereich. *Acta Neuroveg* (Wien), *8:* 219, 1953.

Blom, S., Heijbel, J., and Bergfors, P.G.: Benign epilepsy of children with centrotemporal EEG foci. Prevalence and follow-up study of 40 patients. *Epilepsia, 13:*609-619, 1972.

Bochnik, H.J.: Klinische Elektrophysiologie des Zentralnervensystems. In Cobet, Gutzeit, Bock (Eds.): *Klinik der Gegenwart.* 33 München, Urban und Schwarzenberg, vol. V, 1957.

Bochnik, H.J. and Spiegelberg, U.: Klinische und experimentelle EEG-Untersuchungen bei Epileptikern und Gesunden mit Perludin (2 Phenyl-3-methyl-tetrahydro-1, 4-oxazin-hydrochlorid). *Nervenarzt, 28*:425, 1957.

Boerner, D., Jovanović, U.J. and Henschler, D.: Beeinflussung der Hirnfunktion durch Alkalisierung bei der Behandlung von Schlafmittelvergiftungen mit forcierter Diurese. *Z Gese Exp Med, 152*:223, 1970.

Bogacz, J. and Yanicelli, E.: Vegetative phenomena in petit mal epilepsy. *World Neurol, 3*:195, 1962.

Bogina, F.M.: Gaz metabolism in experimental epilepsy. In *To the Knowledge of the Mechanisms of Pathological Reactions.* (Russ) Kievuan, pp. 57-61, 1942.

Bogoch, S.: Studies on the neurochemistry of schizophrenic and affective disorders. *Am J Psychiatry, 116*:743, 1960.

Bogue, J.Y. and Carrington, H.C.: The evaluation of "Mysoline." A new anticonvulsant drug. *Br J Pharmacol, 8*:230, 1953.

Bokonjić, N. and Trojaborg, W.: The effect of meprobamate on the electroencephalogram during treatment, intoxication and after abrupt withdrawal. *Electroencephalogr Clin Neurophysiol, 12*:177, 1960.

Bondyrev, I.M.: Gaz metabolism in traumatic shock. *Collection of the Communications of the Med. Inst., Med. Inst.,* Donezk, 1956, pp. 341-394 (Russ).

Bonnet, H., Laroche, B. and Bonnet, V.: Wirkung verschiedener Phenotiazinderivate auf die Anfälle und Geistesstörungen bei Epileptikern. In Therapeutische Gespräche deutscher und französischer Psychiater. *Rev. Lyon Méd, 121*:1, 1960.

Bonnet, V. and Bremer, F.: Action de potassium, du calcium et de l' acetylcholine sur les activités électriques spontanées et provoquées de l'écorce cérébrale. *C R Soc Biol, 126*:1271, 1937.

Bonnin, A.L.: Effets d'un dérive de la benzodiazepine le Ro 4-5360 sur le système nerveux central et le comportement. Med. Diss., Bordeaux, 1965.

Bonvallet, M., Dell, P. and Hiebel, G.: Tonus sympathique et activité électrique corticale. *Electroencephalogr Clin Neurophysiol, 6*:119, 1954.

Booker, H.E., Hosokowa, K., Burdette, R.D., and Darcey, B.: A clinical study of serum primidone levels. *Epilepsia, 11*:395-402, 1970.

Boone, I.U., Magge, M. and Turney, D.F.: Metabolism of C^{14}-labelled isoniazid in vitamin B_6-deficient rats. *J Biol Chem, 221*:781, 1956.

de Boor, W.: *Pharmacopsychologie und Psychopathologie.* Berlin, Springer, 1956.

Borison, H.L. and Wang, S.C.: Physiology and pharmacology of vomiting. *Pharmacol Rev, 5*:193, 1953.

Bornmann, H. and Schiefer, W.: Krampfanfälle bei Tumoren des Grosshirns. *Dtsch Z Nervenheilkd, 166*:1, 1951.

Borsook, H. and Deasy, C.: The metabolism of proteins and amino acids. *An Rev Biochem, 209,* 1951.

Borsunova, A.S.: On pathogenesis of epilepsy and schizophrenia with regard to treatment with anticonvulsants. (Russ) Diss., UFA, 1952.

Boscott, R.J. and Bickel, H.: Detection of abnormal metabolites in the urine of phenylketonurics. *Scand J Clin Lab Invest, 5*:380, 1953.

Bouchet, B. and Cazauvielh, L.: De l' epilepsie considérée dans ses rapports avec l' aliénation mentale. *Arg Gén Méd, 9*:510, 1825.

Bowers, M., Hartmann, E. and Freedman, D.X.: The effect of dream deprivation on brain acetylcholine levels in the rat. *Report to the Assoc. for the Psychophysiological Study of Sleep.* Manuscript, Gainesville, 1966.

Bowes, H.A.: The role of librium in an outpatient psychiatric setting. *Dis Nerv Syst, 21:*20, 1960.

Bradley, P.B. and Elkes, J.: The effect of amphetamine and D-lysergic acid diethylamide (LSD 25) on the electrical activity of the brain of the conscious cat. *J Physiol (Lond), 120:*13P, 1953.

Bradley, P.B., Elkes, C. and Elkes, J.: On some effects of lysergic acid diethylamide (LSD 25) in normal volunteers. *J Physiol (Lond), 121:*50, 1953.

Bradley, P.B. and Key, B.J.: The effect of drugs on arousal responses produced by electrical stimulation of the reticular formation of the brain. *Electroencephalogr Clin Neurophysiol, 10:*97, 1958.

Bradley, P.B., Wolstencroft, J.H., Hösli, L. and Avanzino, G.L.: Neuronal basis for the central action of Chlorpromazine. *Nature, 22:*1425, 1966.

Bräutigam, W.: Zur epileptischen Wesensveränderung *Psyche, 5:*523, 1951.

Braganca, B.M., Faulkner, P. and Quastel, J.H.: Effects of inhibitors of glutamine synthesis on the inhibition of acetylcholine synthesis in brain slices. *Biochim Biophys Acta, 10:*83, 1953.

Brams, E.A.: *Problems of Medical Chemistry.* (Russ), Moscow, Medgiz, 1955.

Bratz, E.: Das Ammonshorn bei Epileptikern, Paralytikern, Senildementen und anderen Hirnkranken. *Mschr Psychiatr Neurol, 47:*56, 1920.

Braunhofer, J.: Klinische Erfahrungen mit Tegretal®, 5-Carbamyl-5H-dibenzo (b,f) azepin (G 32883-Geigy), einer neuen antiepileptischen Substanz. *Med Klin, 60:*9, 1965.

Brazier, M.A.B.: The action of anesthetics on the nervous system with special reference to the brain stem reticular system. In Adrian, Bremer, Jasper (Eds.): *Brain Mechanisms and Consciousness.* Oxford, Blackwell, pp. 163-193, 1954.

Brazier, M.A.B.: The historical development of neurophysiology. In *Hb. of Physiol.* Neurophysiol. I, 1, Amer. Physiol. Soc., 1959.

Brazier, M.A.B.: Some actions of anesthetics on the nervous system. *Fed Proc, 19:*626, 1960.

Brazier, M.A.B.: The electrophysiological effects of the barbiturates on the brain. In Root, Hofmann (Eds.): *Physiological Pharmacology.* The Nervous System, part A. New York-London, Academic Press vol. I, pp. 219-238, 1963.

Brazier, M.A.B. and Finesinger, J.E.: Action of barbiturates on the cerebral cortex. Electroencephalographic studies. *Arch Neurol Psychiatr, 53:*51, 1945.

Brdička, R.: Polarographic studies with the dropping mercury kathode. Pt. XXXI, XXXII, XXXIII. *Coll Teav Chim Československ, 5:*112a., 148a. 238, 1933.

van Breemen, V.L. and Clemente, C.D.: Silver deposition in the central nervous system and the hematoencephalic barrier studied with the electron microscope. *J Biophys Biochem Cytol, 1:*161, 1955.

Breitner, C.: Drug therapy in obsessional states and other psychiatric problems. *Dis Ner Syst, 21:*31, 1960.

Bremer, F.: Cerveau "isolé" et physiologie du sommeil. *CR Soc Biol, 118:*1235, 1935.

Bremer, F.: Différence d' action de la narcose éthérique et du sommeil barbiturique sur les réactions sensorielles acoustiques du cortex cérébral. Signification decette différence en ce qui concerne le méchanisme du sommeil. *CR Soc Biol, 124:*848, 1937.

Bremer, F.: The neurophysiological problem of sleep. In Adrian, Bremer, Jasper (Eds.): *Brain Mechanisms and Consciousness.* Oxford, Blackwell, pp. 137-158, 1954.

Brenner, C. and Merritt, H.H. Effect of certain choline derivates on electrical activity of the cortex. *Arch Neurol Psychiatr* (Chic), 48: 382, 1942.

Brentano, C.: Weitere Untersuchungen über die Beziehungen der Keatinurine zum Muskelglycogen. III. Mitt. *Arch Exp Pathol Pharmacol, 163:*156, 1931.

Breyer, U., and K. Kanig: Cerebrospinal fluid electrolyte disturbances in neurological disorders/With special reference to inorganic phosphate. *Neurology 20,* 247-253, 1970.

Britanishski, G.R.: Electrocardiographic studies in electrically induced epilepsy. In *Mechanism of Pathological Reactions* (Russ), *9:*10, 1947.

Broca, P.: Anatomie comparée des circonvolutions cérébrales. *Rev d' Anthropologie, 3:* 385, 1878.

Brockhaus, J.: Zur normalen und pathologischen Anatomie des Mandelkerngebietes. *J Psychol Neurol, 49:*136, 1938.

Brodal, A.: The hippocampus and the sense of smell. A review. *Brain, 70:*179, 1947.

Brodie, B.B. and Shore, P.A.: A concept for a role of serotonine and norepinephrine as chemical mediators in the brain. *Ann NY Acad Sci, 66:*631, 1957.

Brodie, B.B., Spector, S. and Shore, P.A.: Interactions of drugs with noradrenaline in the brain. *Pharmacol Rev, 11:*548, 1959.

Broman, T.: On basic aspects of the blood-brain-barrier. Acta *Psychiat Scand, 30:*115, 1955.

Bronk, D.W. and Brink, F.: Mechanism connecting impulse conduction and oxygen metabolism in peripheral nerve. *Fed Proc, 10:*19, 1951.

Brookhart, J.M., Arduini, A., Mancia, M. and Moruzzi, G.: Thalamocortical relations as revealed by induced slow potential changes. *J Neurophysiol, 21:*499, 1958.

Broser, F.: Die moderne Behandlung der verschiedenen Formen epileptischer Anfälle und anderer Symptome epileptischer Erkrankungen. *Nervenarzt, 37:*25, 1966.

van Bruggen, K.T., Hutchens, T.T., Claycomb, C.K. and West, E.S.: Time course of lipid labeling. *J Biol Chem, 200:*31, 1953.

Brunia, C.H.M., and Buyze, G.: Serum copper levels and epilepsy. *Epilepsia, 13:*621-625, 1972.

Brunnemann, A. and Coper, H.: Die Aktivität NAD- und NADP-abhängiger Enzyme in verschiedenen Teilen des Rattengehirns. *Arch Exp Path Pharmakol, 246:*493, 1964a.

Brunnemann, A. and Coper, H.: Vergleichende Untersuchungen über die Biosynthese der NAD(P)-Analogen des 3-Acetylpyridins, 4-Acetylpyridins, 6-Amino-nicotinamids und Isonicotinsäurehydrazids. *Arch Exp Path Pharmakol, 248:*514, 1964b.

Brunnemann, A. and Coper, H.: Hydrolyse von NAD(P) und Biosynthese von 3-APAD (P) durch Hirnmikrosomen verschiedener Tierarten. *Arch Exp Path Pharmakol, 250:* 469, 1965.

Buchner, M. and Gabsch, H.: *Moderne Chemische Methoden in der Klinik.* Leipzig, F. A. Barth, 1956.

Bucy, P.C. and Klüver, H.: An anatomical investigation of the temporal lobe in the monkey (Macaca mulatta). *J Comp Neurol, 103:*151, 1955.

Budanova, A.H.: Edit. *A H SSR, 75:*875, 1950; cit. by: Lando, L.J. and Krupenina, L.B.: Comparative data of the ammonia blood content of schizophrenic and epileptic patients. In *Problems of Schizophrenia.* (Russ) Moscow, Medgit, 1962.

Budanova, A.H. Zh. higher nervous function, 7:544, 1957 (Russ) cited by Pogodaev 1964.

Bürgi, S. and Bucher, V.M.: Über einige rhinencephale Verbindungen des Zwischen-und Mittlhirns. *Dtsch Z Nervenheilkd, 174:*89, 1955.

Bureš, J. and Petran, M.: Über die Bestimmung der Krampfbereitschaft beim Elektroschock. *Cesk Fysiol, 1*:24, 1952.

Burn, J.H. and Rand, M.J.: The relation of circulating noradrenaline to the effect of sympathetic stimulation. *J Physiol* (Lond), *150*:295, 1960.

Burns, J.J. and Conney, A.H.: Enzyme stimulation and inhibition in the metabolism of drugs. *Proc Roy Soc Med, 58*:955, 1965.

Burton, R.M., Salvador, R.A., Goldin, A. and Humphreys, S.R.: Interaction of nicotinamide with reserpine and chlorpromazine. II. Some effects on the central nervous system of the mouse. *Int Pharmacodyn, 128*:253, 1960.

Buscaino, G.A.: Esistono differenze biologico-umorali fra le diverse varieta cliniche della schizophrenia? *Acta Neurol* (Nap), *8*:475, 1953.

Buscaino, G.A. and Rapisarda, A.: -ketoglutaric acid in the blood in dementia praecox —its changes from administration on nicotinic acid and nicotinamide. *Acta neurol* (Nap), *3*:251, 1948.

Buscaino, V.M.: Ammine tossiche present in circolo, in dementi precoci, mancanti in maniaci e in melancolici. *Rass Stud Psichiatr, 12*:245, 1923.

Buscaino, V.M.: Nuovi dati sulla genesi patologica delle zolle di disintegrazione a grappolo. Reperti in un caso di demenza precoce catatonica. *Riv Patol Nerv Ment, 29*: 93, 1924.

Buscaino, V.M.: Distribuzione geografica dell'epilessia e del gozzo endemico nella Svizzera. *Riv Patol Nerv Ment, 30*:131, 1925.

Buscaino, V.M.: Risultati delle richerche d' istopatologia del sistema nervoso di dementi precoci fatte nel beiennio 1924-1925. (Con un' appendice sulle "zolle di disintegrazione a grappolo") Rivista sintetico-critica. *Riv Patol Nerv Ment, 31*:329, 1926.

Buscaino, V.M.: Componenti enterogene della demenza precoce. II. *Schizophrenie, 2*:3, 1932.

Buscaino, V.M.: Componenti enterogene della demenza precoce. I. Dati anatomo-patologici. *Riv Patol Nerv Ment, 41*:483, 1933.

Buscaino, V.M. and de Giacomo, U.: Azione catalettogena del somnifen nell' uomo. Utnema di patogenesi amminica delle sindromi schizophreniche. *Boll Soc Ital biol Sperim, 5*:38, 1930.

Busche, E.K.A:. Die krampferregenden Eigenschaften des Penicillins bei unmittelbarer Einwirkung auf die nervöse Substanz. *Acta Neurochir* (Wien), *5*:391, 1957.

Butler, T.C. and Waddell, W.J.: Metabolic conversion of Primidone (Mysoline) to phenobarbital. *Proc Soc Exp Biol Med, 93*:544, 1956.

Buttenworth, K.R. and Mann, M.: The release of adrenaline and noradrenaline from the adrenal gland of the cat by acetylcholine. *Brit J Pharmacol, 12*:422, 1957.

Buzard, J.A. and Nytch, P.D.: Some characteristics of rat kidney 5-hydroxy-tryptophan decarboxylase. *J Biol Chem, 227*:225, 1957.

Cade, J.J.J.: Lithium salts in the treatment of psychotic excitement. *Med J Aust, 36*:349, 1949.

Cadilhac, J.: *Hippocame et Epilepsie.* A propos d'une série d'experiences sur le cobaye et le chat et de l'exploration électrique de la corne d'ammon chez l'homme. Montpellier, P. Déhan, 1955.

Cahn, J., Herlod, M., Dubrasquet, M., Alano, J., Barre, N. and Buret, J.P.: Contribution à un concept biochimique des psychoses expérimentales. *C R Soc Biol, 151*:11, 1820, 1957. a. *151*:12, 2079, 1958.

Cajal, S.R.: *Studien über die Hirnrinde des Menschen.* Leipzig, Barth, 1900.

Caliezi, J.M.: Beitrag zur Frage der Wirkung von Librium bei Epileptikern. *Schweiz Med Wochenschr, 92*:520, 1962.

Canger, R. and Wahl, L.: Die Behandlung der Epilepsie mit Maliasin®. *Nervenarzt, 39:* 10, 1956.

Canzanelli, A., Bogers, G. and Rapport, D.: Effects of inorganic ions on respiration of brain cortex. *Amer J Physiol, 135:*309, 1942.

Careddu, P.: Veränderungen des Tryptophanstoffwechsels bei den BNS-Krämpfen des Kindesalters. *Helv Paediat Acta, 18:*398, 1963.

Cares, R. and Buckmann, C.: Comparative review of the structure and side-effects of newer psychotropic agents. *Dis Nerv Syst, 24:*92, 1963.

Cartellieri, L.: Klinische Erfahrungen mit dem Antiepilepticum Mylepsin. *Med Klin, 51:*986, 1956.

Casamajor, G.: Bromide intolerance and bromide poisoning. *J Nerv Ment Dis, 1:* 345, 1911.

Caspers, H. Die Beeinflussung der corticalen Krampferregbarkeit durch das aufsteigende Reticulärsystem des Hirnstamms. II. Narkosewirkungen. *Z Ges Exp Med, 129:*582, 1958.

Caspers, H., and Speckmann, E.-J.: Cerebral pO_2, pCO_2 and pH: Changes during convulsive activity and their significance for spontaneous arrest of seizures. *Epilepsia, 13:* 699-725, 1972.

Caspersson, T.O.: *Cell Growth and Function.* New York, 1950.

Cassiano, P.: Applicazioni della reazione di Takata in psichiatria. *Schizophrenie, 5:*151, 1935.

Castells, C., Fuster, B. and Maslenikov, V. :Crisis disfásicas de origen temporal. *Acta Neurol Lat Am, 3:*172, 1957.

Castells, C. and Maslenikov, V.: as crisis epilepticas en los tumors temporales. *Arch Urug Med, 50:*741, 1957.

del Castillo, J. and Engbaek, L.: Neuromuscular block produced by MG. *J Physiol* (Lond), *124:*370, 1954.

Catania, E. and Nigro, A.: *Arch. Atti. Soc. Med. Chir. Messina, 8,* fasc. 4th 1964; cit. by Nigro, A.: Kybernetische Mechanismen bei Epilepsie. In *Clinical Neurophysiology EEG-EMG.* 6th Int. Congr. Electroencephalogr Clin Neurophysiol, Vienna 81, 1965.

Cavanagh, J.B. and Meyer, A.: Aetiological aspects of ammon's horn sclerosis associated with temporal lobe epilepsy. *Br Med J, 5006:*1403, 1956.

Ceccarelli, G. and Coen-Giordana, C.: Influenza della promazina sulla sintomatologica psichica e sul numero delle crisi convulsive di ammalati epilettici degenti in ospedale psichiatrico. Osservazioni su 50 casi. *Neuropsichiatr.* (Geneva), *16:*327, 1960.

Cereghino, J.J., and Dow, R.S.: Effect of cobalt applied to the cerebellum on cobalt experimental epilepsy in the cat. *Epilepsia, 11:*413-421, 1970.

Chafetz, M.E. and Cadilhac, J.: A new procedure for a study of barbiturate effect and evoked potentials in the EEG. *Electroencephalogr Clin Neurophysiol, 6:*565, 1954.

Chain, E.B.: Recent studies on carbohydrate metabolism. *Br Med J, 2:*709, 1959.

Chain, E. and Duthie, E.S.: Myclocytic enzyme in testis extracts. *Nature* (Lond), *144:*977, 1939.

Chain, E. and Duthie, E.S.: Identity of hyaluronidase and spreading factor. *Br J Exp Path, 21:*324, 1940.

Chang, H.T.: Similarity in action between curare and strychnine on cortical neurons. *J Neurophysiol, 16:*221, 1953.

Chapman, W.P., Livingston, K.E. and Poppen, J.L.: Effect upon blood pressure of electrical stimulation of tips of temporal lobes in man. *J Neurophysiol, 13:*65, 1950.

Charatan, F.B.E.: An evaluation of chlorpromazine (Largactil) in psychiatry. *J Ment Sci, 100:*882, 1954.

Charcot, I.N.: *Klinische Vorträge über Krankheiten des Nervensystems.* 13: Vorlesung: Hysteroepilepsie. Stuttgart 1874, übers. von Fetzer.

Charman, L.F. and Wolff, H.G.: Proteolytic enzymes in cerebrospinal fluid. Capacity of incubated mixtures of cerebrospinal fluid and plasma to form vasodilator substances that contract the isolated rat uterus. *Arch Int Med, 103:*86, 1959.

Charonnat, R., Lechat, P. and Chareton, J.: Recherches sur le choc provoqué par les injections intravéineuses de Vitamine B_1. *Ann Pharm Franc, 11:*17, 1953a.

Charonnat, R., Lechat, P. and Chareton, J.: Etude clinique de l'origine du choc thiaminique. *Ann Pharm Franc, 11:*26, 1953b.

Charonnat, R., Lechat, P. and Chareton, J.: Recherches biologiques sur la nature du choc thiaminique. *Ann Pharm Franc, 11:*735, 1953c.

Charonnat, R., Lechat, P. and Chareton, J.: Etude du choc provoqué par injection intravéineuse de Chlorhydrate de Thiamine. *Acta Vitamin* (Milano), *131:*91, 1953d.

Charonnat, R., Lechat, P. and Chareton, J.: Passage d' un convulsivant dans la série de la thiamine. *Thérapie, 11:*261, 1956.

Charonnat, R., Lechat, P. and Chareton, J.: Sur les propriétés pharmacodynamiques d'un dérivé thiazolique. 2ème note, Toxicité. *Thérapie, 12:*954, 1957b.

Charonnat, R., Lechat, P. and Chareton, J.: Sur les propriétés pharmacodynamiques d'un dérivé thiazolique. 3ème note: Action sur le système nerveux central. *Thérapie, 13:*1, 1958.

Chatfield, P.O. and Dempsey, E.W.: Some effects of prostigmine and acetylcholine on cortical potentials. *Am J Physiol, 135:*633, 1942.

Chen, G., Ensor, C.R., and Bohner, B.: A facilitation action of reserpine on the central nervous system. *Proc Soc Exp Biol, 86:*507, 1954.

Cheraskin, E. and Ringsdorf, J.R.: Epilepsy and the cortisone-glucose-tolerance test. *Lancet, 83:*248-275, 1963.

Chevrie, J.J., and Aicardi, J.: Childhood epileptic encephalopathy with slow spike-wave. *Epilepsia, 13:*259-271 1972.

Chirigos, M., Greengard, P. and Udenfriend, S.: Uptake of tyrosine by rat brain. *J Biol Chem, 235:*2057, 1960.

Chow, K.L.: A retrograde cell degeneration study of the cortical projection field of the pulvinar in the monkey. *J Comp Neurol, 93:*313, 1950.

Chowdhury, A.K., Skinner, A., Spector, R.G. and Yap, S.L.: Effect of chlorpromazine on glucose and nucleotide metabolism in mouse brain. *Br J Pharmacol, 33:*218, 1968.

Christ, W., Coper, H., and Schmidt, D.: On the mode of action of nicotinic acid selenoamine (some pharmacological and biochemical findings). *Naunyn-Schmiedebergs Arch Pharmak,* Suppl. Vol. *270,* R 19, 1971.

Christ, W., Schmidt, D., and Coper, H.: Comparison of Thio-$NADP^+$ and Seleno-$NADP^+$ in $NADP^+$-Dependent Oxidoreductases. *Hoppe-Seyler's Z Physiol Chem, 351:*427-434, 1970a.

Christ, W., Schmidt, D., and Coper, H.: Versuche zur enzymatischen Dephosphorylisierung von NADP-Analogen durch die alkalische Phosphatase aus Kälberdarm. *Hoppe-Selyer's Z Physiol Chem, 351:*803-808, 1970b.

Christ, W., Schmidt, D., and Coper, H.: Gel filtration behaviour of sulphur and selenium-containing nicotinamide-analogues on sephadex G-25. *J Chromatog, 51:*537-538, 1970c.

Christian, W.: EEG Befund bei einem Fall von epileptischer Halluzinose. *Dtsch Z Nervenheilkd, 176:*693, 1957.

Christian, W.: Bioelektrische Charateristik tagesperiodisch gebundener Verlaufsformen epileptischer Erkrankungen. *Dtsch Z Nervenheilkd, 181:*413, 1960.

Christian, W.: Schlaf-Wach-Periodik bei Schlaf-und Aufwachepilepsien. *Nervenarzt, 32:* 438, 1961.

Christian, W.: EEG Veränderungen bei der psychomotorischen Epilepsie. *Dtsch Z Nervenheilkd, 183:*218, 1962.

Christian, W.: *Klinische Elektroencephalographie.* Stuttgart, Thieme, 1968a.

Christian, W.: Pathogenese und Ätiologie der Epilepsien. *Hippokrates, 39:*157, 1968b.

Christian, W. and Hallen, O.: Über Ausolösung und Provokation epileptischer Anfälle durch Aneuxol-(Aminophenazon-) Injektion. *Nervenarzt, 28:*160, 1957.

Chusid, J.G., and Kopeloff, L.M.: Use of chronic irritative foci in laboratory evaluation of antiepileptic drugs. *Epilepsia, 10:*239-262, 1969.

Cicardo, V.H.: Physico-chemical mechanisms. *J Nerv Ment Dis, 101:*527, 1945.

Civilko, V.S.: *Pathoanatomical studies of the brain in experimental seizures.* (Russ) Moscow, Medgiz, 1947.

Clark, C.T., Weisbach, H. and Udenfriend, S.: 5-hydroxytryptophan decarboxylase – preparation and properties. *J Biol Chem, 210:*139, 1954.

Clark, W.G.: Electrophysiological correlates of chlordiazepoxide. *Dis Nerv Syst, 22:*16, 1961.

Claude, H. and Baruk, H.: Les crises de catalepsie. Leur diagnostic avec le sommeil pathologique. Leurs rapports avec l'hysterie et al catatonie. *Encéphale 23:*373, 1928.

Clausen, J.: The beta-lipoprotein of cerebrospinal fluid. *Acta Neurol Scand, 42:*153, 1966.

Clemente, C.H. and Holst, E.A.: Pathological changes in neurons, neuralgia and blood-brain barrier induced by X-irradiation of heads of monkeys. *Arch Neurol Psychiat* (Chic), *71:*66, 1954.

Cochrane, W.A.: Idiopathic hypoglycemia and leucine sensitivity. *Metabolism, 9:*386, 1960.

Cochrane, W.A., Payne, W.W., Simpkiss, M.J. and Woolf, I.: Familial hypoglycemia praecipitated by amino acid. *J Clin Invest, 35:*411, 1956.

Coggeshall, R.E. and MacLean, P.D.: Hippocampal lesion following administration of 3-acetypyridine. *Proc Soc Exp Biol, 98:*687, 1958.

Cohen, N.H., McAuliffe, M. and Aird, R.B.: "Startle" epilepsy treated with chlordiaze-poxide (Librium). *Dis Nerv Syst, 22:*20, 1961.

Colfer, H.F. and Essex, H.E.: Distribution of total electrolyte potassium and sodium in cerebral cortex in relation to experimental convulsions. *Am J Physiol, 150:*27, 1947.

Collens, W.S. and Banovitch, M.M.: Insulin resistance; report of an unusual case with requirements up to 7840 units in 24 hours. *Metabolism, 4:*355, 1955.

Collier, G. and Martin, A.: Les effets secondairs du trofanil. Revue générale à propos de trois cas de polynévrite des membres inférieurs. *Ann Med Psychol* (Paris), *118:* 719, 1960.

Collins, W.F. and O'Leary, J.L.: Study of somatic evoked response of midbrain reticular substance. *Electroencephalogr Clin Neurophysiol, 6:*619, 1954.

Colombati, S. and Canestrari, R.: L'azione tranquillante di un nuovo farmaco neurolet-tico. *Minerva Med* (Torino), *47:*2175, 1956.

Conrad, K.: Aphasie, Agnosie, Apraxie. *Fortschr Neurol Psychiat, 19:*291, 1951.

Conrad, K., Domanowsky, K. and Wieser, S.: Über extrapyramidale Anfallszustände bei Behandlung mit Phenothiazinen. *Fortschr Neurol Psychiatr, 24:*505, 1956.

Conrad, K. and Ule, G.: Ein Fall von Korsakow-Psychose mit anatomischen Befund und klinischen Betrachtungen. *Dtsch Z Nervenheilkd, 165:*430, 1951.

Contini, M.: Ricerche sulla protidemia nella demenza precoce. *Rass Stud Psichiatr, 25:* 223, 1936a.

Contini, M.: I protidiplasmatici nell' epilessia e lor variazioni in rapporto all' acceso. *Rass Stud Psichiatr, 25:*813, 1936b.

Coombs, J.S., Eccles, J.C. and Fatt, P.: Excitatory synaptic action in motoneurons. *J Physiol* (Lond), *130:*374, 1955.

Cooper, J.: The role of ascorbic acid in the oxidation of trytophane to 5-hydroxytryptophane. *Ann NY Acad Sci, 92:*208, 1961.

Cooper, J. and Melcer, I.: Enzymic oxidation of trytophan in the biosynthesis of serotonine. *J Pharmacol Exp Ther, 132:*265, 1961.

Cooper, J.R., Roth, R.H. and Kini, M.N.: Biochemical and physiological function of thiamine in nervous tissue. *Nature, 199:*609, 1963.

Copelman, L.-S.: Etudes et recherches au sujet de l'action cholenergique de la folliculine, de l'influence épileptogène de l'acéthylcholine et du rôle favorable des androgènes dans le traitement de l'épilepsie ovarienne. *Rev Path Gén, 63:*515-519, 1963.

Coper, H.: Der Gehalt an NAD, NADP und Nicotinsäureamid im Gehirn von Ratten nach Einwirkung zentral wirksamer Pharmaka. *Arch Exp Path Pharmakol, 224:*420, 1963.

Coper, H.: Stoffwechselstörungen durch Antimetaboliten des Nicotinamids. In v. Kress Blum (Eds.): *B-Vitamine.* Stuttgart, Schattauer, 1966.

Coper, H.: Disturbances in pyridine nucleotide metabolism of the central nervous system caused by nicotinamide antimetabolites. *Biochem J, 106:*7, 1967.

Coper, H.: Pharmakologische Aspekte der Therapieresistenz. Möglichkeiten der pathologischen Erregungsausbreitung und der medikametösen Erregungsbegrenzung im ZNS. In Kruse, Rolf, (Ed.) *Epilepsie. Therapie-Indikationen. Neue Antiepileptika. Therapie-Resistenz.* Georg Thieme Verlag, Stuttgart, pp. 87-93, 1971.

Coper, H., Deyhle, G., Fähndrich, Ch., Fähndrich, E., Rosenberg, L., Strauss, S., (in cooper. with), Blum, A. and Dufour H.: Excretion of vanillyli- mandelic acid, homovanillic acid, N-Methyl-Nicotinamide, and N-Methyl-2-Pyridone-5-Carboxamide in urine of voluntary test persons and psychiatric patients before and after administration of methionine. *Pharmakopsychiat, 5:*177-187, 1972.

Coper, H., Deyhle, G. v. Herrath, D. and Veit, J.: Zum Mechanismus der Schlafverlängernden Wirkung verschiedener Pharmaka. *Arch Exp Path Pharmakol, 260:*366, 1968.

Coper, H., Hadass, H. and Lison, H.: Untersuchungen zum. Mechanismus zentralnervöser Funktionsstörungen durch 6-Aminonicotinaid. *Arch Exp Path Pharmakol, 255:*97, 1966.

Coper, H. and Herken, H.: Schädigung des Zentralnervensystems durch Antimetaboliten des Nikotinsäureamids. *Dtsch Med Wochenschr, 88:*2025, 1963.

Coper, H., v. Herrath, D. and Veit, J.: On the mechanism of the sleep prolonging effect of antimetabolites of nicotinamide. *Arch Exp Path Pharmakol, 259:*161, 1968.

Coper, H., Lison, H., Rommelspacher, H., Schulze, G., and Strauss, S.: The influence of adrenergic receptor-blocking agents, Amphetamine, and 6-Aminonicotinamide on thermoregulation. *Naunyn-Schmiedebergs Arch Pharmak, 270:*378-391, 1971.

Coper, H., and Selbach, H.: Zur Wirkungsweise von Antiepileptika. *Therapiewoche, 20:* 16, 657, 1970.

Coppen, A.: Biochemistry of affective disorders. *Proc. 4th World Congr. Psychiatr.* 1966, Part 1, Amsterdam, Excerpta Med. p. 506, 1967.

Cordeau, J.P., Beaulness, A., Laurin, C. and Moreau, A.: EEG and behavioral changes following micro injections of acetylcholine and adrenaline in the brain stem of cats *Arch Ital Biol, 101:*30, 1963.

Cori, T.G. and Cori, C.F.: Glucose-6-phosphatase of the liver in glycocen-storage disease. *J Biol Chem, 199*:661, 1952.
Cornforth, J.W.: Biosynthesis of fatty acids and cholesterol considered as a chemical process. *J Lipid Res, 1*:3, 1959.
Cornu, F.: Medikamentöser Schlaf mit paradoxem EEG. Schweiz. *Schweiz Arch Neurol Neurochir Psychiatr, 96*:164, 1965.
Corsellis, J.A.N.: The incidence of ammon's horn sclerosis. *Brain, 80*:193, 1957.
Costa, E. and Brodie, B.B.: Concepts of the neurochemical transducer as an organized molecular unit at sympathetic nerve endings. *Progr Brain Res,* New York, Elsevier, vol. VIII, 1964.
Costa, E., Gessa, G.L., Hirsch, C., Kuntzman, R. and Brodie, B.B.: On current status of serotonine as a brain neurohormone and in action of reserpinelike drugs. *Ann NY Acad Sci, 96*:118, 1962.
Costa-Foru, D.: Modificarile cuprului din creier, fiçat, rinichi, splina şi single determinate de accesul convulsiv experimental la şobolani. *Stud Cercet Neurol, 6*:125, 1961.
Coursin, D.B.: Convulsive seizures in infants with pyridoxine-deficient diet. *JAMA, 154*: 406, 1954.
Coursin, D.B.: Vitamin B_6 deficiency in infants. *JAMA, 154*:406, 1954.
Coursin, D.B.: Seizures in vitamin B_6 deficiency. In Roberts, E. (Ed.): *Inhibition in the Nervous System and Gamma-Aminobutyric Acid.* Oxford, Pergamon Press, pp. 294-301, 1960.
Courvoisier, S., Fournel, J., Ducrot, R., Kolsky, M. and Koltscheck, P.: Propriétés pharmacodynamiques du chlorhydrate de choloro-3 (diethylamino-3-propyl)-10 phenothiazine (4,560 RP). *Arch Int Pharmacodyn, 92*:305, 1953.
Cramer, H.: Die Pyridoxin-abhängigen Säuglingskrämpfe. *Dtsch Med Wochenschr, 85,* 1577, 1962.
Cramer, H.: Krampfanfälle im frühen Kindesalter und Vitamin B_6. In v. Kress, Blum (Eds.): *B-Vitamine.* Stuttgart, Schattauer, pp. 333-348, 1966.
Cravioto, R.O., Massieu, G. and Izquierdo, J.J.: Free amino acids in rat brain during insulin shock. *Proc Soc Exp Biol, 78*:856, 1951.
Creutzfeldt, O.: Der elektrisch ausgelöste Ammonshornkrampf und seine Ausbreitung in andere Hirnregionen. Diss. Freiburg/Br. 1953.
Creutzfeldt, O.: Die Kramfausbreitung im Temporallappen der Katze. Die Krampfentladungen des Ammonshorns und ihre Beziehungen zum übrigen Rhinencephalon und Isocortex. *Schweiz Arch Neurol Neuochir Psychiatr, 77*:163, 1956.
Creutzfeldt, O.: Neurophysiologische Grundlagen der elektrischen Reizung des Gehirns. *Neurochirurgia, 1*:38, 1958.
Creutzfeldt, O. and Meyer-Mickeleit, R.W.: Patterns of convulsive discharges of the hippocampus and their propagation. *Electroencephalogr Clin Neurophysiol, 3*:43, 1953.
Crighel, E. and Stoica, E.: Cercetari asupra focarului meascalinic sigmoidian. *Stud Cercet Neurol, 6*:547, 1961.
de Crinis, M.: Epilepsie. In Kraus, Brugsch (Eds.): *Spezielle Pathologie und Therapie innerer Krankheiten.* Nervenkrankheiten III. Berlin-Wien, Urban & Schwarzenberg vol. X, 3, 1924.
de Crinis, M.: Über die Beeinflussung des histologischen Bildes des Zentralnervensystems durch humorale Veränderungen. *Mschr Psychiatr Neurol, 58*:185, 1925.
Crocker, A.C. and Mays, V.B.: Sphingomyelin synthesis in Nieman-Pick disease. *Am J Clin Nutr, 9*:63, 1961.
Crossland, J.: The significance of brain acetylcholine. *J Ment Sci, 99*:247, 1953.

Crossland, J. and Mitchell, J.F.: Effect of electrical activity of cerebellum of a substance present in cerebral extracts. *J Physiol* (Lond), *132:*391, 1956.

Cumings, J.N.: Chemistry of disease of the central nervous system. Symposium. *Metabolism, 9:*219, 1960.

Cummins, J.E. and Hydén, H.: Adenosine triphosphate (ATP) levels and adenosine triphosphatases in neuron, glia and neuronal membranes of the vestibular nucleus. *Biochem Biophys Acta, 60:*271, 1962.

Curran, F.J.: A study of fifty cases of Bromide psychosis. *J Nerv Dis, 88:*163, 1938.

Curtis, H.J.: Intercortical connections of corpus callosum as indicated by evoked potentials. *J Neurophysiol, 3:*401, 1940a.

Curtis, H.J.: An analysis of cortical potentials mediated by the corpus callosum. *J Neurophysiol, 3:*414, 1940b.

Curtis, H.J. and Cole, K.S.: Membrane resting and action potentials from the squid giant axon. *J Cell Comp Physiol, 19:*135, 1942.

Cushing, H.: *Pituitary Body, Hypothalamus and Parasympathetic Nervous System.* Baltimore, Thomas, 1932.

Cvetkova, M.B.: Dynamics of protein metabolism in alcohol delirium. In *Obm Veshtch Psikhiat Zabol,* Moscow, Medgiz, pp. 200-204, 1960.

Dahlström, A. and Fuxe, K.: Evidence for the existence of monoamines containing neurons in the central nervous system. *Acta Physiol Scand, 62:*232, 1964.

Dalby, M.A.: Antiepileptic and psychotropic effect of carbamazepine (Tegretol) in the treatment of psychomotor epilepsy. *Epilepsia, 12:*325-334, 1971.

Dalby, M.A.: The anticonvulsant and psychotropic effect of Tegretol in the treatment of psychomotor epilepsy. Skand. epilept. arsmøde Helsingør, Denmark, 1972.

Dale, H.H.: Adventures in Physiology with Excursions Into Autopharmacology. London, F A. Chirchill Ltd., 1953.

Dalgliesh, C.E. and Dutton, R.W.: Biogenesis of 5-hydroxytryptophan. *Br J Cancer, 11:* 296, 1957.

Dam, Mogens: Number of Purkinje cells in patients with grand mal epilepsy treated with diphenylhydantoin. *Epilepsia, 11:*313-320, 1970.

Danielson, B.G., Bittar, E.E., Chen, S., and Tong, E.Y.: The effect of diphenylhydantoin on sodium efflux from single barnacle muscle fibres. *Life Sciences, X.,* Part I, pp. 437-443, 1971.

Dancis, J., Hutzler, J. and Levitz, M.: Metabolism of the white blood cells in maple-syrup urine disease. *Biochem Biophys Acta, 43:*342, 1960.

Dancis, J., Jansen, V., Hutzler, J. and Levitz, M.: The metabolism of leucine in tissue culture of skin fibroblasts of maple-syrup urine disease. *Biochem Biophys Acta, 77:* 523, 1963.

Danilenko, V.I.: *Zh Nevropatol Psikhiatr,* "Korsakoff" 9, 1954 cit. by: Krasilinovka, M.N.: Dysfunction of liver in schizophrenia (Russ). In *Obm Veshtch Psikhiat Zabol* Moscow, Medgiz, pp. 154-158, 1960.

Danillo, S.: The visual cortex—can it be explained as initial point of the epileptic seizure? *J Clin Forens Psychiatr Pathol, 2:*216, 1883 (Russ).

Danillo, S.: On the stimulation of the visual cortex. (Russ) *Vrač, 13:*88, 1889.

Das, N.N., Dasgupta, S.R. and Werner, G.: Changes of behavior and electroencephalogram in rhesus monkeys caused by chlorpromazine. *Arch Int Pharmacodyn, 99:*451, 1954.

Dasgupta, S.R., Killam, E.K. and Killam, K.F.: Drug action on rhinencephalic seizure activity in the cat. *J Pharmacol, 122:*16A, 1958.

David, J.: *L'épilepsie du Réveil.* (A propos de 100 observations). Thesis, Lyon, 1955.

Davidov, I.N.: Reflectorial Regulation of Blood Circulation in Experimental Epilepsy. (Russ) Diss, Swerdlovsk, 1950.

Davidson, G.M.: Concerning the causes of death in certain psychoses. *Am J Psychiatry, 91:*41, 1934.

Davies, E.W., McCulloch, W.W. and Roseman, E.: Rapid changes in the O_2 tension of cerebral cortex during induced convulsions. *Am J Psychiatry, 100:*805, 1944.

Davies, P.W. and Rémond, A.: Oxygen consumption of the cerebral cortex of the cat during metrazol convulsions. A. *Res Nerv Ment Dis Proc, 26:*205, 1947.

Davis, H. and Wallace, W.M.: Factors affecting changes produced in electroencephalogram by standardized hyperventilation. *Arch Neurol* (Chic), *47:*606, 1942.

Davis, P.W. and Brody, T.M.: Inhibition of NA+ K+–activated adenosine triphosphatase activity in rat brain by substituted phenothiazines. *Biochem Pharmacol, 15:* 703, 1966.

Davison, A.N.: Pyridoxal phosphate as coenzyme of diamine oxidase. *Biochem J, 64:* 546, 1956.

Dawson, J., Hullin, R.P. and Pool, A.: Variations in the blood levels of acetone and butane-2,3-diol in normal individuals and mental patients. *J Ment Sci, 100:*536, 1954.

Dawson, R.M.C.: Cerebral amino acids in fluoroacetate poisoned, anesthetized and hypoglycemic rats. *Biochem Biophys Acta, 11:*548, 1953.

Dawson, R.M.C. and Richter, D.: Effect of stimulation on the phosphate esters of brain. *Am J Physiol, 160:*203, 1950.

Dazzi, P. and Lugaresi, E.: Sullo "stato di piccolo male". *Riv Neuropsichiatr, 2:*144, 1956.

Decsi, L. and Méhes, J.: The action of tranquilizing drugs on brain metabolism. *Experientia, 14:*145, 1958.

Dekaban, A.S.: Plasma lipids in epileptic children treated with the high fat diet. *Arch Neurol* (Chic), *15:*177, 1966.

Delay, J., Verdeaux, G., Verdeaux, J., Mordret, M. and Quétin, A.M.: Contrôle EEG du traitement par le G 22355 (Tofranil). *Rev Neurol, 102:*345, 1960.

Delgado, J.M.R. and Mihailović, L.: Use of the intracerebral electrodes to evaluate drugs that act on the central nervous system. *Ann NY Acad Sci, 64:*644, 1956.

Dell, M.B., Dreyfus-Brisac, G.C. and Lairy-Bounes, C.: Le problème des complexes pointe-onde dans l' épilepsie. *Encéphale, 42:*353, 1953.

Dell, P., Bonvallet, M. and Hugelin, A.: Mechanisms of reticular deactivation. In *The Nature of Sleep.* London, Churchill, 1961.

Delmas, A.: Lobe ou complexe temporal. Considérations anatomiques et embryologiques sur le démembrement du lobe temporal. In Alajouanine, T.: *Les Grandes Activités du Lobe Temporal.* Paris. Masson & Cie, 1955.

Delorme, F., Froment, J.L. and Jouvet, M.: Suppression du sommeil par la P. Chlorométhamphétamine et la P. Chlorophényllalanine. *C R Soc Biol, 160:*2347, 1966.

Delorme, F., Jeannerod, M. and Jouvet, M.: Effets remarcable de la Réserpine sur l' activité phasique pontogéniculo-occipitale. *C R Soc Biol, 159:*900, 1965.

Delorme, F., Jouvet, M. and Riotte, M.: Conditions de déclenchement du sommeil paradoxal par les acides gras à chaine courte chez le chat pontique chronique. *C R Soc Biol, 160:*1457, 1966.

Dempsey, E.W. and Morison, R.S.: The electrical activity of a thalamo-cortical system. *Am J Physiol, 138:*283, 1942.

Denny-Brown, D.: Diseases of basal ganglia. Their relation to disorders of movement. *Lancet, 2:*1155, 1960.

Denys, W.J.: L'épilepsie clinique. *Acta Neurol Psychiatr belg, 63*:892, 1963.

Derdyshire, A.J., Rempel, B., Forbes, A. and Lampert, E.F.: The effects of anesthetics on action potentials in the cerebral cortex of the cat. *Am J Physiol, 116*:577, 1936.

Desani, G.: La reazione di Takata-Ara nelle malatie mentali. *Note psichiatr, 64*:115, 1935.

Dettbarn, W.D. and Stämpfli, R.: Die Wirkung von 2,4-Dinitrophenol auf das Membranpotential der markhaltigen Nervenfaser. *Helv Physiol Acta, 15*:25, 1957.

Dewar, A.J., Dow, R.C., and McQueen, J.K.: RNA and protein metabolism in cobalt-induced epileptogenig lesions in rat brain. *Epilepsia, 13*:552-560, 1972.

Diamant, E.J. and Guggenheim, K.: Electrolyte metabolism in pyridoxine, riboflavin and pathotenic acid-deficient rats. *Am J Physiol, 91*:108, 1957.

Dieke, S.H.: Thiosemicarbazid: A new toxic derivative of thiourea. *Proc Soc Exp Biol Med, 70*:688, 1949.

Diethelm, O.: On bromide intoxication. *J Nerv Dis, 71*:151, 1930.

Dimitrov, G.A. and Kolotilova, A.A.: Effect of chlorpromazine on respiration and oxidative phosphorylation of the mitochondria of the cerebral hemispheres of rats. (Russ) *Biokhimya, 32*:156, 1967.

Dingmann, W. and Sporn, M.B.: The penetration of proline and proline derivates into brain. *J Neurochem, 4*:148, 1959.

v. Ditfurth, H.: Zur Frage der sogenannten Epilepsiepsychosen. *Nervenarzt, 24*:348, 1953.

v. Ditfurth, H.: Zur Frage des Wirkungsmechanismus psychotroper Pharmaka, speziell des Tofranil. *Med Exp* (Basel), *2*:147, 1960.

Dobrynina, W.I.: Influence of Protein-Deficiency in Nutrition on the Chemical Compound and Certain Metabolism in Brain. (Experimental study). (Russ), Diss., Moscow, 1955.

Döring, G.: Zur Histologie und Pathogenese des tödlichen Insulinschocks. *Dtsch Z Nervenheilkd, 147*:217, 1938.

Dolenko, L.I.: *Collected Writings on the Problem of Schizophrenia-Therapy in Pathophysiological View*. (Russ), Charkov, Akademija Nauk, 1958.

Dolin, A.O.: Induced Epileptiform Seizure. *Theses of the 3rd Conference on Problems of Higher Nervous Function*. (Russ), Moscow, 1938.

Dolin, A.O.: Conditioned Reflectory Triggering and Suppression of Pathological States of the Organism. (Russ) . Diss., Moscow, Akademija Nauk, 1952.

Domino, E.F.: A pharmacological analysis of the functional relationship between the brain stem arousal and diffuse thalamic projection systems. *J Pharmacol, 115*:449, 1955.

Domino, E.F. and Ueki, S.: Differential effects of general anesthetics on spontaneous electrical activity of neocortical and rhinencephalic brain systems of the dog. *J Pharmacol, 127*:288, 1959.

Doose, H.: Verlaufsformen kindlicher Epilepsien. *Fortschr Neurol Psychiatr, 35*:148, 1967.

Doose, H. and Scheffner, D.: Über die Beziehung zwishcen Absencen, psychomotorischen und fokalen Anfällen. *Arch Psychiatr Z Neurol, 206*:504, 1965.

Dott, N.M.: In: Le Gros Clark, Beathie, Riddoch a. Dott (Eds.) *The Hypothalamus: Morphological, Functional, Clinical and Surgical Aspects*. Edinburg, Oliver & Boyd, 1938.

Dow, C.R., McQueen, J.K., and Townsend, H.R.A.: The production and detection of epileptogenic lesions in rat cerebral cortex. *Epilepsia, 13*:459-465, 1972.

Dresse, A.: Influence de 15 neuroleptiques (Butyrophenones et Phenothiazines) sur les variations de la teneur du cerveau en noradrenaline et l'activité du rat dans le test d'autostimulation. *Arch Int Pharmacodyn, 159:*353, 1966.

Dreyer, R.: Klinische Erfahrungen mit neueren antiepileptischen Mitteln. *Vortag zur Tagung d. Nord und Nordwestdeutschen Neurologen u. Psychiater,* Lübeck, Unpubl. Congr. Presentation, 1953.

Dreyer, R.: Erfahrungen mit Mylepsin in der Epilepsiebehandlung. *Dtsch Med Wochenschr, 81:*1681, 1956.

Dreyer, R.: Die Differentialtypologie des kleinen epileptischen Anfalls. *Fortschr. Neurol Psychiatr, 30:*289, 1962.

Dreyer, R.: Die Behandlung der Epilepsien im Erwachsenenalter. In Schulte, W. (Ed.): *Epilepsie und ihre Randgebie in Klinik und Praxis.* München, Lehmann, 1964.

Dreyer, R.: Erfahrungen mit Tegretal. *Nervenarzt, 36:*10, 1965.

Dreyer, R.: Zur Frage des Status epilepticus mit psychomotorischen Anfällen. *Nervenarzt, 36:*221, 1965.

Drooglever-Fortuyn, J.: Introduction à l'anatomie du rhinencéphale. *Acta Neurol Psychiat Belg, 56:*115, 1956.

Drury, K.K. and Farran-Ridge, C.: Some observations on the type of blood sugar curves found in different forms of insanity. *J Ment Sci, 71:*8, 1925.

Duiju, van, H., and Visser, S.L.: The action of some anticonvulsant drugs on cobalt-induced epilepsy and on the begemide threshold in alert cats. *Epilepsia, 13:*409-420, 1927.

Dumermuth, G.: Photosensible Epilepsie und Television. *Schweiz Med Wochenschr, 91:* 1633, 1961.

Dunlop, C.W.: Effect of carbon dioxide on deep structures of temporal lobe of brain in the marsupial phalanger. *Am J Physiol, 190:*172, 1957a.

Dunlop, C.W.: Effect of carbon dioxide in the rhinencephalon on the marsupial phalanger. *Am J Physiol, 191:*200, 1957b.

Duran-Reynals, F. Exaltation de l'activité du virus vaccinal par les extraits de certains organs. *C R Soc Biol* (Paris), *99:*6, 1928.

Duran-Reynals, F.: The effect of extracts of certain organs from normal and immunized animals on the infecting power of vaccine virus. *J Exp Med, 50:*327, 1929.

de Duve, C., Pressmann, B.C., Gianetto, R. Wattiaux, R. and Applemans, F.: Tissue fractionation studies. VI. Intracellular distribution patterns of enzymes in rat liver tissue. *Biochem J, 60:*604, 1955.

Earle, K.M., Baldwin, M. and Penfield, W.: Incisural sclerosis and temporal lobe seizure produced by hippocampal herniation at birth. *Arch Neurol, 69:*27, 1953.

Ebert, A.G. and Hess, S.M.: The distribution and metabolism of fluphenazine enanthate. *J Pharmacol Exp Ther, 148:*412, 1965.

Eccles, J.C.: *The Neurophysiological Basis of Mind: The Principles of Neurophysiology.* Pergamon Press, Oxford, 1953.

Eccles, J.C.: *The Neurophysiology of Nerve Cells.* Baltimore, Hopkins, 1957.

Eccles, J.C.: Der Mechanismus der postsynaptischen Hemmung. *Angew Chemie, 76:*674, 1964.

Eccles, J.C.: The control of neuronal activity by postsynaptic inhibitory action. *Proc. XXIIIrd. Congr. Physiol. Sci.* Tokyo, 1965.

Eccles, J.C., Katz, B. and Kuffler, S.W.: Nature of the "endplate potential" in curarized muscle. *J Neurophysiol, 4:*362, 1941.

Eccles, J.C., LLinas, R. and Sasaki, K.: Golgi cell inhibition in the cerebellar cortex. *Nature* (Lond), *204:*1265, 1964.

Eccles, R.M. and Lundberg, A.: Significance of supraspinal control of reflex actions by impulses in muscle afferents. *Experientia* (Basel), *14*:197, 1958.

Echlin, F.A.: Vasospasm and focal cerebral ischemia. *Arch Neurol Psychiatr, 47*:77, 1942.

Echlin, F.A. and McDonald, J.: The supersensitivity of chronically isolated cerebral cortex as a mechanism in focal epilepsy. *Trans Am Neurol Ass, 79*:75, 1954.

v. Economo, G.: *Zellaufbau der Grosshirnrinde.* Wien, Springer, 1927.

Edström, J.E.: Quantitative determination of ribonucleic acid from individual nerve cells. *Biochem Biophys Acta, 11*:301, 1953.

Edström, J.E.: Extraction hydrolysis and electrophoretic analysis of ribonucleic acid (RNA) from microscopic tissue units (microphoresis). *J Biophys Biochem Cytol, 8*: 39, 1960.

Eeg-Olofsson, R.: Über Plasmaeiveiss bei Epilepsie. Acta *Med Scand* (Stockh), *103*-111, 1940.

Egyhazi, N. and Hydén, H.: Experimentally induced changes in the base composition of the ribonucleic acids isolated nerve cells and their oligodendroglial cells. *J Biophys Biochem Cytol, 10*:403, 1961.

Ehlers, G.: Über die Anwendbarkeit von Cosaldon bei der Behandlung des zerebralsklerotischen Parkinsonismus. *Munch Med Wochenschr, 101*:1355, 1959.

Ehringer, H. and Hornykiewicz, O.: Verteilung von Noradrenalin und Dopamin (3-Hydroxytryptamin) in Gehirn des Menschen und ihr Verhalten bei Erkrankungen des extrapyramidalen Systems. *Klin Wochenschr, 38*:1236, 1960.

Eichhorn, O.: Die Bedeutung der Gefässpermeabilität im Gehirn. *Wien Klin Wochenschr, 237*:1956.

Eidelberg, E.: Hippocampal "dendritic" responses in rabbits. *J Neurophysiol, 24*:521, 1961.

Eidelberg, E., White, J.C. and Brazier, M.A.B.: The hippocampal arousal pattern in rabbits. *Exp Neurol, 1*:483, 1959.

Elian, M.: The long-term oral use of valium (Diazepam) in epilepsy. *Epilepsia, 10*:487-493, 1969.

Elian, M.: Aussichten der Epilepsiebehandlung mit Carbamazepin. *Harefuah, 82* (4), 200, 1972.

Elliott, K.A.C.: Chemical studies in relation to convulsive conditions. In Elliott, Page, Quastel (Eds.): *Neurochemistry.* Springfield, Thomas 1955.

Elliott, K.A.C. and van Gelder, N.M.: Occlusion and metabolism of gamma-aminobutyric acid by brain tissue. *J Neurochem, 3*:28, 1958.

Elliott, K.A.C. and Heller, I.H.: Metabolism of neurons and glia. *Metabol. Nerv. System.* London-New York, Pergamon Press, p. 286, 1957.

Elliott, K.A.C. and Henderson, N.: Metabolism of brain tissue slices and suspensions from various mammals. *J Neurophysiol, 11*:485, 1948.

Elliott, K.A.C. and Jasper, H.H.: Gamma-aminobutyric acid. *Physiol Rev, 39*:383, 1959.

Elliott, K.A.C., Swank, R.L. and Henderson, N.: Effect of anesthetic on acetylcholine content of brain. *Am J Physiol, 162*:469, 1950.

Elmadijan, F., Lamson, E.T. and Neri, R.: Excretion of adrenaline in human subjects. *J Clin Endocrinol Metab, 16*:222, 1956.

Embden, G. and Baldes, K.: Über den Aufbau des Phenylalanins im tierischen Organismus. *Biochem Z, 55*:301, 1913.

Empey, L.W., Patterson, H.A. and McQuarrie, I.: The pH and CO_2 content of cerebrospinal fluid in epilepsy. *Proc Soc Exp Biol Med, 29*:1003, 1932.

Engel, R.: Die praktische Bedeutung des Wasserhaushalts in der Epilepsie, zugleich ein Beitrag zur Permeabilitätstheorie. *Nervenarzt, 6*:120, 1933.

Ephimovitch, N.G.: Theses—Proceedings to the conference on problems of metabolism in patients with psychic disorders. (Russ), Moscow, Medgiz, 1958.

Epstein, A.A.: Acid-base reciprocal effect in brain tissue. (Russ) unpublished presentations Univer. of Leningrad, Leningrad, 1947.

Erickson, T.C.: Spread of the epileptic discharge. An experimental study of the after discharge induced by electrical stimulation of the cerebral cortex. *Arch Neurol Psychiatr* (Chic), *43*:429, 1940.

Erspamer, V.: Observations on the metabolism of endogenous 5-hydroxpamine (enteramine) in the rat. *Experientia, 10*:471, 1954.

Erspamer, V., Glasser, A., Pasini, C. and Stoppani, G.: *In vitro* decarboxylation of tryptophan by mammalian decarboxylase. *Nature* (Lond), *189*:483, 1961.

Ervin, F.A., Epstein, W. and King, H.E.: Behavior of epileptic and nonepileptic patients with "temporal spikes". *Arch Neurol Psychiatr, 74*:488, 1956.

Espinosa, J.C.: Tégrétol dans les troubles du caractère et du comportement chez les enfants et adolescents épileptiques. *Méd Campagne, 7, 7*:26-39, 1972.

Esquiriol, F.E.D.: *Maladies Mentales.* 1838; cit. by Adrin-Delteil, P.: *L'épilepsie Psychique* Bern, Huber, 1898.

Essig, C.F.: Withdrawal convulsions in dogs following chronic meprobamate intoxication. *Arch Neurol Psychiatr, 80*:649, 1958.

Essig, C.R. and Ainslie, J.D.: Addiction to meprobamate. *JAMA, 164*:1382, 1957.

Etling, N.: Action des hypnotiques sur le métabolisme hydrocarboné du cerveau. III. Action des hypnotiques sur la dégradation de l'héxose monophosphate. *Bull Soc Chim Biol, 36*:567, 1954.

v. Euler, H., Günther, G. and Vestin, R.: Glycolyse und Phosphataustausch in zellfreien Hirnextrakten normaler Säugetiere. *Hoppe Seylers Z Physiol Chem, 240*:265, 1963.

v. Euler, U.S. and Gaddum, J.H.: Unidentified depressor substance in certain tissue extracts. *J Physiol* (Lond), *72*:74, 1931.

v. Euler, U.S. and Hillarp, N.A.: Evidence of presence of noradrenaline in submicroscopic structures of adrenergic axons. *Nature* (Lond), *177*:44, 1956.

Evarts, E.V.: A review of the neurophysiological effects of lysergic acid diethylamide (LSD) and other psychomimetic agents. *Ann NY Acad Sci, 66*:479, 1957.

Ewalt, J.R. and Bruce, E.I.: Newer concepts of schizophrenia. *Texas Rep Biol Med, 6*:97, 1948.

Fabisch, W.: The effect of chlorpromazine on the electroencephalogram of epileptic patients. *J Neurol Neurosurg Psychiatr, 20*:185, 1957.

Faddeev, V.K.: The influence of phenamine on the action of higher parts of CNS in animals (albino rats). (Russ) *Zh Vyssh Nerv Deiat, 1*:165, 1951.

Faerø, O., Kastrup, K.W., Nielsen, E.L., Melchiar, J.C., and Thron, J.: Successive Prophylaxis of Febrile Convulsions with Phenobarbital. Epilepsia, *13*:279-285 (1972).

Falconer, M.A.: Die chirurgische Behandlung der Temporallappenepilepsie. *Vortrag z. Tagung d. Int. Liga gegen Epilepsie,* Dtsch, Sektion, 1965.

Falconer, M.A.: Genetic and Related Aetiological Factors in Temporal Lobe Epilepsy. A Review. Epilepsia, *12*:13-31 (1971).

Falconer, M.A., Glasgow, G.L. and Cole, D.S.: Sensory disturbances occurring in sciatica due to intervertebral disc potusions: some observations on the fifth lumbar and first sacral dermatomes. *J Neurol, 10*:72, 1947.

Falconer, M.A., Hill, D., Meyer, A., Mitchell, W. and Pond, O.A.: Treatment of temporal lobe epilepsy temporal lobectomy. *Lancet, 219*:827, 1955.

Falconer, M.A., McFarlan, A.M. and Russel, D.S.: Experimental brain abscesses in rabbit. *Br J Surg, 30*:245, 1943.

Falconer, M.A., McGeorge, M. and Begg, A.C.: Surgery of lumbar intervertebral disc protusion. A study of principles and results based upon one hundred consecutive cases submitted to operation. *Br J Surg, 35:*225, 1948.

Falconer, M.A., McGeorge, M. and Begg, A.C.: Observations on the cause and mechanism of symptom production in sciatica and low-back pain. *J Neurol, 11:*13, 1948.

Falconer, M.A., Meyer, A. and Beck, E.: Pathological findings in temporal lobe epilepsy. *J Neur NS, 17:*276, 1954.

Falconer, M.A., Pond, D.A., Meyer, A. and Woolf, A.L.: Temporal lobe epilepsy with personality and behavior disorders caused by an unusual calcifying lesion. *J Neurol Neurosurg Psychiatry, 16:*234, 1953.

Farb, H.H.: Experience with librium in clinical psychiatry. *Dis Nerv Syst, 21:*27, 1960.

Farstad, M.: Determination of fatty acids in cerebrospinal fluid: III Quantitative and qualitative studies on some neurological and psychiatric disorders. *Scand J Clin Lab Invest, 16:*554, 1964.

Fatt, P. and Katz, B.: An analysis of the end-plate potential recorded with an intracellular electrode. *J Physiol* (Lond), *115:*320, 1951.

Fattovich, G.: Osservazioni capillaroscopiche negli epilettici. *Note Riv Psichiatr, 60:*47, 1931.

Fattovich, G.: Ricerche sulla funzionalita epatica negli ammalati di mente. *Note Riv Psichiatr, 62:*431, 1933.

Fattovich, G.: Ricerche sulle siero-globuline nei malati di mente. *Riv Sper freniatr, 58:*150, 1934.

Faure, J., Vincent, D. and Bensch, C.: Etude électroencéphalographique et neurophysiologique des effets du Ro 4-5360 chez le lapin. *Rev Neurol, 112:*275, 1965.

Fay, T.: Some factors in the "mechanical theory of epilepsy" with special reference to the influence of fluid and its control in the treatment of certain cases. *Am J Psychiatry, 8:*783, 1929.

Feath, W.H., Warner, W.A. and Walker, A.E.: Electroencephalographic changes in experimental psychomotor seizures in the monkey. *Electroencephalogr Clin Neurophysiol, 6:*339, 1954.

Fedorov, I.I.: *On the Central Control of Metabolism.* (Carbohydrate metabolism and oxydation reduction processes). Experimental studies. (Russ) Leningrad, WMMA, 1941.

Feindel, W. and Gloor, P.: Comparison of electrographic effects of stimulation of the amygdala and brain stem reticular formation in cats. *Electroencephalogr Clin Neurophysiol, 6:*389, 1954.

Feldberg, W.: The role of acetylcholine in the central nervous system. *Brit Med Bull, 6:*312, 1950.

Feldberg, W.: Some aspects in pharmacology of central synaptic transmission. *Arch Int Physiol, 59:*544, 1951.

Feldberg, W.: Acetylcholine. In Richter, D. (Ed.): *Metabolism of the Nervous System.* New York, Pergamon Press, 1957.

Feldberg, W., Fessard, A. and Nachmansohn, D.: The cholinergic nature of the nervous supply to the electrical organ of torpedo (Torpedo marmorata). *J Physiol (Lond), 97:*3P 1940.

Feldmann, S.: Electrical Activity of the Brain following Cerebral Microninfusion of Cortisol. Epilepsia, *12:*249-262 (1971).

Feldmann, S. and Porter, R.W.: Long latency responses evoked in the anterior brain stem under pentobarbital anesthesia. *Electroencephalogr Clin Neurophysiol, 12:*111, 1960.

Feldmann, S., van der Heyde, C.S. and Porter, R.W.: Evoked potentials in the hypothalamus. *Am J Physiol, 196:*1163, 1959.

Fellman, J.H. and Devlin, M.K.: Concentration and hydroxylation of free phenylalanine in adrenal glands. *Biochem Biophys Acta, 28:*328, 1958.

Felstein, I.L.: The value of cosaldon in cerebral sclerosis. *Clin Practice, 17:*448, 1963.

Ferdmann, D.L.: Annual *"Advances in Biochemistry"*. Vol. 1 1950, pp. 216 (Russ); cit. by Lando, L.I. and Krupenina, L.B.: Comparative data of the ammonia blood content of schizophrenic and epileptic patients. In *Problems of Schizophrenia.* Moscow, Medgiz, 1962.

Ferdmann, D.L. and Feinschmidt, O.J.: On the biochemistry of hibernators. *Notes of the ukr biochem Institute, 5:*20, 1932 (Russ).

Féré, C.: *Les épilepsies et les épileptiques.* Paris, Alcan, 1890. Transl. by P. Ebers, Leipzig, Engelmann, 1896.

Ferrari, V., Campagnari, F. and Guida, A.: Oligofrenia fenilpiruvica: nuovi reperti chimico-patologici. *Minerva Med, 46:*119, 1955.

Ferse, H.: Behandlung der Cerebralsklerose. Ärztl, *Praxis, 8:*32, 1956.

Fessard, A. and Posternak, J.: Les mécanismes élémentaires de la transmission synptique. *J Physiol* (Paris), *42:*319, 1950.

Feuchtwanger, E.: Anfallsäquivalente und psychische Dauerveränderungen bei der Epilepsie nach Hirnverletzung. *Nervenarzt, 3:*577, 1930.

Fieser, L.F. and Fieser, M.: *Organische Chemie.* 2nd Edit. Weinheim/Bergstr. Verlag, Chemie, 1968.

Fincle, L. and Reyna, L.J.: cit. by Sourkes, T.L.: *Biochemistry of Mental Disease.* New York, Horecker, p. 55, 1962.

Fine, E.A., Kunkel, A.M. and Will, J.H.: *Fed Proc, 9:*272, 1950; cit. by. Kanig, K.: *Die Bedeutung der B-Vitamine für das Nervensystem.* Wiss. Berichte, E. Merck, Darmstadt, 1968.

Fischer, R.: Factors involved in drug-produced model psychoses. *J Ment Sci, 100:*623, 1954.

Fischer, R., Zeman, W. and Irons, I.: Differential dye uptake in excited and non excited nervous tissue after treatment with pepsin and neotetrazolium chloride. *J Histochem Cytochem, 9:*103, 1961.

Fischer, S.: Gassttoffwechselveränderungen bie Schizophrenen, III. Mitt. *Z Neurol, 147:* 109, 1933.

Fisher, C., Ingram, W.P. and Ranson, S.W.: Relation of hypothalamicohypophyseal system to diabetes insipidus. *Arch Neurol Psychiatr, 34:*124, 1935.

Flack, B.: Cellular localization of monoamines. *Progr. Brain Res.* New York, Elsevier, vol. VIII, 1964.

Flanigan, S., Gabrieli, E.R. and Mac Lean P.D.: Cerebral changes revealed by radioautography with S35-labeled L-methionine. *Arch Neurol Psychiatr, 77:*588, 1957.

Fleck, U.: Über die Malaria- und Recurrensbehandlung der Paralyse. *Arch Psychiatr Nervenkr, 75:*562, 1925.

Fleck, U.: Über das Epileptoid und den epileptischen Charakter. *Arch Psychiatr Nervenkr, 102:*283, 1934.

Fleckenstein, A.: *Die periphere Schmerzauslösung und Schmerzschaltung.* Frankfurt, Steinkopff, 1950.

Fleischhauer, K.: Zur Chemoarchitektonik der Ammonsformation. *Nervenarzt, 30:*305, 1959.

Fleischhauer, K. and Horstmann, E.: Intracorticale Dithizonfärbung homologer Felder der Ammonsformationen von Säugern. *Z Zellforsch, 46:*598, 1957.

Flexner, L.B., Flexner, I.B., de la Haba, G. and Roberts, R.B.: Loss of memory as related to inhibition of cerebral protein synthesis. *J Neurochem, 12:*535, 1965.

Flink, E.B.: Magnesium deficiency syndrome in man. *JAMA, 160:*1406, 1956.

Flor-Henry, P.: Psychosis and temporal lobe epilepsy. *Epilepsia, 10:*363-395, 1969.

Flor-Henry, P.: Ictal and interictal psychiatric manifestations in epilepsy: Specific or non-specific ? A critical review of some of the evidence. *Epilepsia, 13:*773-783, 1972.

Fölling, A.: Über Ausscheidung von Phenylbenztraubensäure in den Harn als Stoffwechselanomalie in Verbindung mit Imbezilität. *Hoppe-Selyers Z Physiol Chem, 227:*169, 1934.

Foerster, O.: Die Pathogenese des epileptischen Krampfanfalls. *Dtsch Z Nervenheilk, 94:*15, 1926.

Foerster, O.: Motorische Felder und Bahnen. In Buhmke-Foerster (Eds.): *Hb. d. Neurologie.* Berlin, Springer, vol. VI, 1936.

Folch-Pi, J.: Brain cephalin mixture of phosphatides. Separation from it of phosphatidyl serine, phosphatidyl ethanolamine and fraction containing inositol phosphatide. *J Biol Chem, 146:*35, 1942.

Folch-Pi, J.: Complete fractionation of brain cephalin: isolation from it of phosphatidyl serine, phosphatidyl ethanolamine and diphosphoinositide. *J Biol Chem, 177:*487, 1949.

Folch-Pi, J. and Lees, M.J.: Proteolipids a new type of tissue lipoproteins. Their isolation from brain. *J Biol Chem, 191:*807, 1951.

Fomin, S.W.: Influence on the function of the acoustic and optic centres of the cortex in the dog by protolysis. *Notes of the Ukr Biochem Institute* (Russ), *3:*143, 1928.

Forbes, A. and Morison, B.R.: The cortical responses to sensory stimulation under deep barbiturate narcosis. *J Neurophysiol, 2:*112, 1939.

Forbes, H.S., Wolff, H.G. and Cobb, S.: The cerebral circulation. X. The action of histamine. *Am J Physiol, 89:*266, 1929.

Forster, F.M.: Action of acetylcholine on motor cortex. *Arch Neurol Psychiatr, 54:*391, 1945.

Fox, C.A.: Amygdalo-thalamic connections in macaca mulatta. *Anat Rec, 103:*121, 1949.

Fox, C.A. and Schmitz, J.T.: A marchi study of the distribution of the anterior comissure in the cat. *J Comp Neurol, 79:*297, 1943.

Fox, J.C. and German, W.I.: Observations following left (dominant) temporal lobectomy. Report of a case. *Arch Neurol, 33:*791, 1935.

Frain, M.M.: Preliminary report on Melleril in epilepsy. *Am J Psychiatry, 117:*547, 1960.

Frankel, S.I.: Dilantin sodium in treatment of epilepsy. *JAMA, 114:*1320, 1940.

French, J.D., Verzenao, M. and Magoun, H.W.: A neural basis of the anesthetic state. *Arch Neurol Psychiatr, 69:*519, 1953.

Frey, H.H. and Hahn, J.: Untersuchungen über die Bedeutung des durch Biotransformation gebildeten Phenobarbital für die antikonvulsive Wirkung von Primidon. *Arch Int Pharmacodyn, 128:*281, 1960.

Frid, P., Green, J.R., and Pupferberg, H.J.: Simultaneous determination of sulthiame and diphenylhydantoin serum levels by gas-liquid chromatography. *Epilepsia, 13:* 273-277, 1972.

Friede, R.L. and Knoller, M.: A quantitative mapping of acid phosphatase in the brain of the rhesus monkey. *J Neurochem, 12:*441, 1965.

Friedländer, W.J.: Electroencephalographic changes in acute brain stem vascular lesions. *Neurology* (Minneap), *9:*24, 1959.

Frigerio, L.: *Arch di Psych di Lombroso, 1*:305, 1899; cit. by Hallen, O.: Das Oral-Petit Mal. *Dtsch Z Nervenheilkd, 171*:236, 1954.

Frisch, F.: *Die Epilepsie*. Leipzig, Weidmann, 1937.

Frisch, F. and Fried, E.: Die Serumeiweisskörper bei Epilepsie. *Z Ges Exp Med, 56*:766, 1927.

Frohmann, C.E., Goodman, M. and Beckett, P.G.S.: The isolation of an active factor from serum of schizophrenic patients. *Ann NY Acad Sci, 96*:438, 1962.

Frolkis, W.W.: Über den Mechanismus des Krampfanfalls. (Russ.) *Vopr Fiziol, 5*:21, 1953.

Frolkis, W.W.: On the mechanism of circulation change in convulsive seizures. In *Problems of Clinical Neuropathol. a. Psychiat* (Russ). Kiev, Ukerainian Sci. Acad., pp. 334-356, vol. II, 1958.

Fumi, S.: La carbamazepina nel trattamento della epilessia e delle sue manifestazioni psichiche. *Gazzetta Medica Italiana, 131*:(1), 25-28, 1972.

Füngfeld, E.W.: Zur Frage der Megaphenprovokation bei der Elektroencephalographie. *Arch Psychiatr Nervenkr, 194*:517, 1956.

Füngfeld, E.W.: "Morbus Sacer". Ein Überblick vom Altertum bis zur Gegenwart. *Med Welt, 5*:258, 1966.

Füngfeld, E.W.: Zerebrale Krampfanfälle im Erwachsenenalter unter Piperazin-Kur. *Med Klin, 63*:137, 1968.

Funderburk, W.H., Finger, K.F., Drakontides, A.B. and Schneider, J.A.: EEG and biochemical findings with MAO inhibitors. *Ann NY Acad Sci, 96*:289, 1962.

Fuster, B., Castells, C. and Rodriguez, B.: Psychomotor attacks of subcortical origin. *Arch Neurol Psychiatr, 71*:466, 1954.

Gabay, S. and Harris, S.R.: Proc. 5th Internat. Congr. C.I.N.P., Washington, 1966, Internat. Congr. Ser. 129, pp. 1180-1183, Amsterdam, Excerpta Med. (in press) cit. by Kanig, K., *Arzneim Forsch, 19*:397, 1969.

Gabka, J.: Pathologie unde Therapie der Trigeminusneuralgie. *Z ärztl Fortbild, 50*:910, 1961.

Gaddum, J.H.: Beiträge zum Histaminproblem. *Acta Neurovegetativa* (Wien), *4*:268, 1952.

Gänshirt, H.: Das Elektroencephalogramm in Diagnose und Behandlung der Epilepsie. *Nervenarzt, 32*:262, 1961.

Gänshirt, H.: Die Behandlung der Epilepsie in der nervenärztlichen Sprechstunde. *Nervenarzt, 38*:429, 1967.

Gänshirt, H.: Konservative Therapie der Epilepsie bei Erwachsenen. Ärztl, *Praxis, 19*: 3108, 1967.

Gänshirt, H., Poeck, K., Schliep, H., Vetter, K. and Gänshirt, L.: Durchblutung und Sauerstoffversorgung des Gehirnes im Elektrokrampf bei Katze und Hund. *Arch Psychiatr Nervenkr, 198*:601, 1959.

Gänshirt, H. and Vetter, K.: Schlafelektroencephalogramm und Schlaf-Wachperiodik bei Epilepsien. *Nervenarzt, 32*:275, 1961.

Gaitonde, M.K., Dahl, D.R. and Elliott, K.A.C.: Entry of glucose carbon into amino acids of rat brain and liver *in vivo* after injection of uniformly ^{14}C-labelled glucose. *Biochem J, 94*:345, 1965.

Gaitonde, M.K. and Richter, D.: Metabolic activity of proteins of the brain. *Proc Roy Soc Biol, 145*:83, 1956.

Gal, E.M., Proczik, M. and Marshal, F.D.jr.: Hydroxylation of trytophan to 5-hydroxytryptophan by brain tissues *in vivo*. *Biochem Biophys Res Commun, 12*:39, 1963.

Gallenko, V.E.; Osberg, I.J. and Azbukina, V.D.: Aminazine in psychiatric clinic. (Russ.) *Zh Nevropatol Psikhiatr, 56:*162, 1956.
Gangloff, H. and Monnier, M.: The action of anticonvulsant drugs tested by electrical stimulation of the cortex, diencephalon and rhinencephalon in the unanesthetized rabbit. *Electroencephalogr Clin Neurophysiol, 9:*43, 1957a.
Gangloff, H. and Monnier, M.: Topische Wirkung des Phenobarbitals auf Cortex, Rhinencephalon, Nucleus caudatus, Thalamus und Substantia reticularis des Kaninchens. *Arch Exp Path Pharmakol, 231:*211, 1957b.
Gangloff, H. and Monnier, M.: Effect of phenobarbital on evoked activity following stimulation of cortical and subcortical structures in the unanesthetized rabbit. *J Pharmacol, 122:*23A, 1958.
Ganner, H. and Stiefler, G.: Zur Symptomatologie der Schläfenlappentumoren. *Arch Psychiatr, 101:*399, 1934.
Garsche, R. and Schönfelder, T.: Zur Klinik der psychomotorischen Epilepsie im Kindesalter. *Arch Kinderh, 184:*241, 1954.
Gastager, H., Haas, J. and Weinkamer, E.: Erfahrungsbericht über die Anwendung von Ditraneurin in der Psychiatrie. *Wein Klin Wochenschr, 76:*639, 1964.
Gastaut, H.: Corrélations entre le système nerveux végétativ et le système de la vie de relation dans le rhinecéphale. *J Physiol* (Paris), *44:*431, 1952.
Gastaut, H.: So called "psychomotor" and "temporal" epilepsy. *Epilepsia* (Boston), *2:* 59, 1953.
Gastaut, H.: *The Epilepsy.* Springfield, Thomas, 1954.
Gastaut, H.: Etat actuel des connaissances sur l' anatomie pathologique des épilepsies. *Acta Neurol Psychiatr Belg, 56:*5, 1956.
Gastaut, H.: Sémiologie et physiopathogémie des crises épileptiques généralisées. *Helv med Acta, 30:*319, 1963.
Gastaut, H.: Comment on petit mal variant revisited. *Epilepsia, 12:*97-99, 1971.
Gastaut, H., Bernard, R. and Giraud, P.: Les convulsions de l'enfance, étude clinique et pathogémique. *Pédiatrie, 8:*591, 1953.
Gastaut, H., Courjon, J., Poire, R., and Weber, M.: Treatment of status epilepticus with a new benzodiazepine, more active than diazepam. *Epilepsia, 12:*197-214, 1971.
Gastaut, H. and Gastaut, Y.: Corrélations électroencépalographiques et clinques à propos de 100 cas d'épilepsie dite "psychomotrice" avec foyers sur la région temporale du scalp. *Rev Oto-Neuro-Ophtal, 23:*257, 1951.
Gastaut, H., Morin, G. and Lesèvre, N.: Etude du comportement des épileptiques psyco-moteurs dans l'intervalle de leurs crises. Les troubles de l'activité globale et de la sociabilité. *Ann Med Psychol* (Paris), *113:*1, 1955.
Gastaut, H., Naquet, R. and Roger, A.: Etude des postdécharges électriques provoquées par stimulation du complexe nucléaire amygdalien chez le chat. *Rev Neurol, 87:*224, 1952.
Gastaut, H., Naquet, R. Vigouroux, R. and Corriol, J.: Provocation de comportements émotionels divers par stimulation rhinencéphalique chez le chat avec électrodes à demeure. *Rev Neurol, 86:*319, 1952.
Gastaut, H., Naquet, R., Vigouroux, R., Roger, A. and Badier, M.: Etudes életrographiques chez l'homme et chez l'animal des décharges épileptiques dites "psychomotrices". *Rev Neurol, 88:*310, 1953.
Gastaut, H. and Poirier, F.: Experimental or reflex induction of seizures. *Epilepsia, 5:* 256, 1964.
Gastaut, H. and Roger, A.: Origine et propagation des décharges épileptiques tempo-

rales provoquées. In Alajouanine, T. (Ed.): *Les grandes activités du lobe temporal.* Paris, Masson 1955.

Gastaut, H., Terzian, H., Naquet, R. and Luschnat, K.: Corrélations entre les "automatismes" des crises temporales et les phénomènes électroencéphalographiques qui les accompagnent. *Rev Neurol, 86:*678, 1952.

Gastaut, H., Toga, M., Roger, F. and Gibbson, W.C.: A correlation of clinical, electroencephalographic and anatomical findings in nine autopsied cases of "temporal lobe epilepsy". *Epilepsia, 4:*56, 1959.

Gastaut, H., Vigouroux, R., Corriol, J. and Badier, M.: Effets de la stimulation électrique (par électrodes à demeure) du complex amygdalien chez le chat non narcotisé. *J Physiol, 43:*740, 1951.

Geese, K.: Epilepsie. *Mat med Nordm, 13:*261, 1961.

Geets, W. and Leotard, G.: L'EEG et l'équilibre acide base du sang. *Clin. Neurophysiol.,* 6th Int. Congr. Vienna, Congr. Organization, 1965.

Geiger, A.: Glycolysis in cell-free extracts of brain. *Biochem J, 34:*465, 1940.

Geiger, A.: Chemical changes accompanying activity in the brain. In Richter, K. (Ed.): *Metabolism of the Nervous System.* Oxford-London, Pergamon Press, 1957.

Geiger, A., Dobkin, J. and Magnes, J.: Accumulation of acid soluble nitrogen in the brain cortex of cats during stimulation. *Science, 118:*655, 1953.

Geiger, A., Kawakita, Y., Barkulis, S.S., Nebel, L., Stephenson, R., Ling, D., Scruggs, W. and Sandberg, G.H.: Major pathways of glucose utilization in the brain in brain perfusion experiments *in vivo* and *in situ. J Neurochem, 5:*323, 1960.

Geiger, A., Magnes, J. and Geiger, R.S.: Survival of the perfused cat's brain in the absence of glucose. *Nature* (Lond), *170:*754, 1952.

Geiger, A., Magnes, J., Samra, D. and Zlotnik, A.: The isolation of the cerebral circulation and the perfusion of the brain in the living cat. *Am J Physiol, 149:*517, 1947.

Geiger, W.: Über Brompsychosen. *Nervenarzt, 26:*99, 1955.

Gellhorn, E.: *Physiological Foundations of Neurology and Psychiatry.* Minneapolis, U of Minn Pr, 1953.

Gellhorn, E. and Heymans, C.: Differential action of anoxia, asphyxia and carbon dioxide on normal and convulsive potentials. *J Neurophysiol, 11:*261, 1948.

Gellhorn, E. and Kessler, M.: Interaction of electric shock and insulin hypoglycemia. *Arch Neurol Psychiatr, 49:*808, 1943.

Gellhorn, E. and Yesinick, L. :The significance of carotid sinus reflexes for the effect of anoxia and carbon dioxide on convulsions. *Am J Physiol, 137:*404, 1942.

Genes, S.G.: *The Nervous System and Increation.* (Russ) Moscow, Medgiz, 1955.

Georgi, F.: Zur Genese des epileptischen Anfalls (ionogene Kolloidstabilitätsstörung. Theorie der Faktorenkoppelung). Klin Wochenschr, *4:*2053, 1925.

Georgi, F.: Pathogenese des epileptischen Anfalls (Humoralpathologie). *Z Ges Neurol Psychiatr, 106:*751, 1926.

Gerard, R.W., Marshall, W.H. and Saul, L.J.: Electrical activity of the cat's brain. *Arch Neurol Psychiatr, 36:*675, 1936.

Geratz, H.J.: Die klinische Anwendung von Meprobamat bei Säuglingen. Kindarärztl, *Praxis, 27:*67, 1959.

Gerebetzoff, M.A.: Apport de l'histochimie â la connaissance de l'écorce cérébrale. In Tower, Schadé (Eds.): *Structure and Function of the Cerebral Cortex.* Amsterdam. Elsevier, p. 334, 1960.

Gerschenfeld, H.M., Wald, F., Zadunaisky, J.A. and de Robertis, E.: Function of astroglia in the water metabolism of the central nervous system. An electron microscope study. *Neurology, 9:*412, 1959.

Gershenovitch, Z.S., Krichevskaya, A.A. and Kolousek, J.: The effect of raised oxygen pressure and of methionine sulfoximine on the glutamine activity of rat brain. *J Neurochem, 10*:79, 1963.
Gershoff, E.N., Newell, G.W. and Stone, W.E.: Chemical studies of the brain in dogs with "running fits". *Arch Biochem, 21*:74, 1949.
Gesenway, D. and Cohen, K.D.: Report of a case of convulsion and skin reaction following brief oral administration of imipramine (tofranil). *Am J Psychiatry, 116*: 1027, 1960.
Gey, K.F. and Pletscher, A.: Effects of chlorpromazine on the metabolism of dl-2-C14-DOPA in the rat. *J Pharmacol Exp Ther, 145*:337, 1964.
Gey, K.F., Rutishauser, M. and Pletscher, A.: Suppression of glycolysis in rat brain *in vivo* by chlorpromazine, reserpine and phenobarbital. *Biochem Pharmacol, 14*:507, 1965.
Giacobini, E. and Salum, J.: Treatment of delirium tremens. A comparative study of different therapeutic methods in 434 cases. *Acta Psychiat Scand, 37*:198, 1961.
de Giacomo, U.: Fisiopatologia del nucleo rosso. *Riv Pat Nerv Ment, 36*:26, 1930.
Gibbs, E.L., Fuster, B. and Gibbs, F.A.: Peculiar low temporal localization of sleep; induced seizure discharges of psychomotor type. *Arch Neurol Psychiatr, 60*:95, 1948.
Gibbs, E.L., Gibbs, F.A. and Fuster, B.: Psychomotor epilepsy. *Arch Neurol Psychiatr, 60*:331, 1948.
Gibbs, E.L. and Lennox, W.G.: Epilepsy, a paroxysmal cerebral dysrhythmia. *Brain, 60*:377, 1937.
Gibbs, E.L., Lennox, W.G., Nims, L.F. and Gibbs, F.A.: Arterial and cerebral venous blood-arterial-venous differences in man. *J Biol Chem, 144*:325, 1942.
Gibbs, F.A.: Ictal and nonictal psychiatric disorders in temporal lobe epilepsy. *J Nerv Ment Dis, 113*:522, 1951.
Gibbs, F.A.: Petit mal variant revisited. *Epilepsia, 12*:89-96, 1971.
Gibbs, F.A. and Gibbs, E.L.: *Atlas of Electroencephalography*. 2nd Ed. *Epilepsy*. Cambridge, Addison-Wesley Press, vol. II, 1952.
Gibbs, F.A., Gibbs, E.L. and Lennox, W.G.: Epilepsy: A paroxysmal cerebral dysrhythmia. *Brain, 60*:377, 1937.
Gibbs, F.A., Gibbs, E.L. and Lennox, W.G.: Cerebral dysrhythmias of epilepsy. *Arch Neurol Psychiatr, 39*:298, 1938.
Gibbs, F.A., Lennox, W.G. and Gibbs, E.L.: Cerebral blood flow proceeding and accompanying epileptic seizures in man. *Arch Neurol Psychiatr, 32*:257, 1934.
Gibbs, F.A., Lennox, W.G. and Gibbs, E.L.: Variations in the carbon dioxide content of the blood in epilepsy. *Arch Neurol Psychiatr, 43*:223, 1940.
Gibbs, F.A. and Maltby, G.L.: Effect on the electrical activity of the cortex of certain depressant and stimulant drugs, barbiturates, morphine, caffeine, benzedrine and adrenaline. *J Pharmacol Exp Ther, 78*:1, 1943.
Gibbs, F.A., Maxwell, H. and Gibbs, E.L.: Volume flow of blood through the human brain. *Arch Neurol Psychiatr, 57*:137, 1947.
Gibson, F.D. and Philips, S.: Peripheral neuritis after long-term isoniazid. *Geriatrics, 21*:178, 1966.
Gjessing, R.: Beiträge zur Kenntnis der Pathophysiologie der katatonen Erregung. III. Mitt. Über periodisch rezidivierende katatone Erregung mit kritischem Beginn und Abschluss. *Arch Psychiatr Nervenkr, 104*:355, 1935.
Gjessing, R.: Disturbances of somatic functions in catatonia with a periodic course and their compensation. *J Ment Sci, 84*:608, 1938.
Gjessing, R.: Beiträge zur Kenntnis der Pathophysiologie periodisch katatoner Zustände.

IV. Mitt. Versuch einer Ausgleichung der Funktionsstörungen. *Arch Psychiatr Nervenkr, 109*:525, 1939.

Gjessing, R.: Beiträge zur Somatologie der periodischen Katatonie. *Arch Psychiatr Nervenkr, 191*:191, 1953.

Gejessing, R.: A review of the biochemistry of periodic catatonia. *Proc. 4th World Congr. Psychiatr. 1966;* Part 1, Amsterdam, Excerpta Med. p. 516, 1967.

Glaser, G.H.: Sodium and seizures. *Epilepsia, 5*:97, 1964.

Glaser, G.H. and Golub, L.M.: The electroencephalogram of psychomotor seizures in childhood. *Electroencephalogr Clin Neurophysiol, 7*:329, 1955.

Glasov, V.A.: *Nevropatol Psikhiatr, 6*:9, 1937; cit. by Krasnova, A.I.: The polarographic activity of blood-serum of schizophrenics and epileptics. In *Obm Veshtch Psikhiat Zabol.* Moscow, Medgiz, pp. 114-119, 1960.

Glasov, V.A.: Catatonia. (Experimental study) (Russ) Diss. 1940.

Glees, P. and Griffith, F.: Bilateral destruction of the hippocampus in a case of dementia. *Psychiatria et Neurologia* (Basel), *123*:193, 1952.

Glezer, I.I. and Jakobson, I.S.: Données histochimiques et électronomicroscopiques sur l'action de la stelazine sur le cerveau des rats blancs. (Russ.) *Zh Nevropatol Psikhiatr, 67*:567, 1967.

Gloor, P.: The pattern of conduction of amygdaloid seizure discharge. An experimental study in the cat. *Arch Neurol, 77*:247, 1957.

Glusman, M., Ransohoff, J., Pool, L. and Sloan, N.: Electrical excitability of human uncus. *J Neurophysiol, 16*:528, 1953.

Gmellin, L.: Über einige im Gehirn der Menschen und Tiere vorkommende Fettarten. *Z Physiol* (Heidelberg), *1*:119, 1824.

Gogolak, G. and Pillat, B.: Effect of Mogadon on the arousal reaction in rabbits. In Akert, Bally, Schadé (Eds.): *Sleep Mechanisms. Progr. Brain Res.* Amsterdam, Elsevier, vol. XVIII, pp. 229-230, 1965.

Goldman, D.: Reserpine and chlorpromazine. Psychiat. Res. Rep. No. 4, *Am Psychiatr Ass, 79*:1956.

Goldsmith, G.A.: Niacin: antipellagra factor, hypocholesterolemic agent. Model of nutrition research yesterday and today. *JAMA, 194*:167, 1965.

Goldstein, B.I.: *Studies on the Biochemistry of Tissue Proteins.* (Catepsin). (Russ) Kiev, Ukrain. Sci. Acad., 1938.

Goldstein, B.I.: *On the Influence of Sulfhydryl-Groups on the Biological Quality of Tissue Proteins.* (Russ) Kiev, Ukrain. Sci. Acad., 1955.

Gomes, O.: Klinischer und forensischer Wert der Hyperventilation bei Epilepsie. *Arch Manic Judic Rio, 1*:55, 1930.

Goodman, L.S. et al.: Anticonvulsant properties of 5-phenyl-5-ethyl-hexahydropyrimidin-4, 6-dione (Mysoline), a new antiepileptic drug. *J Pharmacol, 108*:428, 1953.

Gordon, A.: Epilepsy and arteriosclerosis. *J Nerv Dis, 113*:170, 1951.

Gordon, M.T. and Waelsch, H.: Electrolytes and nerve function. In Elliott, Page, Quastel (Eds.): *Neurochemistry.* Springfield, Thomas, 1955.

Gore, M.B.R. and McIlwain, H.: Effects of some inorganic salts in the metabolic response of section of mammalian cerebral cortex to electrical stimulation. *J Physiol (Lond), 117*:471, 1952.

Gorodiskaya, G.J.: Papers on the problem of the chemical topography of the brain. (Russ) *Med Biol Zh, 2*:61a. *1*:77, 1926.

Gorodiskaya, G.J. and Hvatova, E.M. *Byull eksp biol Med, 4*:31, 1951; cit. by Lando, L.I.: The hyaluronidase in blood serum of schizophrenics during treatment. In *Obm. Veshtch. Psikahiat. Zabol.* Moscow, Medgiz, pp. 66-75, 1960.

Gorodisskaya, G.J. and Karlik, L.D.: Nitrogen metabolism in brain under action of ether and strychnine. In *Biochemistry of the Brain.* (Russ) R.A.N., Gorki, p. 123, 1941.

Gorodkova, T.M.: Vopr. Fiziol. 4, Kiev, 1953; cit. by Wolfsohn, H.M.: On the signification of some biochemical shifting to prognosis and effect of schizophrenia therapy. In *Obm Veshtch. Psikhiat. Zabol.* Moscow, Medgiz, pp. 128-145, 1960.

Gortner, R.A.: The water content of medusae. *Science* (NY), *1*:282, 1933.

Gosh, J.J.: Drug action and brain ribonucleoproteins. *J Indian Chem Soc, 44*:872, 1967.

Gosh, J.J. and Quastel, H.J.: Narcotics and brain respiration. *Nature* (Lond), *174*:28, 1954.

Goshev, A.I.: Influence of epileptogenic substances on the activity of cholinesterase in animals and epileptics. (Russ) Diss. Leningrad, 1955.

Gottstein, U.: Klinik und Therapie der Zerebralsklerose. *Z ärztl Fortbild, 11*:797, 1967.

Gowers, W.R.: *Epilepsy and Other Chronic Convulsive Diseases.* London, Churchill, 1901.

Grafe, E.: *Ernährungs- und Stoffwechselkrankheiten und ihre Behandlung.* Berlin-Göttingen-Heidelberg, Springer, 2. Aufl. 1958.

Grashtchenkov, N.I.: Physiological mechanisms of the epileptic seizure. (Russ) *Arch Biol Sci, 38*:49, 1935.

Grashtchenkov, N.I.: Experimental studies on the pathogenesis of epilepsies. (Russ) Diss. *Fiziol Zh, 21*:702, 1936.

Grashtchenkov, N.I. and Fiedelholz, L.G.: Neurological mechanisms of the epileptic seizure. (On the problem of epilepsy.) *Sovj Neuropathol Psychiatr a Psychogenesis, 3*: 2, 1934 (Russ).

Grastyán, E.: The central nervous system and behavior. 2. *Macy Conference 119,* Princeton, Congr. Presentation (Unpubl.) 1959.

Grastyán, E., Hori, Y. and Roger, A.: Etude électroencéphalographique temporo-spatiale d'un conditionnement moteur chez le chat. *Ier Congr. Int. des Sci. Neurol.* Bruxelles, Acta med. belg. p. 464, 1957.

Grastyán, E.: Lissák, K. and Kédesi, F.: Facilitation and inhibition of conditioned alimentary and defensive reflexes by stimulation of the hypothalamus and reticular formation. *Acta Physiol Hung, 9*:133, 1956.

Grastyán, E., Lissák, K., Kédesi, F., Madarász, I. and Vereby, G.: Beiträge zur Physiologie des Hippocampus. *Physiol Bohemoslov, 7*:9, 1958.

Grastyán, E., Lissák, K., Madarász, I. and Donhoffer, H.: Hippocampal electrical activity during the development of conditioned reflexes. *Electroencephalogr Clin Neurophysiol, 11*:409, 1959.

Grastyán, E., Lissák, K., Szabo, J. and Vereby, G.: Über die funktionelle Bedeutung des Hippocampus. In *The Problems of the Modern Physiology of the Nervous and Muscle System.* In honour of Beritashvili. Acad. Sci. Georgian SSR, Tbilisi, p. 67, 1965.

Green, A.L.: Activity correlations and the mode of action of aminoalkylphenothiazine tranquilizers. *J Pharm Pharmacol, 19*:207, 1967.

Green, D.E., Leloir, L.F. and Nocito, V.: *J Biol Chem, 161*:559, 1945; cit. by Kanig, K.: *Die Bedeutung der B-Vitamine für das Nervensystem.* Wiss. Berichte, E. Merck, Darmstadt, 1968.

Green, H. and Sawyer, J.L.: Biochemical - pharmacological studies with 5-hydroxytryptophan, precusor of serotonine. In Humwich, E. (Ed.): *Biogenic Amines.* Amsterdam, Elsevier, 1964.

Green, J.D.: The hippocampus. *Physiol Rev, 44*:561, 1964.

Green, J.D. and Adey, W.R.: Electrophysiological studies of hippocampal connections and excitability. *Electroencephalogr Clin Neurophysiol, 8*:245, 1956.

Green, J.D. and Arduini, A.A.: Hippocampal electrical activity in arousal. *J Neurophysiol, 17*:533, 1954.

Green, J.D., Clemente, C.D. and de Groot, J.: Experimentally induced epilepsy in the cat with injury of cornu ammonis. *Arch Neurol Psychiatr, 78*:259, 1957.

Green, J.D., Duisberg, R.E.H. and McGrath, W.B.: Focal epilepsy of psychomotor type. *J Neurosurg, 8*:157, 1951.

Green, J.D. and Shimamoto, T.: Hippocampal seizures and their propagation. *Arch Neurol, 70*:687, 1953.

Gregoriades, A.D.: A medical and social survey of 231 children with seizures. *Epilepsia, 13*:13-20, 1972.

Greville, G.D. and Heppenstall, M.E.: Pharmacology. In Hill, Parr (Eds.): *Electroencephalography*. London, Macdonald, New York, Macmillan, 1952.

Griffel, A.: Über mensuell gebundene epileptische Anfälle. Diss. Bern, 1953.

Gross, H.P. and Schulte, F.J.: Polygraphische Ableitungen bei Kindern mit Phenylketonurie. Sitzungsberichte Dtsch.EEG.Ges., 14.Jahrestagung, Münster, 1968.

Grühle, H.W.: Rhythmus epileptischer Anfälle. *Nervenarzt, 8*:624, 1935.

Grünthal, E.: Über das klinische Bild nach umschriebenem beidseitigem Ausfall der Ammonshornrinde. *Psychiatr Neurol* (Basel), *113*:1, 1947.

Grünthal, E. and Walther-Büel, H.: Über Schädigung der Oliva inferiori durch Chlorphenazin (Trilafon). *Psychiatr Neurol* (Basel), *140*:249, 1960.

Grüsser, O.J., Gaedt, C. and Lunkenheimer, H.-U.: Die funktionelle Organisation rezeptiver visueller Felder: Neuere Untersuchungen über laterale Inhibition in einem humoralen Netzwerk. *Zbl Ges Neurol Psychiatr, 191*:149, 1968.

Grüttner, R. and Bonkalo, A.: Über Ermüdung und Schlaf auf Grund hirnbioelektrischer Untersuchungen. *Arch Psychiatr, 111*:652, 1940.

Grumbach, M.M. and Kaplan, S.L.: Amino acid and α-keto acid induced hyperinsulinism in the leucine-sensitive type of infantile and childhood hypoglycemia. *Pediatrics, 57*:346, 1960.

Grundfest, H.: Synaptic and ephaptic transmission. In Field, J. et al. (Eds.): *Hb. of Physiol.*, Sect. 1, Vol. 1, Amer.Physiol.Soc. p. 147, 1959.

Grundfest, H. and Grasser, H.S.: Properties of mammalian nerve fibres of slowest conduction. *Am J Physiol, 123*:307, 1938.

Gubar, V.A.: On the nature of phenamine. (Russ.) *Byull Eksp Biol Med, 18*:51, 1944.

Guerrero-Figueroa, R., Barros, A., Heath, R.G. and Gonzales, G.: Experimental subcortical epileptiform focus. *Epilepsia, 5*:112, 1964.

Guggenheim, K.: Studies on water metabolism of pyridoxine and pantothenic acid-deficient rats. *Endocrinology, 55*:156, 1954.

Guirard, B.M. and Snell, E.E.: Pyridoxal phosphate and mental ions as cofactors for histidine decarboxylase. *J Am Chem Soc, 76*:4745, 1955.

Guldberg, H.C. and Yates, C.M.: Effects of chorpromazine on the metabolism of catecholamines in dog brain. *Brit J Pharmacol, 34*:233P, 1968.

Gulotta, S.: Il glutatione nel sangue di alcuni malati di mente e dei dementi precoci in ispecie. *Boll Soc Ital Biol Sper, 6*:499, 1931.

Gurdjan, E.S., Webster, J.E. and Stone, W.E.: Cerebral metabolism in metrazol convulsions in the dog. *Res Publ Ass Nerv Ment Dis, 26*:184, 1947.

Gurin, S. and Delluva, A.M.: The biological synthesis of radioactive adrenaline from phenylalanine. *J Biol Chem, 170*:545, 1945.

Gutnikoff, Z.V.: Experimental studies of epilepsy. (Russ.) *Arkh Psikhiatr Nevrol Psikhopatol, 17*:75, 1891.

Haas, H.: Der Wirkungsmechanismus des 1-1Cyclohexyl-2-methyl-aminopropan-5,5-phenylacetylbarbiturats und seine Eignung als Antiepilepticum. *Arzneim Forsch, 13*: 613, 1963.

Haase, H..: *Neuroleptica, Tranquilizer and Antidepressiva in Klinik and Praxis.* Düsseldorf, Jansen 1966.

Haber, C. and Saidel, L.: Glutamic acid in neural activity. *Fed Proc, 7*:47, 1948.

Haberland, C.: Histological studies in temporal lobe epilepsy based on biopsy material. *Psychiatr Neurol* (Basel), *135*:12, 1958.

Hackstock, H. and Bielinski, C.: Zur Therapie verschiedener Hirnfunktionsstörungen. *Ther Umsch, 18*:241, 1961.

Haessle, H., Corrodi, H., Fuxe, K. and Hokfelt, T.: The effect of neuroleptics on the acitvity of central catecholamine neurons. *Life Sci, 7*:767, 1967.

Hagberg, B., Hamfelt, A. and Hansson, O.: Epileptic children with disturbed tryptophan metabolism treated with vitamin B_6. *Lancet I, 145*:1964.

Haikina, B.I. and Gontcharova, E.E.: Annual of biochemistry of the central nervous system. 1954; cit. by Tchalissov, M.A.: Carbon-phosphate metabolism and its importance in psychiatry. (Russ.) In *Obm. Veshtch. Psikhiat. Zabol.* Moscow, Medgiz, pp. 14-20, 1960.

Haimovitch, L.A.: *Theses and Writings to the 20th Congress.* UNIPNI, Charkov, 1956, (Russ).

Haimovitch, L.A. and Podkamenii, B.N.: The reaction of schizophrenics dependent on the period of disease and somemetabolic processes. (Russ) In *Obm. Veshtch. Psikhiat. Zabol.* Moscow, Medgiz, pp. 47-55, 1960.

Haizlip, T.M. and Ewing, J.A.: Meprobamate habituation. *New Engl J Med, 258*:1181, 1958.

Hajnsek, F. and Sartorius, N.: A case of intoxication with Tegretol. *Epilepsia, 5*:371, 1964.

Hallen, O.: Zur Differentialdiagnose von Jackson-Anfällen. *Dtsch Med Wochenschr, 78*: 260, 1953.

Hallen, O.: Das Oral-Petit Mal. *Dtsch Z Nervenheilkd, 171*:236, 1954a.

Hallen, O.: Zur Lokalisation des Oral-Petit Mal. *Zbl Neurol Psychiatr, 130*:3, 1954b.

Hallen, O.: Zur Frage des Oral-Petit Mal. (Entgegnungen auf die Bemerkungen von E. Niedermeyer) *Dtsch Z Nervenheilkd, 172*:535, 1955.

Hallen, O.: Die Klinik, Diagnose und Differentialdiagnose der kleinen epileptischen Anfälle. *Dtsch Z Nervenheilkd, 176*:321, 1957.

Hallen, O.: Die Psychiatrie der Oral-Petit Mal Epilepsie. *Psychiat Neurol (Basel), 134*: 43, 1957.

Hallen, O.: Zur Differenzierung der psychomotorischen Anfälle in Klinischen Formen. *Dtsch Z Nervenheilkd, 183*:199, 1962.

Hamberger, A.: Oxidation of tricarboxylic acid cycle intermediates by nerve cell bodies and glial cells. *J Neurochem, 8*:31, 1961.

Hamfelt, A.: Pyridoxine metabolism in the human being at different ages. In v. Kress, Blum (Eds.): *B-Vitamine.* Stuttgart, Schattauer, p. 305, 1966.

Hance, J.A.: The effects of chlorpromazine, thiopentone, amphetamine and d'lysergic acid diethylamide on conduction within an extralemniscal system in the brain stem of the cat. *J Physiol* (Lond), *145*:41, 1959.

Haneke, K.: On the treatment of the blitz-nick-salaam convulsions with ACTH. *Kinderärztl Praxis, 29*:471, 1961.

Haneke, K.: Erfahrungen mit Mylepsinum bei der Behandlung cerebraler Anfälle im Kindesalter. *Mschr Kinderheilkd, 113*:652, 1965.

Haneke, K.: Tegretal® bei kindlichen Anfallsleiden. *Med Klin, 61*:20, 1966.

Hansen, H.E., Wiese, H.F., Adam, D.J.D., Bussey, D.R. and Worsham, A.G.: Influence of pyridoxine on mineral balance in infant maintained on a convulsigenic milk preparation. *Fed Proc, 13*:460, 1954.

Hanson, A.: Inhibition of brain glutamic acid decarboxylase by phenylalanine metabolites. *Naturwissenschaften, 45*:423, 1958.

van Harrefeld, A. and Kok, D.J.: A propos de la nature de la catalepsie expérimentale. *Arch Neurol Physiol, 20*:411, 1935.

Hartchenko, S.I.: On the problem of pathogenesis of epilepsy. (Russ.) Diss. Igevsk, 1942.

Hartchenko, S.I.: The development mechanisms of epileptic seizures. (Russ.) *Proc of the Med Inst Kursk, 2*:167, 1948.

Hartmann, E.L.: *The Biology of Dreaming*. Springfield, Thomas, 1967.

Hartmann, K. and Simma, K.: Untersuchungen über die Thalamusprojektionen beim Menschen. *Psychiatr Neurol* (Basel), *123*:329, 1952.

Hartsook, E.W., Hershberger, T.V. and French, C.E.: A study of the effect of desoxypyridoxine or isoniazid upon mineral retention and liver enzyme activities of pyridoxine-deficient male rats. *J Nutr, 65*:547, 1958.

Hasselbach, H. and Schwabe, K.: A new polarographic cancer reaction. *Pharmazie, 10*:310, 1955.

Hassler, C., Hassler, R., Okada, Y. and Bak, I.J.: Pre-Ictal and ictal changes of serotonin, GABA and glutamate contents in different regions of rabbit brain during methoxypyridoxine-induced seizures. *Acta Neurol Latinoamer 17*:595-611, 1971.

Hassler, R.: Zur Pathologie der Paralysis agitans und des postencephalitischen Parkinsonismus. *J Psychol Neurol* (Lpz), *48*:387, 1938.

Hassler, R.: Extrapyramidal-motorische Syndrome und Erkrankungen. In v. Bergmann, Frey, Schwiegk (Eds.): *Hb. inn. Med.* 4th Ed. Berlin, Springer, vol. V/3, 1953.

Hassler, R.: Motorische und sensible Effekte umschriebener Reizungen und Ausschaltungen im menschlichen Zwischenhirn. *Dtsch Z Nervenheilkd, 183*:148, 1961.

Hassler, R.: *Limbische und diencephale Systeme der Affektivität und Psychomotorik.* Muskel und Psyche. Symp. Wien 1963; Basel-New York, Karger, pp. 3-33, 1964a.

Hassler, R.: Zur funktionellen Anatomie des limbischen Systems. *Nervenarzt, 35*:386, 1964b.

Hassler, R.: *Das Schmerzerlebnis in Abhängigkeit von neuronalen Systemen.* Basel-New York, Karger, 1968.

Hassler, R.: Saggittal thalamotomy for relief of motor disorders in cases of double athetosis and cerebral palsy. *Conf Neurol, 34*:18-28, 1972.

Hassler, R., Dalle, G., Ore, A., Bricolo, G., Dieckmann, G. and Dolce, G.: EEG and clinical arousal induced by bilateral long-term stimulation of pallidal systems in traumatic vigil coma. In Electroencephalography and clinical Neurophysiology. *27:* 689-690, 1969.

Hassler, R., Dalle, G., Ore, A., Dieckmann, G., Bricolo, A. and Dolce, G.: Behavioural and EEG arousal induced by stimulation of unspecific projection systems in a patient with post-traumatic apallic syndrome. *Electroenceph clin Neurophysiol, 27:* 306-310, 1969.

Hassler, R. and Dieckmann, G.: Reizexperimente zur Funktion des Putamen der Katze. *J Hirnforsch 10*:187-225, 1968.

Hassler, R. and Dieckmann, G.: Traitement stéréotaxique des tics et des cris inarticulés ou copralaliques considérés comme phénomène d'obsession motrice au cours denla maladie de Gilles de la Tourette. *Rev Neurol, 123*:89-100, 1970.

Hassler, R. and Dieckmann, G.: Violence against oneself and against others as a target for stereotaxic psychosurgery (Erethismic imbecility and temporal lobe epilepsy). In "Present Limits of Neurosurgery" (Ed.) I. Fusek and Z. Kunc. Proc. Fourth Europ. Congr. Neurosurg. Avicenum, Czechoslovak Medical Press, Prague, 477-482, 1972.

Hassler, R. and Walker, A.E.: Trigeminal Neuralgia, Pathogenesis and Pathophysiology, Stuttgart, Georg Thieme Verlag, pp. 124-137, 1970.

Hassler, R. and Riechert, T.: Beitrag zur stereotaktischen Fornicotomie bei temporaler *Epilepsie Zbl Ges Neurol Psychiatr, 140*:10, 1957.

Hastert, F.: Emploi de la thiopropérazine dans les troubles caractériels chez les épileptiques, les débiles et les psychopathes. Acta Neurol. Belg. *62*:509-513, 1962.

Hauschild, F.: Pharmakologie und Grundlagen der Toxikologie. 2nd Ed. Leipzig, F. A. Barth, 1960.

Havliček, V.: The effect of dihydroxyphenylserine on the ECOG of unrestrained rats. *Int J Neuropharmacol, 6*:81, 1967.

Hawkins, J.E.jr. and Sarett, L.H.: On the efficacy of asparagine, glutamine, gamma-aminobutyric acid and 2-pyrolidinone in preventing chemically induced seizures in mice. *Clin Chem Acta, 2*:481, 1957.

Hayashi, S., (Japanese) *Nôshinkeiryôiki, 7*:73 and 132, 1954; cit. by Sperling, E. and Creutzfeldt, O.: Der Temporallappen. *Fortschr Neurol Psychiat, 27*:296, 1959.

Health, R.G. and Guerrero-Figueroa, R.: Psychotic behavior with evoked septal dysrhythmia: effects of intracerebral acetylcholine and gamma aminobutyric acid. *Am J Psychiatr, 121*:1080, 1965.

Heath, R.G. and Leach, B.E.: Brain recordings with schizophrenic behavior: Some metabolic factors responsible for physiological alteration. *Ann NY Acad Sci, 96*:425, 1962.

Heath, R.G., Martens, S., Leach, B.E., Cohen, M. and Angel, C.: Effect on behavior in humans with the administration of taraxein. *Am J Psychiatry, 114*:14, 1957.

Heath, R.G., Martens, S., Leach, B.E., Cohen, M. and Feigley, C.A.: Behavioral changes in nonpsychotic volunteers following the administration of taraxein, the substance extracted from the serum of schizophrenic patients. *Am J Psychiatry, 114*:917, 1958.

Heathcote, J.G.: Toxic effect of the crystals from "agenized" zein on certain acid producing bacteria. *Nature* (Lond), *164*:439, 1949.

Heathcote, J.C. and Pace, J.: Inhibition of the growth of Leuconostoc mesenteroides by the toxic factor from agenized zein: reversal by L-glutamine. *Nature* (Lond), *166*: 353, 1950.

Hebb, C.D. and Waites, G.M.H.: Choline acetylase in antero- and retro-grade degeneration of cholinergic nerve. *J Neurophysiol* (Lond), *132*:667, 1956.

Hebb, C.D. and Whittacker, V.P.: Intracellular distribution of acetylcholine and choline acetylase. *J Physiol* (Lond), *142*:187, 1958.

Hécaen, H. and Angelergues, R.: Epilepsie et troubles de langage. *Encéphale, 49*:138, 1960.

Hecker, A., Andermann, F., and Rodin, E.A.: Spitting Automatism in Temporal Lobe Seizures, with a Brief Review of Ethiological and Phylogenetic Aspects of Spitting. *Epilepsia, 13*:767-772, 1972.

v. Hedenström, I.: Bedeutung der Wesensänderung für die Diagnose der kryptogenetischen und symptomatischen Epilepsie. *Arch Psychiatr Neurol, 206*:599, 1965.

v. Hedenström, I. and Dreyer, R.: Gleichzeitiges Vorkommen von Absencen und psychomotorischen Anfällen bei einer Patientin. *Nervenarzt, 38*:68, 1967.

v. Hedenström, I. and Schorsch, G.: EEG Befunde bei epileptischen Dämmer- und Verstimmungszuständen. *Arch Psychiatr Nervenkr, 191*:311, 1959.

Hellström, B. and Vassella, F.: Tryptophan metabolism in infantile spasm. *Acta Paediat.* (Stockh), *51*:665, 1962.

Helmchen, H.: Beitrag zur konstitutionellen Differenenzierung im Bereich genuiner Epilepsien. *Dtsch Z Nervenheilkd, 178*:541, 1958.

Helmchen, H.: *Bedingungskonstellationen Paranoid-Halluzinatorischer Syndrome.* (Zugleich ein methodischer Beitrag zur Untersuchung psychopathologischelektroencephalographischer Korrelationen.) Berlin-Heidelberg-New York, Springer, 1968.

Helmchen, H., Kanowski, S. and Künkel, H.: Die Altersabhängigkeit der Lokalisation von EEG-Herden. *Arch Psychiat Z Neurol, 209*:474, 1967.

Helmchen, H. and Künkel, H.: Möglichkeiten quantitativer Auswertung elektroencephalographischer Verlaufsuntersuchungen bei neuroleptischer Behandlung. *Med Exp:* (Basel), *2*:95, 1960.

Helmchen, H. and Künkel, H.: Pneumencephalographische und elektroencephalographische Untersuchungen bei Phenothiazin-Behandelten. I. Mitt.: Herdbefunde. *Med Exp, 5*:406, 1961a.

Helmchen, H. and Künkel, H.: Pneumencephalographische und elektroencephalographische Üntersuchungen bei Phenothiazin-Behandelten. II. Mitt.: Paroxysmale Dysrhythmie. *Med Exp, 4*:412, 1961b.

Helmchen, H. and Künkel, H.: Der Einfluß von EEG-Verlaufsuntersuchungen unter psychiatrischer Pharmakotherapie auf die Prognostik von Psychosen. *Arch Psychiatr Z Neurol, 205*:1, 1964a.

Helmchen, H. and Künkel, H.: EEG-Längsschnittuntersuchungen bei der Pharmakotherapie von Psychosen. In Bradley, Flügel, Hoch (Eds.): *Neuropsychopharmacology.* Amsterdam, Elsevier, vol. III, 1964b.

Helmchen, H. and Künkel, H.: Die prognostische Bedeutung elektroencephalographischer Veränderungen unter psychiatrischer Pharmakotherapie. *Arzneim Forsch, 14*:595, 1964c.

Helmchen, H., Künkel, H. and Selbach, H.: Periodische Einflüsse auf die individuelle Häufigkeit cerebraler Anfälle. *Arch Psychiatr Neurol, 206*:293, 1964.

Helmholtz, H.F. and Keith, H.M.: Eight years' experience with the ketogenic diet in the treatment of epilepsy. *JAMA, 95*:707, 1930.

Hemkes, F.: Über Atrophie und Sklerose des Ammonshorns bei Epileptischen. *Algg Z Psychiatr, 34*:678, 1878.

Hempel, J.: Zur Frage der morphologischen Hirnveränderungen im Gefolge von Insulinschock- und Cardiazol und Azomankrampfbehandlung. *Z Ges Neurol Psychiatr, 173*:210, 1941.

Henatsch, H.D.: Allgemeine Elektrophysiologie der erregbaren Strukturen. In Landois-Rosemann: *Lehrbuch der Physiologie des Menschen.* 28th Ed. München, Urban & Schwarzenberg, vol. II, 1962.

Hendriksen, V.: Hyperventilation bei Epilepsie. *Hospitalstidene, 70*:263, 1927.

Hennemann, D.H., Altschule, M.D. and Goncz, R.M.: Carbohydrate metabolism in brain diseases: II. Glucose metabolism in schizophrenic, manic-depressive and involutional psychosis. *Arch Int Med, 94*:402, 1954.

Hennemann, D.H., Altschule, M.D., Goncz, R.M. and Davis, P.: Carbohydrate metabolism in brain disease. V. Effect of epinephrine on intermediary carbohydrate metabolism in schizophrenic and manic depressive psychoses. *Arch Int Med, 95*:594, 1955.

Henry, C.E., Obrist, W., Porter, P. and Anglas, R.: Effect of Equantil on the EEG. *Electroencephalogr Clin Neurophysiol, 9*:172, 1957.

Henry, G.W. and Magnum, E.: Blood in personality disorders. *Arch Neurol Psychiatr* (Chic), *13*:743, 1925.

Heppenstall, M.E.: Relation between the effects of the bloodsugar levels and hyperventilation on the electroencephalography. *J Neurol Neurosurg Psychiatr, 7*:112, 1944.

Herberg, D.: Alveolare Hypoventilation und chronisches Cor Pulmonale. *Hippokrates, 35*:337, 1965.

Herken, H. and Neuhoff, V.: Mikroanalytischer Nachweis von Acetylpyridin-adenin-dinucleotid und Acetylpyridin-adenin-dinucleotid-phosphat im Gehirn. *Hoppe Seylers Z Physiol Chem, 331*:85, 1963.

Herken, H. and Timmler, R.: Kinetik der Dihydrofolsäurereduktase aus Rattenleber und -gehirn mit 3-APA, DPH + H^+ als Wasserstoffdonator. *Arch Exp Path Pharmacol, 250*:293, 1965.

Hernández-Peón, R.: Sleep induced by localized electrical or chemical stimulation of the forebrain. *Electroencephalogr Clin Neurophysiol, 14*:423, 1962.

Hernández-Peón, R.: Fisiología del sistema nervioso autónomo. *Acta neurol Latinoamer, 9*:260, 1962.

Hernández-Peón, R.: Neurophysiological correlates of EEG patterns during wakefulness and sleep. *Electroencephalog Clin Neurophysiol, 17*:469, 1964.

Hernández-Peón, R.: Psychiatric implications of neurophysiological research. *Bull Menninger Found, 28*:165, 1964.

Hernández-Peón, R.: Neurophysiological mechanisms of wakefulness and sleep. *Acta Psychol, 23*:271, 1964.

Hernández-Peón, R.: A cholinergic hypnogenic limbic forebrain-hindbrain circuit. In Jouvet, M. (Ed.): *Aspects Anatomo-Fonctionnels de la Physiologie du sommeil.* A Symposium. Paris, Masson, pp. 63-84, 1965a.

Hernández-Peón, R.: Die neuralen Grundlagen des Schlafes. *Arzneim Forsch, 15*:1099, 1965b.

Hernández-Peón, R.: Cholinergic and other humoral mechanisms: The problem of chemical specificity in the neural substratum of the sleep-wakefulness cycle. *Neurosc Res Progr Bull, 4*:43, 1966.

Hernández-Peón, R. and Rojas-Ramirez, J.A.: Central mechanisms of tranquilizing, anticonvulsant and relaxant actions of Ro 4-5360. *Int J Pharmacodyn, 5*:263, 1966.

Hernández-Peón, R. and Scherrer, H.: "Habituation" to acoustic stimuli in choclear nucleus. *Fed Proc, 14*:71, 1955a.

Hernández-Peón, R. and Scherrer, H.: Inhibitory influence of brain stem reticular formation upon synaptic transmission in trigeminal nucleus. *Fed Proc, 14*:71, 1955b.

Herzberg, M.O.: *Nevropatol Psikhiat, 6*: 7, 1937; cit. by Wolfson, H.M.: On the signification of some biochemical shifting to prognosis and effect of schizophrenia therapy. In *Obm. Veshtch. Psikhiat. Zabol.* Medgiz, Moscow, pp. 128-145, 1960.

Hess, A.: Blood-brain barrier and ground substance of central nervous system: Similarities in development. *Arch Neurol Psychiatr,* (Chic), *73*:380, 1955a.

Hess, A.: Blood-brain barrier and ground substance of central nervous system. *Arch Neurol Psychiatr,* (Chic), *74*:149, 1955b.

Hess, A.: The ground substance of the developing central nervous system. *J Comp Neurol, 102*:65, 1955c.

Hess, W.R.: Das Schlafsyndrom als Folge dienzephaler Reizung. *Helv Physiol Pharmacol Acta, 2*:305, 1944.

Hess, W.R.: *Die funktionelle Organisation des vegetativen Nervensystems.* Basel, Schwabe, 1948.

Hess, W.R.: *Das Zwischenhirn.* Basel, Schwabe, 1954.

Hess, W.R.: *Hypothalamus und Thalamus.* Stuttgart, Thieme, 1956.

Hicks, S.P.: Pathologic effects of antimetabolites. I. Acute lesions in the hypothalamus, peripheral ganglia and adrenal medulla caused by 3-acetyl-pyridine prevented by nicotinamide. *Am J Path, 31:*189, 1955.

Hill, D.: The electroencephalographic concept of psychomotor epilepsy. A summary. *IV Congr Neurol Internat, 1:*27, 1949.

Hill, D.: EEG in episodic psychotic and psychopathic behavior. *Electroencephalogr Clin Neurophysiol, 4:*419, 1952.

Hill, D., Pond, D.A., Mitchell, W. and Falconer, M.A.: Personality changes following temporal lobectomy for epilepsy. *J Ment Sci, 103:*18, 1957.

Hillarp, N.A., Lagerstedt, S. and Nicholson, B.: Isolation of granular fraction from suprarenal medulla, containing sympathomimetic catechol amines. *Acta Physiol Scand, 29:*251, 1953.

Hillbom, E.: Schizophrenia-like psychoses after brain trauma. *Acta Psychiat Sncad, 60:* 1951.

Himwich, H.E.: *Brain Metabolism and Cerebral Disorders,* Baltimore, Hopkins, 1951.

Hippius, H. and Jantz, H.: Die heutige Behandlung der Depressionen. *Nervenarzt, 30:* 466, 1959.

Hippius, H., Mellin, P. and Rosenkötter, L.: Megaphenwirkung im EEG des Kaninchens. *Z Exp Med, 2:*128, 1955.

Hippius, H., Rosenkötter, L. and Selbach, H.: Untersuchungen zur Verlaufsdynamik corticaler Krampfpotentiale. *Arch Psychiatr Nervenkr, 196:*379, 1957.

Hodgkin, A.L.: The ionic basis of electrical activity in nerve and muscle. *Biol Rev 26:*339, 1951.

Hodgkin, A.L. and Huxley, A.F.: Action potentials recorded from inside a nerve fibre. *Nature* (Lond), *144:*710, 1939.

Hodgkin, A.L. and Huxley, A.F.: Resting and action potentials in single nerve fibers. *J Physiol* (Lond), *104:*176, 1945.

Hodgkin, A.L. and Keynes, R.D.: Active transport of cations in giant axons from sepia and logio. *J Physiol* (Lond), *128:*28, 1955.

Hodgkin, A.L. and Keynes, R.D.: Movements of labeled Ca in squid giant axons. *J Physiol* (Lond), *138:*253, 1957.

Höber, R.: Beiträge zur physikalischen Chemie der Erregung und der Narkose. *Pflügers Arch, 120:*492, 1907.

Höber, R.: *Physikalische Chemie der Zelle und der Gewebe.* Leipzig, Engelmann, 1926.

Hoff, H.: *Lehrbuch der Psychiatrie.* Basel-Stuttgart, Schwabe, 1956.

Hoffer, A.: In Martin, G.J. and Kisch, B. (Eds.): *Enzymes and Mental Health.* Toronto, Lippincott, 1966; cit. by Kanig, K.: *Arzneim Forsch, 19:*397, 1969.

Hofmann, G. and Kryspin-Exner, K.: Klinische Erfahrungen mit einem neuen Neurolepticum (TP 21, Melleril). *Wein Med Wochenschr, 110:*897, 1960.

Hollister, L.E. and Glazener, F.S.: Withdrawal reactions from meprobamate, alone and combined with promazine: a controlled study. *Psychopharmacol* (Berlin), *1:*336, 1960.

Holm, E.: Eine Faktorenanalyse von evoked-potential-Schwellen nach der Hauptachsenmethode. *Pflüg Arch, 291:*28, 1966.

Holm, E.: Schlafmittelwirkungen auf subkortikale Hirngebiete. In Jovanović, U.J. (Ed.): *Der Schlaf. Neurophysiologische Aspekte.* München, Barth, 1969.

Holm, E., Kelleter, A., Heinemann, H and Hamann, K.F.: Wirkungen von Tegretal® auf das Zentralnervensystem der Katze. (Elektrophysiologische Untersuchungen). Unpublished (personal correspondence) 1970.

Holm, E. and Schaefer, H.: Eine Faktotrenanalyse von Schwellen subkortikaler Reizantworten. *Exp Brain Res, 8:*79, 1969.

Holmden, F. E.: Bromomania. *Lancet, 2:*816, 1890.

v. Holst, E. and Mittelstaedt, H.: Das Reafferenzprinzip. *Naturwissenschaften, 37:*464, 1950.

Holtz, P. and Heise, R.: Fermentativer Abbau von 1-Dioxyphenylalanine (DOPA) durch die Niere. *Arch Exp Path Pharmakol, 191:*87, 1938.

Holtz, P. and Westermann, E.: Über die DOPA-decarboxylase und Histidindecarboxylase des Nervengewebes. *Arch Exp Path Pharmakol, 277:*538, 1956.

Horecker, B.L.: Glucose-6-phosphate dehydrogenase, the pentose phosphate cycle and its place in carbohydrate metabolism. *Am J Clin Path, 47:*271, 1967.

Hornykiewicz, O.: Dopamin (3-hydroxytryptamin) im Zentralnervensystem und seine Beziehung zum Parkinsonsyndrom des Menschen. *Dtsch Med Wochenschr, 87:*1807, 1962.

Horstmann, E. and Meves, H.: Die Feinstruktur des molekularen Rindengraues und ihre physiologische Bedeutung. *Z Zellforsch, 49:*569, 1959.

Horstmann, W. and Wegener, K.: Atmung und alveolarer Kohlensäuregehalt anfallskranker Kinder. *Z Kinderheilkd, 95:*291, 1966.

Horyd, W. and Patelska, T.: Leczenie zachowawcze padaczki skroniowej. *Neurol Neurochir Psychiat Pol, 15:*433, 1965.

Hoskins, R.G.: Oxygen metabolism in schizophrenia. *Arch Neurol, 38:*1261, 1937.

Houben, P.F.M., Hommes, O.R., and Knaven, P.J.H.: Antitconvulsant drugs and folic acid in young mentally retarded epileptic patients. *Epilepsia, 12:*235-247, 1971.

Hramcova, N.S.: On the problem of protein metabolism in postinfectious psychoses. In *Obm Veshtch. Psikhiat. Zabol. Moscow,* Medgiz, pp. 194-199, 1960.

Hsia, D.Y.Y. et al: A one-year controlled study of the effect of low phenylalanine diet on phenylketonuria. *Pediatrics, 21:*178, 1958.

Hsu, J.M., Davis, R.L. and Chow, B.F.: Electrolyte imbalance in vitamin B_6 deficient rats. *J Biol Chem, 230:*889, 1958.

Hubach, H.: Veränderungen der Krampferregbarkeit unter Einwirkung von Medikamenten und während der Entziehung. *Fortschr Neurol Psychiatr, 31:*4, 1963.

Huber, G.: Typen und Korrelate organischer Abbausyndrome. In Kranz, H. (Ed): *Psychopathologie Heute.* Stuttgart, Thieme, 1962.

Huber, G.: Pneumencephalographischer Befund bei idiopathischer Epilepsie. *Dtsch Z Nervenheilkd, 183:*1962.

Hunsperger, R.W.: Affektreaktionen auf elektrische Reizung im Hirnstamm der Katze. *Helv Physiol Pharmacol Acta, 14:*70, 1956.

Hunsperger, R.W.: Les représentations centrales des réactions affectives dans le cerveau antérieur et dans le tronc cérébral. *Neurochirugia, 5:*207, 1959.

Hunt, D.A.jr., Stokes, J.jr., McCrory, W.W. and Stroud, H.H.: Pyridoxine dependency: report of a case of intractable convulsions in an infant controlled by pyridoxine. *Pediatrics, 13:*140, 1954.

Hunter, J.: Further observations on subcortically induced epileptic attacks in unanesthetized animals. *Electroencephalogr Clin Neurophysiol, 2:*193, 1950.

Hutt, S.J.: Experimental analysis of brain activity and behaviour in children with minor seizures. *Epilepsia, 13:*520-534, 1972.

Hutton, J.Th., Trost, J.D., and Foster, J.: The influence of the cerebellum in cat penicillin epilepsy. *Epilepsia, 13:*401-408, 1972.

Hydén, H.: Protein metabolism in the nerve cell during growth and function. *Acta Physiol Scand, 6:*67, 1943.

Hydén, H.: Automatisering inom cellforskningen. *Sven Läk, 54:*1825, 1957.

Hydén, H.: Biochemical changes in glial cells and nerve cells of varying activity. In Brücke, F. (Ed.): *Biochemistry of the Central Nervous System.* New York, Pergamon Press, 1959.

Hydén, H.: *The Cell.* Brachet, Mirsky (Eds.) New York, Academic Press, vol. IV, 1960.

Hydén, H.: Neuron und seine Gliazellen als biochemische und funktionelle Einheit. *Endeavour, 21:*144, 1962.

Hydén, H. and Egyhazi, E.: Nuclear RNA changes of nerve cells during learning experiments in rats. *Proc Nat Acad Sci* (Wash), *48:*1366, 1962.

Hydén, H. and Egynazi, E.: Changes in RNA content and base composition in cortical neurons of rats in a learning experiment involving transfer of handedness. *Proc Nat Acad Sci, 52:*1030, 1964.

Ignatova, N.I.: Studies of end-products of metabolism in involutional psychoses. (Russ) In *Obm. Veshtch, Psikhiatr. Zabol.* Moscow. Medgiz, pp. 178-184, 1960.

Ilina, W.N.: Clinical experimental conditions to the elaboration of the method of electroshock-therapy. (Russ.) Diss., Jaroslavid, 1953.

Ilyuchenok, R.J.: The role of cholinergic systems of the brain stem reticular formation in the mechanism of central effects of anticholinesterase and cholinolytic drugs. *I Int Pharmacol Meeting Oxford,* (London), *8:*211, 1962.

Ilyuchenok, R.J.: Problems of chemical perceptibility of the brain stem reticular formation. *Psychopharmacol Methods,* Prague *2:*115, 1963.

Ilyuchenok, R.J.: Hemato-encephalic barrier and EEG changes in effects of cholinergic substances. *6th Int Congr Electroencephalogr Clin Neurophysiol, Wien,* p 513, 1965.

Ilyuchenok, R.J. and Mateeva, R.B.: Participation of M-cholinoreactive systems in the mechanism concerning the central action of chlorpromazine. (Russ) *Farmakol Toksikol, 28:*643, 1965.

Ingenito, A.J. and Bonnycastle, D.D.: On the relationship between drug-induced changes in brain amines and body temperature. *Can J Physiol Pharmacol, 45:*723, 1967.

Ingvar, D.H.: Experimental data on the effects of chlorpromazine on the central nervous system. *Nord Med, 58:*1611, 1957.

Isaacson, R.L., Schwartz, H., Persoff, N., and Pinson, L.: The role of the corpus callosum in the establishment of areas of secondary epileptiform activity. *Epilepsia, 12:*133-146, 1971.

Isler, W. and Dumermuth, G.: Fieberkrämpfe. Pädiat *Praxis, 7:*105, 1968.

Itil, T.M.: Die Veränderungen der Pentothal-Reaktion im Elektroencephalogramm bei Psychosen unter der Behandlung mit psychotropen Drogen. In *Proc III World Congr Psychiat.* Toronto, Univ. Toronto Press, p. 947, 1961.

Ivanenko, E.F. and Dunaeva, V.F.: The swelling of colloides in the brain at stimulation of the CNS. (Russ) *Biokhimia, 20:*636, 1955.

Iwama, K. and Jasper, H.H.: The action of gamma-amino-butyric acid on cortical electrical activity in the cat. *J Physiol, 138:*365, 1957.

Jackson, J.H.: Writings 1872-1899. In Taylor, Holmes, Walshe (Eds.): *Selected Writings of J.H. Jackson.* New York, Basic Books, Inc., vol. I. a. II, 1958.

Jackson, J.H. and Beevor, C.: Case of a tumour of the right temporosphenoidal lobe bearing on the localization of the sense of smell and on the interpretation of a particular variety of epilepsy. *Brain, 12:*346, 1890.

Jackson, J.H. and Stewart, J.P.: Epileptic attacks with a warning of a crude sensation of smell and with the intellectual aura (dreamy state) in a patient who had symptoms pointing to gross organic disease of the right temporo-spenoidal lobe. *Brain, 22:*534, 1899.

Jacobs, R.: The anti-epileptic Tegretol from the point of view of child-psychiatry and neurology. *Med Klin, 59:*1070, 1964.

Jaenicke, L.: Folsäurefermente und Einkohlenstoffeinheiten. In v. Kress, Blum (Eds.): *B-Vitamine.* Stuttgart, Schattauer, pp. 35-64, 1966.

Jaenicke, L. and Lynen, F.: Coenzyme A. In Boyer, Lardy, Myrbäk (Eds.): *The Enzymes.* New York, Academic Press, 1960, vol. III.

Jänkälä, E.O. and Näätänen, E.K.: Brain capillary permeability. An experimental study carried out with rabbits to determine the effect of psychic stress, insulin, adrenaline, corticoids and a sympathicolytic drug on the trypan blue vital staining method. *Ann Acad Sci fenn A, 50:*1, 1955.

Järnefelt, J.: Sodium-stimulated adenosin-triphosphastase in microsomes from rat brain. *Biochem Biophys Acta, 48:*104, 1961.

Jahn, D. and Greving, H.: Untersuchungen über die körperlichen Störungen bei katatonen Stuporen und der tödlichen Katatonie. *Arch Psychiatr, 105:*105, 1936.

Jantz, H.: Über Elektrophoreseuntersuchungen bei symptomatischen Psychosen. *Nervenarzt, 27:*193, 1956.

Janz, D.: Epilepsiebehandlung mit Hydantoinpräparaten. *Nervenarzt, 21:*3, 1950.

Janz, D.: "Nacht"-oder "Schlaf"-Epilepsien als Ausdruck einer Verlaufsform epileptischer Erkrankungen. *Nervenarzt, 24:*361, 1953a.

Janz, D.: "Aufwach"-Epilepsien (als Ausdruck einer den "Nacht"-oder "Schlaf"-Epilepsien gegenüberzustellenden Verlaufsform epileptischer Erkrankungen.) *Arch Psychiatr Z Neurol, 191:*73, 1953b.

Janz, D.: "Diffuse" Epilepsien, als Ausdruck einer Verlaufsform vorwiegend symptomatischer Epilepsien im Vergleich zu "Nacht"-und "Aufwach"-Epilepsien. *Dtsch Z Nervenheilkd, 170:*486, 1953c.

Janz, D.: Anfallsbild und Verlaufsform epileptischer Erkrankungen. *Nervenarzt, 26:*20, 1955.

Janz, D.: *Die Petit-Mal-Epilepsien.* (Habil. Schrift), Unpublished Dissertation, University Library, Heidelberg, 1955.

Janz, D.: Die klinische Stellung der Pyknolepsie. *Dtsch Med Wochenschr, 80:*1392, 1955.

Janz, D.: Wegweisung zur differenzierten Behandlung der Epilepsien. *Nervenarzt, 28:* 145, 1957.

Janz, D.: Gezielte Therapie der Epilepsien. *Dtsch Med Wochenschr, 82:*1158, 1957.

Janz, D.: Moderne Differentialdiagnostik und Therapie der Epilepsie. *Medizinische, 42:* 1517, 1957.

Janz, D.: Rehabilitation von Epileptikern im Rahmen einer Ambulanz. *Ärztl Mitt, 43:* 1227, 1958.

Janz, D.: Was sind eigentlich Epilepsien? Symptomatik einer alten Krankheit in neuem Licht. *Umschau, 22:*677, 1958.

Janz, D.: Moderne Epilepsie-Behandlung. *Umschau, 3:*68, 1959.

Janz, D. Die medikamentöse Behandlung der epileptischen Anfallserkrankungen. *Landarzt, 36:*271, 1960.

Janz, D.: Status epilepticus und Stirnhirn. *Dtsch Z Nervenheilkd, 180:*562, 1960.

Janz, D.: Condition and causes of status epilepticus. *Epilepsia, 2:*170, 1961.

Janz, D.: Gezielte Therapie bei Epilepsien. *Med Welt, 12:*629, 1962a.

Janz, D.: The Grand mal epilepsy and the sleeping waking cycle. *Epilepsia, 3:*69, 1962b.

Janz, D.: Differentialtypologie der idiopathischen Epilepsien. In *Psychopathologie Heute*. Stuttgart, Thieme, 1962.

Janz, D.: *Wegweisung zu einer differenzierten Behandlung der Epilepsien*. 3rd Ed. Dtsch. Sektion d. Intern. Liga gegen Epilepsie, 1962.

Janz, D.: Epilepsie-Ambulanz als Institution. *Dtsch med Wochenschr, 87*:953, 1962.

Janz, D.: Verlaufsgestalten idiopathischer Epilepsien. *Nervenarzt, 34*:333, 1963.

Janz, D.: Soziale Aspekte der Epilepsie. *Psychiatr Neurol Neurochir, 66*:240, 1963.

Janz, D.: Status epilepticus and frontal lobe lesions. *J Neurol Sci, 1*:446, 1964.

Janz, D.: Über das Suchtmoment in der Epilepsie. *Nervenarzt, 39*:350, 1968a.

Janz, D.: Zur Abgrenzung verschiedener Psychosyndrome bei Epilepsie. *Hippokrates, 39*: 402, 1968b.

Janz, D.: Anfalls-Syndrome. Psychiatrie der, Gegenwart, Forschung und Praxis, Vol. II/2. Kilnische Psychiatrie 2. (Eds.) K. P. Kisker, Meyer, J.-E., Müller, M., and E. Strömgren. Springer-Verlag Berlin-Heidelberg-New York, pp. 565-630, 1972.

Janz, D. and Christian, W.: Impulsiv-Petit mal. *Dtsch Z Nervenheilkd, 176*:346, 1957.

Janz, D. and Matthes, A.: *Die Propulsiv-Petit-mal-Epilepsie*. Basel-New York, Karger, 1955.

Janz, H.W.: Zur diagnostischen Verwertbarkeit der Cardiazolkrämpfe. *Munch Med Wochenschr, 1*:471, 1937.

Janz, H.W.: Die diagnostische Verwertbarkeit einiger Methoden zur Provokation epileptischer Anfälle. *Arch Psychiatr, 106*:267, 1937.

Janzen, R., Magun, R. and Becher, F.: Tierexperimentelle Untersuchungen über die Ausbreitung der epileptischen Erregung. I. Mitt. *Dtsch Z Nervenheilkr, 166*:223, 1951.

Janzen, R. and Müller, E.: Tierexperimentelle Untersuchungen über die Ausbreitung der epileptischen Erregung. II. Mitt. *Dtsch Z Nervenheilkr, 169*:181, 1952.

Janzen, R., Müller, E. and Becher, F.: Tierexperimentelle Studien über die Ausbreitung der epileptischen Erregung. III. Mitt. *Dtsch Z Nervenheilkr, 172*:259, 1954.

Jasper, H. and Drooglever-Fortuyn, J.: Experimental studies on the functional anatomy of petit mal epilepsy. *Res Publ Ass Nerv Ment Dis, 26*:272, 1947.

Jasper, H. and Erickson, T.C.: Cerebral blood flow and pH in excessive cortical discharge induced by metrazol and electrical stimulation. *J Neurophysiol, 4*:333, 1941.

Jasper, H., Naquet, R. and King, E.E.: Thalamocortical recruiting responses in sensory receiving areas in the cat. *Electroencephalogr Clin Neurophysiol, 7*:99, 1955.

Jasper, H., Pertuisset, B. and Flanigan, H.: EEG and cortical electrograms in patients with temporal lobe seizures. *Arch Neurol Psychiatr* (Chic), *65*:272, 1951.

Jatzkewitz, H.: Zwei Typen von Cerebrosidschwefelsäureestern als sogenannte "Prälipide" und Speichersubstanzen bei Leukodystrophie Typ Scholz (metachromatische Form der diffusen Sklerose). *Hoppe Seylers Z Physiol Chem, 311*:259, 1958.

Jelinski, J. and Kierzkowska-Dobrowolska, J.B.: Kozweinikow epilepsy in the case of tumor of frontal lobe. *Neurol Neurochir Psychiat Pol, 10*:541, 1960.

Jenney, E.H. and Pfeiffer, C.C.: The convulsant effect of hydrazides and the antidotal effect of anticonvulsants and metabolites. *J Pharmacol Exp Ther, 122*:110, 1958.

Jensen, H.P.: Die Behandlung der Trigeminusneuralgie mit Diphenylhydantoin. *Ärztl Wschr, 9*:5, 1954.

Jensen, H.P.: Die Behandlung der Trigeminusneuralgie mit Diphenylhydantoin. *Therapiewoche, 5*:345, 1955.

Jensen, H.P.: Behandlungsschema der genuinen Trigeminusneuralgie mit Zentropil. *Mat Med Nordm, 8*:13/14, 1956.

Jervis, G.A.: Phenylpyruvic oligophrenia; deficiency of phenylalanine oxidising system. *Proc Soc Exp Biol* (NY), *82*:514, 1953.

Jessel, H.J.: Erfahrungen mit Prothinpendyl in der Psychiatrie. *Dtsch Med Wochenschr, 85:*192, 1960.

Jörgensen, R.S. and Wulff, M.H.: The effect of orally administered chlorpromazine on the electroencephalogram of man. *Electroencephalogr Clin Neurophysiol, 10:*325, 1958.

John, K.: Zur Beurteilung psychischer Krankheitserscheinungen bei rechtsseitiger Schläfenlappenaffektion. *Z Neurol Psychiatr, 127:*569, 1930.

Johnston, J.B.: Further contributions to the study of the evolution of the forebrain. *J Comp Neurol, 35:*337, 1923.

Jonas, W. and Scheel-Krueger, J.: Amphetamine induced stereotyped behavior correlated with the accumulation of O-methylated Dopamine. *Arch Int Pharmacodyn, 177:*379, 1969.

de Jong, R.N.: "Psychomotor" or "temporal lobe" epilepsy. A review of the development of our present concepts. *Neurology* (Minneap), *7:*1, 1957.

Jongsmann, J.W.M.: Report on the anti-epileptic actions of Tegretol. *Epilepsia, 5:* 73, 1964.

Joss, J.C.: Traumatische Trigeminusneuralgie. *Mat Med Nordm, 9:*409, 1957.

Jouvet, M.: Paradoxical sleep. In Sleep Mechanisms. *Progr Brain Res, 18:*20, 1965.

Jouvet, M.: Neurophysiologische Mechanismen im Schlaf. In Jovanović, U.J. (Ed.): *Der Schlaf. Neurophysiologische Aspekte.* München, Barth, 1969.

Jouvet, M.: The Role of Monoamines and Acetylcholine-Containing Neurons in the Regulation of the Sleep-Waking Cycle. In "Review of Physiology" "(Neurophysiology and Neurochemistry of Sleep and Wakefulness)." With Contributions by M. Jouvet and G. Moruzzi. Springer-Verlag, Berlin-Heidelberg-New York. Vol. 64, pp. 166, 1972.

Jouvet, M., Delorme, F. and Jouvet, D.: Evolution des signes électriques du sommeil paradoxal au cours de la narcose au pentobarbital. *C R Soc Biol, Paris, 159:*387, 1965.

Jovanović, U.J.: Über die Allergie. Vortrag im Fachklub d. med. Fakultät Sarajewo, Oktober, 1959.

Jovanović, U.J.: Über die Rolle der biogenen Amine in der Allergie. *Sarajevski Medicinar, 1:*1, 1960.

Jovanović, U.J.: Das Elektrenzephalogramm des Menschen unter Wirkungvon 2-Diäthylamino-5-Phenyl-Oxazolinon-(4). *Ärztl Forsch, 19:*640, 1965.

Jovanović, U.J.: Experimentelle Untersuchungen über die Wirkung des 2-Diäthylamino-5-Phenol Oxazolinon-(4) (Ha 94) auf das EEG der Epileptiker. *Ärztl Forsch, 20:*98, 1966a.

Jovanović, U.J.: Elektroencephalographische und klinische Betrachtungen über die Wirkung des 2-Diäthylamino-5-Phenyl-Oxazolinon-(4) beim Menschen. *Ärztl Forsch, 20:*121, 1966b.

Jovanović, U.J.: Die diagnostische Bedeutung des Schlafelektroencephalogramms. *Dtsch Med Jour, 17:*121, 1966c.

Jovanović, U.J.: Natürlicher Schlaf als beste diagnostische Provokationsmethode bei Epileptikern. Schweiz. *Arch Neurol Psychiatr, 98:*244, 1966d.

Jovanović, U.J.: Forcierte Normalisierung im EEG (Landolt) und forcirte Pathologisierung des Schlaf-Elektroencephalogramms. *Psychiatr Neurol* (Schweiz), *152:*370, 1966e.

Jovanović, U.J.: Das Schlafelektroencephalogramm als spezielle diagnostische Methode. *Landarzt, 43:*600, 1967a.

Jovanović, U.J.: Schlaf und Epilepsie. *Therapiewoche, 17:*95, 1967b.

Jovanović, U.J.: Neure Aspekte zur Einteilung der Epilepsie aufgrund von Schlafuntersuchungen. *Zbl Neurol Psychiatr, 188:*22, 1967c.

Jovanović, U.J.: Das Schlafverhalten der Epileptiker. I. Schlafdauer, Schlaftiefe und Besonderheiten der Schlafperiodik. *Dtsch Z Nervenheilkd, 190:*159, 1967d.

Jovanović, U.J.: Das Schlafverhalten der Epileptiker. II. Elemente des EEG, Vagetativum und Motorik. *Dtsch Z Nervenheilkd, 191:*257, 1967e.

Jovanović, U.J.: Prüfung eines barbitursäurehaltigen Schlafmittels. Die Wirkung von 5-Vinyl-5-(1-Methylbutyl)-barbitursäure. *Arnzneim Forsch, 17:*365, 1967f.

Jovanović, U.J.: Das Schlafverhalten der Epileptiker. III. Epileptische Anfälle und Äquivalente. *Dtsch Med Jour, 19:*67a. 112, 1968a.

Jovanović, U.J.: Zur Vermeidung von Nebenwirkungen der Behandlung mit Elektrokrampf. *Arzneim Forsch, 18:*417, 1968b.

Jovanović, U.J.: Die sich aus dem natürlichen Schlaf der Epileptiker, ergebenden therapeutischen Konsequenzen. *Nervnarzt, 39:*199, 1968c.

Jovanović, U.J.: Das Schlafverhalten der Epileptiker. IV. Psycho-physiologische Korrelate des Traums. Unpublished. (1968d).

Jovanović, U.J.: Das Schlafverhalten der Epileptiker. V. Konsequenzen und Schulssfolgerungen. Unpubl. (1968e).

Jovanović, U.J. (Ed.): *Der Schlaf—Neurophysiologische Aspekte.* München, Barth, 1969.

Jovanović, U.J.: Schlafforschung und ihre klinischen Aspekte. *Nervenarzt, 41:*5, 1970a.

Jovanović, U.J.: Somnambule psychomotorische Epilepsie. *Dtsch Z Nervenheilkd, 197:* 181, 1970b.

Jovanović, U.J.: *Cosaldon und Elektroschock.* In Press. 1970c.

Jovanović, U.J.: *Elektrokrampf bei zusätzlicher Gabe von SK-7 und Nikotinsäure.* In Press, 1970d.

Jovanović, U.J.: *Serum-Elektrophorese bei Epilepsien.* Unpublished manuscript 1970e.

Jovanović U.J.: *Normal Sleep in Man,* (Monograph). Hippokrates Verlag, Stuttgart, 1971a.

Jovanović, U.J.: Zur Frage der Differenzierung der psychomotorischen Epilepsie von den anderen Epilepsieformen aufgrund von Befunden mittels Serum-Elektrophorese. Unpublished Manuscript, 1971b.

Jovanović, U.J.: Disturbed Sleep in Man. (Monograph), Unpublished Manuscript 1972a.

Jovanović, U.J.: Polygraphische registrierungen nach parenteraler applikation von 3-7-Dimethyl-1-(5-oxo-hexyl)-xanthin (BL 191). *Arzneim Forsch (Drug Res), 22:*994-999, 1972b.

Jovanović, U.J.: Die Beeinflussbarkeit der spezifischen Krampfelemente im Elektroencephalogramm der Epileptiker durch eine intravenöse Applikation von 3,7-Dimethyl-l-(5-oxo-hexyl)-xanthin (BL 191). Unpublished Manuscript, 1972c.

Jovanović, U.J.: Beziehungen der epileptischen Anfälle zu den Schlafstadien. Polygraphische Untersuchungen während des Anfalls und in den Intervallen. Unpublished Manuscript, 1972d.

Jovanović, U.J.: *Die Behandlung der Kranken mit Enuresis nocturna mit Monochlorimipramin (Anafranil®).* In Press, 1972e.

Jovanović, U.J., Boerner, D. and Henschler, D.: Veränderungen der Hirnaktivität nach experimentell verabreichten Barbituraten in toxischen Dosen. Sitzungsber. Dtsch. EEG-Ges., *EEG-EMG, 1:*119, 1970.

Jovanović, U.J. and Sattes, H.: Die Behandlumg der endogenen Depressionen mit Chlorimipramin (Anafranil). *Schweiz Med Wochenschr, 97:*1917, 1967.

Jovanović, U.J. and Schäfer, E.-R.: Elektroencephalogramm und Klinik der Schlafepileptiker unter Berücksichtigung des Schlafes vor und nach der Behandlung. *Nervenarzt, 37:*290, 1966.

Jovanović, U.J. and Tan-Eli, B.: Penile erection during sleep. *Arzneim Forsch, 19:*966, 1968.

Juchlov, A.K.: Histological changes in the CNS in experimental epilepsiy. II. In *Mechanisms of Pathological Reactions.* (Russ) VMMA, pp. 395-397, 1952.

Julian, R.M., and Halperin, L.M.: Effects of diphenylhydantoin and other antiepileptic drugs on epileptiform activity and purkinje cell discharges rates. *Epilepsia, 13:*384-400, 1972.

Jung, R.: Hirnelektrische Untersuchungen über den Elektrokrampf. *Arch Psychiatr Neurol, 183:*206, 1949.

Jung, R.: Neurophysiologische Untersuchungsmethoden. In *Hb. d. Inn. Med.* Berlin-Heidelberg-Wien, Springer, vol. V, pp. 1206, 1953.

Jung, R.: Neuropharmakologie: Zentrale Wirkungsmechanismen chemischer Substanzen und ihre neurophysiologischen Grundlagen. *Klin Wochenschr, 36:*1153, 1958.

Jung, R.: *EEG-Korrelate von Bewuss tseinsveränderungen: Tierexperimentelle Grundlagen. EEG-*Untersuchungen bie Bewusstseinsveränderungen des Menschen ohne neurologische Erkrankungen. I. Congr. Int. Sci. Neurol. Bruxelles, pp. 147, a. 208, 1957.

Jung, R.: *Hirnpotentialwellen, Neuronenentladungen und Gleichspannungsphänomene.* Jenenser EEG-Symposium, 1959, VEB-Verlag, pp. 54-81, 1963.

Jung, R.: Physiologie und Pathophysiologie des Schlafes. *Verh. Dtsch. Ges. Inn. Med.,* 71. Kongr. München, Bergmann, 1965.

Jung, R. and Kornmüller, A.E.: Eine Methodik der Ableitung lokalisierter Potentialschwankungen aus subkortikalen Hirngebieten. *Arch Psychiatr Nervenkr, 109:*1, 1938.

Jung, R. and Tönnies, J.F.: Über Entstehung und Erhaltung von Krampfentladungen. Die Vorgänge am Reizort und die Bremsfähigkeit des Gehirnes. *Arch Psychiatr, 185:*701, 1950.

Kaada, B.R.: Somato-motor, autonomic and electrocorticographic responses to electrical stimulation of "rhinencephalic" and other structures in primates, cats and dogs. *Acta Physiol Scand, 24:*suppl. 83, 1951.

Kaada, B.R.: Cingulate, posterior orbital, anterior insular and temporal pole cortex. In Field, J. (Ed.): *Hb.of.Physiology.Sect.I.,* (Am Physiol. Soc.) Washington, vol. II, pp. 1345, 1960.

Kaada, B.R., Andersen, P. and Jansen, J.: Stimulation of the hippocampus and medical cortical areas in unanesthetized cats. *Neurology (Minneap), 3:*844, 1953.

Kaada, B.R., Andersen, P. and Jansen, J.: Stimulation of the amygdaloid nuclear complex in unanesthetized cats. *Neurology,* (Minneap), *4:*48, 1954.

Kaada, B.R. and Jasper, H.: Respiratory response to stimulation of temporal pole, insula and hippocampal and limbic gyri in man. *Arch Neurol, 68:*609, 1952.

Kaada, B.R., Pribram, K.H. and Epstein, J.A.: Respiratory and vascular responses in monkeys from temporal pole, insula, orbital surface and cingulate gyrus. *J Neurophysiol, 12:*347, 1949.

Kaim, S.C. and Rosenstein, I.N.: Anticonvulsant properties of a new psychotherapeutic drug. *Dis Nerv Syst, 21:*46, 1960.

Kajtor, F.: Experimentelle Untersuchungen über die Hemmungswirkungen von Histamin und anderen gefässerweiternden Mitteln auf die Krämpfe im Cardiazol- und Elektroschock am Menschen. *Arch Psychiatr Z Neurol, 186:*46, 1951.

Kalinowsky, L.B.: Entziehungskrämpfe und Entziehungspsychosen. *Nervenarzt, 29:*465, 1958.

Kamrin, R.P. and Kamrin, A.A.: The effects of pyridoxine antagonists and other convulsive agents on amino acid concentrations of the mouse brain. *J Neurochem, 6:* 219, 1961.

Kanai, T. and Szerb, J.C.: Mesencephalic reticular activating system and cortical acetylcholine output. *Nature, 205:*80, 1965.

Kanig, K.: *Der Einfluss zentral wirksamer Substanzen auf den Nucleotid-Stoffwechsel des Gehirns.* Habil. Schrift, Freie Universit. Berlin, 1963.

Kanig, K.: Experimental and clinical biochemistry; energy metabolism. In Bente, Bradley (Eds.): *Neuro-Psychopharmacology.* Amsterdam, Elsevier, vol. IV, pp. 27-30, 1965.

Kanig, K.: Zur Biochemie psychotischer Erkrankungen. *Hippokrates, 36:*457, 1966.

Kanig, K.: Die Neurochemie als Grundlagenforschung und ihre Bedeutung für die Klinik. *Med Welt, 18:*23, 1967.

Kanig, K.: *Die Bedeutung der B-Vitamine für das Nervensystem.* Wiss. Berichte, E. Merck, A.G., Darmstadt, 1968.

Kanig, K.: Der Einfluβ von Pharmaka auf den Nucleotid-Stoffwechsel des Gehirns. Beitrag zur Theorien-Bildung in der Schizophrenie-Forschung. *Arzneim Forsch, 19:* 397, 1969.

Kanig, K.: Biocehmische Aspekte bei symptomatoischen Psychosen. Janssen Symposien, Weinsberg 1970. In Reimer, F. (Ed.): *Zur diagnostischen und therapeutischen Problematik symptomatischer Psychosen.* Janssen Düsseldorf, 1970.

Kanig, K.: Die Rolle des Aminosäuren- und Aminostoffwechsels bei endogenen Psychosen. *Hippokrates, 42:*393-394, 1971a.

Kanig, K.: Zum Stoffwechsel der Psychopharmaka. Enzyme und Pharmaka, Editiones "Roche" Basel, pp. 289-303, 1971b.

Kanig, K.: Erforschung der bichemischen Grundlagen der Schizophrenien. In "Äthiologie der Schizophrenien. Bestandsaufnahme und Zukunftsperspektiven". 1. Weissenauer Schizophreniesynposion. (Ed.) G. Huber, F.K. Schattauer Verlag, Stuttgart-New York, pp. 127-156, 1971c.

Kanig, K.: Biocehmische Aspekte bei endogenen Psychosen. *Münchner Med Wochenschrift, 114:*422-423, 1972.

Kanig, K., and W. Oesterle: Der Einfluss von Psychopharmaka auf den Gehirnstoffwechsel. *Pharmakopsychiatrie/Neuro-Psychopharmakologie, 4:*105-122, 1971.

Kanig, K., W. Oseterle and N. Rubly: Nucleinsäuren im Rattengehirn, II. Stoffwechsel einezlner RNA-Fraktionen. *Hoppe-Seyler's Z Physiol Chem 352:* 977-983, 1971.

Kaps, G.: Über elektrophoretische Untersuchungen an Hirngewebe, insbesondere aus der Umgebung von Tumoren — zugleich ein Beitrag zur Pathogenese von Hirnschwellung und Hirnödem. *Arch Psychiatr Nervenkr, 192:*115, 1954.

Karcher, D., van Sande, M. and Lowenthal, A.: Micro-electrophoresis in agar gel of proteins of the cerebrospinal fluid and central nervous system. *J Neurochem, 4:*135, 1959.

Karlson, P.: Biochemistry of morphogenesis. *Dtsch Med Wochenschr, 88:*1029, 1963.

Kashiwagi, S., Hiramatsu, H., Wada, M. and Sugiura, M.: The action of adrenaline on the cyclophorase system. *Jap J Pharmacol, 7:*16, 1957.

Kasimirova, Z.N.: Carbohydrate-phosphor metabolism in the brain of mice at stimulation and inhibition of the cortex. *Theses to the Conference L.O.L.G.U., Biol.Sect.* Leningrad, 1953-54 (Russ).

Kasimirova, Z.N.: cit. by Prochorovoy, M.I., 1956.

Kass, E.H., Geiman, Q.M. and Finland, M.: Effects of ACTH on induced malaria in man. *N Engl J Med, 245:*1000, 1951.

Kassil, G.N.: Brain metabolism at different states of the blood-brain barrier. IV. Nitrogen metabolism in brain. (Russ.) *Byull Eksp Biol Med, 3:*226, 1937.

Kassil, G.N.: Metabolism in the CNS. *Advances of modern biology, 9:*434, 1938 (Russ.).

Kassil, G.N. and Plotitzina, T.G.: Rapports entre le métabolisme du cerveau et l' état de la barriére hématoencéphalique. I. II, III. *Byull Biol Med eksp SSSR, 1:* 73 a. 368, a. 415, 1936.
Kaufmann, M.: *Beiträge zur Pathologie des Stoffwechsels bei Psychosen.* 3. Teil. 1941.
Kaufmann, S.: The enzymatic conversion of phenylalanine to tyrosine. *Biochem Biophys Acta, 23:*445, 1957a.
Kaufmann, S.: The enzymatic conversion of phenylalanine to tyrosine. *J Biol Chem, 226:*511, 1957b.
Kaufmann, S.: A new factor required for the enzymatic conversion of phenylalanine to tyrosine. *J Biol Chem, 230:*931, 1958.
Kaufmann, S.: Studies on the mechanism of the enzymatic conversion of phenylalanine to tyrosine. *J Biol Chem, 234:*2677, 1959.
Kaufmann, S.: The nature of the primary oxidation product formed from tetrahydropteridines during phenylalanine hydroxylation. *J Biol Chem, 236:*804, 1961.
Kaufmann, S.: On the structure of the phenylalanine hydroxylation cofactor. *J Biol Chem, 237:*PC2712, 1962.
Kaufmann, S.: The structure of the phenylalanine hydroxylation cofactor. *Proc Nat Acad Sci, 50:*1085, 1963.
Kaufmann, S., Bridgers, W.F., Eisenberg, F. and Freidman, S.: The source of oxygen in the phenylalanine hydroxylase and the dopamine-β-hydroxylase catalysed reactions. *Biochem Biophys Res Commun, 9:*497, 1962.
Kaul, C.L., Lewis, J.J., Livingstone, S.D.: Influence of chlorpromazine on the levels of adenine nucleotides in the rat brain and hypothalamus *in vivo. Biochem Pharmacol, 14:*165, 1965.
Keith, F.E. and Ardoline, G.A.: Anticonvulsant action of Methaminodiazepoxide hydrochloride. *Fed Proc, 19:*263, 1960.
Kelentei, B. and Földes, J.: Haemato-encephalic barrier. I. Effects of hyaluronidase with special reference to the passage of antibiotics. *Acta Physiol Acad Sci Hung, 5:*139, 1954.
Keller, E.B., Boisonnas, R.A. and du Vigneaud, V.: Origin of methyl group epinephrine. *J Biol Chem, 183:*627, 1950.
Kelmischkeut, E.G.: Comparative biochemical studies in involutional psychoses und schizophrenia of old people. In *Obm. Veshtch. Psikhiatr. Zabol.* Moscow, Medgiz, pp. 94-98, 1960.
Kelmischkeut, E.G. and Sigrist, A.V.: Proteins and their fractions in blood serum of sane persons and schizophrenics dependent on the biological development. (Russ.) In *Obm. Veshtch. Psikhiat. Zabol.* Moscow, Medgiz, pp. 85-93, 1960.
Kemali, D. and Romano, G.: Ulteriori dati cromatografici sul dismetabolismo indolico in schizofrenici. *Acta neurol* (Napoli), *11:*959, 1956.
Kendrick, J.F. and Gibbs, F.A.: Origin, spread and neurosurgical treatment of the psychomotor type of seizure discharge. *J Neurosurg, 14:*270, 1957.
Kennard, M.A.: The electroencephalogram and disorders of behavior. A review. *J Nerv Ment Dis, 124:*103, 1956.
Kety, S.S.: Biochemical theories of schizophrenia. A two-part critical review of current theories and of the evidence used to support them. *Science, 129:*1528, a. 1590, 1959.
Kety, S.S.: Current biochemical approaches to schizophrenia. *Proc. 4th World Congr. Psychiat, 1966;* Part 1 Amsterdam, Excerpta Med. Found., pp. 501, 1967.
Kety, S.S. and Schmidt, C.F.: Effects of altered arterial tensions of CO_2 and O on cerebral blood flow and cerebral O consumption. *J Clin Invest, 27:*476, 1948.

Ketz, E.: Status epilepticus—Aktuelles an Erscheinungsbild, Ursache und zeitgemässer Therapie. *Therapie d Gegenw, 106:*741, 1967.

Keynes, R.D. and Maisel, G.W.: The energy requirement for sodium extrusion from a frog muscle. *Proc Roy Soc* (Lond), Ser. B., *142:* 383, 1954.

Kiessling, H.: Auswirkungen des Fluphenazins "Lyogen" auf die seelischen Veränderungen, die Anfallshäufigkeit und das EEG von Epileptikern. *Nervenarzt, 35:*543, 1964.

Killam, E.K.: Drug action on the brain stem reticular formation. *Pharmacol Rev, 14:* 175, 1962.

Killam, E.K. and Killam, K.F.: The influence of drugs on central afferent pathways. In Fields, W.S. (Ed.): *Brain Mechanisms and Drug Action.* Springfield, Thomas, 1957.

Killiam, E.K., Killam, K.F. and Shaw, T.: The effect of psychotherapeutic compounds on central afferent and limbic pathways. *Ann NY Acad Sci, 66:*784, 1957.

Killam, K.F.: Convulsant hydrazides. II. Comparison of electrical changes and enzyme inhibition induced by the administration of thiosemicarbazide. *J Pharmacol Exp Ther, 119:*263, 1957.

Killam, K.F.: Possible role of gamma-aminobutyric acid as an inhibitory transmitter. *Fed Proc, 17:*1018, 1958.

Killam, K.F. and Bain, J.A.: Convulsant hydrazides: I. *in vitro* and *in vivo* inhibition of vitamin B_1 enzymes by convulsant hydrazides. *J Pharmacol Exp Ther, 119:*255, 1957.

Killam, K.F. and Killam, E.K.: Drug action on pathways involving the reticular formation. In Jasper, Proctor, Knighton, Noshay, Costello (Eds.): *Reticular Formation of the Brain.* Henry Ford Hospital Symposium. Boston, Little, Brown & Co., pp. 111-122, 1958.

Kimball, O.P.: The treatment of epilepsy with sodium diphenyl hydantoinate. *JAMA, 112:*1244, 1939.

King, E.E., Naquet, R. and Magoun, H.W.: Action of pentobarbital on somatic afferent conduction in the cat with special reference to the thalamic relay. *J Pharmacol, 113:* 31, 1955.

King, E.E., Naquet, R. and Magoun, H.W.: Alterations in somatic afferent transmission through the thalamus by central mechanisms and barbiturates. *J Pharmacol, 119:*48, 1957.

King, G. and Weeks, S.D.: Pyribenzamine activation of the electroencephalogram. *Electroencephalogr Clin Neurophysiol, 18:*503, 1965.

Kini, M.M. and Quastel, J.H.: Carbohydrate-amino acid irrelations in brain cortex *in vitro. Nature* (Lond), *184:*252, 1959.

Kirk, R.Th.: Amino acid and ammonia metabolism in liver diseases. 1936.

Kirshner, N.: Biosynthesis of adrenaline and noradrenaline. *Pharmacol Rev, 11:*350, 1959.

Kirshner, N. and McGoodall, C.: Formation of adrenaline from noradrenaline. *Biochem Biophys Acta, 24:*658, 1957a.

Kirshner, N. and McGoodall, C.: Biosynthesis of adrenaline and noradrenaline *in vitro. J Biol Chem, 226:*213, 1957b.

Kishimoto, Y. and Ralin, N.S.: cit. by Rossiter, R.J.: Chemical constituents of brain and nerve. In Elliott, Page. Quastel (Eds.) *Neurochemistry.* 2nd Ed. Springfield, Thomas, 1962.

Kitay, J.I. and Altschule, M.D.: Blood ketone concentration in patients with mental and emotional disorders. *Arch Neurol Psychiatr* (Chic), *68:*506, 1952.

Kiyota, K.: Electrophoretic protein fractions and the hydrophilic property of brain tissue. II. The protein of brains with edema. *J Neurochem, 4:*209, 1959.

Kiyota, K.: Abnormality of protein distribution on the epileptic brain and its significance. *Fol Psychiatr Neurol Jap, 15:*10, 1961.

Klapetek, J.: Induction of latent epileptic activity with megimide in temporal epilepsy (Czech). *26:*160-164, 1963.

Klapetek, J.: Alteration of latent epileptic activity in the EEG with chlorpromazine (Czech). *Cas Lek Cesk 103:*742-745, 1964.

Klein, J.R. and Olsen, N.S.: Effect of convulsive activity upon the concentration of brain glucose, glycocen, lactate and phosphate. *J Biol Chem, 167:*746, 1947.

Klein, K.E.: Die sensible Chronaxie in der Klinik. *Dtsch Z Nervenheilkd, 176:*25, 1957.

Klenk, E.: Über die Natur der Phosphatide der Milz bei der Niemann-Pick'schen Krankheit. 10. Mitt. über Phosphatide. *Hoppe Seylers Z Physiol Cheme 229;*151, 1934.

Klenk, E.: Beiträge zur Chemie der Lipoidosen. 3. Mitt. Niemann-Pick'sche Krankheit und amaurotische Idioten. *Hoppe Seylers Z Physiol Chem, 262:*128, 1939.

Klenk, E.: The pathological chemistry of the developing brain. In Waelsch, H. (Ed.): *Biochemistry of the Developing Nervous System.* New York, Academic Press, 1955.

Kletzkin, M. and Swan, K.: The effects of meprobamate and pentobarbital upon cortical and subcortical responses to auditory stimulation. *J Pharmacol, 125:*35, 1959.

Klimes, K. and Lang, A.: Serumeiweiβuntersuchungen bei Epileptikern. *Arch Psychiatr D, 114:*691, 1942.

Klingler, J.: Die makroskopische Anatomie der Ammonshornformation. *Denkschr d Schweiz Naturforsch Ges Bd, 78:*33, 1948.

Klüver, H.: Brain mechanisms and behavior with special reference to the rhinencephalon. *Lancet* (Minneap), *72:*567, 1952.

Klüver, H. and Bucy, P.C.: "Psychic blindness" and other symptoms following bilateral temperal lobectomy in Rhesus monkey. *Am J Physiol, 119:*352, 1937.

Klüver, H. and Bucy, P.C.: Preliminary analysis of functions of the temporal lobes in monkeys. *Arch Neurol Psychiatr* (Chic), *42:*979, 1939.

Knapp, A.: *Die Geschwülste des rechten und linken Schläfenlappens.* Wiesbaden, Bergmann, 1905.

Knapp, A.: Die Tumoren des Schläfenlappens. *Z Neurol, 42:*226, 1918.

Knauel, H. and Grüter, W.: Über psychotrope Wirkungen von Tegretal. *Votr. vor d. Int. Liga gegen Epilepsie Dtsch. Sekt.,* Tübingen, Unpublished Congr. Report, 1966.

Kobinger, W.: Beeinflussung der Cardiazolkrampfschwelle durch veränderten 5-Hydroxytryptamingehalt des Zentralnervensystems. *Arch Exp Path Pharmakol, 233:*559, 1958.

Koe, B.K. and Weissman, A.: Chlorphenylalanine: a specific depletor of brain serotonine. *J Pharm Exp Ther, 154:*499, 1966.

Koelle, G.B.: Neurohumoral functions of acetylcholine and acetylcholinesterase. *J Pharm Pharmacol, 14:*65, 1962.

Koenig, H.: Epileptogenic action of substances that interact with gangliosides. *Trans Amer Neurol Ass, 87:*57, 1962.

Koenig, J.Q.: A study of pulvinar-cortical interaction in acute acid-induced epilepsy in the cat. *Epilepsia, 13:*445-457, 1972.

Kogan, R.: Über das Eindringen von Jodionen in die Schädelhöhle bei Ionisierung. *Zh nevropatol Psikhiatr, 20:*239, 1927.

Kogan, S.A. and Moskovich, E.G.: Epileptic seizures in patients suffering from diabetes mellitus. (Russ) *Klin Med, 43:*60, 1965.

Koikegami, H. and Fuse, S.: Studies on the functions and fiber connections of the amygdaloid nuclei in periamygdaloid cortex. Experiments on the respiratory movements. *Folia Psychiatr Neurol Jap, 6*:94, 1952.

Koikegami, H., Kushiro, H. and Kimoto, A.: Studies on the functions and fiber connections of the amygdaloid nuclei and periamygdaloid nuclei and periamygdaloid cortex. *Folia Psychiatr Neurol Jap, 6*:76, 1952.

Koikegami, H., Yamada, K. and Usui, K.: Stimulation of amygdaloid nuclei and periamygdaloid cortex with special reference to its effects on uterine movements and ovulation. *Folia Psychiatr Neurol Jap, 8*:7, 1954.

Kolle, K.: *Psychiatrie.* 4th Ed. Munich, Urban & Schwarzenberg, 1955.

Kolousek, J., Herab, F. and Jiraček, V.: Beitrag zur Kenntnis des Stickstoffmetabolismus des Gehirns der Ratten, die einem akustischen epileptitogenen Reiz gegenüber empfindlich oder unempfindlich sind. *J Neurochem, 4*:175, 1959a.

Kolousek, J. and Jiraček, V.: Stickstoffmetabolismus des Gehirns und der Leber bei Ratten nach einer Applikation von Methioninsulfoximin. *J Neurochem, 4*:178, 1959b.

Kolousek, J. and Lodin, Z.: Effect of D, L-methionine sulfoximide on metabolism of ^{35}S-D, L-methionine in organs of the dog and the rat. *Physiol Bohemoslov, 8*:129, 1959.

Kopeloff, L.M., Barrera, J.E. and Kopeloff, N.: Recurrent convulsive seizures in animals produced by immunological and chemical means. *Am J Psychiatry, 98*:881, 1942.

Koresner, P.E.: Some observations on the hippuric acid test in schizophrenia. *Acta Psychiatr* (Kopenh), *47*:145, 1947.

Kornmüller, A.E.: *Die bioelektrischen Erscheinungen der Hirnrindenfelder.* Leipzig, Thieme, 1937.

Kornmüller, A.E.: Erregbarkeitssteuernde Elemente und Systeme des Nervensystems. *Fortschr Neurol Psychiatr, 18*:437, 1950.

Koschtojanc, H.S.: *Akad Nauk SSSR, 6*:60. 1948; cit. by Lando, L.I.: The hyaluronidase in blood serum of schizophrenics during treatment. (Russ.) In *Obm Veshtch. Psikhiat. Zabol.* Moscow, Medgiz, pp. 65-75, 1960.

Koschtojanc, H.S.: *Proteins, Metabolism and Neuro-Regulation.* (Russ), Moscow, Acad. Nauk SSSR., 1951.

Kovaleva, E.J.: The glycemic curve after load with saccharose in schizophrenic and manic depressive psychoses. (Russ) In *Obm. Veshtch. Psikhiat. Zabol.* Moscow, Medgiz, pp. 62-65, 1960.

Kraepelin, E.: *Einführung in die Psychiatrische Klinik,* 1st. Ed. Leipzig, Barth, 1900.

Kraepelin, E.: *Psychiatrie. Ein Lehrbuch für Studierende und Ärzte.* 8th. Ed. Leipzig, Barth, vol. II, 1909.

Kraepelin, E.: *Das epileptische Irresein. Lehrbuch der Psychiatrie.* part II, Leipzig, Barth, vol. III, 1913.

Krainski, N.N.: On the signification of nitrogen of carbamic acid in the organism and its action on the development of the epileptic seizure. (Russ) *Zh Psikhait Nevrol eksp Psikhol, 6*:435 a. *8*:603, 1896.

Kramer, S.Z. and Seifter, J.: The effects of GABA and biogenic amines on behavior and brain electrical activity in chicks. *Life Sci, 5*:527, 1966.

Krasilinovka, M.N.: Dysfunction of liver in schizophrenia. (Russ) In *Obm. Veshtch. Psikhait. Zabol.* Moscow, Medgiz, pp. 154-158, 1960.

Krasnova, A.I.: The polarographic activity of blood serum of schizophrenics and epileptics. (Russ) In *Obm. Veshtch. Psikhiat. Zabol.* Moscow, Medgiz, pp. 114-119, 1960.

Krasnova, A.I. and Pogodaev, K.I.: Protein metabolism in the brain in experimentally induced epileptic seizures. In *Problems of Epilepsy.* (Russ), pp. 302-319, 1959.

Kraus, P. and Simane, Z.: The influence of perathiepine and chlorpromazine on some enzyme reactions in rat brain preparations. *Experientia, 23*:90, 1967.

Krause, G.: Klinische Erfahrungen mit Distraneurin. *Med Klin, 59*:1550, 1964.

Krayenbühl, H., Hess, R. and Weber, G.: Elektroencephalographische und therapeutische Ergebnisse bei der chirurgischen Behandlung von 21 Fällen mit sogenannter Schläfenlappenepilepsie. *Zbl Neurol Psychiatr, 128*:327, 1954.

Krebs, H.A. and Johnson, W.A.: Metabolism of ketonic acids in animal tissues. *Biochem J, 31*:645, 1937.

Kreienberg, W. and Erhardt, H.: Die Gehirndurchblutung im Elektroschock. *Nervearzt, 18*:154, 1947.

Kreindler, A.: Recherches expérimentales sur les rélations entre le sinus carotidien et le système nerveux central. *Bull Soc Sci Acad Roum, 28*:448, 1946.

Kreindler, A.: *Epilepsia.* Bucuresti, Acad. R.P.R., 1955.

Kreindler, A.: *Epilepsia.* Kliniceskie i experimentalnyie issledovania. Moskova, Medgiz, 1960.

Kreindler, A.: *Experimental epilepsy. Progr. Brain Res.* Amsterdam, Elsevier, Vol. 19, 1965.

Kreindler, A., Brosteanu, R. and Poilici, J.: Coreltii electroencefalografice şi vegetative. *Stud Cercet Neurol, 2*:462, 1957.

Kreindler, A., Crighel, E. and Tudor, L.: Mechanisme reflexie si anoxice în modificarile electrocorticografice produse de insuficienta circulatorie cerebrala acuta. *Stud Cercet Neurol, 8*:93, 1963.

Kreis, A.: Reflexepilepsie. Diss. Zürich, 1968.

Krings, F.: Trigeminusneuralgie. *Mat Med Nordm, 7*:472, 1955.

Krischek, J.: Die Schlaf-Wach-Periodik der Grand-mal Epilepsie und die sich daraus ergebenden therapeutischen Konsequenzen. *Dtsch Med Wochenschr, 78*:2528, 1962.

Kristiansen, K. and Courtois, G.: Rhythmic electrical activity from isolated cerebral cortex. *Electroenceph Clin Neurophysiol, 1*:265, 1949.

Kröber, E.: Die Praxis der Epilepsiebehandlung. *Dtsch Med Wochenschr, 76*:10, 1951.

Kröber, E.: Über Monoaminoxydase-Hemmer. *Psychiatr Neurol,* (Basel), *140*:92, 1960.

Kronenberg, G.: Pharmakologische Grundlagen der Kombination Reserpin-Mephenamin (Phasein), *Nervenarzt, 29*:266, 1958.

Kroth, H. and Hopf, H.C.: Status psychomotorischer Anfälle. *Dtsch Z Nervenheilkd, 189*:67, 1966.

Krüger, H.J.: Katamnestische Erhebungen üben einen Zeitraum von 9 Jahren zur Therapie der Epilepsie mit Carbamazepin. *Med Welt 23:* Heft 24, 1972.

Krüger, H.J. and Schwarz, H.: Klinische Mitteilung zur Epilepsie-Therapie mit Maliasin. *Med Welt, 14*:690, 1965.

Krupenina, L.B.: Electrophoretic studies of serum-proteins in patients with epilepsy. (Russ) In *Obm. Veshtch. Psikhiat. Zabol.* Moscow, Medgiz, pp. 159-166, 1960.

Kruse, H.D., Orent, E., and McCollum, E.V.: Studies on magnesium deficiency in animals. I. Symptomatology resulting from magnesium deprivation. *J Biol Chem, 96:* 519, 1932.

Kruse, R.: Schlafepilepsie im Kindesalter. *Nervenarzt, 35*:200, 1964.

Kruse, R.: Osteopathien bei antieplieptischer Langzeittherapie. (Vorläufige Mitteilung). *Mschr Kinderheilkd, 116*:378, 1968.

Kuchinskas, E.J., Horvath, A. and du Vigneaud, V.: An antivitamin B_6 action of L-penicillamine. *Arch Biochem Biophys, 68*:69, 1957.

Kuchinskas, E.J. and du Vigneaud, V.: An increased vitamin B_6 requirement in the rat on a diet containing L-penicillamine. *Arch Biochem Biophys, 66*:1, 1957.

Kudravčeva, A.I. and Kudravčeva, N.G.: On the biochemistry of the brain in experimental epilepsy. The action of experimental epilepsy on the acido-basic processes in brain. (Russ) *Ukr Biokhim Zh, 22*:435, 1950.

Kühnau, J.: Die Biochemie der Wirkstoff-Hemmstoff Antagonismen. *Verh Dtsch Ges Inn Med, 58*:30, 1952.

Küppers, K.: Vergleichende Untersuchungen über die Hämatologie und den Purinstoffwechsel bei Schizophrenen und Epileptikern. *Allg Z Psychiatr, 97*:354, 1932.

Kuhlenbeck, H.: *Vorlesungen über das Zentralnervensystem der Wirbeltiere.* Jena, G. Fischer, 1927.

Kukoleva, I.I.: *Actual Writings on the Problem of Neurology and Psychiatry.* (Russ), Kuibishev, Acad. Nauk SSSR., 1957.

Kulenkampff, H.: Das Verhalten der Neuroglia in den Vorderhörnern der weiβen Maus unter dem Reiz physiologischer Tätigkeit. *Z Anat Entwickl Gesch,* 116, 304, 1952.

Kunz, A. and Sulcin, N.M.: The neuroglia in the autonomic ganglion cytologic structures and reaction to stimulation. *J Comp Neurol, 85*:467, 1947.

Kunz, H.A.: Über die Wirkung von Antimetaboliten des Aneurins auf die einzelne markhaltige Nervenfaser. *Helv Physiol Acta, 14*:411, 1956.

Kuschmann, M.I.: The action of novocaine on the acido-basic processes in nervous tissue. *Papers of the Tchicaloff Med Inst, 5*:212, 1956 (Russ).

Kusnecov, A.I.: *Materials on the Pharmacology of Sympaticomimetical Amines.* Theses on the 25th anniversary of the Ukr. Inst. of exp. Endocrinology. (Russ), Charkov, pp. 38-41, 1945.

Kusnecov, A.I.: *The Action of Narcotics on Vegetative Nervous System.* VII. meeting of physiologists, biochem. a. pharmacol. Medgiz, pp. 675, a. 677, 1947. (Russ).

Laborit, H.: Les rapports neurono-névrogliques. Interprétations sur les bases expérimentales de leurs rôles en neurophysiologie et dans mécanisme d'action des drogues psychotropes. *Presse Méd, 72*:1, 1964.

Laborit, H., Broussolle, B. and Perrimon-Tronchet, R.: Essais pharmacologiques concernant le mècanisme des convulsions dues à l'oxygène pur en pression oliez lessouris. *J Physiol* (Paris), *49*:963, 1947.

Laborit, H., Coirault, R., Damasio, R., Gaujard, R., Laborit, G., Fabrizy, P., Charonnat, R. Lechat, P. and Chareton J.: Sur un type nouveau d'anesthésie chirurgicale et sur, l'emploi en thérapeutique d'un dépresseur du cortex cérébral. *Anesth Analg Réanim, 14*:384, 1957a.

Laborit, H., Coirault, R. Damasio, R., Gaujard, R., Laborit, G., Fabrizy, P., Charonnat, R., Lechat, P. and Chareton, J.: Sur un type nouveau d'anesthésie chirurgicale et sur l'emploi en thérapeutique d'un dépresseur du cortex cérébral. (S.C.T.Z.) *Presse Med, 65*:1051, 1957b.

Lajtha, A.: Protein metabolism of the nervous system. *Int Rev Neurobiol, 6*:1, 1964a.

Lajtha, A.: Alteration and pathology of cerebral protein metabolism. *Int Rev Neurobiol, 7*:1, 1964b.

Lajtha, A. and Toth, J.: The effect of drugs on uptake and exit of cerebral amino acids. *Biochem Pharmacol, 14*:729, 1965.

Lando, L.I.: Zh.nevropatol. psikhiat. "Korsakoff" 2, 1957; cit. by: Wolfsohn, H.M.: On the signification of some biochemical shifting to prognosis and effect of schizophrenia therapy. In *Obm. Veshtch. Psikhiat. Zabol.* Moscow, Medgiz, pp. 128-145, 1960.

Lando, L.I.: The hyaluronidase in blood serum of schizophrenics during treatment. (Russ) In *Obm. Veshtch. Psikhiat. Zabol.* Moscow, Medgiz, pp. 66-75, 1960.

Lando, L.I.: and Krupenina, L.B. Comparative tests of the ammonia blood content of schizophrenic and epileptic patients. In *Problems of Schizophrenia* (Russ) Moscow, pp. 232-240, 1962.

Landolt, H.: Über Verstimmungen, Dämmerzustände und schizophrene Zustandsbilder bei Epilepsie. Schweiz. *Arch Neurol Psychiatr, 76:*313, 1955.

Landolt, H.: *Die Temporallappenepilepsie und ihre Psychopathologie.* Basel-New York, Karger 1960.

Landolt, H.: Psychische Störungen bei Epilepsie. *Dtsch Med Wochenschr, 79:*446, 1962.

Landolt, H.: Über einige Korrelationen zwischen Elektroencephalogramm und normalen und pathologischen psychischen Vorgängen. *Schweiz Med Wochenschr, 93:*107, 1963.

Landolt, H.: Die Dämmer- und Verstimmungszustände bei Epilepsie und ihre Elektroencephalographie. *Dtsch Z Nervenheilk, 185:*411, 1963.

Lang, K.: Der intermediäre Stoffwechsel. In Trendelenburg, Schütz (Eds.): *Lehrbuch der Physiologie.* Berlin-Göttingen-Heidelberg, Springer, 1952.

Langdon-Down, M. and Brain, W.R.: Time of day in relation to convulsions in epilepsy. *Lancet, 3:*1029, 1929.

Lanoir, J., Dolce, G. and Chirnos, E.: Etude neurophysilogique du Ro 4-5360. Soc. Biol. de Marseille, 1965a.

Lanoir, J. and Killam, E.K.: Action de deux diazepines sur le cycle "veille-sommeil" de chats en préparation chronique. *34e réunion de l'association des physiologistes de langue française.* Orsay, 1966.

Lanoir, J., Requin, S., Dolce, G. and Chirinos, E.: Etude neurophysilogique comparative de deux drogues anticonvulsantes: Le Valium et le Mogadon. Comm. 6th. Int. Congr. Electroenceph. clin. Neurophysiol. 1965; Vienna, Verlag, Wien.Med.Akad. pp. 49-51, 1965b.

Lapinski, M.N.: On the problem of cortex stimulation in relation to epileptic seizures in lower animals. (Russ). *Nevrol Zh, 7:*59, 1899.

Lapinski, M.N.: On the problem of the part of temporal lobe in epileptic seizure. (Russ) *Vrač Gaz, 14:*179, 1913.

Lapteva, H.H.: Zh. Nevropatol. Psikhiat. "Korsakoff" 2, 1956; cit. by Kelmischkeut, E.G.: Comparative biochemical studies in involutional psychoses and schizophrenia of old people. In: *Obm. Veshtch Psikhiat. Zabol.* Moscow, Medgiz, pp. 94-98, 1960.

Larrabee, M.G. and Bronk, D.W.: Metabolic requirements of sympatic neurons. *Cold Spring Harbor Symp on Quant Biol,* 17, 1952.

Laruelle, L.: Le repérage des ventricules cérébraux par un procédé de routine. *Presse Med, 39:*1888, 1931.

Lascar, E.: Influenta hiperglicemei provocate asupra modificarilor, activityltii, citrocromoxidazei şi succinidehidrazei din cortexul motor al iepulerui dupa accessul convulsive experimental. *Stud Cercet Neurol, 3:*85, 1958.

Lasich, A.J. and Psych, F.F.: Clinical evaluation of a new anticonvulsant drug effective against epilepsy and trigeminal neuralgia. *S Afr Med J, 40:*308, 1966.

Lasslo, A. and Meyer, A.L.: *Nature, 184:* 1922, 1951; cit. by Kanig, K.: *Arzneim Forsch, 19:*397, 1969.

Lausberg, G. and Calatayud-Maldonado, V. Die differential-diagnostische Bedeutung cerebraler Ansfallsformen bei temporalen Tumoren. *Dtsch Z Nervenheilkd, 191:*1, 1967.

Lauter, H.: Lithiumbehandlung manisch-depressiver Psychosen. *Med Klin, 64:*348, 1969.

Lavy, S., Carmon, A., and Yahr, J.: Assessment of a clinical and electroencephalographic classification of epileptic patients everyday neurological practice. A survey of 450 cases. *Epilepsia, 13:*498-508, 1972.

Lavy, S., and Herishann, Y.: The effect of tharacic spinal cord transection of alertness in cats. *Epilepsia, 13*:287-293, 1972.
Laxenaire, M., Tridon, P. and Poiré, P.: Effect of chlormethiazole in treatment of delirium tremens and status epilepticus. *Acta Psychiatr Scand, 42*:87, 1966.
Leach, B.E., Cohen, M. Heath, R.G. and Martens, S.: Studies of the role of ceruloplasmin and albumin in adrenaline metabolism. *Arch Neurol, 76*:635, 1956.
Le Beau, J.: *Psycho-chirurgie et fonctions mentales*. Paris, Masson, 1954.
Lechat, P.: The pharmacology of vitamin B_1: *Wien Klin Wochenschr, 73*:42, 1961.
Leder, A.: Zur Testpsychologischen Abgrenzung und Bestimmung der Aufwachepilepsie vom Pyknolepsie-Typ. Diss. Zürich, 1966.
Leder, A. Zur Psychopathologie der Schlaf- und Aufwachepilepsie. *Nervenarzt, 38*:434, 1967.
Leder, A.: *Tegretol: Zum Problem der psychotropen Wirkung*. Bulletin 1, Psychol. Institut d. Univers. Zürich, 1968.
Leder, A. and Timäeus-Wolf, S.: Bericht über psychodiagnostische Untersuchungen zur Frage der psychotropen Wirkung von Tegretal. Sitzungsberichte *Dtsch Ges Psychiatr Nervenheilkd*, ref. *Zbl Ges Neurol Psychiatr, 188*:19, 1967.
Leemann, H. and Pichler, E.: Über den Lactoflavingehalt des Zentralnervensystems und seine Bedeutung. *Arch Psychiatr D, 114*:265, 1942.
Leeper, L.C. and Udenfriend, S.: Studies on the metabolism of noradrenaline, adrenaline and their O-methyl analogs by partially purified enzyme preparations. *Fed Proc, 15*:298, 1956.
Le Gros Clark, E.W.: The connexions of the frontal lobes of the brain. *Lancet, 254*: 353, 1948.
Le Gros Clark, E.W. and Meyer, M.: The terminal connexions of the olfactory tract in the rabbit. *Brain, 70*:304, 1947.
Le Gros Clark, E.W. and Northfield, D.W.C.: The cortical projection of the pulvinar in the macaque monkey. *Brain, 60*:126, 1937.
Lehmann, A.: Action de crises répétées d'épilepsie acoustique sur le taux de noradrenaline des zones corticales et sous-corticales du cerveau de souris. *Compt Rend Soc Biol, 159*:62, 1965.
Lehmann, H.E. and Hanrahan, G.E.: Chlorpromazine. *Arch Neurol Psychiatr* (Chic), *71*:227, 1954.
Lehmann-Facius, H.: Über die Liquordiagnose der Schizophrenien. *Klin Wochenschr, 2*: 1646, 1937.
Lehninger, A.L.: *The Mitochondrion*. New York-Amsterdam, Benjamin Inc., 1964.
v. Lehoczký, T. and Doboš, A.: Die moderne Behandlung der Epilepsie. *Wein Med Wochenschr, 2*:849, 1941.
Leloir, L.F., Olivarria, J.M., Goldemberg, S.H. and Carminatti, H.: Biosynthesis of glycocen from uridine diphosphate glucose. *Arch Biochem, 81*:508, 1959.
Lemere, F.: Habit-forming properties of meprobamate. *Arch Neurol Psychiatr* (Chic), *76*:1431, 1956.
Lemke, R.: Über die Indikationen zur Insulinschockbehandlung bei Schizophrenie. *Arch Psychiatr, 107*:223, 1938.
Lennox, M.: Effects of sedative drugs on the electroencephalogram. *Am J Psychiatry, 102*:799, 1946.
Lennox, W.G.: Constancy of the cerebral blood flow. *Arch Neurol Psychiatr* (Chic), *36*: 375, 1936.
Lennox, W.G.: Drug therapy for epileptic children. *Nerv Child, 6*:1, 1947.

Lennox, W.G.: Childhood epilepsy. *NYJ Med, 50:*2263, 1950.
Lennox, W.G.: Phenomena and correlates of the psychomotor triad. *Neurology, 1:*356, 1951.
Lennox, W.G.: *Epilepsy and Related Disorders.* Boston, Little, Brown & Co., 1960.
Lennox, W.G. and Allen, M.B.: cit. by Klimes, K. a. Lang, A.: Serumeiweiβuntersuchungen bei Epileptikern. *Arch Psychiatr D, 114:*693, 1942.
Lennox, W.G. and Gibbs, E.L.: Oxygen saturation of arterial blood in epilepsy. *Arch Neurol Psychiatr, 35:*1198, 1936a.
Lennox, W.G. and Gibbs, E.L.: Oxygen saturation of blood draining the brain and the limbs of patients with epilepsy. *Arch Neurol Psychiatr, 36:*13, 1936b.
Lennox, W.G., Gibbs, F.A. and Gibbs, E.L.: Effect on the electroencephalogram of drugs and conditions which influence seizures. *Arch Neurol Psychiatr, 36:*1236, 1936.
Lennox, W.G. and Merritt, H.H.: The cerebrospinal fluid in "essential" epilepsy. *J Neurol Psychopath, 17:*97, 1936.
Lenz, H.: Ambulante Behandlung der Depression. *Wien Med Wochenschr, 111:*421, 1961.
Leonhard, K.: Die Klinik des Thalamus opticus. *Arch Psychiatr Z Neurol, 184:*256, 1950.
Lerner, A.M., Decarli, L.M. and Davidson, C.S.: Association of pyridoxine deficiency and convulsions in alcoholics. *Proc Soc Exp Biol Med, 98:*841, 1958.
Leshtschinski, A.L.: *Papers of the Psychoneurological Central Institute SSSR, 10:*173, 1938; cit. by Lando, L.I. a, Krupenina, L.B.: Comparative tests of the ammonia blood content of schizophrenic and epileptic patients. In *Problems of Schizophrenia.* (Russ), Moscow, pp. 232-240, 1962.
Leshtschinski, A.L. and Brodskij, F.I.: *Problems of Pathophysiology and Therapy in Schizophrenics.* (Russ), Vol. 2, Kiev, 1947.
Leube, H.: Beitrag zur Therapie der Zerebralsklerose. Ärztl. *Praxis, 11:*388, 1959.
Leuner, H.C.: *Die experimentelle Psychose.* Ihre Psychopharmakologie. Phänomenologie und Dynamik in Beziehung zur Person. Berlin-Göttingen-Heidelberg, Springer, 1962.
Leusen, J.: Monoamin-Freisetzer und Monoaminoxydase-Hemmer. Psychiatr Neurol (Basel), *12:*154-164, 1960.
Levin, M.: Bromide hallucinosis. *Arch gen Psychiatr, 2:*429, 1960.
Levtova, F.A.: L'influence de l'aminazine et du tofranil sur le comportement alimentaire des chiens normaux et au cours de la névrose experimentale. (Russ) *Zh Nevropat Psikhiatr, 66:*1658, 1966.
Lewis, J.J. and van Petten, G.R.: *Brit J Pharmacol, 20:*462, 1963; cit. by Kanig, K.: *Arzneim Forsch, 19:*397, 1969.
Lewis, J.J. and Pollock, D.: Effects of d-amphetamine and chlorpromazine on oxidised (NAD) and reduced $NADH_2$) nicotinamide adenine dinucleotide levels in rat brain. *Biochem Pharmacol, 14:*636, 1965.
Ley, H.: Differentialdiagnose der zerebralen Vergiftung. In Bodechtel, G. (Ed.) : *Differentialdiagnose neurologischer Krankheitsbilder.* 1st. Ed. Stuttgart, Thieme, 1958.
Liberson, W.T. and Akert, K.: Hippocampal seizure status in guinea pigs. *Electroenceph Clin Neurophysiol, 7:*211, 1955.
Liberson, W.T. and Cadilhac, J.G.: Electroshock and rhinencephalic seizure states. *Confinia Neur* (Basel), *13:*278, 1953.
Liberson, W.T., Scoville, W.B. and Dunsmore, R.H.: Stimulation studies of the prefrontal lobe and uncus in man. *Electroenceph Clin Neurophysiol, 3:*1, 1951.
Liddel, D.W. and Retterslöh, N.: The occurrence of epileptic fits in leucotomized patients receiving chlorpromazine therapy. *J Neurol Psychiatr, 20:*105, 1957.

Lien, J.B.: Depth-EEG of two schizophrenic patients under Marsilid-medication. *Psychiatr Neurol* (Basel), *140:*133, 1960.

Lindsley, D.B.: Attention, consciousness, sleep and wakefulness. In Field, Magoun, Hall (Eds.): *Hb. of Physiology*. Sec. I. Washington, Drechsler vol. III, 1960.

Lingjaerde, O.: Investigations of the liver function in mental diseases. (With special regard to the relation between liver affection, intestinal intoxication and malnutrition in schizophrenics) *Acta Psychiatr* (Kopenh), *8:*421, 1933.

Lingjaerde, O.: Investigations of the basal metabolism of schizophrenics. Effects of thyroid treatment. *Acta Psychiatr* (Kopenh), *8:*573, 1933.

Lingjaerde, O.: Ein Fall von hepato-lentikulärer Degeneration. *Norsk Mag Laegevidensk, 98:*1267, 1937.

Lingjaerde, O.: Beiträge zur somatologischen Schizophrenieforschung. Bedeutung des Kohlenhydratdefizits. *Arch Psychaitr Z Neurol, 191:*114, 1953.

Lipman, F.: Development of acetylation problems, a personal account. *Science, 120:* 855, 1954.

Livencev, N.M.: Study of some reactions of the organism by influence of current on the CNS. (Russ) Diss. Moscow, 1952.

Livingston, S.: Abdominal pain as manifestation of epilepsy (abdominal epilepsy) in children. *J Pediat, 38:*687, 1951.

Livingston, S.: *The Diagnosis and Treatment of Convulsive Disorders in Children.* Springfield, Thomas, 1954.

Livingston, S.: General principles of antiepileptic drug therapy. *Clin Pediat 2:*233-237, 1963.

Livingston, S., Villamater, C., Sakata, Y. and Pauli, L.L.: Use of carbamazepine in epilepsy. Results in 87 patients. *JAMA, 200:*204, 1967.

Lockard, J.S., Dendell, L., Uhlir, W., and Uhlir, V.: Spontaneous seizures frequency and avoidance conditioning in monkeys. *Epilepsia, 13:*437-444, 1972.

Löfvendahl, H. and Valatin, T.: Glucide metabolism in schizophrenia. *Acat Med Scand, 106:*70, 1941.

Loiseau, P., and Beaussart, M.: Hereditary factors in partial epilepsy. *Epilepsia, 10:*23-31, 1969.

Loiseau, P. and Cohadon, S.: Activité antiépileptique du trinuride. *Presse Méd, 72:* 1969, 1964.

Longo, V.G. and Silvestrini, B.: Contribution à l' étude des rapports entre le potentiel réticular évoqué, l'état d'anesthésie et l'activité électrique cérébrale. *Electroenceph Clin Neurophysiol, 10:*111, 1958.

Looney, J.M. and Childs, H.M.: The lactic acid and glutathione content of the blood of schizophrenic patients. *J Clin Invest, 13:*963, 1934.

Lorente de Nó, R.: Studies on the structures of the cerebral cortex. *J Psychol Neurol, 45:*381, 1933.

Lorente de Nó, R.: Studies on the structures of the cerebral cortex. II. Continuation of the study of the ammonic system. *J Psychol Neurol, 46:*113, 1934.

Lorente de Nó, R.: Analysis of the activity of chains of internuncial neurons. *J Neurophysiol, 1:*207, 1938.

Lorente de Nó, R.: Transmission of impulses through cranial nerve nuclei. *J Neurophysiol, 2:*402, 1939.

Lorente de Nó, R.: Cerebral cortex: architecture, intracortical connexions, motor projections. In Fulton, J.F. (Ed.): *Physiology of the Nervous System.* 2nd Ed. Oxford, 1943, pp. 286.

Lorento de Nó, R.: Correlation of nerve activity with polarization phenomena. *Harvey Lect, 42:*43, 1947.

Lorenz, W.F.: Sugar tolerance in Dementia praecox and other mental disorders. *Arch Neurol Psychiatr* (Chic), *8:*184, 1922.

Lorgé, M.: Klinische Erfahrungen mit einem neuen Antiepilepticum Tegretol (G 32883), mit besonderer Wirkung auf die epileptische Wesensveränderung. *Schweiz Med Wochenschr, 93:*30, 1963.

Lotspeich, W.: The role of insulin in the metabolism of amino acids. *J Biol Chem, 179:* 175, 1949.

Lowell, O. and Randall, L.O.: Pharmacology of methaminodiazepoxide. *Dis Nerv Syst, 21:*7, 1960.

Lowry, O.H., Roberts, N.R., Leiner, K.J., Wu, M.L., Farr, A.L. and Alpers, R.W.: Quantitative biochemistry of brain: III Ammon's horn. *J Biol Chem, 207:*39, 1954.

Lugaresi, E., Pazzaglia, P., and Tassinari, C.A.: Differentiation of absence status and temporal lobe status. *Epilepsia, 12:*77-87, 1971.

Lumsden, C.E.: Functional aspects of the glial apparatus. *Acta Neurol Psychiat Belg, 57:*472, 1957.

Lunde, F.: Pyridoxine deficiency in chronic alcoholism. *J Nerv Ment Dis, 131:*77, 1960.

Lundquist, G.: The clinical use of chlormethiazole. *Acta Psychiat Scand, 42:*113, 1966a.

Lundquist, G.: The risk of dependence on chlormethiazole. *Acta Psychiat Scand, 42:*203, 1966b.

Luse, S.: Histochemical implications of electron microscopy of the central nervous system. *J Histochem Cytochem, 8:*398, 1960.

Lustig, B. and May, J.: Über die Behandlung der Epilepsie mit Zentronal compositum. *Mat Med Nordm, 7:*6, 1955.

Lyberi, G. and Last, S.L.: The use of chlorpromazine as an activating agent. *Electroenceph Clin Neurophysiol, 8:*711, 1956.

Lynen, F.: Der Weg von der "aktivierten Essigsäure" zu den Terpentinen und Fettsäuren. *Angew Chemie, 77:*929, 1965.

Lyon, J.B., Bain, J.A. and Williams, H.L.: Distribution of vitamin B_6 in the tissue of two inbred strains of mice fed complete and vitamin B_6-deficient rations. *J Biol Chem, 237:*1989, 1962.

Mac Farlane, M.G. and Weill-Malherbe, H.: Changes in phosphate distribution during anaerobic glucolysis in brain slices. *Biochem J, 35:*1, 1941.

Mac Kenzie, D.Y. and Woolf, L.I.: Maple syrup urine disease, an inborn error of the metabolism of valine, leucine and isoleucine associated with gross mental deficiency. *Br Med J, 1:*90, 1959.

Mac Lardy, T.: Thalamic projection to the frontal cortex in man. *J Neurol N.S., 13:* 198, 1950.

Mac Lean, P.D.: A new nasopharyngeal lead. *Electroenceph Clin Neurophysiol, 1:*110, 1949.

Mac Lean, P.D.: Psychosomatic disease and the visceral brain. Recent developments bearing on the Papez theory of emotion. *Psychosom Med, 11:*338, 1949.

Mac Lean, P.D.: Some psychiatric implications of physiological studies on frontotemporal portion of limbic system (visceral brain). *Electroenceph Clin Neurophysiol, 4:* 407, 1952.

Mac Lean, P.D.: The limbic system and its hippocampal formation. Studies in animals and their possible application to man. *J Neurosurg, 11:*29, 1954.

Mac Lean, P.D.: The limbic system (visceral brain) and emotional behavior. *Arch Neurol Psychiatr, 73:*130, 1955.

Mac Lean, P.D.: Chemical and electrical stimulation of hippocampus in unrestrained animals. Part I/II. *Arch Neurol Psychiatr* (Chic), *78*:113 a., 128 1957.

Mac Lean, P.D.: The limbic system with respect to self-preservation and the preservation of the species. *J Nerv Ment Dis, 127*:1, 1958.

Mac Lean, P.D.: The limbic system with respect to two basic life principles. In Brazier, M.A.B. (Ed.): *The Central Nervous System and Behavior.* Madison, N.J., Madison Printing Comp., pp. 31-118, 1959.

Mac Lean, P.D.: Psychosomatics. In Field, Magoun, Hall (Eds.): *Hb. of Physiology.* Amer, Physiol. Soc., Washington, III, pp. 1723-1744, 1960.

Mac Lean, P.D.: New findings relevant to the evolution of psychosexual functions of the brain. *J Nerv Ment Dis, 135*:289, 1962.

Mac Lean, P.D. and Arellano, J.A.P.: Basal lead studies in epileptic automatisms. *Electroenceph Clin Neurophysiol, 2*:1, 1950.

Mac Lean, P.D. and Delgado, J.M.R.: Electrical and chemical stimulation of frontotemporal portion of limbic system in the waking animal. *Electroenceph Clin Neurophysiol, 5*:91, 1953.

Mac Lean, P.D., Denniston, R.H. and Dua, S.: Further studies on cerebral representation of penile erection: caudal thalamus, midbrain, pons. *J Neurophysiol* (Springfield), *26*:273, 1963.

Mac Lean, P.D., Denniston, R.H., Dua, S. and Ploog, D.W.: Hippocampal changes with brain stimulation eliciting penile erection. In Passouant, P. (Ed.): *Physiologie de l'hippocampe. Centre de la recherche scientifique Paris, 107*:389, 1962.

Mac Lean, P.D., Dua, S. and Denniston, R.S.: Cerebral localization of scratching and seminal discharge. *Arch Neurol* (Chic), *9*:485, 1963.

Mac Lean, P.D., Flanigan, S., Flynn, P., Kim, C. and Stevens, J.R.: Hippocampal function: tentative correlations of conditioning, EEG drug and radioautographic studies. *Yale J Biol Med, 28*:380, 1955/56.

Mac Lean, P.D., Horwitz, N.H. and Robinson, F.: Olfactory-like responses in pyriform area to non-olfactory stimulation. *Yale J Biol Med, 25*:159, 1952.

Mac Lean, P.D. and Ploog, D.: Cerebral representation of penile erection. *J Neurophysiol, 25*:29, 1962.

Mac Lean, P.D., Ploog, D.W. and Robinson, B.W.: Circulatory effects of limbic stimulation with special reference to the male genital organ. *Physiol Rev, 40*:105, 1960.

Mac Lean, P.D., Robinson, B.W. and Ploog, D.W.: Experiments on localization of genital function in the brain. *Trans Am Neurol Ass, 84*:105, 1959.

Mac Lean, P.D., Rosner, B.S. and Robinson, F.: Pyriform responses to electrical stimulation of olfactory fila, bulb and tract. *Am J Physiol, 189*:395, 1957.

Mac Quarrie, I.: Determination of blood pH without transfering sample. *Proc Soc Exp Biol Med, 25*:134, 1927.

Mac Quarrie, I.: Epilepsy in children. The relationship of water balance to the occurrence of seizures. *Am J Dis Child, 38*:451, 1929.

Mac Quarrie, I.: Some recent observations regarding the nature of epilepsy. *Ann Intern Med, 6*:497, 1932.

Mac Quarrie, I. and Keith, H.M.: Epilepsy in children. *Am J Dis Child, 34*:1013, 1927.

Mac Quarrie, I., Manchester, R.C. and Husted, C.: Study of the water and mineral balances in epileptic children. I. Effects of diuresis, catharsis, phenobarbital therapy and water storage. *Am J Dis Child, 43*:1519, 1932.

Mac Quarrie, I. and Peeler, D.B.: The effect of sustained pituitary antidiuresis and forced water drinking in epileptic children. A diagnostic and eitologic study. *J Clin Invest, 10*:915, 1931.

Magnes, J., Moruzzi, G. and Pompeiano, O.: Synchronization of the EEG produced by low-frequency electrical stimulation of the region of the solitary tract. *Arch Ital Biol, 99:*33, 1961a.

Magnes, J., Moruzzi, G. and Pompeiano, O.: Electroencephalogram-synchronizing structures in the lower brain stem. In Wolstenholme, O'Connor (Eds.): *Ciba Foundation Symposium on the Nature of Sleep*. London, Churchill, pp. 57-78, 1961b.

Magni, F., Moruzzi, G., Rossi, G.F., and Zanchetti, A.: EEG arousal following inactivation of the lower brain stem by selective injection of barbiturate into the vertebral circulation. *Arch Ital Biol, 97:*33, 1959.

Magnus, O. and Lammers, H.J.: The amygdaloid nuclear complex. *Fol Psychiatr Neurol Neurochir Neerl, 59:*555, 1956.

Magnus, O., Penfield, W. and Jasper, H.: Mastication and consciousness in epileptic seizures. *Acta psychiat* (Kopenh), *27:*91, 1952.

Magoun, F.W. and Rhines, R.: An inhibitory mechanism in the bulbar reticular formation. *J Neurophysiol, 9:*165, 1946.

Maj, J. and Przegalinski, E.: Disulfiran and the effect of catecholamines on neuroleptic-induced catalepsy in mice and rats. *J Pharm Pharmacol, 19:*69, 1967.

Makarova, K.M. and Mittelstedt, A.A.: Glutamine content in blood serum of patients suffering from hepatocerebral dystorophy. (Russ). *Zh Nevropatol Psikhiatr, 66:*55, 1966.

Malaguzzi-Valeri, C.: On the zumohexase of nervous tissue. *Arch Sci Biol* (Napoli), *22:* 77, 1936.

Malpas, J.S., Spray, G.H. and Witts, L.J.: Serum folic-acid and vitamin B_{12} levels in anticonvulsant therapy. *Br Med J, 1:*955, 1966.

Malzone, W.F., Wilder, B.J., and Mayersdorf, A.: A methtod of modifying the rapidity of cobalt-induced epileptogenesis in the cat. *Epilepsia, 13:*643-648, 1972.

Mamoli, A.: La carbamazepina (Tegretol) nel trattamento prolungato dell'epilessia nelle sue manifestazioni sia comiziali che psicopatologiche. *Rivista Neurol, XLII,* fasc. 1, 1972.

Mandel, P., Bieth, R. and Weill, J.D.: Recherches sur le métabolisme énergétique du cerveau au cours du dévelopement chez le rat. I. Consommation d'oxygène. II. Composés phosphorés acidosolubles. *Bull Soc Chem Biol, 37:*4, 1955.

Mandel, P., Bieth, R. and Weill, J.D.: General metabolism of the rat brain during post-natal development. Metabolism nervous system. London-New York, Pergamon Press, 1957.

Manery, J.F.: Water and electrolyte metabolism. *Pyhsiol Rev, 34:*334, 1954.

Mann, P.J.G., Tennenbaum, M. and Quastel, J.H.: Acetylcholine metabolism in the central nervous system. The effect of potassium and other cations on acetylcholine liberation. *Biochem J, 33:*822, 1939.

Mann, S.A.: Blood sugar studies in mental disorders. *J Ment Sci, 71:*443, 1925.

Marazzi, A.S. and Hart, E.R.: The possible role of inhibition at adrenergic synapses in the mechanism of hallucinogenic and related drug actions. *J Nerv Dis, 122:*453, 1955.

Marazzi, A.S., Hart, E.R. and Rodriguez, J.M.: Action of blood-borne gamma-aminobutyric acid on central synapses. *Science, 127:*284, 1958.

Marburg, O.: Die Tumoren der Schläfenlappen. *Hb. d. Neurol. d. Ohres,* Berlin, Urban & Schwarzenberg, vol. I, pp. 1864, 1929.

Marchini, E. and Severini, P.: L'azione dell' acetazolamide (diamox) sui tracciati elettroencefalografici di epilettici. *Riv Neur* (Napoli), *27:*583, 1957.

Margerison, J.H. and Corsellis, J.A.N.: Epilepsy and the temporal lobes. A clinical, elec-

troencephalographic and neuropathological study of the brain in epilepsy with particular reference to the temporal lobes. *J Neurophysiol, 89:*499, 1966.
Marinacci, A.A.: A special type of temporal lobe (psychomotor) seizures following ingestion of alcohol. *Bull Los Angeles Neurol Soc 28:*241-250, 1963.
Markova, E.I.: Problems of psychiatry and neuropathology. (Russ), *UFA, 4:*19, 1944.
Markovits, G.: Leberfunktionsprüfungen bei versichiedenen Geisteskrankheiten. *Mschr Psychiatr, 88:*248, 1934.
Marks, N. and Lajtha, A.: Subcellular distribution and properties of neutral and acid proteinases. *Biochem J, 89:*438, 1963.
Marshall, J. and Whitty, C.W.M.: Value of pneumoencephalography in diagnosis of fits. *Br Med J, vol. I.* 847, 1952.
Martin, H., Rodhight, R., McIlwain, H. and Tresize, M.A.: A second major constituent of the blood exidized at the brain. *Nature, 179:*419, 1957.
Martin, W.R., Demaar, E.W.J. and Unna, K.R.: Chlorpromazine. I. The action of chlorpromazine and related phenothiazines on the EEG and its activation. *J Pharmacol Exp Ther, 122:*343, 1958.
Martinengo, V.: Le globuline nel siero di sangue dei malati di mente. *Note Psichiatr, 61:*405, 1932.
Martinson, E.E. and Tjahepild, L.J.: *Vopr Med Chim, 1:*4, 1955; cit. by Krasilinovka, M.N.: Dysfunction of liver in schizophrenia. (Russ.) In *Obm Veshtch. Psikhiat. Zabol.* Moscow, Medgiz, pp. 154-158, 1960.
Maske, H.: Über den topochemischen Nachweis von Zink im Ammonshorn verschiedener Säugetiere. *Naturawissenschaften, 42:*424, 1955.
Mason, C.R., and Cooper, R.M.: A permanent change in convulsive threshold in normal and brain-damaged rats with repeated small doses of pentylentetrazol. *Epilepsia, 13:*663-674, 1972.
Maspers, P.E., Grattarola, F.R. and Marossero, F.: Etude anatomopathologique de 36 cas d'epilepsie temporale opérés. Essai de corrélations anatomo-électrocliniques. *Acta Neurol Psychiatr Belg, 56:*103, 1956.
Maspers, P.E. and Marossero, F.: L'epilesia temporale et il suo trattamento chirurgico. *Chirurgia* (Milano), *9:*171, 1954.
Máthé, V. and Kassay, G.: Die Wirkung von Psychopharmaka auf den energetischen Stoffwechsel des Hirngewebes, *Arzneim Forsch, 19:*419, 1969.
Matsuda, M. and Makino, K.: D-penicillamine as an antidote to 8-hydroxyquinoline and alloxan. *Nature, 192:*261, 1961.
Matsumoto, J. and Jouvet, M.: Effets de réserpine, DOPA et 5 HTP sur les deux états de sommeil. *C R. Soc Biol* (Paris), *158:*2137, 1964.
Matthes, A.: Die psychomotorische Epilepsie im Kindesalter. *Z Kinderheilkd, 85:*455, a. 472, a. 668, 1961a,b,c.
Matthes, A.: Béhandlung kindlicher Epilepsien. *Dtsch med Wochenschr, 92:*1079, 1967.
Matthews, C.G. and Klove, H.: Differential psychological performances on major motor, psychomotor and mixed seizure classifications of known and unknown etiology. *Epilepsia* (Aust.), *8:*117, 1967.
Matusis, I.I. and Matusis, Z.S.: *Byull eksp Biol Med, 4:*31, 1951; cit. by Lando, L.I.: The hyaluronidase in blood serum of schizophrenics during treatment. (Russ) In *Obm. Veshtch. Psikhiat. Zabol.* Moscow, Medgiz, pp. 66-75, 1960.
Matussek, N.: Neuro-Biologie. In Wieland, Pfleiderer (Eds.): *Molekular-Biologie.* Frankfurt (M), Umschau-Verlag 3rd. Ed. pp. 245-257, 1969.
Matussek, N.: Biochemie des Schlafes. In Baust, W. (Ed.): *Ermüdung, Schlaf und Traum.* Stuttgart, Wiss. Verlagsges. pp. 205-216, 1970.

Matussek, N. and Patschke, U.: Beziehungen des Schlaf-Wach-Rhythmus zum Noradrenalin- und Serotoningehalt im Zentralnervensystem von Hamstern. *Med Exp, 11*:81, 1964.

Mauceri, J. and Strauss, H.: Effects of chlorpromazine on the electroencephalogram with report of a case of chlorpromazine intoxication. *Electroenceph Clin Neurophysiol, 7*:671, 1956.

di Mauro, S.: La prova del Förster nella diagnosi di epilessia. *Osp Psichiatr, 2*:481, 1934.

Mauz, F.: *Die Veranlagung zu Krampfanfällen*. Leipzig, Thieme, 1937.

Maxion, H.: Erfahrungen mit Tegretal im polygraphischen Schlaf-EEG. *Nervenarzt, 39*: 547, 1968.

Maxion, H., Schneider, E., Haiss, V., and Seuthe, V.: Polygraphische Nachtschlafuntersuchungen bei Schlaf- und Aufwachepilepsien. Intern. Symposium September 1971 (Würzburg/W. Germany), Jovanovic, U.J. (Ed.): *The Nature of Sleep,* Stuttgart, Gustav Fisher Verlag, pp. 235, 1973.

May, C.D.: Vitamin B_6 in human nutrition: A critique and object lesson. *Pediatrics, 14*: 269, 1954.

Mayer-Gross, W.E. and Walker, J.: Effect of l-glutamic acid and other amino acids in hypoglycemia. *Biochem J, 44*:92, 1949.

Maynert, E.W.: The role of biochemical and neurohumoral factors in the laboratory evaluation of antiepileptic drugs. *Epilepsia, 10*:145-162, 1969.

McCormick, D.B., Gregory, M.E. and Snell, E.E.: Pyridoxal phosphokinases. I. Assay, distribution, purification and properties. *J Biol Chem, 236*:2076, 1961.

McCormick, D.B., Guirard, B.M. and Snell, E.E.: Comparative inhibition of pyridoxal kinase and glutamic acid decarboxylase by carbonyl reagents. *Proc Soc Exp Biol Med, 104*:554, 1960.

McCormick, D.B. and Snell, E.E.: Pyridoxal kinase of human brain and its inhibition by hydrazine derivates. *Proc Nat Acad Sci* (Wash), *45*:1371, 1959.

McCormick, D.B. and Snell, E.E.: Pyridoxal phosphokinases. II. Effects of inhibitors. *J Biol Chem, 236*:2085, 1961.

McCowan, P.K. and Quastel, J.H.: Blood-sugar studies in abnormal mental states. *J Ment Sci, 77*:525, 1931.

McFarland, R.A. and Goldstein, H.: The biochemistry of Dementia praecox. *Am J Psychiatry, 95*:509, 1938.

McIlwain, H.: Glutamic acid and glucose as substrates for mammalian brain. *J Ment Sci, 97*:674, 1951.

McIlwain, H.: Effect of depressants on the metabolism of stimulated cerebral tissue. *Biochem J, 53*:403, 1953a.

McIlwain, H.: Substances which support respiration and metabolic response to electrical impulses in cerebral tissues. *J Neurol Neurosurg Psychiatr, 16*:257, 1953b.

McIlwain, H.: Glucose level, metabolism and response to electrical pulses in cerebral tissues from man and laboratory animals. *Biochem J, 55*:618, 1953c.

McIlwain, H.: *Biochemistry and the Central Nervous System.* London, Churchill, 1955.

McIlwain, H.: *Chemotherapy and the Central Nervous System.* Boston, Little, Brown & Co. 1957.

McIlwain, H.: Electrical pulses and the *in vitro* metabolism of cerebral tissues. In Elliott, Page, Quastel (Eds.): *Neurochemistry,* 2nd Ed. Springfield, Thomas, 1962.

McIlwain, H.: *Chemical Exploration of the Brain.* London, Elsevier, 1963.

McIlwain, H.: *Biochemistry and the Central Nervous System,* 3rd. Ed. London, Churchill, 1966.

McIntosh, F.C. and Oborin, P.E.: Release of actetylcholine from intact cerebral cortex. *Abstr Comm 19th Int Physiol Congr,* p. 580, 1953.

McKenzie, B.W. and McChesney, E.W.: Proteins of the blood serum in cases of essential epilepsy. *Arch Neurol, 34*:764, 1935.

McKenzie, J.S.: The influence of morphine and pethidine on somatic evoked responses in the hippocampal formation of the cat. *Electroenceph Clin Neurophysiol, 17*:428, 1964.

McKerracher, D.W., McGuire, W.A. and Aronson, A.: Pseudocholinesterase and the prediction of stability in subnormal and psychopathic offenders. *Br J Psychiatr, 112*:717, 1966.

McKhann, G.M., Albers, R.W., Sokoloff, L. and Mickelsen, O.: The quantitative significance of the gammaminobutyric acid pathway in cerebral oxidative metabolism. In Roberts, E. (Ed.): *Inhibition in the Nervous System and Gamma-Aminobutyric Acid.* New York, Pergamon Press, 1960.

McLardy, T.: Zinc enzymes and the hippocampal mossy fibre system. *Nature* (Lond), *194*:300, 1962.

McLennan, H.Y.: A comparison of some physiological properties of an inhibitory factor from brain (Factor I) and of gamma-aminobutyric acid and related compounds. *J Physiol* (Lond), *139*:79, 1957.

McMillan, P.J., Douglas, G.W. and Mortensen, R.A.: Incorporation of ^{14}C, of acetyl-l-^{14}C and pyruvate-2-^{14}C into brain cholesterol. *Proc Soc Exp Biol,* (NY), *96*:738, 1957.

Meggendorfer, F.: Intoxikationspsychosen. In Bumke, O. (Ed.): *Hb. d. Geisteskrankheiten.* Part 3, Berlin, Springer, vol. VII, 1928.

Meijer, J.W.A.: Simultaneous quantitative determination of anti-epileptic drugs, including carbamazepine, in body fluids. *Epilepsia, 12*:341-352, 1971.

Meister, A.: Enzymatic transfer of alpha amino groups. *Science, 120*:43, 1954.

Mekler, L.B., Pogodaev, K.L. and Hatchaturayan, A.A.: Study of the isoelectrical point of brain proteins in the frog during the locomotor and excomatose phase of electrical convulsion. *Problems in Epilepsy.* Moscow, Medgiz, 1959.

Menkes, J.H., Hurst, P.L. and Craig, J.M.: Progressive familial infantile cerebral dysfunction associated with unusual urinary substance. *Pediatrics, 14*:462, 1954.

Mellick, R.S. and Bassett, R.L.: The cerebrospinal-fluid glutamic oxaloacetic transaminase activity in neurological diseases. *Lancet, I*:904, 1964.

Menšikova, Z., Polak, O., Röschova, H. and Škrivanova, S.: Die Aktivierung des EEG durch Chlorpromazin und dessen Einfluß auf die hirnelektrische Aktivität bei sensiblen Reizen. ref. *Zbl Ges Neurol Psychiatr, 149*:34, 1959.

Mercer, M.D.A.: Analytical methods for the study of periodic phenomena obscured by random fluctuations. *Cold Spring Harb Symp Quant Biol, 25*:73, 1960.

Merlis, S.: Psychopharmacology in rehabilitation of the chronic psychotic. *Dis Nerv Syst, 22*:143, 1961.

Merritt, H.H. and Putnam, T.J.: Sodium diphenyl hydantoinate in the treatment of convulsive disorders. *JAMA, 111*:1068, 1938.

Mertens, H.G.: Das Syndrom "kontinuierlicher Muskelfaseraktivität" von Isaacs als Modell einer gestörten Synapsenfunktion. *Zbl Ges Neurol Psychitr, 180*:220, 1965.

Mets, J.: The clinical treatment of depressives with tofranil. *Ned T Geneesk, 104*:815, 1960.

Mettler, F.A.: *Neuroanatomy,* 2nd. Ed. St. Louis, Mosby & Co., 1948.

Meves, H.: Die Funktion erregbarer Membranen. Neue Erkenntnisse über die Elektrophysiologie des Nervensystems. *Umschau, 62*:299, a. 341, a. 367, 1962.

Meyer, A.: Lésions observées sur les pieces opératives prévelées chez les epileptiques timporaux. *Acta Neurol Psychiatr Belg, 56:*21, 1956.
Meyer, A.: Hippocampal lesions in epilepsy. In Williams, D. (Ed.): *Modern Trends in Neurology*. London, Butterworth, pp. 301, 1957.
Meyer, A., Falconer, M.A. and Beck, E.: Pathological findings in temporal lobe epilepsy. *J Neurol Neurosurg Psychiatr, 17:*267, 1954.
Meyer, J.S. and Waltz, A.G.: Arterial oxygen stauration and alveolar carbon dioxide during electroencephalography. I. *Arch Neurol* (Chic), *2:*631, 1960.
Meyerhof, O.: Isolation of 3-glyceraldehyde phosphoric acid during the enzymic degradation of hexosediphosphoric acid. II. *Bull Soc Chem Biol, 20:*1345, 1938.
Meyer-Mickeleit, W.R.: Über atypische Krampfanfälle und epileptische Äquivalente in EEG. *Verh Dtsch Ges Inn Med,* 56. Kongr. *9:*5, 1950.
Meyer-Mickeleit, W.R.: Die Dämmerattacken als charakteristischer Anfallstyp der temporalen Epilepsie. (Psychomotorische Anfälle, Äquivalente, Automatismen). *Nervenarzt, 24:*331, 1953.
Meynell, M.J.: Megaloblastic anaemia in anticonvulsant therapy. *Lancet, 1:*487, 1966.
Meynert, T.: Studien über das pathologisch-anatomische Material der Wiener Irrenanstalt. *Dtsch Vjschr Psychiatr, 1:*395, 1868.
Mezei, B.: Behandlung der Epileptiker mit 5-5'-Diphenylhydantoin. *Psychiatr-neur Wschr, 115:*1941.
Michaelis, R.: "Herzanfälle" und Schläfenlappenepilepsie. *Dtsch Med Wochenschr, 92:* 152, 1967.
Michnev, A.L.: *Klinische Studien des veränderten Metabolismus bei Lebererkrankungen.* Kiev, Acad. Nauk USSR., 1950.
Michon, P., Larcan, A., Huriet, C., Beaudonin, D. and Berthier, D.V.: Intoxication volontaire mortelle par imipramine (g 22-355). *Bull Soc Med (Paris), 75:*989, 1959.
Mignone, R.J., Donnelly, E.F., and Sadowsky, Doris: Psychological and neurological comparisons of psychomotor and non-psychomotor epilepsy. *Epilepsia, 11:*345-359, 1970.
Miletti, M.: Die Lokalisierung der epileptischen Foci in 20 Fällen von Temporallappenepilepsie. *Zbl Neurol Psychiatr, 140:*8, 1957.
Millen, J.W. and Hess, A.: Blood-brain-barrier–study with vital dyes. *Brain, 81:*248, 1958.
Millichap, J.G.: Relation of laboratory evaluation to clinical effectiveness of antiepileptic drugs. *Epilepsia, 10:*315-328, 1969.
Milner, B.: Psychological defects produced by temporal lobe excision. *Res Publ Ass Nerv Ment Dis, 36:*244, 1958.
Minz, B.: Aspects neuro-humoraux de l'épilepsie. *Thérapie, 20:*1329, 1965.
Minz, B. and Noel, P.: On the presence of adrenaline sensitive receptors at the cerebral cortex of the rabbit. *Experientia, 19:*102, 1963.
Mishkinsky, J., Lajtos, Z.K. and Sulman, F.G.: Initiation of lactation by hypothalamic implantation of perphenazine. *Endocrinology, 78:*919, 1966.
Mison-Crighel, N.: Actiunea miocainei asupra modificarilor determinate de accesul convulsiv experimental în substanta cerebrala. *Stud Cercet Neurol, 2:*361, 1957.
Mison-Crighel, N., Constantinescu, E. and Crighel, E.: Vliane predconvulsivnovo funcionalnovo sostoiania na razvetryvanie sudorojnovo pripadka i byzyvaemye. *Ukr Biokhim Zh, 31:*834, 1959.
Mison-Crighel, N., Constantinescu, E., Costa-Foru, D. and Crighel, E.: Changes in the activity of some enzyme systems determined in the cortical scar and at the level of secondary degenerative lesions. *Acta Neurol Scand, 38:*81, 1962.

Mison-Crighel, N., Crighel, E. and Costa-Foru, D.: Actiunea insuficientei circulatorii cerebrale acute asupra unor leziuni din cortexul cerebral. Correlatii cu date electroencefalografice. *Stud Cercet Neurol, 8:*105, 1963.

Mison-Crighel, N., Lazar, D., Lascar, E. and Giosan, E.: Modificarile metabolismului minerali si echilibrului acidobazic determinante de accesul convulsiv experimentae. *Stud Cercet Fiziol Neurol, 6:*373, 1955.

Mison-Crighel, N., Luca, N. and Crighel, E.: Effect of epileptogenic focus induced by topical application of mescaline on glutamic acid, glutamine and GABA in the neocortex of cats. *J Neurochem, 11:*333, 1964.

Mison-Crighel, N., Pintilie, C. and Crighel, E.: Glutaminase activity and neocortical excitability. *Nature, 206:*1257, 1965.

Mitev, I.P. and Kharizanova, M.S.: Polarographic analysis of the sulfhydryl activity of blood proteins in x-irradiated cancer patients. (Russ) *Arkh Pat Moscow, 20:*17, 1958.

Mölbert, E., Baumgartner, G. and Ketelsen, U.P.: Elektroenmikroskopische Untersuchungen an der Grosshirnrinde der Katze nach Elektrokrämpfen. *Ditsch Z Nervenheilkd, 190:*295, 1967.

Möllenhoff, F.: Ein Fall von Brompsychose. *Mschr Psychiatr Neurol, 67:*364, 1928.

Moeller, K.O.: *Pharmakologie,* 3rd. Ed. Basel, Schwabe, 1958.

Moldave, K., Winzler, R.J. and Pearson, H.E.: Incorporation *in vitro* of ^{14}C into amino acids of control and virus-infected mouse brain. *J Biol Chem, 200:*357, 1953.

Molony, C.J. and Parmelee, A.H.: Convulsions in young infants as a result of pyridoxine (vitamin B_6) deficiency. *JAMA, 154:*405, 1954.

Monnier, M.: Actions électro-physiologiques des stimulants du système nerveux central. I. Systèmes adrénergiques, cholinergiques et neurohumeurs sérotoniques. *Arch Int Pharmacodyn, 124:*281, 1960.

Monnier, M.: Der Schlaf als trofotrope Leistung. *Physiologie und Pathophysiologie des vegetativen Nervensystems.* Stuttgart, vol. I, pp. 263, 1962.

Monnier, M.: *Physiologie und Pathophysiologie des vegetativen Nervensystems.* Stuttgart, Hippokrates, vol. II, 1963.

Monnier, M.: Biochemische, pharmakologische und humorale Aspekte des Schlaf-Wachseins. In Jovanović, U.J. (Ed.): *Der Schlaf. Neurophysiologische Aspekte.* München, Barth, 1969.

Monnier, M. and Krupp, P.: Elektrophysiologische Analyse der Wirkung verschiedener Neuroleptica (Chlorpromazin, Reserpin, Tofranil, Meprobamat). *Schweiz Med Wochenschr, 53:*89, 1959.

Monnier, M. and Romanowski, W.: Les systèmes cholinoceptifs cérébraux. Actions de l'acétylcholine, de la physiostigmine, pilocarpine et de GABA. *Electroenceph Clin Neurophysiol, 14:*486, 1962.

Monnier, M. and Tissot, R.: L'action de la réserpine-sérotonine sur le cerveau; suppression par les antagonistes de la réserpine: iproniazid (Marsilid) et L.S.D. *Schweiz Arch Neurol Psychiatr, 82:*218, 1958.

Montanelli, R.P. and Hassler, R.: Stimulation effects of the globus pallidus and nucleus entopeduncularis of the cat. *Excerpta Med, 48:*Nr. 1091, 1962.

Montanelli, R.P. and Hassler, R.: Motor effects elicited by stimulation of the pallidothalamic system in the cat. In Bargmann, Schadé (Eds.): *Progr Brain Res.* Amsterdam, Elsevier, vol. V, pp. 56, 1964.

Montedoro, A. and Buttighone, M.: Intorno alla comparsa di manifestazioni convulsive in corso di terapia promazinica in campo psichiatrico. *Acta Neurol* (Napoli), *14:* 680, 1959.

Moore, M.T.: Symptomatic abdominal epilepsy. *Am J Surg, 72:*883, 1946.

Moran, N.C. and Butler, W.M.: The pharmacological properties of chlorpromazine sulfoxide, a major metabolite of chlorpromazine; a comparison with chlorpromazine. *J Pharmacol Exp Ther, 118:*328, 1956.

Morel, B.A.: *Gaz hébd méd et chir, 7:*773, 1850; cit. by: Landolt, H.: *Die Temporallappenepilepsie und ihre Psychopathologie.* Basel-New York, Karger, 1960.

Morel, F. and Wildi, E. Sclérose ammonienne et épilepsie. *Acta Neurol Belg, 56:*61, 1956.

Morell, F. and Florenz, A. Modification of the freezing technique for producing experimental epileptogenic lesions. *Electroenceph Clin Neurophysiol, 10:*187, 1958.

Morell, F. and Torres, F.: Electrophysiological analysis of a case of Tay Sachs disease. *Brain, 83:*213, 1960.

Morillo, A.: Effects of benzodiazepines upon amygdala and hippocampus of the cat. *Int J Neuropharm, 1:*353, 1962.

Morison, R.S. and Dempsey, E.W.: A study of thalamo-cortical relations. *Am J Physiol, 135:*281, 1942.

Morrell, F.: Cellular pathophysiology of focal epilepsy. *Epilepsia, 10:*495-505, 1969.

Morris, A.A.: Temporal lobectomy with removal of uncus, hippocampus and amygdala, results for psychomotor epilepsy three to nine years after operation. *Arch Neurol, 76:*479, 1956.

Mortillaro, M., Kanig, K., and Emser, W.: Der Einfluss von Harmin auf die bioelektrische Aktivität des Rattengehirns. *Arch Psychiat Nervenkr 213,* 327-344, 1970.

Moruzzi, G.: Synchronizing influences of the brain stem and the inhibitory mechanisms underlying the production of sleep by sensory stimulation. In Jasper, Smirnov (Eds.): The Moscow colloquium on electroencephalography of higher nervous activity. *Electroenceph Clin Neurophysiol, 13:*231, 1960.

Moruzzi, G.: The Sleep-Waking Sycle. In *Review of Physiology* (Neurophysiology and Neurochemistry of Sleep and Wakefulness). With Contributions by M. Jouvet and G. Moruzzi. Springer-Verlag, Berlin-Heidelberg-New York, *64:*1, 1972.

Moruzzi, G. and Magoun, H.W.: Brain stem reticular formation and activation of the EEG. *Electroenceph Clin Neurophysiol, 1:*455, 1949.

Moser, H.W. and Karnovsky, M.L.: Biosynthesis of glycolipids and other lipids of the brain. *J Biol Chem, 234:*1990, 1959.

Mosinger, B.: Some metabolic manifestations of central electrotonus. *Physiol Bohemoslov Fremdspr Ausg, 6:*156, 1957.

Müller, D., Müller, J., and Hoppe, W.: Dosierungsprobleme bei der medikamentösen Behandlung der Epilepsien. *Therapiewoche, 22:*39, 1972.

Müller, H.R., Klingler, M., Kaeser, H.E., Wurmser, P. and Hirt, H.R.: Zur Behandlung des Status epilepticus mit Diazepam (Valium). *Schweiz Med Wochenschr,* 121, 1966.

Müller, J., and Müller, D.: Hirnelektrische Korrelate bei Überdosierung von antikonvulsiven Medikamenten. *Nervenarzt, 43:*270-272, 1972.

Müller, O. and Müller, G.: Synthesis in the vitamin B_{12} series. XIV On the synthesis of corrinoids with cobalt-carbon binding. *Biochem Zschr, 336:*299, 1962.

Müller, P.B. and Langemann, H.: Distribution of glutamic acid decarboxylase activity in human brain. *J Neurochem, 9:*399, 1962.

Mulder, D.W. and Daly, D.: Psychiatric symptoms associated with lesions of temporal lobe. *JAMA, 150:*173, 1952.

Mulder, D.W., Daly, D. and Bailey, A.A.: Visceral epilepsy. *Arch Int Med, 93:*481, 1954.

Mumenthaler, M.: Anfälle im Kindesalter in der Sicht des Neurologen. *Praxis, 56:* 1586, 1967.

Munch-Petersen, C.J.: Beitrag zur Pathogenese der Epilepsie und zur Genese des durch Hyperventilation hervorgerufenen epileptischen Anfalls. *Hosp Tid, 1:*418, 1931.

Munkvad, I.: Determinations of glutamine and glutamic acid in a material of mental patients. Preliminary report. *Acta Psychiat Scand, 25*:269, 1950.

v. Muralt, A.: Role of thiamine in nervous excitation. *Exp Cell Res, 5*:72, 1958.

v. Muralt, A.: *Neue Ergebnisse der Neurophysiologie*. Berlin-Göttingen-Heidelberg, Springer, 1958.

Murphy, Q.R. (Ed.): Metabolic aspects of transport across cell membranes. Madison, U of Wis Pr, 1957.

Mustard, D.H.: Treatment of Parkinsonism in elderly patients with Cosaldon. *Br J Clin Pract, 18*:537, 1964.

Mutani, R., Bergamini, L., Fariello, R., and Quattrocolo, G.: An experimental investigation on the mechanisms of interaction of asymmetrical acute epileptic foci. *Epilepsia, 13*:597-608, 1972.

Nachmansohn, D.: Die Rolle des Acetylcholins in den Elementarvorgängen der Nervenleitung. *Ergeb Physiol, 48*:575, 1955.

Nachmansohn, D.: Chemical and molecular basis of nerve activity. In Elliott, Page, Quastel (Eds.): *Neurochemistry*, 2nd Ed. Springfield, Thomas, 1962.

Nachmansohn, D. and Feld, E.A.: Studies on cholinesterase; on mechanism of diisoporyl fluorophosphate action *in vivo*. *J Biol Chem, 171*:715, 1947.

Náhunek, K., Bojanowský, J. and Rybáková, V.: Excitomotor preparkinsonian symptoms in the ataractic treatment. *Csl Psychiatr, 55*:377, 1959.

Naquet, R. and King, E.E.: Central influences on somatic afferent transmission through the thalamus. *Am J Physiol, 179*:659, 1954.

Natalevitch, E.S.: Theses—Proceedings to the conference on problems of metabolism in patients with psychic disorders. (Russ) Moscow, 1958.

Natalevitch, E.S.: Exploration of products of phosphorilization in schizophrenics with sitophobia. (Russ.) In *Obm Veshtch Psikhiat Zabol*. Moscow, Medgiz, pp. 40-46, 1960.

Naumova, O.A.: Study on the cerebral convulsibility. (Russ) L.M.I., 1940.

Nauta, W.J.H.: An experimental study of the fornix in the rat. *J Comp Neurol, 104*: 247, 1956.

Nauta, W.J.H.: Hippocampal projections and related neural pathways to the midbrain in the cat. *Brain, 81*:319, 1958.

Nayrac, P. and Beaussart, M.: Concerning 4 c/sec rhythmus in posterior head regions in old head injuries. *Electroenceph Clin Neurophysiol, 8*:730, 1956a.

Nayrac, P. and Beaussart, M.: A propos des rhythmes à 4 c/sec postérieurs chez les anciens traumaticés cranies. *Rev Neurol, 94*:849, 1965b.

Neimanis, G.: Klinische und morphologische Befunde bei vier Fällen von psychomotorischer Epilepsie. *Dtsch Z Nervenheilkd, 183*:258, 1962.

Nellhaus, G.: Experimental epilepsy in rabbits: Failure to detect a difference in phenylalanine metabolism in convulsant rabbits. *Proc Soc Exp Biol Med, 120*:259, 1965.

Neri, A.: Il comportamento del metabolismo basale negli epilettici allo stato di riposo e sotto l'azione delle sostanze farmacodinamiche. *Rass Stud Psichiatr, 23*:1148, 1934.

Nesorova, T.A.: *Aminazine in Clinical and Ambulant Practice*. (Russ) Moscow, Medgiz, 1961.

Netter, H.: *Theoretische Biochemi* Berlin-Göttingen-Heidelberg, Springer, 1959.

Neubauer, H.: Die Langzeitbehandlung mit Cosaldon bei Durchblutungsstörungen der Netz- und Aderhaut. *Klin Monatsbl Augenheilkd, 146*:646, 1965.

Neubauer, O.: Über den Abbau der Aminosäuren im gesunden und kranken Organismus. *Dtsch Arch Klin Med, 95*:211, 1909.

Neuhoff, V. and Harris, T.: Isolierung und Identifizierung von Metaboliten des 3-Acetylpyridins. *Arch Exp Path Pharmakol, 249*:11, 1964.

Nicholas, H.J. and Thomas, B.E.: Metabolism of cholesterol and fatty acids in the central nervous system. *J Neurochem, 4*:42, 1959a.

Nicholas, H.J. and Thomas, B.E.: Metabolism of cholesteral and fatty acids in the central nervous system. *Biochem Biophys Acta, 36*:583, 1959b.

Niebeling, H.G.: Die Provokationsmethoden im EEG. In Niebeling, G. (Ed.): *Einführung in die Elektroencephalographie*. Leipzig, Barth, pp. 160-165, 1968.

Niedermeyer, E.: Psychomotor seizure with generalized synchronous spike and wave discharge. Report of a case. *Electroenceph Clin Neurophysiol, 6*:49, 1954.

Niedermeyer, E.: Verlauf und Prognose der psychomotorischen Epilepsie. Klinische und elektroencephalographische Gesichtspunkte. *Schweiz Arch Neurol Neurochir Psychiatr, 76*:382, 1955.

Niedermeyer, E.: Zur Frage der psychomotorischen Epilepsie des Kindesalters. *Zbl Neurol Psychiatr, 140*:3, 1957.

Nigro, A.: 3rd Int. Congr. Cyber. Med., Napoli 1964; cit. by Nigro, A.: Kybernetische Mechanismen bei Epilepsie. In *Clinical Neurophysiology EEG-EMG*. 6th Int. Congr. EEG Clin. Neurophysiol. Vienna, p. 81, 1965.

Nigro, A.: Kybernetische Mechanismen bei Epilepsie. In *Clinical Neurophysiology EEG-ENG. 6th Int. Congr. EEG Clin. Neurophysiol.* Vienna, p. 81, 1965.

Niklowitz, W.: Elektronenmikroskopische Untersuchungen am Ammonshorn. II. *Z Zellforsch Mikrosk Anat, 70*:220, 1966.

Niklowitz, W., Bak, I.J. and Hassler, R.: Electronmicroscopial observations of pyramidal cells in the hippocampus after 3-Acetylpyridine treatment. II. *Int. Congr. Histo-Cytochem.* 172, 1964.

Nissen, G.: Klinik and Therapie der Epilepsie im Kindesalter. Monatschrift Kinderheilk., *118*:624-629, 1970.

Northcote, M.L.M.: Somatic changes in the psychosis. A comprehensive investigation of the bodily functions of thirty psychotic patients by means of clinical, pathological, biochemical, pharmacological and radiological methods. *J Ment Sci, 78*:263, 1932.

Novikoff, A.B., de The, G., Beard, D. and Beard, J.W.: Electron microscopic study of the ATPase activity of the BAI strain A (myeloblastosis) avian tumor virus. *J Cell Biol, 15*:451, 1962.

Novlanskaya, K.A.: Clinical application of calcium salts of glutamic acid in epilepsy. Conference on the amino acids in medicine. (Russ) MGU, pp. 50-52, 1956.

O'Brien, J.L. and Goldensohn, E.S.: Paroxysmal abdominal pain as a manifestation of epilepsy. *Neurology* (Minneap), *7*:549, 1957.

Ochoa, S.: "Coupling" of phosphorilation with oxidation of pyruvic acid in bran tissue. *J Biol Chem, 138*:751, 1941a.

Ochoa, S.: Glycolysis and phosphorilation in brain extracts. *J Biol Chem, 141*:245, 1941b.

Oeriu, S.: Tanaescu, G., Dimitriu, M., Siminoscu-Grigorescu, G., Manescu, M., Costescu, G. et al.: Biochimia creerului. VII. Procesul de transaminase in cerierul de sobolan supuse actiunii luminalului sau benezedrinei. Studii şi cercetari viochem. *Acad R P R, 1*:213, 1958.

Oesterle, W., Kanig, K., Büchel, W. and Nickel, A.-K.: Preparation of DNA and four different RNAs from rat brain. A new RNA fraction and a new characteristic of the various RNAs. *J Neurochem 17*:1403-1419, 1970.

Oesterle, W., K. Kanig and P. Johann: Nucleinsäuren im Rattengehirn, I. In-vivo-Markierung mit$^{32}P_i$; Präparation von DNA und vier verschiedenen RNA-Fraktionen in einem Arbeitsgang. *Hoppe-Seyler's Z Physiol Chem 352*:959-976, 1971.

Oettinger, L.jr. and Simonds, R.: A new anticonvulsant (1-methyl-5-5-phenylethylhydantoin) in treatment of epilepsy in children. *Dis Nerv Syst, 23*:403, 1962.

Ogata, K.: Experimental study on the genesis of swelling of the brain. Electrophoretic analysis of proteins of the brain tissue. *Tukushima J Exp Med, 1:*138, 1954.
Okumura, M., Kawaki, K., Kawada, S., Fujita, S., Morisada, A. and Kobayashi, S.: cit. in *RJHJM Bioch, 15:*524, 1960.
Oles, M.: Klinische Erfahrungen mit dem Neuroleptikum Haloperidol (R 1625) *Acta Neurol Belg, 60:*100, 1960.
Omorikov, N.: Über Indikanurie bei Geisteskrankheiten. *Obosrenije psikh, 9:*36, 1909.
Ortmann, R.: Über die chemische Spezifität von Neuronensystemen. In *Progr. Brain Res.,* Amsterdam, Elsevier., vol. VI, p. 4.
Ostermann, E., Bellander, S., Löfvenberg, S. and Lassenius, B.: SCTZ. A new sedative and hypnotic related to thiamine. *Acta Psychiatr Scand, 34:*56, 1959.
Oswald, I.: Human brain protein, drugs and dreams. *Nature* (Lond), *223:*893, 1969.
Oswald, I., Berger, R.J., Jaramillo, R.A., Keddie, R.M., Olley, P.C. and Plunkett, G.B.: Melancholia and barbiturates: A controlled EEG, body and eye movement study of sleep. *Br J Psychiatry, 109:*66, 1963.
Paal, G.: Zur Frühdiagnose von Hirntumoren. *Hippokrates, 36:*185, 1965.
Paal, G.: Zur klinischen Diagnose von Hirntumoren. *Hippokrates, 36:*387, 1965.
Pace, J. and McDermott, E.E.: Methionine sulfoximine and enzyme systems involving glutamine. *Nature* (Lond), *169:*145, 1952.
Pache, H.-D. and Stolecke, H.: Zur Behandlung von BNS-Krämpfen mit ACTH. *Mschr Kinderheilkd, 110:*105, 1962.
Pache, H.D. and Tröger, H.: Das West-Syndrom und seine Behandlung mit ACTH. *Munch Med Wochenschr, 109:*2408, 1967.
Padovani, G.: L'aspetto biologico del problema. *Lav Nevropsichiatr* (Roma), *14:*359, 1954.
Padovani, V.: Le alterazioni funzionali del sistema reticolo-endoteliale nelle schizofrenie rivelate dalla "prova del Rosso Congo". *Note Psichiat, 64:*265, 1935.
Paffrath, F.: Das Problem des psychiatrischen Alterns vom Kreislauf und einem Durchblutung fördernden Mittel her aufgerollt. *Die Medizinische, 11:*388, 1959.
le Page, G.A.: Biological energy transformations during shock as shown tissue analysis. *Am J Physiol, 146:*267, 1946.
Page, I.H.: Serotonin (5-hydroxytryptamin). *Physiol Rev, 34:*563, 1954.
Pagniez, P.: Contribution à l'étude des effets de l'hypernée chez les épileptiques. *Bull Acad Natl Med* (Paris), *3:*419, 1933.
Paine, R.S., Hsia, D.Y.-Y., Hsia, H.H. and Driscoll, K.: Dietary phenylalanine requirements and tolerances of phenylketonuric patients. *Am J Dis Child, 94:*224, 1957.
Palladin, A.V.: Brain metabolism at stimulation. (Russ) *J High Nerv Syst, 3:*801, 1953.
Palladin, A.V.: Biochemia Nervnoi Sistemy (monograph) *Tsv Akad Nauk SSSR,* 1954.
Palladin, A.V.: Functional biological chemistry of the brain. (Russ) *Suppl. 20th Int. Congr. Physiol.* Burxelles, 1956.
Palladin, A.V.: Biochemical characteristics of the functional different parts of the nervous system. (Russ) *Ukr Biokhim Zh, 31:*756, 1959.
Palladin, A.V.: Brain metabolism at stimulation and inhibition. (Russ) *Ukr Biokhim Zh, 34:*621, 1962.
Palladin, A.V., Belik, Y.V. and Krachko, L.S.: The rate of protein renewal in the brain in states of stimulation and inhibition of different ages of the test animal. *Biokhimia* (Moscow), *22:*359, 1957.
Palladin, A.V., Belik, Y.V., Polyakova, N.M. and Silich, T.P.: Proteins of the nervous system. (Russ) *Vopr. Biokhim. Nerv. Sist.,* Kiev, Acad. Nauk USSR., pp. 9-30, 1957.
Palladin, A.V. and Vladimirov, G.E.: Application of radioactive isotopes in the explora-

tion of the functional biological chemistry of the brain. In *Application of Isotopes in Technic, Biology and Other Sciences* (Russ) . Moscow, Medgiz, pp. 227-242, 1955.
Paludan, J.: Autoptic findings in a child with infantile spasms with a survey of the effect of ACTH. *Dan Med Bull, 8:*128, 1961.
Pampiglione, G. and Falconer, M.A.: Some observations upon stimulation of the hippocampus in man. *Electroenceph Clin Neurophysiol, 8:*718, 1956.
Pampiglione, G. and Falconer, M.A.: Electrical stimulation of the hippocampus in man. In Field, Magoun, Hall (Eds.): *Hb. of Physiology,* Sect. I. Baltimore, Williams & Wilkins, vol. II, p. 1391, 1960.
Pampiglione, G. and Kerridge, J.: EEG abnormalities from the temporal lobe studied with sphenoidal electrodes. *J Neurol NS, 19:*117, 1956.
Pampus, F.: Der Gesichtsschmerz und seine Behandlung. *Münch Med Wochenschr, 100:* 1292 ,1958.
Papadopulos, F.F.: The glycemic curve after two loads with saccharose in schizophrenics. In *Obm. Veshtch. Psikhiat. Zabol.* Moscow, Medgiz, pp. 56-61, 1960.
Papez, J.W.: A proposed mechanism of emotion. *Arch Neurol, 38:*725, 1937.
Pappius, H.M. and Elliott, K.A.C.: Adenosine triphosphatase electrolytes and oxygen uptake rates of human normal and epileptogenic cerebral cortex. *Can J Biochem Physiol, 32:*481, 1954.
Pappius, H. M. and Elliott, K.A.C.: Water distribution in incubated slices of brain and other tissues. *Can J Biochem Physiol, 34:*5, 1956.
Paquay, M.M., Arnould Burton, Tinant and Piersotte: Untersuchung der Wirksamkeit von Cosaldon auf die Cerebralsklerose auf psychiatrischem Gebiet. *Acta Neurol Psychaitr Belg, 62:*1069, 1962.
Pare, C.B.M., Sandler, M. and Stacey, R.S.: 5-hydroxytryptamine deficiency in phenylketonuria. *Lancet, I:*551, 1957.
Paritchenko, E.V.: *Collected Writings on the Problem of Schizophrenia Therapy in Pathophysiological View.* (Russ) Charkov, Acad. Nauk SSSR., 1958.
Parks, R.E.jr., Kidder, G.W. and Dewey, V.C.: Thiosemicarbazide toxicity in mice. *Proc Soc Exp Biol Med, 79:*287, 1952.
Parsonage, M.J. and Norris, J.W.: Use of diazepam in treatment of severe convulsive status epilepticus. *Br Med J, 3:*85, 1967.
Pasolini, F. and Dede, G.: Studio della protidemia, con metodo elettroforetico nel siero di sangue di epilettici. Nota II. *Acta Neurol* (Napoli), 11, 111, 1956.
Passouant, P., Passouant-Fontaine, T. and Cadilhac, J.: Hippocampe et réaction d'eveil. *C R Soc Biol,* (Paris), *149:*164, 1955.
Patry, F.L.: The relation of time of day, sleep and other factors to the incidence of epileptic seizures. *Am J Psychiatry, 10:*798, 1931.
Pauig, P.M., Deluca, M.A. and Osterheld, R.G.: Thirodiazine hydrochloride in the treatment of behavior disorders in epileptics. *Am J Psychiatry, 117:*832, 1961.
Paulusch, R.: Behandlung peripherer Durchblutungsstörungen. Arztl. *Praxis, 12:*1151, 1960.
Pavlov, P.I.: *Psychiatry as Term of Physiological Changes in the Great Brain Hemispheres.* Petersburg, Acad. Nauk, Russ. pp. 274-275, 1919.
Pavlov, P.I.: *Selected Writings.* Moscow, Acad. Nauk SSSR., 1951.
Peiffer, J.: Probleme der pathologischen Anatomie der Temporallappenepilepsie. *Dtsch Z Nervenheilkd, 183:*245, 1962.
Peiffer, J.: Morphologische Aspekte der Epilepsien. *Monographien aus dem Gesamtgebiet der Neurologie und Psychiatrie.* Berlin-Göttingen-Heidelberg, Springer, 1963.

Peiffer, J.: Morphologische Gesichtspunkte zur Ursache und Pathogenese der Epilepsie. *Therapiewoche, 17:*63, 1967.
Peiffer, J.: Zur Neuropathologie der Epilepsie. *Epilepsy Mod Probl Pharmacopsychiat* IV:42-50, 1970.
Penachietti, M.: Esami biopsici del fetago nelle schizofrenie. I., II. *Schizophrenie, 5:* 247 a. 401, 1935.
Penfield, W.: Classification of the epilepsies. *Arch Neurol Psychiatr, 60:*107, 1948.
Penfield, W.: Memory mechanisms. *Arch Neurol Psychiatr, 67:*178, 1952.
Penfield, W.: Vestibular sensation and the cerebral cortex. *Annals of Otol Rhinol Laryngol, 66:*691, 1957.
Penfield, W.: Centrencephalic integrating system. *Brain, 8:*231, 1958.
Penfield, W.: The interpretive cortex; the stream of consciousness in the human brain can be electrically reactivated. *Science, 129:*1719, 1959.
Penfield, W. and Erickson, T.C.: *Epilepsy and Its Cerebral Localization.* Moscow, Medgiz 7, 1949 (Russ).
Penfield, W. and Faulk, M.E.jr.: The insula. Further observation of its function. *Brain, 78:*445, 1955.
Penfield, W. and Flanagin, H.: Surgical therapy of temporal lobe seizures. *Arch Neurol Psychiatr, 64:*491, 1950.
Penfield, W. and Jasper, H.H.: *Epilepsy and the Functional Anatomy of the Human Brain.* Boston, Little, Brown & Co., 1954.
Penfield, W. and Milner, B.: Memory deficit produced by bilateral lesions in the hippocampal zone. *Arch Neurol Psychiatr, 79:*475, 1958.
Penfield, W. and Rasmussen, T.: The Cerebral Cortex of Man. Fed. Proc. *6:*452-460, New York, 1950.
Penfield, W. and Ward, A.: Calcifying epileptogenic lesions (hemangioma calcifians). *J Neuropath Exp Neurol, 7:*111, 1948.
Penin, H.: Wirkung und Indikation eines neuen Antiepilepkums. *Dtsch Med Wochenschr, 89:*1638, 1964.
Penin, H.: Die Epilepsietherapie im Erwachsenenalter. *Therapiewoche, 17:*171, 1967.
Pennel, R.B. and Savaris, C.A.: A human factor inducing behavioral and electrophysiological changes in animals. I. Isolation and chemical nature of the agent. *Ann NY Acad Sci, 96:*462, 1962.
Penta, P.: Orientamenti terapeutici nelle schizophrenie *Riforma Med, 53:*1817, 1937.
Perlstein, M.A.: Use of meprobamate (Miltown) in convulsive and related disorders. *JAMA, 161:*1040, 1956.
Peter, A.L., Holden, B. and Jirout, J.: The efferent intercortical connections of the superficial cortex of the temporal lobe (Macaca mulatta). *J Neuropath Exp Neurol, 8:* 100, 1949.
Petermann, M.G.: The ketogenic diet in the treatment of epilepsy. A preliminary report. *Am J Dis Child, 28:*28, 1924.
Peters, E.L. and Tower, D.B.: Glutamic acid and glutamine metabolism in cerebral cortex after seizures induced by methionine sulphoximine. *J Neurochem, 5:*80, 1959.
Peters, R.A.: Significance of thiamine in the metabolism and function of the brain. In Elliott, Page, Quastel (Eds.): *Neurochemistry.* Springfield, Thomas, 1962.
Petersén, I. and Hambert, O.: Klinisk och elektroencephalografisk studie av affekten av Chlormethiazole och Lignocaine vid myoklonus epilepsi. 1966a cit. by Petersén, I. and Liessner, P.: *Acta Psychiatr Scand, 42:*103, 1966.
Petersén, I. and Hambert, O.: Clinical and electroencephalographic studies of responses

to lidocaine and chlormethiazole in progressive myoclonus epilepsy. *Acta Psychiatr Scand, 42:*45, 1966b.

Petersén, I. and Leissner, P.: Effect of intravenous injection of chlormethiazole in spasticity, rigidity and tremor. Preliminary comm. *Acta Psychiatr Scand, 42:*103, 1966.

Petrilowitsch, N.: *Psychiatrische Krankheitslehre und psychiatrische Pharmakotherapie.* Basel-New York, Karger, 1966.

Petsche, H., Marko, A. and Monnier, M.: Mikrozeitliche toposkopische Analyse bioelektrischer Hirnwellen beim Kaninchen. II. *Helv Physiol Acta, 14:*169, 1956.

Petsche, H. and Monnier, M.: Die elektrische Aktivität der Hirnrinde und des Zwischenhirns bei Reizung von Cortex, Rhinencephalon und Diencephalon. *Helv Physiol Acta, 12:*123, 1954.

Pette, H.: Über den vegetativen Anfall. *Zschr Neurol, 165:*320, 1939.

Pette, H. and Janzen, R.: Das Verhalten vegetativer Regulationen in der Anfallsbereitschaft bei Epileptikern. *Dtsch Z Nervenheilkd, 145:*1, 1938.

Peyrethon, J., Dusan, D. and Jouvet, M.: Suppression élective du sommeil paradoxal par Alpha-methyl DOPA. *Experientia, 14:*2B, 1967.

Pfeiffer, C.C., Jenney, E.H. and Marshall, W.H.: Experimental seizures in man and animals with acute pyridoxine deficiency produced by hydrazides. *Electroenceph Clin Neurophysiol, 8:*307, 1956.

Pflanz, M. and Schrader, A.: Experimentelle Untersuchung über den Einfluß zentraler Stimulantien auf das Elektroencephalogramm des Menschen. *Klin Wochenschr, 37:* 483, 1959.

Pfleger, L.: Beobachtungen über Schrumpfung und Sklerose des Ammonshorns bei Epilepsie. *Allg Z Psychiatr, 36:*359, 1880.

Philippopoulou, G.S. et al.: Klinische Beobachtungen und Resultate bei der Anwendung eines neuen Vasodilators bei frischen und chronischen Fällen von cerebralen vaskulären Affektionen. *Iatrica Chronica* (Med. ann. Athen), *2:*1, 1963.

Pia, H.W.: Klinik und Syndrom der Schläfenlappengeschwülste. *Fortschr Neurol Psychiatr, 12:*555, 1953.

Pieril, L. and Hürlimann, A.: Zur Pharmakologie des Schlafes. *Arzneim Forsch, 15:*1134, 1965.

Pilcz, A.: *Lehrbuch der speziellen Psychiatrie.* Jena, Fischer, 1901.

Pile, W.J.: Effect of glutamic acid on chronic psychotic patients. *Dis Nerv Syst, 13:*106, 1952.

Pincus, J.H., Grove, I., Marino, B.B., and Glaser, G.E.: Studies on the mechanism of action of diphenylhydantoin. *Arch Neurol 22:*566-571, 1970.

Pintilie, C., Mison-Crighel, N., and Crighel, E.: Mescaline-Spikes and amino acids in the cortex of cats pretreated with caffeine and pentetrazol. *Epilepsia, 11:*303-311, 1970.

Pisano, J.J., Mitoma, C. and Udenfriend, S.: Biosynthesis of gamma-guanidino-butyric acid from gamma-amino-butyric acid and arginine. *Nature* (Lond), *180:*1125, 1957.

Plaa, G.L. et al.: Intoxication from Primidone due to its biotransformation to phenobarbital. *JAMA, 168:*1769, 1958.

Pleasure, H.: Psychiatric and neurological side-effects of isoniazid and iproniazid. *Arch Neurol Psychiatr, 72:*313, 1954.

Pletscher, A., Bruderer, H., Burkard, W.P. and Gey, K.F.: Decrease of cerebral 5 HT and 5 HIAA by an arylalkylamine. *Science, 11:*828, 1963.

Pletscher, A. and da Prada, M.: Veränderung des cerebralen Dopaminmetabolismus durch Psychopharmaka. *Helv Physiol Pharmacol Acta, 24:*C45, 1966.

Plischevskaya, E.G.: Stable isotopes. In *Methods of Marked Atomes in Biology.* MGU, pp. 178-207, 1955, (Russ).

Plotnikoff, N.: *Science, 151:*703, 1966; cit. by Kanig, K. *Arzneim Forsch, 19:*397, 1969.

Podoprigora, V.D.: Protein fractions in blood-serum of schizophrenic patients (polarographic method). (Russ) In *Obm. Veshtch. Psikhiat. Zabol.* Moscow, Medgiz, pp. 107-113, 1960.

Poeck, K.: Die Formatio reticularis des Hirnstamms. (Physiologie und Klinik). *Nervenarzt, 30:*289, 1959.

Pöldinger, W.: *Kompendium der Psychopharmakotherapie.* Dtsch. Hoffman-La Roche AG, Grenzach, Baden, 1967.

Pogodaev, K.I.: On nature and mechanisms of viscous acidobasic potentials of the blood and certain tissues. "Nature and method of study of bioelectrical potentials". *Annual of Physiological Exploration Methods in Biology.* (Russ) Acad. Sci. SSSR, Moscow, pp. 50-54, 1954.

Pogodaev, K.I.: Vopr. Psikhiat. Moscow 1956; cit. by Krasnova, A.I.: The polarographic activity of blood-serum of schizophrenics and epileptics. In *Obm. Veshtch. Psikhiat. Zabol.* Moscow, Medgiz, pp. 114-119, 1960.

Pogodaev, K.I.: *Biochemistry of the Epileptic Seizure.* (Russ) Moscow, Medicina, 1964.

Pogodaev, K.I. and Galenko, V.E.: Vopr. Psikhiat. 1956; cit. by Podoprigora, V.D.: Protein fractions in the blood-serum of schizophrenic patients (polarographic method). In *Obm. Veshtch. Psikhiat. Zabol.* Moscow, Medgiz, pp. 107-113, 1960.

Pogodaev, K.I. and Krasnova, A.I.: Antiepileptic action of Karamanoff-mixture in experimentally explored animals. *XIX. session of the Ukr. Inst. of Research of Psychoneurology.* Charkov, Acad. Nauk SSSR., pp. 109-111, 1954.

Pogodaev, K.I. and Krasnova, A.I.: Acido-basic processes and metabolism in schizophrenic patients dependent on the method of therapy. *Proc. of the Confer. Dedicated to the 100th birthday of S.S. Korsakoff and Actual Problems of Psychiatry.* (Russ) Moscow, Medgiz, pp. 293-296, 1955.

Pogodaev, K.I. and Krasnova, A.I.: Jodo-metrical determination of sulphur proportion in urine. Actual problems of psychiatry. *Research Report of the Inst. of Psychiatry, Ministery of Health of the SSSR* (1945-1953). (Russ) Moscow, Medgiz, 1956.

Pogodaev, K.I., Krasnova, A.I. and Mekler, L.B.: Acido-basic processes and nitrogen metabolism in brain in experimental epilepsy. In *Vopr. Psikhiat.* Moscow, Medgiz, p 270, 1956.

Pogodaev, K.I. and Mehmedova, A.I.: Protein metabolism and respiration of some brain parts in test animals during and after medicamentally induced sleep. In *Vopr. Biokhim. Nerv. Sist.* Kiev, Acad. Nauk USSR., pp. 40-46, 1957.

Pogodaev, K.I., Savtchenko, Z.I., and Gusyatinskaya, M.I.: Biochemical base of clonic seizures. Research reports of the institute for higher nervous function. *Serie: Physiology, 5:*253, 1960. (Russ)

Pogodaev, K.I., Savtchenko, Z.I., Ossipova, M.S. and Turova, N.F.: Protein metabolism of brain tissue in repeated epileptic seizures. (Russ) *Ukr Biokhim Zh, 32:*808, 1960.

Pogodaev, K.I. and Turova, N.F.: Isolation of radio-methionine and radio-tyrosine in brain tissue in singular and repeated epileptic seizures. *Ukr Biokhim Zh, 31:*849, 1959.

Pogodaev, K.I., Turova, N.F., and Savtchenko, Z.I.: Protein metabolism and energetic changes in brain at inhibition and exhaustion. *5th Intern Biochem Congr, 1:*468, 1961.

Pogrund, R.S., Drell, S.W. and Clark, W.G.: Transamination of 3-hydxoy-phenyl-pyruvic acid *in vivo. Fed Proc, 14:*116, 1955.

Pogrund, R.S., Drell, S.W. and Clark, W.G.: Metabolism of 3-hydroxy- and 3,4-dihydroxy-phenyl-pyruvic avids. *J Pharmacol Exp Ther, 131:*294, 1961.

Pokrovsky, A.A. and Ponomavera, L.G.: Enzyme activities of brain tissues in reflex epilepsy. *Fed Proc 24:* Pt. 2, 995, 1965.

Poli, C.: Sopra un caso di sindrome Cotard incompleta. *Rass Stud Psichait, 31:*394, 1942.

Polishtchuk, I.A.: *Biochemical Advances in Psychiatry.* Kiev, 1937.

Polishtchuk, I.A.: *Nevropatol Psikhiat, 6:*1938; cit. by Sorokina, T.T.: Biochemical and experimental studies of catatonic stupor of schizophrenic kind. In *Obm. Vestch. Psikhiat. Zabol.* Moscow, Medgiz, pp. 77-84, 1960.

Polishtchuk, I.A.: Proc. of the 19th. conference of the Ukr. Inst. 1939; cit. by Sorokina, T.T.: Biochemical and experimental studies of catatonic stupor of schiozphrenic kind. In *Obm. Veshtch. Psikhiat. Zabol.* Moscow, Medgiz, pp. 77-84, 1960.

Polishtchuk, I.A.: *On the Toxic Factors in Schizophrenia.* Kiev, Acad. Nauk USSR., 1940.

Polishtchuk, I.A.: *Problems of Pathophysiology and Therapy in Schizophrenics.* Kiev, Acad. Nauk USSR., vol. II, 1947.

Polishtchuk, I.A. and Sobolevskaya, R.V.: *Problems of Pathophysiology and Therapy in Schizophrenics.* Kiev, Acad. Nauk USSR., vol. II, 1947.

Pollock, G.H. and Bein, J.A.: Convulsions in the cerebellum and cerebrum induced by gamma-chlorinated amines. *Am J Physiol, 160:*195, 1950.

Pope, A., Caveness, W. and Livingston, H.E.: Architectonic distribution of acteylcholinesterase in frontal isocortex of psychotic and nonpsychotic patients. *Arch Neurol Psychiatr, 68:*425, 1952.

Pope, A., Morris, A.A., Jasper, H., Elliott, K.A.C. and Penfield, W.: Histochemical and action potential studies on epileptogenic areas of cerebral cortex in man and monkey. *Res Publ Assoc Nerv Ment Dis, 26:*218, 1947.

Popov, E.A.: *Actual Problems of Neurology and Psychiatry.* Kuibishev, Russ. Acad. Nauk 1957 (Russ.).

Popov, E.A. Epilepsy. In Kerbikoff, M.B., Ozerecki, N.I., Popov, E.A. and Snedznevski, A.B. (Eds.): *Compendium of Psychiatry.* Moscow, Medgiz pp. 231-244, 1958.

Popp, A.: Trigeminusneuralgie. *Mat Med Nordm, 6:*361, 1954.

Poroschina, A.A.: Zh. Nevropatol. Psikhiat. "Korsakoff" 4, 1955; cit. by Wolfsohn, H.M.: On the signification of some biochemical shifting to prognosis and effect of schizophrenia therapy. In *Obm. Veshtch. Psikhiat. Zabol.* Moscow, Medgiz, pp. 128-145, 1960.

Poroschina, A.A., Sokolova, L.P. and Ballantin, I.G.: *Proceedings of the Sci. Conference.* Location of Rostow, 1957.

da Prada, M. and Pletscher, A.: On the mechanism of chlorpromazine-induced changes of cerebral homovanillic acid levels. *J Pharm Pharmacol, 18:*628, 1966.

Pravditchneminski, B.B.: *Arch Biolog Sciences, 33:*121, 1933 (Russ.); cit. by Lando, L.I. and Krupenina, I.B.: Comparative tests of the ammonia blood content in schizophrenic and epileptic patients. In *Problems of Schizophrenia.* (Russ) Moscow, Medgiz, pp. 232-240, 1962.

Pravditchneminski, B.B.: Moscow, Medgiz, 1958; cit. by Lando, L.I.: The hyaluronidase in blood-serum of schizophrenics during treatment. (Russ.) In *Obm. Veshtch. Psikhiat. Zabol.* Moscow, Medgiz, pp. 66-75, 1960.

Preston, D.N. and Atack, E.A.: Temporal lobe epilepsy. *Can Med Ass J, 91:*1256, 1964.

Price, J.C., Waelsch, H. and Putnam, T.J.: d. l-glutamic acid hydrochlorid in treatment of petit mal and psychomotor seizures. *JAMA; 122:*1153, 1943.

Prior, P.F., Maclavine, G.N., Scott, D.F., and Laurance, B.M.: Tonic status epilepticus preapitated by intravenous diazepam in a child with petit mal status. *Epilepsia, 13:* 467-472, 1972.

Prochorova, M.I. and Tupikova, Z.N.: Readiness for renewal of carbohydrates and lipids in brain and liver at stimulation and narcotic sleep. *Vopr. Biokhim. Nerv. Sist.* Kiev, pp. 118-130, 1957. (Russ)

Prokop, D.J., Schowe, P.A. and Brodie, B.B.: An anticonvulsant effect of monamine oxidase inhibitors. *Experientia* (Basel), *15:*145, 1959.

Protopopov, V.P.: Pathophysiological bases of rational schizophrenia-therapy. Kiev, Acad Nauk USSR, 1946. (Russ)

Protopopov, V.P. and Polishtchuk, I.A.: *Annual on the Problems of Modern Psychiatry.* (Russ) Moscow, Medgiz 1948.

Protopopov, V.P., Polishtchuk, I.A. and Poznanskii, A.S.: Proceedings of the Central Institute of Neurology Nr. 2 Moscow 1939.

Prüll, G.: Zerebraler Anfall—biochemische Aspekte und allgemeine Prinzipien der antikonvulsiven Therapie. *Therapeut Berichte, 39:*343, 1967.

Pryse-Phillips, W.E.M., and Jeavons, P.M.: Effect of carbamazepine (Tegretol) on the electroencephalograph and ward behaviour of patients with chronic epilepsy. *Epilepsia, 11:*263-273, 1970.

Purpura, D.P.: Further analysis of evoked "secondary discharge"; a study in reticulocortical relations. *J Neurophysiol, 18:*246, 1955.

Purpura, D.P.: Mechanism of the inhibitory action of LSD on cortical dendritic activity. *Ann NY Acad Sci, 66:*515, 1957.

Purpura, D.P.: Properties and activities of dendrites. *Electroenceph Clin Neurophysiol,* (extra number) *27:*645, 1969.

Purpura, D.P. and Callan, D.A.: Electrophysiological analysis of psychogenic drug action. I. Effect of LSD on specific afferent systems in the cat. *Arch Neurol, 75:*122, 1956.

Purpura, D.P. and Callan, D.A.: Electrophysiological analysis of phychogenic drug action. II. General nature of lysergic acid diethylamide (LSD) action on central synapses, *Arch Neurol, 75:*132, 1956.

Purpura, D.P., Girado, M. and Grundfest, H.: Mode of action of aliphatic aminoacids on cortical synaptic activity. *Proc Soc Exp Biol Med, 95:*791, 1957.

Purpura, D.P., Girardo, M., Smith, T.G., Callan, D.A. and Grundfest, H.: Structure activity determinant of pharmacological effects of amino acids and related compounds on central synapses. *J Neurochem, 3:*238, 1959.

Purpura, D.P. and Gonzales-Monteagudo, O.: Acute effects of methoxypyridoxine on hippocampal end-blade neurons, an experimental study of "special pathoclisis" in the cerebral cortex. *J Neuropath Exp Neurol, 19:*421, 1960.

Purpura, D.P. and Grundfest, H.: Comparative pharmacological analysis of different hippocampal synaptic organizations (Cat). *Fed Proc, 18:*123, 1959.

Purpura, D.P., Smith, T. and Gomez, J.A.: Synaptic effects of systemic gamma-aminobutyric acid in cortical regions of increased permeability. *Proc Sov Exp Biol Med, 79:*348, 1958.

Quadbeck, G.: Blut-Hirnschranke und Hirnernährung. *Münch Med Wochenschr, 104:* 24, 1962.

Quadbeck, G.: In Bente, Bradley (Eds.): Neuro-Psychopharmacology. Amsterdam, Elsevier 1966, vol. IV, pp. 11-15; cit. by Kanig, K.: *Arzneim Forsch, 19:*397, 1969.

Quadbeck, G. and Helmchen, H.: Bluthirnschranke und Krampfbereitschaft. *Dtsch Z Nervenheilkd, 177:*295, 1958.

Quadbeck, G., Landmann, H.R., Sachsse, W. and Schmidt, J.: Der Einfluβ von Pyrithoxin auf die Bluthirnschranke. *Med Exp, 7:*144, 1962.

Quadbeck, G. and Randerath, K.: Wirkung von Rutin auf die Bluthirnschranke. *Zschr Naturforsch, 8b:*370, 1953.

Quadbeck, G. and Röhm, E.: Zur Konstitutionsspezifität der antikonvulsiven Wirkung von 5-p-Chlorphenyl-5-methyl-hydantoin beim audiogenen Krampf der Ratte. *Arzneim Forsch, 6:*531, 1956.

Quadbeck, G., Sachsse, W. and Hess, O.: Über die antikonvulsive Wirkung der Nikotinsäure im Tierversuch. *Klin Wochenschr, 39:*599, 1961.

Quadbeck, G. and Sartori, G.D.: Über den Einfluβ von Pyridoxin und Pyridoxal-5-phosphat auf den Thiosemicarbazid-Krampf der Ratte. *Arch Exp Path Pharmacol, 230:* 457, 1957.

Quandt, J. and Sommer, H.: Zur Frage der Hirngewebsschädigung nach elektrischer Krampfbehandlung. Eine tierexperimentelle Studie. *Fortschr Neurol Psychiatr, 34:* 513, 1966 and 1969.

Quastel, J.H.: *The Biology of Mental Health and Diseases.* New York, Pergamon Press, 1952.

Quastel, J.H.: Enzymatic mechanism of the brain and the effect of some neurotropic agents. In Brücke, F. (Ed.): *Biochemistry of the Central Nervous System.* New York, Pergamon Press, 1959.

Quastel, J.H.: Effect of anesthetics, depressants and tranquilizers on brain metabolism. In Elliott, Page, Quastel (Eds.): *Neurochemistry,* 2nd Ed. Springfield, Thomas, 1962a.

Quastel, J.H.: Effects of electrolytes on brain metabolism. In Elliott, Page, Quastel (Eds.): *Neurochemistry,* 2nd Ed. Springfield, Thomas, 1962b.

Quilliam, J.P.: The pharmacology of consciousness. *Med Press, 6169:*121, 1957.

Rabe, F.: Zum Wechsel des Anfallscharakters kleiner epileptischer Anfälle während des Krankheitsverlaufs. *Dtsch Z Nervenheilkd, 182:*201, 1961.

Rabe, F.: Hysterische Anfälle bei Epilepsie. *Nervenarzt, 37:*141, 1966.

Radtke, H.: Die Wirkung von 5-Phenyl-2-imino-4-oxo-oxazolidin auf die Hirnaktion des Menschen. *Nervenarzt, 31:*136, 1960.

Raines, A., and Standaert, F.G.: Effects of anticonvulsant drugs on nerve terminals. *Epilepsia, 10:*211-517, 1969.

Rallo Piqué, E. and Henking, R.: Expérimentation clinque et électroncéphalographique du diazepam intravéineux chez les malades épileptiques. *Psychiatr Neurol* (Basel), 150: 214, 1965.

Ralston, B.L.: The mechanism of transition of interictal spiking foci into ictal seizure discharge. *Electroenceph Clin Neurophysiol, 10:*217, 1958.

Ramos, A.O., Slemer, O., Saraiva, S., Bissetti, P.C. and Ramos, L.: Erweiternde Wirkung von 1-Hexyl-3, 7-dimethylxanthin auf die Piagefäβe. *Arqu Neuro-Psiquiatr, 21:* No. 1, 1963.

Randall, L.C., Schalleck, W., Scheckel, C., Bagdon, R.E. and Rieder, J.: Zur Pharmakologie von Mogadon, einem Schlafmittel mit neuartigem Wirkungsmechanismus. *Schweiz Med Wochenschr, 95:*334, 1965.

Ranke, O.F.: *Physiologie des Zentralnervensystems vom Standpunkt der Regelungslehre.* Keidel, W.D. (Ed.), München-Berlin, Urban & Schwarzenberg, 1960.

Raphael, T., Ferguson, W. and Searle, O.: Long section blood sugar tolerance study in a case of depression. *Arch Neurol Psychiatr, 19:*120, 1928.

Raphael, T. and Parsons, J.P.: Blood sugar studies in dementia praecox and manic depressive insanity. *Arch Neurol Psychiatr, 5:*687, 1921.

Rapoport, S.M.: *Medizinische Biochemie* 2nd. Ed. Berlin, VEB-Verlag, 1964.

Rapport II, R., and Penry, J.K.: Pharmacologic prophylaxis of posttraumatic epilepsy. *Epilepsia, 13*:295-304, 1972.

Raschba, E.A.: Ukr. Biokhim. Zh. 20, 1948; cit. by Tchalissov, M.A.: Carbon. phosphate metabolism and its importance in psychiatry. In *Obm. Veshtch. Psikhiat. Zabol.* Moscow, Medgiz, pp. 14-20, 1960.

Rasin, S.D.: Med. Zh. 18, 1949; cit. by Wolfsohn, H.M.: On the signification of some biochemical shifting to prognosis and effect of schizophrenia therapy. In *Obm. Vestch. Psiakhiat. Zabol.* Moscow, Medgiz, pp. 128-145, 1960.

Rasin, S.D.: Clinical experimental criticism of antiepileptic therapy. (Russ) Diss. Kiev, 1955.

Rasmussen, T.: Surgical therapy of frontal lobe epilepsy. *Epilepsia, 11*:27-28, 1970.

Redlich, E.: Über die Beziehung der genuinen zur symptomatischen Epilepsie. *Dtsch Z Nervenheilkd, 36*:197, 1909.

Reiko, Z.A., Petrov, I.P. and Kudrickaya, T.E.: On the action of hypothermia and ganglion-blockers on the carbohydrate- and phosphor-combinations of test animals during the elimination of heart- and blood-circulation. *Zh Ves Chirurg, 78:* 56, a. 158, 1957.

Reilly, R.H., Killam, K.F., Jenney, E.H., Marshall, W.H., Tausig, T., Apter, N.S. and Pfeiffer, C.C.: *JAMA, 152*:1317, 1953; cit by Kanig, K.: *Die Bedeutung der B-Vitamine für das Nervensystem.* Wiss. Berichte E. Merck AG, Darmstadt, 1968.

Reiner, L., Misani, F. and Weiss, P.: Studies on nitrogen trichloride-treated prolamines, suppression of development of convulsions with methionine. *Arch Biochem, 25*:447, 1950.

Renshaw, B.J.: Activity in the simplest spinal reflex pathways. *J Neurophysiol, 3*:373, 1940.

Renshaw, B.J.: Influence of discharge of motoneurons upon excitation of neighbouring motoneurons. *J Neurophysiol, 4*:167, 1941.

Renson, J., Weissbach, H. and Udenfriend, S.: Hydroxylation of tryptophane by phenylalanine hydroxylase. *J Biol Chem, 237*:18, 1962.

Retzius, G.: *Das Menschenhirn.* Stockholm, Norstedt & Söner, 1896.

Reynolds, E.H., Wrighton, R.J., Johnson, A.L., Preece, J., and Chanarin, I.: Inter-relations of folic acid and vitamin B_{12} in drug-treated epileptic patients. *Epilepsia, 12:* 165-171, 1971.

Ricci, G., Berti, G., and Cherubini, E.: Changes in interictal focal activity and spike-wave paroxysms during motor and mental activity. *Epilepsia, 13*:785-794, 1972.

Richter, D.: Protein Metabolism of the Brain. Proc. 4th Int. Congr. Biochem., Vienna, 1958.

Richter, D.: In F. Brucke, (Ed.): Biochemistry of the Central Nervous System. New York, Pergamon Press, 1959.

Richter, D.: Biochemical aspects of mental retardation. *Proc. 4th World Congr. Psychiatr.* 1966, Excerpta Med. Amsterdam, pp. 523, 1967.

Richter, D. and Crossland, J.: Variation in acetylcholine content of brain with physiological state. *Am J Physiol, 159*:247, 1949.

Richter, D. and Dawson, R.M.C. Ammonia and glutamine content of brain. *J Biol Chem, 176*:119, 1948.

Richter, R.B.: Infantile subacute necrotizing encephalopathy with predilection for the brain stem. *J Neuropath Exp Neurol, 16*:281, 1957.

Riebeling, C.: Chemische Befunde am Hirn und Liquor der Schizophrenen. *Zbl Neurol Psychiatr, 91*:194, 1939.

Riley, J.F.: Tissue mast cells. Distribution and significance. *Can J Biochem, 39*:633, 1961.

Rimbaud, L., Passouant, P. and Cadilhac, J.: Participation de l'hippocampe à la régulation des états de veille et de sommeil. *Rev Neurol, 93*:303, 1952.

Rindi, G., Perry, V. and de Caro, L.: The uptake of pyrithiamine by cerebral tissue. *Experientia, 17*:546, 1961.

Rioch, D. and Brenner, L.: Experiments on the corpus striatum and rhinencephalon. *J Comp Neurol, 68*:491, 1938.

Rittenberg, S., Sproul, E.E. and Shemin, D.: Rate of protein formation in the livers of partially hepatectomized rats. *Fed Proc, 7*:180, 1948.

Rizzati, E.: Ulteriori contributi allo studio dello squilibrio albumino-globulinico nelle schizophrenie. II. Altro mezzo di indagine dello squilibrio albumino-globulinico del siero di sangue negli schizophrenici. *Schizophrenie, 4*:347, 1934.

Rizzatti, E. and Martinengo, V.: Ulteriori contributi allo studio dello squilibrio albumino-globulinico nelle schizophrenie. I. La reazione di Lange applicata aö siero di sangue dei malati di mente e degli schizophrenici in particolare con il metodo di Gerundo. *Schizophrenie, 4*:333, 1934.

de Robertis, E., Gerschenfeld, H.M. and Wald, F.: Cellular mechanism of myelination in the central nervous system. *J Biochem Biophys Cytol, 4*:651, 1958.

Roberts, E.: Free amino acids of nervous tissue: some aspects of metabolism of gamma-aminobutyric acid. In Roberts, E. (Ed.): *Inhibition in the Nervous System and Gamma-Aminobutyric Acid.* Oxford, Pergamon Press, 1960.

Roberts, E.: γ-Aminobutyric acid (γ-ABA)-vitamin B_6 relationship in the brain. *Am J Clin Nutr, 12*:291, 1963.

Roberts, E. and Bregoff, H.M.: Transamination of γ-aminobutyric acid and β-alanine in brain and liver. *J Biol Chem, 201*:393, 1953.

Roberts, E. and Eidelberg, E.: Metabolic and neurophysiological roles of gamma-aminobutyric acid. *Rev Neurobiol, 2*:279, 1960.

Roberts, E., Harman, P.J. and Frankel, S.: Gamma aminobutyric acid content and glutamic decarboxylase activity in developing mouse brain. *Proc Soc Exp Biol Med, 78*:799, 1951.

Roberts, R.B., Flexner, J.B. and Flexner, L.B.: Biochemical and physiological differentiation during morphogenesis. XXVI. Further observations relating to the synthesis of amino acids and proteins by the cerebral cortex and liver of the mouse. *J Neurochem, 4*:78, 1959.

Robins, E., Smith, K. and Lowe, J.P.: cit. by Lajtha, A.: Alteration and pathology of cerebral protein metabolism. *Int Rev Neurobiol, 7*:1, 1964.

Robinson, L.J.: Gingival changes produced by dilantin sodium. *Dis Nerv Syst, 3*:88, 1942.

Rodenhäuser, J.H.: *Uveadurchblutung und Augeninnendruck.* Bücher, d.Augenarztes 42. Heft, Stuttgart, Enke, 1963.

Rodin, E.A., de Jong, R.N., Waggoner, R.W. and Bagehi, B.K.: Relationship between certain formes of psychomotor epilepsy and "Schizophrenia". I. Diagnostic considerations. *Arch Neurol Psychiatr, 77*:449, 1957.

Rodriguez, L.A.: Experiments on the histologic locus of the hemato-encephalic barrier. *J Comp Neurol, 102*:27, 1955.

Roger, A. and Dongier, M.: Corrélations électrocliniques chez 50 épileptiques internés. *Rev Neurol, 83*:593, 1950.

Rommelspacher, F.: Neuere Erfahrungen in der Epilepsiebehandlung. *Ärztl Wschr, 5*: 7, 1950.

Ronco, P.: Il processo di inversione figura-sfondo. La polarizzazzione percettiva verso il colore o la forma e la capicita di integrazione di forma in schizophrenici nella iperpireto-terapia neuro-vaccinica. *Acta Neuol* (Napoli), *11*:316, 1956.

Roos, B.E.: The effect of reserpine, chlorpromazine and haloperidol on the monoamines in central nervous system. *Acta Psychiatr Scand, 180*:421, 1965.

Rose, M.: Der Allocortex bei Tier und Mensch. *J Psychol Neurol, 34*:1, 1926.

Rose, M.: Die sogenannte Reichrinde beim Menschen und beim Affen. *J Physiol Neurol, 34*:261, 1927.

Rose, W.C., Wixom, R.L., Lockhart, H.B. and Lambert, G.L.: Amino acid requirements; summary and final observations. *J Biol Chem, 217*:987, 1955.

Rosen, F., Holland, J.F. and Nichol, F.: Proc. Amer. Ass. Cancer Res. 2, 243, 1957; cit. by Kanig, K.: *Die Bedeutung der B-Vitamine für das Nervensystem.* Wiss. Berichte, E. Merck AG. Darmstadt, 1968.

Rosengardt, V.I., Lebedeva, E.E. and Maslova, M.N.: Physiological changes and phosphor combinations in the brain of rabbits at epileptic stimulation. VII. *Annual Meeting of the Physiol., Biol., Pharmacol. Acad. Sci. SSSR,* pp. 317, 1955. (Russ)

Rosengardt, V.I. and Maslova, M.N.: Action of seizure on the changes of radio-methionine in brain and liver proteins. (Russ) *Dokl Akad Nauk SSSR, 109*:1176, 1956.

Rosengardt, V.I., Maslova, M.N. and Panyukov, A.N.: Physiological changes in the brain of rabbits at epileptic stimulation. (Russ) *Dokl Akad Nauk SSSR, 110*:122, 1956.

Rosenstein, I.N.: A new psychosedative (Librium) as an anticonvulsant in grand mal type convulsive seizures. Dis *Nerv Syst, 21*:57, 1960.

Ross, A.T. and Jackson, V.: Dilantin sodium: its influence on conduct and on psychometric ratings of institutionalized epileptics. *Ann Int Mes, 14*:770, 1940.

Ross, E.M., and Evans, D.: Epilepsy in bristol secondary school children. *Epilepsia, 13*: 7-12, 1972.

Rossi, G.F. and Zanchetti, A.: The brain stem reticular formation. Anatomy and physiology. *Arch Ital Biol, 95*:199, 1957.

Rossiter, R.J.: Discussion of: Elliott, K.A.C.: The relation of ions to metabolism in brain. *Can J Biochem, 33*:477, 1955.

Roth, B.: *Narkolepsie und Hypersomnie.* Berlin, VEB-Verlag, 1962.

Roth, G. Zur Kombinationstherapie epileptischer Anfälle. *Wien Med Wochenschr, 118*: 116, 1968.

Rothballer, A.B.: The effect of phenylpherine, metamphetamine, cocaine and serotonine upon the adrenaline-sensitive component of the reticular activating system. *Electroenceph Clin Neurophysiol, 9*:409, 1957.

Rothballer, R.J.: Studies on adrenaline sensitive components of reticular activating system. *Electroenceph Clin Neurophysiol, 8*:603, 1956.

Rothschuh, K.E.: Vom spiritus animalis zum Nervenaktionsstrom. *Ciba-Zschr, 8*: Nr. 89, 1958.

Roubiček, J.: Laughter in epilepsy with some general introductory notes. *J Ment Sci, 92*:734, 1946.

Rowntree, L.G.: Effects on mammals of administration of excessive quantities of water. *J Pharmacol Exp Ther, 29*:135, 1926.

Royer, P., Colmart, C. and Rayel, L.: Le traitement de l' alcoolisme par l'hemineurine. *Rev Alcool, 409*:411, 1958.

Rozanova, V.D.: On the analysis of the role and nature of cholinergic and adrenergic substances of the reticular formation in dogs of various ages. *Tr Inst Norm Patol Fiziol* (Mosk), *7*:75, 1964.

Rubel, V.M.: On the problem of nitrogen metabolism in brain. *Byull Eks Biol Med, 8:* 345, 1939. (Russ)

Rudoj, H.N.: Some changes of protein fractions of blood serum at different types of tuberculosis studied by electrophoretic method. (Russ) Diss., 1956.

Ruf, H.: Das Elektrencephalogramm beim Hirntumor. *Dtsch Z Nervenheilkd, 162:*60, 1950a.

Ruf, H.: Experimentelle über Stunden dauernde Verlängerung des Elektrokrampfes durch Sauerstoff und Kreislaufmittel. *Nervenarzt, 21:*109, 1950b.

Sacks, W.: Cerebral metabolism of isotopic glucose in normal human subjects. *J Appl Physiol, 10:*37, 1957.

Sacks, W.: Cerebral metabolism of isotopic glucose in chronic mental disease. *J Appl Physiol, 14:*849, 1959.

Sakuragi, T. and Kummerow, F.A.: The vitamin B_6 derivates structurally analogous to thiamine and their biological activity. *Arch Biochem Biophys, 71:*303, 1957.

Salesski, G.D.: Sovj, Med. 12, 1955; cit. by Lando, L.I.: The hyaluronidase in blood serum of schizophrenics during treatment. In *Obm. Vestch. Psikhiat. Zabol.* Moscow, Medgiz, pp. 66-75, 1960.

Salum, I.: The clinical use of Heminevrin. *Nord Psykiatr Tidsskr, 17:*20, 1963.

Sanders, B.E., Smith, E.V.C., Flataker, L. and Winter, C.A.: Fractionation studies of human serum factors affecting motor activity in trained rats. *Ann NY Acad Sci, 96:* 448, 1962.

Sanders, W.: Epileptische Anfälle mit subjektiven Geruchsempfindungen bei Zerstörung des linken tractus olfactorius durch einen Tumor. *Arch Psychiatr, 4:*234, 1874.

Sandler, M. and Close, H.O.: Biochemical effect of phenylacetic acid in patients with 5-hydroxytryptophansecreting carcinoid tumor. *Lancet, 2:*316, 1959.

Sanidés, F.: Die Architektonik des menschlichen Stirnhirns. *Monogr Neurol Psychiat, 98:* 2015, 1962.

Sano, I., Taniguchi, K., Gamo, T., Takesada, M. and Kakimoto, Y.: Die Katechinamine im Zentralnervensystem. *Klin Wochenschr, 38:*57, 1960.

Sano, K. and Malamud, N.: Clinical significance of sclerosis of the cornu ammonis. Ictal "psychic phenomena". *Arch Neurol, 70:*40, 1953.

Santamouris, C. and Heye, D.: Die Unterbrechung des pyknoleptischen Status mit Valium. *Mschr Kinderheilkd, 114:*104, 1966.

Sapirstein, M.R.: Effect of glutamic acid on central action of ammonium ion. *Proc Soc Exp Biol Med, 52:*334, 1943.

Sattes, H.: Die Behandlung des Delirium tremens mit Distraneurin. *Med Klin, 59:*1515, 1964a.

Sattes, H.: Therapeutische Erfahrungen mit Distraneurin. *Therapiewoche, 14:*786, 1964b.

Sattes, H.: Treatment of delirium tremens with chlormethiazole. *Acta Psychiatr Scand, 42:*192, 1966a.

Sattes, H.: Chlormethiazole treatment of abstinence symptoms after drug withdrawal. Preliminary reports. *Acta Psychiatr Scand, 42:*192, 1966b.

Sattes, H.: Distraneurin als Ersatzmittel bei Alokholsucht. In Kranz, H. a. Heinrich, D. (Eds.): *Pharmakopsychiatrie und Psychopathologie.* Stuttgart, Thieme, 1967.

Sawa, M., Ueki, Y., Arita, M. and Harada, T.: Preliminary report on the amygdaloidectomy on the psychotic patients, with the interpretation of the oral-emotional manifestations in schizophrenics. *Folia Psychiatr Neurol Jap, 4:*309, 1954.

Schabelitz, H.: Experimentelle und Selbstbeobachtungen im Bromismus. *Z Ges Neurol Psychiatr, 28:*1, 1915.

Schaefer, H.: Untersuchungen über den Muskelaktionsstrom. *Pflügers Arch, 237*:329, 1936.

Schaefer, H.: Über den "Reizeinbruch" bei Registrierung von Aktionsströmen. *Pflügers Arch, 237*:717, 1936.

Schaefer, H.: Über die mathematischen Grundlagen einer Spannungstheorie der elektrischen Nervenreizung. *Pflügers Arch, 237*:722, 1936.

Schaefer, H.: Grundprobleme der allgemeinen Elektrobiologie. *Klin Wochenschr, 31*:221, 1953.

Schaefer, K., Kraft, D., Herrath, von, D., and Opitz, A.: Intestinal absorption of Vitamin D_3 in epileptic patients and phenobarbital-treated rats. *Epilepsia, 13*:509-519, 1972.

Schallek, W. and Kuehn, A.: An action of Mogadon on the amygdala of the cat. *Med Pharmacol Exp, 12*:204, 1965.

Schallek, W., Thomas, J., Kuehn, A. and Zabransky, F.: Effects of Mogadon on responses to stimulation of sciatic nerve, amygdala and hypothalamus of cat. *Int J Neuropharmacol, 4*:317, 1965a.

Schallek, W., Thomas, J. and Zabransky, F.: Effects of Mogadon on EEG activation. amygdala and hypothalamus of cat. *Abstracts of Papers Presented at the 23rd. Int. Congr. Physiol. Sci.* Tokyo, Jap. p. 448, 1965b.

Schallek, W., Zabransky, F. and Kuehn, A.: Effects of benzodiazepines on central nervous system of the cat. *Arch Int Pharmacodyn Ther, 149*:467, 1964.

Schanberg, S.M., Schildkraut, J.J. and Kopin, I.J.: The effects of psychoactive drugs on norepinephrine-^{3}H metabolism in brain. *Biochem Pharmacol, 16*:393, 1967.

Scharenberg, K.: Histopathology of psychomotor epilepsy. *Arch Neurol Psychiatr, 77*: 595, 1957.

Schechonin, V.P.: On the problem of permeability of capillaries in pathology. (Russ) 1949.

Scheffner, D., and Schiefer, J.: The treatment of epileptic children with carbamazepine. *Epilepsia, 13*:819-828, 1972.

Scheid, W.: *Febrile Episoden bei schizophrenen Psychosen*. Lipzig, Twieme 1937.

Scheid, W. and Huhn, A.: Neuere Wege in der medikamentösen Behandlung des Alkoholdelirs. *Fortschr Neurol Psychiatr, 32*:490, 1964.

Schenk, H.: Lassen sich Cerebralskelorse, Folgeerscheinungen sowie periphere Durchblutungsstörungen melikamentös beeinflussen? *Med Klin, 52*:1885, 1957.

Scherrer, R. and Hernández-Peón, R.: Inhibitory influence of reticular formation upon synaptic transmission in gracilis nucleus. *Fed Proc, 14*:132, 1955.

Schesterikova, P.T., Ignatova, N.I., Schuhhalter, M.W. and Filyanivskii, F.K.: Some metabolic changes of carbohydrates and nitrogen in psychotic patients, resistent and responding to insulin-therapy. (Russ.) In *Obm. Veshtch. Psikhiat. Zabol.* Moscow, Medgiz, pp. 146-153, 1960.

Schildkraut, J.J., Schanberg, S.M. and Breese, G.R.: Norepinephrine metabolism and drugs used in the affective disorders: a possible mechanism of action. *Am J Psychiatr, 124*:600, 1967.

Schindler, R.: The conversion of ^{14}C-labelled tryptophan to 5-hydroxytryptamine by neoplastic mast cells. *Biochem Pharmacol, 1*:323, 1959.

Schleissing, W.: Moderne Epilepsiebehandlung. Ärztl. *Praxis, 3*:36, 1951.

Schmain, K.D. and Arutunov, D.N.: Sovj. Psikhonevr. 511/12 1936; cit. by Wolfsohn, H.M.: On the signification of some biochemical shifting to prognosis and effect of schizophrenia-therapy. (Russ) In *Obm. Veshtch. Psikhiat. Zabol.* Moscow, Medgiz, pp. 128-145, 1960.

Schmalbach, K.: Experimentelle Untersuchungen über epileptische Reaktionen. Chronische Reizungen des sensomotorischen Cortex der Katze und des Kaninchens. In Müller, Spatz, Vogel (Eds.): *Monographien a.d. Gesamtgeb. d. Neurol. u. Psychiat.* Berlin-Heidelberg-New York, Springer, 1968a.

Schmalbach, K.: *Experimentelle Untersuchungen an neugeborenen und jungen Katzen insbesondere an Tieren mit chronischen epileptischen Herden unterschiedlicher Lokalisation.* Sitzungsber. Dtsch. EEG Ges. 14. Münster, Jahrestagung, 1968b.

Schmalbach, K.: Herdaktivation durch Schlaf oder Medikamente. In Jovanović, U.J. (Ed) *Der Schlaf—Neurophysiologische Aspekte.* München, Barth, 1969.

Schmalbach, K. and Steinmann, H.W.: Bioelektrische Untersuchungen mit chronischen epileptogenen Läsionen. *Dtsch Z Nervenheilkd, 173:*377, 1955.

Schmidt, B.: Zur Therapie der Zerebralsklerose. *Med Welt, 4:*1222, 1960.

Schmidt, C.F., Kety, S.S. and Pennes, H.H.: The gaseous metabolism of the brain of the monkey. *Am J Physiol, 143:*33, 1945.

Schneider, J., Thomalske, G., Perrin, J. and Siffermann, A.: Die Modifikationen des EEG unter der Behandlung mit Psychopharmaka. Langzeituntersuchungen an Giesteskranken. *Nervenarzt, 34:*521, 1963.

Schneidermann, B., Isaacson, R.L., and Hartesveldt, van, C.: The effects of spreading depression on penicillin-induced epileptiform activity in rat brain. *Epilepsia, 13:* 675-697, 1972.

Scholz, W.: Histologische Untersuchungen über Form, Dynamik und pathologisch-anatomische Auswirkung funktioneller Durchblutungsstörungen des Hirngewebes. *Z Ges Neurol Psychiat, 167:*424, 1939.

Scholz, W.: *Die Krampfschädigungen des Gehirns.* Berlin, Springer, 1951.

Scholz, W.: Les lésions cérébrales rencontrées chez les épileptiques: Précisions sur la sclérose de la corne d' Ammon. *Acta Neurol Belg, 56:*43, 1956.

Scholz, W.: An nervöse Systeme gebundene (topistische) Kreislaufschäden. In *Hb. Spez. Patrol. Anat. Histol,* part 1, Berlin-Göttingen-Heidelberg, Springer, vol. XII, pp. 1326, 1957.

Scholz, W.: The contribution of patho-anatomical research to the problem of epilepsy. *Epilepsia* (Boston), *1:*36, 1959.

Scholz, W. and Jötten, J.: Durchblutungsstörungen in Katzengehirn nach kurzen Elektrokrampfserien. *Arch Psychiatr Nervenkr, 186:*264, 1951.

Schorsch, G. and v. Hedenström, I.: Die Schwankungsbreite hirnelektrischer Erregbarkeit in ihrer Beziehung zu epileptischen Anfällen und Verstimmungszuständen. *Arch Psychiatr Nervenkr, 195:*393, 1957.

Schou, M.: Lithium: Ein Specificum gegen manisch-depressive Psychose. *Arnzeim Forsch, 17:*172, 1967.

Schou, M. and Baastrup, P.C.: Lithium treatment of manic-depressive disorder. *JAMA, 201:*696, 1967.

Schriyver, D. and Schriyver-Hertzberger, S.: Über die Blut-Eiweisskörper im schizophrenen Formenkreis. *Z Neurol, 140:*252, 1932.

Schumacher, G.A. and Wolff, H.G.: Experimental studies on headache. A. Contrast of histamine headache with the headache of migraine and that associated with hypertension. B. Contrast of vascular mechanisms in preheadache and in headache phenomena of migraine. *Arch Neurol, 45:*199, 1941.

Schuster, P.: *Psychische Störungen bei Hirntumoren.* Stuttgart, Enke, 1902.

Schwalbe, G.: *Lehrbuch der Neurologie.* University Press, Erlangen, 1881.

Schwarz, B.E., Bickford, R.G., Mulder, D.W. and Rome, H.P.: Mescaline and LSD in activation of temporal lobe epilepsy. *Neurology* (Minneap), *6:*275, 1956.

Schwarz, G.A. and Yanoff, M.: Lafora's disease. Distinct clinico-pathologic form of Unverricht's Syndrome. *Arch Neurol, 12:*172, 1965.

Scott, D.F., Moffett, A., and Swash, M.: Observations on the relation of migraine and epilepsy. An electroencephalographic, psychological and clinical study using oral tyramine. *Epilepsia, 13:*365-375, 1972.

Scoville, W.B. and Milner, B.: Loss of recent memory after bilateral hippocampal lesions. *J Neur NS, 20:*11, 1957.

Scoville, W.B. and Ryan, V.G.: Orbital undercutting in the aged limited lobotomy in the treatment of psychoneuroses and depressions in elderly persons. *Geriatrics, 10:* 311, 1955.

Sedina, N.S.: Changes of inner organs in experimental epilepsy. (Russ) Diss., Leningrad, 1945.

Segundo, J.P., Naquet, R. and Arana, R.: Subcortical connections from temporal cortex of monkey. *Arch Neurol Psychiatr, 73:*515, 1955.

Seiler, N.: *Der Stoffwechsel im Zentralnervensystem.* Stuttgart, Thieme, 1966.

Seitz, I.F.: The aerobic and anerobic metabolism and oxydative phophorilization in the cell. (Russ) Diss., Leningrad, 1953.

Seitz, I.F.: The aerobic and anerobic metabolism and oxydative phosphorilization in the cell. (Russ) Leningrad, Dissertation, 1961.

Selbach, H.: Der epileptische Anfall im Krankheitsbild der genuinen Epilepsie. *Klin Wochenschr, 2:*585, 1938.

Selbach, H.: Die cerebralen Anfallsleiden. In *Hb. d. Inn. Med.* 4th. Ed. Berlin-Göttingen-Heidelberg, Springer, vol. V/3, pp. 1082, 1953.

Selbach, H.: Der generalisierte Krampfanfall als Folge einer gestörten Regelkreisfunktion. *Ärztl Wschr, 9:*1117, 1954.

Selbach, H.: The principle of relaxation oxillation as a special instance of the law of initial value in cybernetic functions. *Ann NY Acad Sci, 98:*1221, 1962.

Selbach, H. (Ed.): *Internationales Colloquium über das Antikonvulsivum Ospolot.* Kamp-Lintfort, Berlin 1963.

Selbach, H.: *Klinik der Schlafstörungen.* Verh. Inn. Med. (71. Kongr. 1965), München, Bergmann, p. 827, 1965.

Selbach, H.: Psychogene Anfälle beim Epileptiker. Stellungnahme zum Beitrag von F. Rabe über: "Hysterische Anfälle bei Epilepsie". *Nervenarzt, 37:*147, 1966.

Selbach, H., Helmchen, H. and Künkel, H.: Die Epilepsie. Pathophysiologie, Klinik und Therapie. *Klinik d Gegenw, 5:*E1, 1965.

Selbach, H. and Selbach, C.:; Zur Pathogenese des epileptischen Anfalls. *Fortschr Neurol Psychiatr, 18:*367, 1950.

Seliger, H.: Trigeminusneuralgie. *Mat Med Nordm, 8:*146, 1956.

Selzer, M.L. and Waldmann, H.: The use of doxylamine in schizophrenia. Pitfalls in the evaluation of a new drug. *Br J Med Psychol, 32:*1, 1958.

Sem-Jacobsen, C.W., Petersen, M.C., Dodge, H.W., Lygne, H.N., Lazorte, J.A. and Holman, C.B.: Intracerebral electrographic study of 93 psychotic patients. *Acta Psychiat* (Kopenh), *106:*222, 1956.

Seppäläinen, A.M., and Similä, S.: Electroencephalographic findings in three patients with nonketonic hyperglycinemia. *Epilepsia, 12:*101-107, 1971.

Sereiski, M.: Le mécanisme d'action des procédés actifs du traitment de la schizophrénie. *Sovj Psikhonevr, 15:*99, 1940.

Sereiski, M.J.: The modern tasks of intensive therapy in psychoses. Clinical and therapeutical problems in psychotic patients. (Russ) Moscow, Medgiz, pp. 227-242, 1946.

Sereiski, M.J. and Lando, L.I.: *Nevropatol Psikhiat, 6:*15, 1946; cit. by Papadopoulos,

F.F.: The glycemic curve after two loads with saccharose in schizophrenics. In *Obm Veshtch. Psikhiat. Zabol.* Moscow, Medgiz, pp. 56-61. 1960.
Sereiski,M.J. and Rothstein, G.A. Annaul "Treaty of Schizophrenia". (Russ). Charkov, An, SSSR, 1938.
Sereiski,M.J. and Schneersohn,S.: Neuropathology, psychiatry and mental hygiene. (Russ) Moscow, Medgiz, 1937.
Servit, Z.: Phylogenesis and ontogenesis of the epileptic seizure. A comparative study. *World Neurol, 3:*259, 1962.
Servít, Z.: Focal epileptic activitty and its spread in the brain of lower vertebrates. A comparative electrophysiological study. *Epilepsia, 11:*227-240, 1970.
Servit, Z. and Bureš, J.: Experimentelle epileptische Anfälle bei Reptilien. *Cesk Fysiol, 1:*13, 1952a.
Servit, Z. and Bureš, J.: Die Pathophysiologie experimenteller epileptischer Anfälle bei Mäusen. *Cesk Fysiol, 1:*122, 1952b.
Servit, Z., Bureš, J., Burešova, O. and Petran, M.: Beitrag zur Frage der Elektronarkose. (Russ.) Česk Fysiol, *2:*337, 1953.
Shanes, A.M.: Electrical phenomena in nerve. III. Frog sciatic nerve. *J Cell Comp Physiol, 167:*147, 1951.
Shanes, A.M.: Electrochemical aspects of physiological and pharmacological action in excitable cells. Part II. The action potential and excitation. *Pharmacol Rev, 10:*165, 1958.
Shapot, V.S.: Brain metabolism in relation to the functional state of the central nervous system. In Richter, D. (Ed.): *Metabolism of the Nervous System.* New York, Pergamon Press, 1957.
Sharman, D.F.: A discussion of the modes of action of drugs which increase the concentration of 4-hydroxy-3-methoxyphenylacetic acid (homovanillic acid) in the striatum of the mouse. *Br J Pharmacol, 30:*620, 1967.
Shea, J.G.: Use of promazine in management of medical emergencies. *Milit Med, 119: 221,* 1956.
Shealy, C.N. and Peele, T.L.: Studies on amygdaloid nucleus of cat. *J Neurophysiol, 20:*125, 1957.
Shevko, A.D.: On the phosphor combinations in the blood of schizophrenic patients. (Russ) Diss., 1952.
Shevko, A.D.: Theses and reports, proceedings to the annual meeting of the Ukr. Psychoneurol. Institute, Charkov Acad. Nauk SSSR. 1958.
Shevko, A.D.: Problems of schizophrenia therapy and pathophysiological problems. (Russ) Charkov, Acad. Nauk SSSR. 1958.
Shevko, A.D.: On problems of acidosis in schizophrenia. In *Obm. Veshtch. Psikhiat. Zabol.* Moscow, Medgiz, pp. 21-39, 1960.
Shevko, A.D., Kovtun, O.I., Pogilko, N.I. and Fadeeva, G.G.: Theses on the 18th sci. Congr. of the Ukr. Psychoneurol. Institute (Russ) Charkov Acad. Nauk SSSR. 1953.
Shimizu, A., Hishikawa, Y., Matsumoto, K. and Kaneko, Z.: Electroencephalographic studies on the action of monoamine oxidase inhibitors. *Psychopharmacologia* (Berlin), *6:*368, 1964.
Show, R.F., Gall, J.C., and Schumann, S.A.: Febrile convulsions as a problem in waiting times. *Epilepsia, 13:*305-311, 1972.
Siegel, S., Niswander, D., Sachs, E. and Stavros, D.: Taraxein, fact or artifact. *Am J Psychiatry, 115:*819, 1959.
Sigg, E.B.: Pharmacological studies with tofranil. *Can Psychiatr Assoc J, 4:*75, 1959.
van Sim, M.: Medical aspects of chemical warfare. *JAMA, 175:*1, 1961.

Simma, K.: Die psychischen Störungen bei Läsionen des Temporallappens und ihre Behandlung. *Mschr Psychiatr Neurol, 130:*129, 1956.

Simons, A.J.R.: EEG-activation by means of chlorpromazine. *Electroenceph Clin Neurophysiol, 10:*356, 1955.

Simpson, D.A.: The efferent fibres of the hippocampus in the monkey. *J Neurol Neurosurg Psychiatry, 15:*79, 1952.

Simpson, D.A.: The projection of the pulvinar to the temporal lobe. *J Anat, 86:*20, 1953.

Simpson, J.R., Grabarits, F. and Harvey, J.A.: Differential effects of CNS lesions on brain amines and reserpine action. *Pharmacol, 9:*213, 1967.

Sinclair, H.M.: Nutritional aspects of pyridoxal as a coenzyme. *Proc Ntur Soc, 12:*94, 1953.

Sinclair, L.: The effects of intraventricular iporniazid in the rat. *J Physiol, 153:*47, 1960.

Sinclair, L.: Gamma aminobutyric acid metabolism in cerebral activity and in epileptic disorders. *Dev Med Child Neurol, 4:*620, 1962.

Singh, H.: Atropine-like poisoning due to tranquilizing agents. *Am J Psychiatry, 117:* 360, 1960.

Singh, S.I. and Malhotra, C.L.: Amino acid content of monkey brain. IV. Effects of chlorpromazine on some amino acids of certain regions of monkey brain. *J Neurochem, 14:*135, 1967.

Singhal, B.S., Hansotia, P., Parekh, C.S., and Hawaldar, P.P.: Study of the psychotropic action of Tegretol in patients with epilepsy. *The Bombay Hosp. J.*, 14,:(2), 1972.

Sinitsky, V.N. and Sologuo, N.M.: Changes in the cardiovascular status of patients with epilepsy in various stages of the disease. (Russ) *Zh Nevropatol Psikhiat, 65:*1371, 1965.

Sitinski, I.A.: Changes of adenosine-triphosphoric acid in brain tissue at different functional initial conditions of CNS. (Russ) Diss., Leningrad, 1955.

Sitinski, I.A.: Changes of adenosine-triphosphoric acid in brain tissue at different functional initial conditions of CNS. (Russ) *Biokhim, 21:*359, 1956.

Sjoerdsma, A., Kornetsky, C. and Ewarts, E.V.: Lysergic acid diethylamide in patients with excess serotonine. *Arch Neurol, 75:*488, 1956.

Skuin, E.J.: *Annual of Schizophrenia.* (Russ) Leningrad, Acad Nauk SSSR., 1939.

Skuin, E.J.: Research report of 1946. (Russ) *Akad Med Nauk SSSR, 4:*71, 1948.

Skuin, E.J.: Vopr. Psikhiat., Moscow, 1956; cit. by Skuin, E.J.: The signification of biochemical correlates in urine in the clinical symptomatology of schizophrenics. In *Obm. Veshtch. Psikhiat. Zabol.* Moscow, Medgiz, pp. 120-127, 1960.

Skuin, E.J.: The signification of biochemical correlates in urine in the clinical symptomatology of schizophrenics. In *Obm. Veshtch. Psikhiat. Zabol.* Moscow, Medgiz, 1960. pp. 120-127, 1960.

Slutchevski, I.F.: Problems of psychiatry and neuropathology. (Russ) (Monograph) Moscow, Medgiz, 1944.

Smirnova, L.G.: *Zh Mikrobiol Epidemiol Immunol, 99:*282, 1951; cit. by Lando, I.I.: The hyaluronidase in blood serum of schizophrenics during treatment. In *Obm. Veshtch. Psikhiat. Zabol.* Moscow, Medgiz, pp. 66-75, 1960.

Smirnova, L.G.: *Clin Med, 6:35, 1957* (Russ); cit. by Lando, L.I.: *Obm. Veshtch. Psikhiat. Zabol.* Moscow, Medgiz, pp. 66-75, 1960.

Smirnova, O.A.: *Action of Hypo- and Hyperthermia on Nitrogen Combinations in the Brain.* Gorki, Biokhim. Moz., pp. 68, 1941.

Smith, G. and Purpura, D.P.: Electrophysiological studies on epileptic lesions of cat cortex. *Electroenceph Clin Neurophysiol, 12:*59, 1960.

Snell, E.E.: Summary of known metabolic functions of nicotinic acid, riboflavin and vitamin B_6. *Physiol Rev, 33*:509, 1953.

Soreni, E.I.: *Ukr Biokhim Zh, 1*:18, 1945; cit. by Shevko, A.D.: On problems of acidosis in schizophrenia. In *Obm. Veshtch. Psikhiat. Zabol.* Moscow, Medgiz, pp.21-39, 1960.

Sorokina, T.T.: Biochemical and experimental studies of catatonic stupor of schizophrenic kind. In *Obm. Veshtch. Psikhiat. Zabol.* Moscow, Medgiz, pp. 77-84, 1960.

Sorrell, T.C., Forbes, I.J., Burness, F.R., and Rischbieth, R.H.C.: Depression of immunological function in patients treated with phenytoin sodium (Sodium Diphenylhydantoin), *Lancet,* pp. 1233-1235,December 4, 1971.

Soula, L.C.: Etude de la protéolyse de la substance nerveuse. Analyse d'un cerveau humain. *C R. Soc Biol, 73*:279, a. 404 a, 570; 74, 244a. 476, 1913; *J Phys Pathol, 15*: 267, 1913; *C R Acad Sci* (Paris), *156*:728, 1913.

Soulairac, A., Cahn, J., Foettesmann, C. and Alano, J.: Neuropharmacological aspects of the action of hypnogenic substances on the central nervous system. In Akert, Bally, Schadé (Eds.): *Sleep Mechanisms. Progr. Brain Res.,* Amsterdam, Elsevier, vol. XVIII, pp. 194-220, 1965.

Sourkes, T.L.: Cerebral and other diseases with disturbance of amine metabolism. *Progr. Brain Res.* New York, Elsevier, Vol. VII, 1964.

Sourkes, T.L. and D'Irio, A.: Inhibitors of catecholamine metabolism. In Hochstetter, Quastel (Eds.): *Metabolic inhibitors.* New York, Academic Press, 1963.

Spaans, F.: No effect of folic acid supplement on CSF folate and serum vitamin B_{12} in patients on anticonvulsants. *Epilepsia, 11*:403-411, 1970.

Spatz, H.: Die Bedeutung der vitalen Färbung für die Lehre vom Stoffaustausch zwischen dem Zentralnervensystem und dem übrigen Körper. *Arch Psychiatr Nervenkr, 101*:267, 1934.

Spehlmann, R., Daniels, J.C., and Chang, C.M.: The effects of eserine and atropine on the epileptiform activity of chronically isolated cortex. *Epilepsia, 12*:123-132, 1971.

Speransky, A.D.: The epileptic seizure. (Russ) *Gosud. Med. Izd.* 1932.

Speransky, A.D.: *A Basis for the Theory of Medicine.* New York Internat. Publishers, 1943.

Sperling, E.: Thalamusveränderungen bei Stirnhirnverletzungen. *Arch Psychiat Z Neurol, 195*:589, 1957.

Sperling, E.: Probleme der Hirnpsychopathologie. *Med Klin, 55*:845, 1960.

Sperling, E. and Creutzfeldt, O.: Der Temporallappen. Zur Anatomie, Physiologie und Klinik (mit Ausnahme der Aphasien). *Fortschr Neurol Psychiatr, 27*:296, 1959.

Sperling, E. and Stender, A.: "Tic douloureux" und Gesichtsschmerz. *Dtsch Z Nervenheilkd, 173*: 1955.

Sperry, W.M., Taylor, R.M. and Meltzer, H.L.: Incorporation of carboxyl carbon of octanoic acid into brain lipids. *Fed Proc, 21*:271, 1953.

Spielmeyer, W.: Über einige Beziehungen zwischen Ganglienzellenveränderungen und Erscheinungen, besonders am Kleinhirn. *Z Ges Psychiatr, 54*:1, 1920.

Spielmeyer, W.: Der gegenwärtige Stand der Epilepsieforschung. *Z Neurol Psychiatr, 89*:360, 1924.

Spielmeyer, W.: Die Pathogenese des epileptischen Krampfes. *Z Neurol, 101*:701, 1926.

Spielmeyer, W.: Die Pathogenese des epileptischen Krampfes. Histologischer Teil. *Z Ges Neurol Psychiatr, 105*:501, 1927.

Sporn, M.B., Dingman, W. and Defalco, A.: A method for studying metabolic pathways in the brain of the intact animal. The conversion of proline to other amino acids. *J Neurochem, 4*:141, 1959.

Sprague, J.M. and Meyer, M.: An experimental study of the fornix in the rabbit. *J Anat* (Lond), *84*:354, 1950.

Squires, R.F.: On the interactions of Na^+, K^+, Mg^{++} and ATP with the Na^+ plus K^+ activated ATPase from Rat brain. *Biochem Biophys Res Commun, 19*:27, 1965.

Stalmaster, R.M., and Hanna, G.R.: Epileptic phenomena of cortical freezing in the Cat: persistent multifocal effects of discrete superficial lesions. *Epilepsia, 13*:313-324, 1972.

Stämpfli, R.: Bau und Funktion isolierter markhaltiger Nervenfasern. *Ergeb Physiol, 47*: 70, 1952.

Stauder, K.H.: Epilepsie und Schläfenlappen. *Arch Psychiatr, 104*:181, 1936.

Stauder, K.H.: *Konstitution und Wesensänderung der Epileptiker.* Leipzig, Thieme, 1938.

Stauder, K.H.: Über Fortschritte der Pharmakotherapie in Neurologie und Psychiatrie. *Fortschr Neurol, 19*:3, 1951.

Stebbins, R.B.: Impaired water metabolism in pyridoxine deficiency and effects of pyridoxine and adrenal cortical hormone. *Am J Physiol, 166*:538, 1951.

Steblov, E.M.: The part of neocortex in chronic seizure. (Russ) *Arkh Biol Nauk, 32*: 321, 1932.

Steblov, E.M.: Epileptic seizure in view of modern research. *Problems of Clinical and Experimental Neuropathology and Psychiatry.* (Russ) Charkov, Russ. Akad Nauk, pp. 142-149, 1936.

Stein, W.H., Paladini, A.C., Hirs, C.H.W. and Moore, S.: Phenylacetylglutamine as a constituent of normal human urine. *J Am Chem Soc, 76*:2848, 1954.

Steinberg, D. and Vaugh, M.: Intracellular protein degradation. *Arch Biochem Biophys, 65*:93, 1956.

Steinberg, D., Vaugh, M. and Anfinsen, C.B.: Kinetics of assembly and degradation of proteins. *Science, 124*:389, 1956.

Steinmann, H.: Der Einfluβ von Megaphen auf das Elektrokortikogramm der Katze. *Zbl Neurochir, 14*:233, 1954.

Steinmann, H.: Aktivierungseffekt bei experimentellen epileptogenen Hirnläsionen. *Zbl Neurochir, 25*:61, 1964/65.

Stene, J.: Comments on febrile convulsions as a problem of waiting times. *Epilepsia, 13*: 335-337, 1972.

Stepanenko, A.G.: Gaz metabolism and changes of acido-basic processes in isolated tissue in experimentally induced shocks. (Russ) Diss., Moscow, 1953.

Stepanjan, E.P., Klimova, V.S. and Gorbarenko, N.I.: *Zh Röntgenol Radiol, 1*:49, 1957; cit. by Lando, L.I.: The hyaluronidase in blood serum of schizophrenics during treatment. (Russ) In *Obm. Veshtch. Psikhiat. Zabol.* Moscow, Medgiz, pp. 66-75, 1960.

Stepanjan, E.P. and Pertchikova, T.E.: *Ther Arkh, 5*:28, 1956; cit. by Lando, L.I.: *Obm. Veshtch. Psikhiat. Zabol.* Moscow, Medgiz, pp. 66-75, 1960.

Stephan, H.: Die kortikalen Anteile des limbischen Systems. *Nervenarzt, 35*:396, 1964.

Stepp, W., Kühnau, J. and Schroeder, H.: *Die Vitamine und ihre klinische Anwendung.* Stuttgart, Enke, 1957.

Sterc, J.: The effect of serpasil seizure susceptibility of normal laboratory rats and of rats with experimental epileptogenic focus in the cerebral cortex. *J Exp Med Sci, 2*:34, 1959.

Stern, W.E. and Marshall, C.: Distribution of ^{32}p in normal and diseased brain tissue. *Proc Soc Exp Biol,* (NY), *78*:16, 1951.

Stewart, L.F.: Chlorpromazine: use to activate electroencephalographic seizure patterns. *Electroenceph Clin Neurophysiol, 9*:427, 1957.

Stief, A. and Tokay, L.: Beiträge zur Histopathologie der experimentellen Insulinvergiftung. *Z Ges Neurol Psychiatr, 139*:434, 1932.

Stille, G.: Zur Frage der Wirkung von Diphenylhydantoin (DH) bei Schmerzzuständen. *Nervenarzt, 31*:109, 1960.

Stössel, K.: Die Behandlung der Katatonie mit grossen Wassergaben, zugleich ein Beitrag zur Theorie der Hirnschwellung. *Arch Psychiatr D, 114*:699, 1942.

Stoll, W.A.: Lysergsäure-diäthylamid, ein Phantastikum aus der Mutterkorngruppe. *Schweiz Arch Neurol Neuochir Psychiatr, 60*:279, 1947.

Stone, W.E.: The effects of anesthetics and of convulsants on the lactic acid content of the brain. *Biochem J, 32*:11, 1938.

Stone, W.E., Webster, J.E. and Gurdjan, E.S.: Chemical changes in the cerebral cortex associated with covulsive activity. *J Neurophysiol, 8*:233, 1945.

Stousland, J. and Sigstad, H.: Complications of chlorpromazine treatment in psychotic patients. *T Norske Laegeforen, 77*:636, 1957.

Strickland, K.P.: Energetics and cerebral metabolism. *Guys Hosp Rep, 105*:108, 1956.

Strobos, R.R.J. and Spudis, E.V.: Effect of anticonvulsant drugs on cortical and subcortical seizure discharge in cats. *AMA Arch Neurol, 2*:399, 1960.

Stucke, W.: Zerebrale Anfälle. *Landarzt, 40*:899, 1964.

Sullivan, T.M., Frohman, C.E., Beckett, P.G.S. and Gottlieb, J.: Biochemical studies of families of schizophrenic patients. *Am J Psychiatry, 122*:1040, 1966.

Sulser, F. and Dingell, J.V.: Adrenergic mechanism in the central action of tricyclic antidepressants and substituted phenothiazines. *Agressologie, 9*:281, 1968.

Suter, C. and Klingman, W.O.: Seizure states and pregnancy. *Neurology* (Minneap), *7: 105*, 1957.

Sutherland, B.S., Berry, H.K. and Shirkey, H.C.: A syndrome of phenylketonuria with normal intelligence and behavior disturbances. *Pediatrics, 57*:521, 1960.

Sutherland, E.W. and Rall, T.W.: *Pharmacol Rev, 12*:265, 1960; cit. by Kanig, K., *Arzneim Forsch, 19*:397, 1969.

Svennerholm, L.: The chemical structure of normal human brain and Tay-Sach's gangliosides. *Biochem Biophys Res Commun, 9*:436, 1962.

Svennerholm, L. and Raal, A.: Composition of brain gangliosides. *Biochem Biophys Acta, 53*:422, 1961.

Swinyard, E.A.: Laboratory evaluation of antiepileptic drugs. Review of laboratory methods. *Epilepsia, 10*:107-119, 1969.

Symonds, C.: Classification of the epilepsies with particular reference to psychomotor seizures. *Arch Neurol Psychiatr, 72*:631, 1954.

Syndermann, S.E., Carretero, R. and Holt, L.E.jr.: Pyridoxine deficiency in the human being. *Fed Proc, 9*:371, 1950.

Tagaki, H. and Ban, T.: cit. by Domino, E.F.: Sites of action of some central nervous system depressants. *Ann Rev Pharmacol, 2*:215, 1962.

Taira, M., Kojima, Y., and Takeuchi, H.: A comparative study of the action of actinomycin D and actinomycinic acid on the central nervous system when injected into the cerebrospinal fluid of higher animals. *Epilepsia, 13*:649-662, 1972.

Takagaki, G., Berl, S., Clarke, D.D.: Purpura, D.P. and Waelsch, H.: Glutamic acid metabolism in brain and liver during infusion with ammonia labelled with nitrogen-15. *Nature* (Lond), *189*:326, 1961.

Takagaki, G., Hirano, S. and Tsukada, Y.: Endogenous respiration and ammonia formation in brain slices. *Arch Biochem Biophys* (NY), *68*:196, 1957.

Takahashi, K.: Experiments on the periamygdaloid cortex of cat and dog. *Folia Psychiatr Neurol Jap, 5*:147, 1951.

Takahashi, R., Nasu, N., Tamura, T. and Kariya, T.: Relationship of ammonia and acetylcholine levels to brain excitability. *J Neurochem, 7*:103, 1961.

Takashima, K., Fumimoto, D. and Tamiya, N.: Incorporation of 18_0 from air into tyrosine. *J Biochem* (Tokyo), *55*:122, 1964.

Tallan, H.H.: Distribution of N-Acetyl-l-aspartic acid in brain. *J Biol Chem, 224*:41, 1957.

Tallan, H.H., Moore, S. and Stein, W.H.: L-cystathionine in human brain. *J Biol Chem 230,* 707, 1958.

Tashian, R.E.: Inhibition of brain glutamic acid decarboxylase by phenylalanine, valine and leucine derivates—a suggestion concerning the etiology of the neurological defect in phenylketonuria and branched-chain ketonuria. *Metabolism, 10*:393, 1961.

Tashiro, S.: Studies on alkaligenesis in tissues. I. Ammonia production in the nerve fiber during excitation. *Am J Physiol, 60*:519, 1922.

Tassinari, C.A., Dravet, C., Rober, J., Cano, J.P., and Gastaut, H.: Tonic status epilepticus precipitated by intravenous benzodiazepine in five patients with lennox-gastaut syndrome. *Epilepsia, 13*:421-435, 1972.

Tatarenko, N.P.: *Zh Nevropatol Psikhiat, 5*:9, 1954; cit. by Haimovitch, L.A. and Podkamenii, B.N.: The reaction of schizophrenics dependent on the period of disease and some metabolic processes. In *Obm. Veshtch. Psikhiat. Zabol.* Moscow, Medgiz, pp. 47-55., 1960.

Tauber, C.G.: Librium, ein neues psychotropes Pharmakon. *Schweiz Med Wochenschr, 90:* p. 1065-1070, 1960.

Taylor, D.C.: Mental state and temporal lobe epilepsy. A correlative account of 100 patients treated surgically. *Epilepsia, 13*:727-765, 1972.

Tchalissov, M.A.: Theses—papers to the conference on problems of metabolism of patients with psychic disorders. (Russ) Moscow, 1958.

Tchalissov, M.A.: Carbon-phosphate metabolism and its importance in psychiatry. (Russ) In *Obm. Veshtch. Psikhiat. Zabol.* Moscow, Medgiz, pp. 14-20, 1960.

Tchalissov, M.A. and Wolfsohn, H.M.: Metabolism of aromatic combinations in the brain of schizophrenics. Communications of the lecturers of the med. Inst. IV, *Annual of the communications of the psychiatric clinic,* M.A. Tchalissov (Ed.), *1:* 161, 1940. (Russ)

Tchalissov, M.A., Wolfsohn, H.M. and Arutunov, D.N.: Intermediary metabolism in human brain. *Biokhim. Dost. Psikhiat. Kiev,* Akad. Nauk USSR, 1937a.

Tchalissov, M.A., Wolfsohn, H.M. and Arutunov, D.N.: *Biochemical Advances in Psychiatry.* Kiev, Akad. Nauk USSR, 1937b.

Teglbjaerg, H. and Stubbe, P.: Clinical experiments with McQuarrie's pitressin test. *Acta Psychiat* (Kopenh), *10*:595, 1935.

Teglbjaerg, H. and Stubbe, P.: *Encephalographie bei Epileptikern.* Verh. Neurol. Ges. pp. 43-44, 1936.

Teleschevskaya, M.E. and Plotitcher, M.: Papers on the 15th Congress of the institute of psychoneurology at Charkov. 1949.

Tellenbach, H.: Epilepsie als Anfallsleiden und als Psychose. *Nervenarzt, 36*:190, 1965.

Teller, D.N., Levine, R.J.C. and Denber, H.C.B.: Binding of chlorpromazine and thioproperazine *in vitro.* II. Fluorometric measurement of stoichiometry and alteration of protein structure. *Agressologie, 9*:167, 1968.

Téllez, A.: Die epileptische Wesensänderung. *Nervenarzt, 38*:49, 1967.

Terner, C., Eggleston, L.V. and Krebs, H.A.: Role of glutamic acid in transport of potassium in brain and retina. *Biochem J, 47*:139, 1950.

Terzian, H. and Dalle Ore, G.: Syndrome of Klüver and Bucy. Reproduced in man by bilateral removal of the temporal lobes. *Neurology* (Minneap), *5*:373, 1955.

Theobald, W. and Kunz, H.A.: Zur Pharmakologie des Antiepileptikums 5-Carbamyl-5H-dibenzo (b,f) azepin. *Arzrneim Forsch, 13*:1963.

Thompson, J.W. and Aste-Salazar, J.H.: Ketonemia in cases of mental disorders. *Arch Neurol Psychiatr, 41*:375, 1938.

Thor, C.J.B. and Gortner, R.A.: Sulfur in proteins. V. The effect of alkalies upon cystine, with special reference to the action of sodium hydroxide. *J Biol Chem, 99:* 383, 1933.

Timm, F.: Zur Histochemie des Ammonshorngebietes. *Z Zellforsch Mikvosk Anat, 48:* 548, 1958.

Timm, F.: Der histochemische Nachweis des Kupfers im Gehirn. *Histochemie, 2*:332, 1961.

Tissot, R.: The effects of certain drugs on the sleep cycle in man. In Akert, Bally, Schadé (Eds.): *Sleep Mechanisms. Progr. Brain Res.* Amsterdam, Elsevier, vol. XVIII, 175-177, 1965.

Tolkatchevskaya, N.F.: *Changes in Metabolism of Child in the First Year of Life,* (Russ) Moscow, Medgiz, 1951.

Tolkatchevskaya, N.F. and Wunder, M.A.: Characteristics of asod-metabolism in epilepsy. In *Obm. Veshtch. Psikhiat. Zabol.* Moscow, Medgiz, pp. 167-177, 1960.

Toman, J.E.P. and Davis, J.P.: The effects of drugs upon the electrical activity of the brain. *Pharmacol Rev, 1*:425, 1949.

Toman, J.E.P., and Sabelli, H.C.: Comparative neuronal mechanisms. *Epilepsia, 10:* 179-192, 1969.

Torack, R.M., Terry, R.D. and Zimmermann, H.M.: The fine structure of cerebral fluid accumulation. II. Swelling produced by triethyl tin poisoning and its comparison with that in the human brain. *Am J Path, 36*:273, 1960.

Torda, C.: Ammonium ion content and electrical activity of the brain during preconvulsive and convulsive phases induced by various convulsants. *J Pharmacol Exp Ther, 107*:197, 1953.

Torda, C.: Effect of single injection of corticotropin (ACTH) on ammonium ion and acetylcholine content of brain. *Am J Physiol, 173*:176, 1953.

Torda, C. and Wolff, H.G.: Effect of administration of ACTH on ammonia content of the brain. *Fed Proc, 11*:163, 1952.

Tower, D.B.: Nature and extent of the biochemical lesion in human epileptogenic cerebral cortex. An approach to its control *in vitro* and *in vivo*. *Neurology, 5*:113, 1955.

Tower, D.B.: Symposium on role of some of newer vitamins in human metabolism and nutrition; neurochemical aspects of pyrodoxine metabolism and function. *Am J Clin Nutr, 4*:329, 1956.

Tower, D.B.: The neurochemical substrates of cerebral function and activity. In Harlow, Woolsey (Eds.): *Biological and Biochemical Basis of Behavior.* Madison, U of Wis Pr, 1958a.

Tower, D.B.: Discussion. In Baldwin, Bailey (Eds.): *Temporal Lobe Epilepsy.* Springfield, Thomas, pp. 288-295, 1958b.

Tower, D.B.: The evidence for a neurochemical basis of seizures. In Baldwin, Bailey (Eds): *Temporal Lobe Epilepsy.* Springfield, Thomas, pp. 301-343, 1958c.

Tower, D.B.: *Neurochemistry of Epilepsy.* Springfield, Thomas, 1960.

Tower, D.B. and Elliott, K.A.C.: Activity of acetylcholine system in cerebral cortex of various unanesthetized mammals. *Am J Physiol, 168*:747, 1952a.

Tower, D.B. and Elliott, K.A.C.: Activity of acetylcholine system in human epileptogenic focus. *J App Physiol, 4*:669, 1952b.
Tower, D.B. and Elliott, K.A.C.: Experimental production and control of an abnormality in acetylcholine metabolism present in epileptogenic cortex. *J Appl Physiol, 5*:375, 1953.
Trojaborg, W. and Plum, P.: Treatment of hypsarhythmia with ACTH. *Acta Paediat* (Uppsala), *49*:572, 1960.
Trojanova, A.G.: Some biochemical changes in patients with "removal-psychosis" (Russ.). In *Obm. Veshtch. Psikhiat. Zabol.* Moscow, Medgiz, 1960, pp. 185-193.
Trolle, E.: Diazepam (Valium) in the treatment of epilepsy. *Acta Neurol Scand, 41:* R99/1, 1965.
Tronillas, P., and Courjon, J.: Epilepsy with multiple sclerosis. *Epilepsia, 13*:325-333, 1972.
Tschirgi, R.D.: Chemical environment of the central nervous system. In Field, Magoun, Hall (Eds.): *Hb. of Physiology. Neurophysiology.* Washington, Amer. Physiol. Soc., vol. III, 1960.
Tschumburidze, P.I.: The dynamics of protein-content in blood in schizophrenia-therapy. In *Obm. Veshtch. Psikhiat. Zabol.* Moscow, Medgiz, pp. 99-106, 1960.
Tucker, H. and Wilensky, K.: A clinical evaluation of meprobamate therapy in a chronic schizophrenic population. *Am J Psychiatry, 113*:698, 1957.
Turek, S. and Čižinsky, B.: Influence of ultracentrifugation of blood serums on the polarographic reaction of their deproteinated solutions. *Česk Onkol, 2*:355, 1955.
Turner, M., Bérard, E., Turner, N. and Franco, N.: Etude des modifications électroencéphalographiques, électrodermographiques et électro-myographiques provoquées par la chlorpromazine. *Anesth Analg* (Paris), *12*:777, 1955.
Turova, N.F.: The isoelectrical point of brain proteins at different functional initial conditions. *Patokhim.* Moz. MOLMI, Moscow, 1963.
Tursky, T., Krizko, J. Halcak, L. and Brechtlova, M.: Effects of psychopharmacological agents on brain metabolism-I. Effect of imipramine and prothiadene upon consumption of oxygen and the uptake and incorporation of L-phenyl-alanine into proteins and lipids of brain slices. *Biochem Pharmacol, 14*:1645, 1965.
Udenfriend, S. and Bessmann, S.P.: Hydroxylation of phenylalanine and antipyrine in phenylpyruvic oligophrenia. *J Biol Chem, 203*:961, 1953.
Udenfriend, S., Clark, C.T. and Titus, E.: 5-hydroxytryptophan decarboxylase; a new route of metabolism to trytophan. *Am Chem Soc J, 75*:501, 1953.
Udenfriend, S. and Cooper, J.R.: Enzymatic conversion of phenylalanine to tyrosine. *J Biol Chem, 194*:503, 1952.
Udenfriend, S., Cooper, J.R., Clark, C.T. and Baer, J.E.: Rate of turnover of epinephrine in adrenal medulla. *Science, 117*:663, 1953.
Udenfriend, S. and Creveling, C.R.: Localisation of dopamine-β-oxidase in brain. *J Neurochem, 4*:350, 1959.
Udenfriend, S. and Wyngaarden, J.B.: Precursors of adrenal epinephrine and norepinephrine *in vivo*. *Biochem Biophys Acta, 20*:48, 1956.
Ueki, S., Oda, M. and Iwaki, J.: *Fukuoka Acta Med, 53*:187, 1962.
v. Uexküll, J.: *Theoretische Biologie*. 2nd. Ed. Berlin, 1928.
Ule, G.: Korsakow-Psychose nach doppelseitiger Ammonshornzerstörung mit transneuraler Degeneration der corpora mammilaria. *Dtsch Z Nervenheilkd, 165*:446, 1951.
Ule, G.: Über das Ammonshorn. *Fortschr Neurol Psychiatr, 22*:510, 1954.
Ulrich, J.: Die konservative Therapie der Epilepsie. *Praxis, 51*:62, 1962.

Umbach, W.: Tiefen- und Cortexableitungen während stereotaktischer Operationen am Menschen. 1. Congr. Int. Neurochir. *Acta Med Belg* (Bruxelles), *18*:161, 1957.
Umbach, W.: Versuche zur Epilepsiebehandlung durch gezielte Tiefenausschaltung. *Acta Neurochir, 5*:341, 1958.
Umbach, W.: What conclusions can be drawn from depth recording and depth stimulations for the regulation of the EEG. *Electroenceph Clin Neurophysiol, 11*:609, 1959.
Umbach, W.: Die operative und stereotaktische Behandlung der Epilepsie. *Therapiewoche, 17*:61, 1967.
Umbach, W. and Riechert, T.: Die stereotaktische Ausschaltung der Fornix zur Behandlung der temporalen Epilepsie. *Proc. I. Intern. Congr. Neur. Sci.* London, Pergamon Press, vol. III, pp. 565-578. 1959.
Ungar, G., Aschheim, E., Psychoyos, S. and Romano, D.V.: Reversible changes of protein configuration in stimulated nerve structures. *J Gen Physiol, 40*:635, 1957.
Ungar, G. and Romano, D.V.: Fluorescence changes in nerve induced by stimulation. *J Gen Physiol, 46*:267, 1962.
Unna, K.R.: A review of the neurophysiological effects of psychotherapeutic drugs. *Ann NY Acad Sci, 66*:777, 1957.
Uzunov, G., Atzev, E. and Avramov, S.: Promeni v elektrischotne aktivnost na mozga pri lokalna aplikatizia na atebrin vrhu moztshanata kora na zaitziti. *Soobsch. Nautchn. Sesia EEG Klin. Neurofiziol.* D c. Sofia, 1961.
Uzunov, G., Bojinov, S., Gheorghieff, I.: Eksperimentalnoe issledovanie patogheneza epileptiformnovo pripadka. *J Nevropat Psikhiatr, 57*:731, 1957.
Valkenburg, V.: Contribution à l'étude de la substance blanche temporo-occipitale de l' homme. *Psych,* Bladen, 1911.
Vallee, B.L., Wacher, W.E.C. and Ulmer, D.D.: Magnesium-deficiency tetany syndrome. *New Engl J Med, 262*:155, 1960.
Vaneva, D., Achkova, M.: Effect of tegretol treatment on different forms of epileptic seizures. *Savremenna Medicina* 11, 27-29, 1971.
Varipaeva, I.S.: Different changes of "free" and "bound" colloides in different brain areas. (Russ.). *Reports of the Med. Institute Gorki, 1*:35, 1957.
Vartanian, M.E.: Discussion. *Proc. 4th World Congr. Psychiatr. 1966,* part 1. Excerpta Med., Amsterdam, pp. 537, 1967.
Vasconcelos, D.: Die Behandlung der Epilepsie mit Tegretal®. *Nervenarzt, 38*:11, 1967.
Vieth, J.B., Holm, E. and Knopp, P.R.: Electrophysiological studies on the action of Mogadon® on central nervous structures of the cat. A comparison with pentobarbital. *Arch Int Pharmacodyn, 2*:262, 1969.
Vigouroux, R., Gastaut, H. and Badier, M.: Les formes expérimentales de l'épilepsie. Provocation de principales manifestations clinques de l'épilepsie dite temporale par stimulation des structures rhinencéphaliques chez le chat non anaesthésié. *Rev Neurol, 85*:505, 1954.
Vilter, R.W.: Symposium on role of some newer vitamins in human metabolism and nutrition; metabolism of vitamin B_6 in human beings. *Am J Clin Nutr, 4*:378, 1956.
Vincent, J.-D., Faure, C., Bensch, C. and Quilichini, R.: Effets d'une benzodiazepine (Ro 4-5360) sur le système nerveux central. *J Med* (Bordeaux), *143*:535, 1966.
Vitello, A.: Il comportamento delle lipasi del sangue e dei liquor nella paralisi progressiva. *Pisani, 55*:89, 1935.
Vladimirov, G.E.: The influence of excitation of the central nervous system on some aspects of metabolism in the cerebral hemispheres of animals. *Fiziol Zh, 39*:33, 1953.

Vladimirov, G.E. and Epstein, J.A.: Organic acids of the blood and the problems of their isolation. (Russ) *Fiziol Zh, 26*:287, 1939.

Vladimirov, G.E. and Kolotilova, A.I.: *Biokhimia, 12*:4, 1947; cit. by Shevko, A.D.: On problems of acidosis in schizophrenia. In *Obm. Veshtch. Psikhiat. Zabol.* Moscow, Medgiz, pp. 21-39, 1960.

Vladimirov, G.E. et al.: cit. by. Pogodaev, K.I.: *Biological Chemistry of the Epileptic Seizure.* Moscow, Medicina, 1964.

Vladimirova, E.A.: Uric acid and different fractions of phosphor combinations in CNS by action of some toxins. In *Experimental Explorations of Neurohumoral Combinations.* (Russ) VIEM, Moscow 3, 37, 1937.

Vladimirova, E.A.: On the problem of ammonia formation in brain tissue. IV. The part of glutamine in ammonia formation in brain tissue at stimulation of CNS by camphor. (Russ) *Byull Eskp Biol Med, 29*:219, 1950.

Vladimirova, E.A.: Biochemical processes in brain at conditioned reflectory functional changes of CNS. II. *Byull Eksp Ment Biol Med, 4*:228, 1951.

Vladimirova, E.A.: Formation and excretion of ammonia in the brain of rats at stimulation of CNS combined with no conditioned and conditioned excitation. (Russ) In *Vopr. Fiziol. Morf. Centr. Nerv. Sist.* Moscow, Medgiz, 1953.

Vladimirova, E.A.: Brain-ammonia—specific biochemical guide to the functional initial condition of CNS. (Russ) In *Biokhim. nerv. Sist.* Kiev, pp. 27-63, 1954a.

Vladimirova, E.A.: Metabolism of first steps of ammonia in the brain hemispheres of the rat at inhibition and stimulation. (Russ) *Dok Akad Nauk SSSR, 95*:837, 1954b.

Vladimirova, E.A.: Dependence of different inhibitory processes on the first steps of ammonia in the brain. In *Vopr. Biokhim. Nerv. Sist.* Kiev. Akad. Nauk USSR, pp. 164-176, 1957.

Vladimirova, E.A.: On the mechanisms of cortex inhibition by action of certain biochemical processes. *Reports to 5th intern. Congr. Biochem. Moscow 1961;* Moscow, Medgiz, p. 452, 1961.

Voelkel, A.: Erfahrungen mit Librium bei psychomotorischen Unruhe- und Angstzuständen, *Med Exp* (Basel), *2*:170, 1960.

Vogl, P.: Erfahrungen in der Behandlung der Epilepsie bei Erwachsenen. *Dtsch Gesundh Wes, 19*:1685, 1964.

Vogt, C. and Vogt, O.: *Sitz und Wesen der Krankheiten im Lichte der topistischen Hirnforschung und des Varilierens der Tiere.* 1. Teil. Leipzig, Barth, 1937.

Vogt, C. and Vogt, O.: Morphologische Gestaltung unter normalen und pathogenen Bedingungen. *J Psychol Neurol, 50*:350, 1942.

Vogt, H.: *Die inkretorischen Regulationen und ihre Störungen.* München-Berlin, Urban & Schwarzenberg, 1956.

Vogt, M.: Concentrations of sympathin in different parts of the central nervous system under normal conditions and after the administration of drugs. *J Physiol* (Lond), *123*:451, 1954.

Voinar, A.O.: Papers on the problem of the different changes of colloides in the brain. Communications of the institute of brain research "B.M. Bechterev". In *Physico-Chemical Bases of Nervous Function* 198, 1935 (Russ).

Volanschi, D., Sterescu, N., Voiculet, N. and Lecca, M.: Studiul comparativ al capacitatii convulsivante a creierului imatur si matur (cercetari cu p^{32}). *Stud Cercet Neurol, 6*:291, 1961.

Vollmering, E.F.W.: Drei Gesichtspunkte für die Behandlung der Epilepsie. *Mat Med Nordm, 7*:413, 1955.

Vrba, R.: A source of ammonia and changes of protein structure in the rat brain during physical exertion. *Nature* (Lond), *176:*117, 1955.

Vrba, R.: On the participation of the glutamic acid glutamine system in metabolic processes in the rat brain during physical exercise. *J Neurochem, 1:*12, 1956a.

Vrba, R.: Pripevok ku studiu metabolickej cinnosti mozgu to vzt'aku k telesnep namache. O ucasti glutaminu na obnovych pochdoch v mozgu. *Česk Fysiol, 5:*265, 1956b.

Vrba, R.: On the participation of ammonia in cerebral metabolism and function. *Rev Čzech Med, 3:*81, 1957.

Vrba, R., Gaitonde, M.K. and Richter, D.: The conversion of glucose carbon into protein in the brain and other organs of the rat. *J Neurochem, 9:*465, 1962.

Vrubel, J.: The influence of adrenaline and acetylcholine on the activity of hyaluronidase. *Čas Lek Česk, 95:*981, 1956.

Vysotskaya, N.B., Sharov, P.A. and Shugina, T.M.: Role of noradrenaline in the mechanism of action of psychotropic drugs. (Russ) *Byul Eksp Biol Med, 66:*1109, 1968.

Vysotskaya, N.B. and Shugina, T.M.: Catecholamines content in the brain stem of albino rats and sedative effect of some tranquilizers. (Russ) *Farmakol Toksikol, 30:*553, 1967.

Wada, T. and Lennox, W.G.: So-called "temporal" epilepsy: The clinical and interseizure findings. *Folia Psychiatr Neurol Jap, 8:*294, 1954.

Wada, T. and Snell, E.E.: The enzymatic oxidation of pyridoxine and pyridoxamine phosphates. *J Biol Chem, 236:*2089, 1961.

Waelsch, H.: Compartmentalized biosynthesis reactions in the central nervous system. In Kety, Elkes (Eds.): *Regional Neurochemistry.* Oxford-London, Pergamon Press, 1961.

Waelsch, H.: Amino acids and protein metabolism. In Elliott, Page, Quastel (Eds.): *Neurochemistry.* Springfield, Thomas, 1962.

Waelsch, H., Sperry, W.M. and Stoyanoff, V.A.: Synthesis and deposition of lipids in brain and other tissues with D as an indicator–lipid metabolism in brain during myelin action. *J Biol Chem, 135:*291, 1940.

Walaas, O. and Walaas, E.: NATO Advanced Study Institute, Oslo 1965; cit. by Kanig, K., *Arzneim Forsch, 19:*397, 1969.

Waldron, D.H.: A report on the use of Cosaldon in general practice. *Brit J Clin Pract, 17:*733, 1963.

Walker, A.E.: *The Primate-thalamus.* Chicago, U of Chicago Pr, 1938.

Walker, A.E.: Recent memory impairments in unilateral temporal lesions. *Arch Neurol Psychiatr, 78:*543, 1957.

Walker, A.E. and Ribstein, M.: Enregistrements et stimulations des formations rhincéphaliques avec électrodes profondes à demeure chez l' homme. *Rev Neurol, 96:* 453, 1957.

Wall, P.D. and Davis, G.D.: The cerebral cortical systems affecting autonomic function. *J Neurophysiol, 14:*507, 1951.

Wallace, H.W., Moldave, K. and Meister, A.: Conversion of phenylalanine to tyrosine in phenylpyruvic oligophrenia. *Proc Soc Exp Biol* (NY), *94:*632, 1957.

Walsh, G.O.: Penicillin iontophoresis in neocortex of cat: Effects on the spontaneous and induced activity of single neurons. *Epilepsia, 12:*1-11, 1971.

Walsne, J.M., de Carli, L. and Davidson, C.S.: Some factors influencing cerebral oxidation in relation to hepatic coma. *Clin Sci, 17:*11, 1958.

Wandrey, D. and Leutner, V.: *Neuropsychopharmaka in Klinik und Praxis.* Stuttgart, Schattauer, 1965.

Ward, A.A.jr.: The cingular gyrus: Area 24. *J Neurophysiol, 11:*13, 1948.

Ward, J.A.A., McCulloch, W.S. and Kopeloff, N.: Temporal and spatial distribution of changes during spontaneous seizures in monkey brain. *J Neurophysiol, 11:*377, 1948.

Weil, A.A.: Depressive reactions associated with temporal lobe uncinate seizures. *J Nerv Ment Dis, 121:*505, 1955.

Weil-Liebert, A.: *Arch Neurol Psychiatr (Chic), 42:*1939; cit. by Scholz, W. and Hager, H.: Epilepsie. In *Henke-Lubarsch: Hb. d. Spez. Anat. u. Histol.* Berlin, Springer, vol. VIII/4, 1956.

Weil-Malherbe, H.: Studies on brain metabolism; metabolism of glutamic acid in brain. *Biochem J, 30:*665, 1936.

Weil-Malherbe, H.: Studies on brain metabolism. II. Formation of succinic acid. *Biochem J, 31:*299, 1937.

Weil-Malherbe, H.: The action of glutamic acid in hypnoglycaemic coma. *J Ment Sci, 95:*330, 1949.

Weil-Malherbe, H.: Significance of glutamic acid for the metabolism of nervous tissue. *Physiol Rev, 30:*549, 1950.

Weil-Malherbe, H.: Die Funktion der Glutaminasäure in Nervengewebe. *Naturwissenschaften, 40:*545, 1953.

Weil-Malherbe, H.: Concentration of adrenaline in human plasma and its relation to mental activity. *J Ment Sci, 101:*733, 1955.

Weil-Malherbe, H.: The effect of reserpine on the intracellular distribution of catecholamines in the brain stem of the rabbit. In Brücke, F. (Ed.): *Biochemistry of the Central Nervous System.* New York, Pergamon Press, 1959.

Weil-Malherbe, H.: Ammonia metabolism in the brain. In Elliott, Page, Quastel (Eds.): *Neurochemistry.* 2nd ed. Springfield, Thomas, 1962.

Weil-Malherbe, H., Axelrod, J. and Tomchik, R.: Blood-brain barrier for adrenaline. *Science, 129:*1266, 1959.

Weil-Malherbe, H., Whitby, L.G. and Axelrod, J.: The uptake of circulating (^{3}H) norepinephrine by the pituitary gland and various areas of the brain. *J Neurochem, 8:*55, 1961.

Weinland, W.F. and Kröber, E.: Electroencephalographische Untersuchungen über die Wirkung von Weckaminen (Isophan, Pervitin) bei Epileptikern. *Arch Psych Neurol, 183:*226, 1950.

Weinland, W.L. and Weinland, G.: Über elektrencephalographische Beobachtungen beim Insulinschock. *Arch Psychiatr Nervenkr, 183:*34, 1949.

Weinmann, H.M.: Behandlung von Blitz-Nick-Salaam-Krämpfen mit Mogadon "Roche". *Munch Med Wochenschr, 13:*727, 1966.

Weinmann, H.M.: Psychomotorische Anfälle beim Kind. Internist. *Praxis, 6:*273, 1966.

Wenzel, E.: Neue Ergebnisse der Epilepsietherapie mit Mylepsin einschließlich katamnestischer Erhebungen an länger behandelten Epileptikern. *Z Gesamte Inn Med, 14:*417, 1958.

Werle, E.: Über die Bildung von Histamin und Histidin durch tierische Gewebe. (Vorläufige Mitteilung). *Biochem Zschr, 288:*292, 1936.

Werle, E. and Aures, D.: Über die Reinigung und Spezifität der DOPA-Decarboxylase. *Hoppe Seylers Z Physiol Chem, 316:*45, 1959.

Werle, E. and Mennicken, G.: Bildung von Tyramin aus Tyrosin durch tierische Gewebe. *Biochem Zschr, 291:*325, 1937.

Werner, G.: Die neurophysiologischen Grundlagen der Wirkung von Tranquilisatoren. *Klin Wochenschr, 36:*404, 1958.

Wertheimer-Luca, N.: Modificarile aminoacizilor liberi din organele de sobolan sub actinuea accesului convulsiv experimental. *Stud Cercet Neurol, 2:*413, 1957.

Wertheimer-Luca, N.: Modificarea aminoacizilor liberi din organele de sobolan sub actinuea accesului convulsiv experimental. Nota II. Cercetari cromatografice. *Stud Cercet Neurol, 3:*211, 1958.

White, T.: Formation and catabolism of histamine in brain tissue *in vitro. J Physiol* (Lond), *149:*34, 1959.

White, T.: Formation and catabolism of histamine in cat brain *in vivo. J Physiol* (Lond), *152:*299, 1960.

Whitlock, D.G. and Nauta, W.J.H.: Subcortical projection from the temporal neocortex in Macaca mulatta. *J Comp Neurol, 106:*183, 1956.

Whittacker, V.P.: The isolation and characterisation of acetylcholine-containing particles from brain. *Biochem J, 72:*694, 1959.

Wiechert, P. and Herbst, A.: Provocation of cerebral seizures by derangement of the natural balance between glutamic acid and γ-aminobutyric acid. *J Neurochem, 13:*59, 1966.

Wiegand, R.G.: The formation of pyridoxal and pyridoxal 5-phosphate hydrazones. *J Am Chem Soc, 78:*5307, 1956.

Wiener, N.: Generalized harmonic analysis. *Acta Math, 55:*117, 1930.

Wilder, J.: Zwangslachen mit Erektion als epileptisches Äquivalent (nebst Beobachtungen über Beziehungen von Erektionen zum Fliegen). *Nervenarzt, 4:*75, 1931.

Wilder, R.: *Mayo Clinic Bull, 2:*307, 1921; cit. by Engel, R.: Die praktische Bedeutung des Wasserhaushalts in der Epilepsie, zugleich ein Beitrag zur Permeabilitätstheorie. *Nervenarzt, 6:*120, 1933.

Williams, H.L. and Abdulian, D.H.: *J Pharmacol Exp Ther, 116:*62, 1956; cit. by Kanig, K.: *Die Bedeutung der B-Vitamine für das Nervensystem.* Wiss. Berichte, Darmstadt, E. Merck, 1968.

Williams, J.R., Eakin, R.E., Beerstecher, E. and Shive, W.: *The Biochemistry of B-vitamins.* New York, Reinhold Publ. Corp, 1950.

Willing, F., Neuhoff, V. and Herken, H. Der Austausch von 3-Acetylpyridin gegen Nikotinsäureamid in den Pridinucleotiden verschiedener Hirnregionen. *Arch Exp Path Pharmakol, 247:*254, 1964.

Winemiller, J.L.: Dilantin therapy in treatment of epileptic convulsions. *Med Times, 69:*461, 1941.

Winterstein, H. and Hirschberg, E.: Über Ammoniakbildung im Nervensystem. *Biochem Zschr, 156:*138, 1925.

Wolfe, L.S. and Elliott, K.A.C.: Chemical studies in relation to convulsive conditions. In Elliott, Page, Quastel (Eds.): *Neurochemistry,* 2nd ed. Springfield, Thomas, 1962.

Wolfovski, A.I.: Collected writings on the problem of schizophrenia treatment in pathophysiological view. *Papers on the 20th Congr., dedicated to, the 35th jubilee of the Ukr. Inst. of Psychoneurol.* (Russ) Charkov, Ukrainian Akad. Nauk 1958.

Wolfsohn, H.M.: *Annual Dedicated to the 35th Jubilee of Prof. Yushtchenko.* (Russ) Rostov-on-Don, Russ. Akad. Nauk, 1928.

Wolfsohn, H.M.: *Sovj Psikhonevrol, 5:* 1932; cit. by Wolfsohn, H.M.: On the signification of some biochemical shifting to prognosis and effect of schizophrenia therapy. In *Obm. Veshtch. Psikhiat. Zabol.* Moscow, Medgiz, pp. 128-145, 1960.

Wolfsohn, H.M.: Dissertation 1940; cit. by Wolfsohn, H.M., In *Obm. Veshtch. Psikhiat. Zabol.* Moscow, Medgiz, pp. 128-145, 1960.

Wolfsohn, H.M.: On the signification of some biochemical shifting to prognosis and effect of schizophrenia therapy. In *Obm. Veshtch. Psikhiat. Zabol.* Moscow, Medgiz, pp. 128-145, 1960.

Woodbury, D.M.: Role of pharmacological factors in the evaluation of anticonvulsant drugs. *Epilepsia, 10:*121-144, 1969.

Woodbury, D.M. and Kemp, J.W.: Some possible mechanisms of action of anti-epileptic drugs. *Pharmakopsychiatr. Neuropsychopharmakol, 3:*201, 1970.

Woodbury, D.M., Koch, A. and Vernadakis, A.: Relation between excitability and metabolism in brain as elucidated by anticonvulsant drugs. *Neurology* (Minneap), *8:*113, 1958.

Woodbury, D.M., Rollins, L.T., Gardner, M.D., Hirsch, W.L., Hogan, J.R., Rallison, M.L., Tanner, G.S. and Brodie, D.A.: Effect of carbon dioxide on brain excitability and electrolytes. *Am J Physiol, 192:*79, 1958.

Woodbury, D.M., Timiras, and Vernadakis, A.: cit. by Hoagland, H.: Steroid hormones and events in the nervous system. In Elliott, Page, Quastel (Eds.): *Neurochemistry,* 2nd ed. Springfield, Thomas, 1962.

Woolf, L.I., Griffiths, R. and Moncrief, A.: Treatment of phenylketonuria with diet low in phenylalanine. *Br Med J, 1:*57, 1955.

Woolf, L.I. and Vulliamy, D.G.: Phenylketonuria with study of effect upon it of glutamic acid. *Arch Dis Child, 26:*487, 1951.

Woolley, D.W.: A possible mechanism of action of serotonine. *Proc Natl Acad Sci USA, 44:*197, 1958a.

Woolley, D.W.: Serotonine receptors. I. Extraction and assay of a substance which renders serotonine fat-soluble. *Proc Natl Acad Sci USA, 44:*1202, 1958b.

Woolley, D.W.: Antimetabolites of water-soluble vitamins. In *Metabolic Inhibitors.* New York-London, Academic Press, vol I, pp. 445, 1963.

Woolley, D.W. and van der Hoeven, T.: Prevention of mental defect of phenylketonuria with serotonine conengers such as melantonin or hydroxytryptophan. *Science, 144:* 1593, 1964.

Woolley, D.W. and Shaw, E.: Some neurophysiological aspects of serotonine. *Br Med J, 488:*122, 1954.

Word, A.A., McCulloch, W.S. and Kopeloff, N.: Temporal and spatial distribution of changes during spontaneous seizures in monkey brain. *J Neurophysiol, 11:*377, 1948.

Woronin, L.G., Tolmasskaya, E.S., Guselnikova, K.G. and Guselnikov, V.I.: Electrophysiological studies of action mechanisms of aminazine. (Russ) *Zh Nevropatol Psikhiatr, 61:*208, 1961.

Wortis, H., Bueding, E. and Wilson, W.E.: Bisulfite-binding substances in the blood and cerebrospinal fluid. *Proc Soc Exp Biol* (NY), *43:*279, 1940.

Wortz, E.C., Brown, W.L. and Elam, C.B.: The synergic effect of reserpine and electroconvulsive shock. *J Comp Physiol Psychol, 43:*285, 1957.

Wright, S.W. and Trajan, G.: Phenylketonuria. *Am J Dis Child, 93:*405, 1957.

Wu, R. and Racker, E.: Regulary mechanisms in carbohydrate metabolism. III. Limiting factors in glycolysis of ascites tumor cells. IV. Pasteur effect and crabtree effect in ascites tumor cells. *J Biol Chem, 234:*1029, 1959.

Yagi, K., Ozawa, T. Ando, M. and Nagatsu, T.: *J Neurochem, 5:*304, 1960; cit. by Kanig, K., *Arzneim Forsch, 19:*397, 1969.

Yamaguchi, N., Ling, G.M. and Marczynsky, T.J.: The effects of electrical and chronical stimulation of the preoptic region and some nonspecific thalamic nuclei in unrestrained waking animals. *Electroenceph Clin Neurophysiol, 15:*145, 1963.

Yeager, F.: cit. by Hubach, H.: Veränderungen der Krampferregbarkeit unter Einwirkung von Medikamenten und während der Entziehung. *Fortschr Neurol Psychiatr, 31:*4, 1963.

Yushtchenko, A.: *Arkh Biol Nauk, 1*:12, 1911; cit. by Wolfsohn, H.M.: On the signification of some biochemical shifting to prognosis and effect of schizophrenia therapy. In *Obm. Veshtch. Psikhiat. Zabol.* Moscow, Medgiz, pp. 128-145, 1960.

Zabarenko, R.N. and Chambers, G.S.: Evaluation of glutamic acid in mental deficiency. *Am J Psychiatry, 108*:881, 1952.

Zack, N.N.: On the appearance of seizures in the treatment with aminazine in psychiatry. (Russ) *Zh Nevropatol Psikhiatr, 57*:750, 1957.

Zappoli, R.: La terapia degli stati depressivi con il derivato iminodibenzilico G 22355 (Tofranil). Nota prelim. *Riv Sper Freniatr, 83*:289, 1959.

Zeman, W.: Zur Frage der Hirngewebsschädigung durch Heilkrampfbehandlung. *Arch Psychiatr Nervenkr, 184*:440, 1950.

Zeškov, P. and Hajnšek, F.: Abdominal epilepsy. *Neuropsihijatrija* (Zagreb), *8*:317, 1960.

Zeuner, K.: Epilepsie. *Mat Med Nordm, 11*:142, 1959.

Ziegler, H.K.: Morphologische Untersuchungen zur Nebennierenfunktion beim Epileptiker. *Nervenarzt, 35*:79, 1964.

Ziehen, V.: Neuere Wege der Epilepsiebehandlung. *Münch Med Wochenschr, 92*:25 a. 27, 1950.

Ziem, M., Coper, H., Broermann, I., and Strauss, S.: Vergleichende Nntersuchungen über einige Wirkungen des Amphetamins bei Ratten verschiedenen Alters. *Naunyn-Schmiedebergs Arch Pharmak, 267*:208-223, 1970.

Zimmermann, F.T. and Burgemeister, B.B.: Effect of glutamic acid on borderline and high-grade defective intelligence. *NY St J Med, 50*:693, 1950.

Zimmermann, F.T. and Burgemeister, B.B.: Permancy of glutamic acid treatment. *Arch Neurol Psychiatr, 65*:291, 1951.

Zimmermann, F.T. and Burgemeister, B.B.: Preliminary report upon the effect of reserpine on epilepsy and behavior problems in children. *Ann NY Acad Sci, 61*:215, 1955.

Zimmermann, F.T. and Burgemeister, B.B.: A controlled experiment of glutamic acid therapy. First report summarizing 13 years of study. *Arch Neurol Psychiatr, 81*:639, 1959.

Zimmermann, F.T., Burgemeister, B.B. and Putnam, T.J.: Group study of effect of glutamic acid upon mental function in children and adolescents. *Psychosom Med, 9*:175, 1947.

Zislina, N.N., Novikova, L.A. and Tkacenko, N.M.: Elektrofiziologhiceskoe issledovanie tormoznîh i vozbujdainscih vliianii. *Fiziol Zh* (Kiev), *49*: 5, 1963.

Zuckerkandl, E.: *Über das Riechzentrum. Eine vergleichend-anatomische Studie.* Stuttgart, Enke, 1887.

Zülch, K.J.: *Die Hirngeschwülste in biologischer und morphologischer Darstellung.* Leipzig, Barth, 1956.

Zurabashvili, A.D.: K teoretitcheskin osnovam elektroskoka. *Zh Nevropat Psikhiatr, 52*: 15, 1952.

Zurabashvili, A.D.: A propos d'une architéctonique pathologique de la schizophrénie à la lumière de nouvelles donnes (Russ.) *Zh Nevropatol Psikhiat, 61*:1241, 1961.

AUTHOR INDEX

E

F

G

H

L

M

N

SUBJECT INDEX

B

E

F

R

S